Choosing Effective Laboratory Tests

Carl E. Speicher, M.D.

Professor of Pathology
College of Medicine
Director of Clinical Laboratories
University Hospitals
The Ohio State University
Columbus, Ohio

Jack W. Smith, Jr., M.D., M.S.

Instructor of Pathology
College of Medicine
Associate Director of Clinical Chemistry
University Hospitals
The Ohio State University
Columbus, Ohio

W. B. Saunders Company   1983

Philadelphia London Toronto Mexico City Rio de Janeiro Sydney Tokyo

W. B. Saunders Company: West Washington Square
Philadelphia, PA 19105

1 St. Anne's Road
Eastbourne, East Sussex BN21 3UN, England

1 Goldthorne Avenue
Toronto, Ontario M8Z 5T9, Canada

Apartado 26370—Cedro 512
Mexico 4, D.F., Mexico

Rua Coronel Cabrita, 8
Sao Cristovao Caixa Postal 21176
Rio de Janeiro, Brazil

9 Waltham Street
Artarmon, N.S.W. 2064, Australia

Ichibancho, Central Bldg., 22-1 Ichibancho
Chiyoda-Ku, Tokyo 102, Japan

Library of Congress Cataloging in Publication Data

Speicher, Carl E.

Choosing effective laboratory tests.

1. Diagnosis, Laboratory—Problems, exercises, etc.   I. Smith,
   Jack W.   II. Title. [DNLM: 1. Diagnosis, Laboratory. QY
   4 S742s]

RB37.S667 1983   616.07′5   82–48504

ISBN 0–7216–8533–1

Choosing Effective Laboratory Tests   ISBN 0-7216-8533-1

Last digit is the print number: 9   8   7   6   5   4   3   2   1

To our wives
and children

Mary Louise   Kathy
Carl Jr., Gregory, and Erik   and Michael

ACKNOWLEDGMENT

This book would not have been possible without the encouragement and support of Donald A. Senhauser, M.D. Special thanks are in order to John B. Henry, M.D., for his tables of reference intervals in the Appendix and for his organ panels throughout the book. John C. Neff, M.D. contributed to many important concepts, and Joel G. Lucas, M.D., kindly read our galley proofs. B. Chandrasekaran, Ph.D., John A. Lott, Ph.D., Robert V. O'Toole, M.D., Thomas D. Stevenson, M.D., and Gregory L. Trzebiatowski, Ph.D., gave us valuable assistance and suggestions. Gratitude is also due to the entire pathology faculty, fellows, residents, graduate students, medical technologists, medical students, and clinical colleagues for the manner in which they continuously educate us.

Deep appreciation is extended to Kay Cook and Linda Wentz for keeping our schedules straight during the writing of this book, and who, together with Christy Anderson and Cindy Berner, accomplished the monumental task of putting our ideas on paper.

To the entire staff of W. B. Saunders Company, Thanks! Albert Meier, Don Abbott, Mary Cowell, Frank Polizzano, George Vilk, and Carol Robins Wolf have given us special guidance and support.

Jack Smith has been partially supported during the writing of this book by a training grant from the National Library of Medicine (LM-00159).

PREFACE

Laboratory medicine is on the threshold of an exciting new phase in its development. For the past three decades laboratory professionals have struggled to assimilate remarkable advances in automation, computers, and management. Now the challenge is to orchestrate these tools for the patient's benefit at a cost that is affordable. And so, we turn our attention increasingly to the bedside.

Technology has increased the number and variety of laboratory studies to the point where they outstrip our ability to keep informed about their use and interpretation. Patients' charts bulge with laboratory reports. These reports usually segregate chemistry, hematology, microbiology, immunology, and other test results and create difficulty in locating, collating, and interpreting data. Busy professionals waste time on clerical tasks. Physicians can overlook important information.

An inability to order and interpret laboratory and other studies in optimal ways can be detrimental to patient care. Inappropriate use of the laboratory can interfere with diagnosis and management. Misuse of the laboratory can consume health care dollars by lengthening patients' stays and increasing the number of laboratory studies.

Collectively, these laboratory and other studies are called tests. In addition to laboratory studies, tests can include such things as diagnostic maneuvers (e.g., sigmoidoscopy and biopsy), radiologic procedures, pulmonary function studies, and even signs and symptoms. Not only individual tests but also test strategies can be used to solve clinical problems. Strategies can be composed entirely of laboratory studies. Strategies can also be made up of test sequences: A physical finding is determined before a laboratory study (digital examination of the prostate followed by measurement of serum acid phosphatase—see prostatic carcinoma, Chapter 12); a laboratory study is followed by determining a physical finding (measurement of serum ceruloplasmin followed by slit-lamp examination of the eye for Kayser-Fleischer rings—see Wilson's disease, Chapter 17); a laboratory study is followed by a radiographic procedure (measurement of arterial blood Po_2 followed by pulmonary angiography—see pulmonary embolism, Chapter 11).

The value of combination testing was recognized by Feinstein,* who said that diagnostic tests are used for three different purposes: discovery (screening), confirmation, and exclusion. Furthermore, he said that single tests are seldom excellent for multiple purposes, such as detection and confirmation; hence, the necessity to use tests "in tandem," which is a test sequence, a strategy.

It may be useful to view patients' illnesses as being composed of clinical

---

*Feinstein AR: Clinical Biostatistics. St. Louis, C. V. Mosby Company, 1977, pp 221–222.

subproblems that often are largely or entirely dependent on laboratory data for their solution. For example, the diagnosis of multiple myeloma entails the solution of several subproblems. Radiologic studies address the subproblem of determining the presence of bone lesions, and laboratory studies address the subproblems of determining the existence of pathologic serum proteins, anemia, and infiltration of the bone marrow by immature, atypical plasma cells.

In this book we have attempted to identify the best available strategies for solving a number of clinical subproblems by reviewing the literature and surveying practicing pathologists. This information was tempered and expanded by our experience. The suggestions and ideas of our associates were freely used. Because medicine is not an exact science, there is no one "correct" strategy and there is always room for alternatives. Our emphasis is clearly on the problem-solving approach. We review the clinical contexts in which the subproblems arise, and after discussing strategies for their solution, we elucidate principles for the interpretation of results. Methods of requesting tests and interpretive reporting of test results are included. The choice of subproblems is selective rather than comprehensive. This book categorizes clinical subproblems and the strategies for their solution on a traditional systemic basis and includes common and important examples in each category. We trust this will enable readers not only to use the strategies we discuss, but also to design and evaluate their own strategies.

We believe this book will interest three groups of readers: physicians, medical students, and laboratory-based consultants. For medical students, we present information essential for learning effective problem solving through the use of laboratory and other studies in patient care. For physicians, we suggest a way of thinking about tests, not simply as individual measurements, but as components of strategies for solving patients' problems. For laboratory-based consultants, such as pathologists, we suggest an approach whereby they can offer problem-solving test sequences as an alternative to a conventional menu of individual laboratory measurements. These test sequences represent effective strategies for given clinical subproblems. Consultative interpretive reports of test results may then be sent to the attending physician when appropriate.

This book is divided into three parts. Part 1, Rationale and Useful Concepts, discusses the logic of the problem-solving method together with necessary background information. Part 2, Clinical Subproblems, covers the clinical contexts, strategies, and interpretations of a series of subproblems. Part 3, Unexpected Test Results, contains tables of potential drug interferences and differential diagnoses for common tests, as well as comments about patient preparation, specimen collection and handling, and methodology. These tables can be used to construct patterns of test results in a variety of diseases and disorders. The tables in Part 3 can also be used to evaluate test results that are unexpectedly within the usual reference intervals.

Readers may be able to use the problem-solving strategies and the tables without covering all of Part 1. However, we recommend reading at least Chapter 1 of Part 1 as a preliminary guide.

Our use of selected older terminology (e.g., CPK, LDH, and SGOT for CK, LD, and AST, respectively) is by design and represents an attempt to bridge the language gap.

CARL E. SPEICHER
JACK W. SMITH, JR.

CONTENTS

PART 1

RATIONALE AND USEFUL CONCEPTS

THE PROBLEM-SOLVING APPROACH TO LABORATORY STUDIES

THE CASE FOR IMPROVING THE USE OF LABORATORY STUDIES IN PATIENT CARE

We believe that the use of the clinical laboratory in health care delivery can be improved. This book describes a problem-solving approach to using laboratory studies, with information on laboratory studies organized in a way that should help the reader to make improvements in providing patient care. This book describes strategies designed to solve common and important clinical subproblems. We are convinced that these strategies constitute a powerful and efficient way of using the clinical laboratory. Some reasons for improving the use of laboratory studies follow.

COMMUNICATION GAP

Benson (1978) recognized the need for improving the role of the laboratory, especially in the area of communication.

A gap has appeared and is growing in breadth between the clinic and the laboratory. This has certainly been due in large measure to the expanded and expanding technology of laboratory medicine. The needs of this day call for a major attempt to bridge the gap by those of us in laboratory medicine. This effort will require new and resourceful means of communication and interaction. It may require a major shift in emphasis away from such a heavy commitment to our tools, our engineering skills,

3

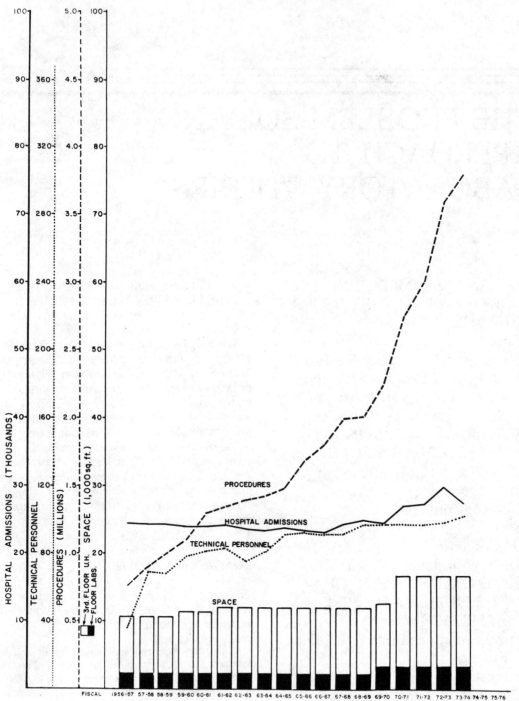

Figure 1–1. Increasing number of procedures per patient at the Ohio State University Hospitals, Columbus, Ohio.

and our management problems and more toward a concern and an occupation with how these tools can most effectively be used to solve actual clinical problems.

INCREASE IN LABORATORY STUDIES

The number of laboratory studies performed each year in the United States has been increasing at the compound rate of 15 per cent per year (Cole, 1980; Conn, 1978) and has been estimated to be 4.0 billion (Kosowsky, 1976). A feature of this increase is that the number of procedures per patient is also growing (Fig. 1–1). This pattern has also been reported in Great Britain (Barnard, 1976). Unfortunately, it is speculative whether this trend is bringing about a proportional improvement in patient care.

Finkelstein (1978) concluded that no single determinant itself can account for the large increases that were observed between 1969 and 1977. However, a number of factors are worth noting. These are enumerated in Table 1–1.

Physicians not only order more tests; they also require the results in a shorter turn-around time; hence, the growth in Stat tests. Viewed from the perspective of life-threatening patient needs, Stat test requests are essential. Viewed from the perspective of laboratory efficiency and cost controls, Stat test requests are disastrous (Barnett, 1978) (see Chapter 6).

The proliferation of laboratory tests has increased the opportunity for their excessive, unnecessary, and unwise use (Russe, 1969). Too much data can interfere with patient care. The technologic revolution in the laboratory has led to a flood of available data and to an information crisis. Better means of data presentation to physicians may help to condense the large volumes of test results currently produced (Connelly and Steele, 1980). (See Chapters 7 and 8.)

Yet, it is inappropriate to accuse physicians of overusing or misusing laboratory tests in every case. First, we are unaware of any widely accepted criteria that define optimal use of laboratory testing in truly objective terms. Second, certain advances in cardiovascular, orthopedic, and transplantation surgery, as well as new therapies for malignant tumors and leukemia, have resulted in a legitimate increase in demand for laboratory studies. Therapeutic drug monitoring represents a

Table 1–1. FACTORS CONTRIBUTING TO THE ANNUAL INCREASE IN LABORATORY STUDIES

1. A greater availability of routine laboratory tests as a result of advances in technology
2. A constantly increasing variety of available tests
3. The capability of diagnosing and defining an increasing number of diseases in terms of laboratory tests
4. The increased number of diseases being managed by laboratory tests
5. The advent of therapeutic drug monitoring and toxicology
6. An increased amount of testing for medicolegal reasons
7. The reluctance of physicians to give up obsolescent tests even though new tests are providing better information
8. A greater reliance by younger physicians on laboratory tests
9. Increased testing to follow up unexplained "abnormal" results discovered by screening (see Chapter 9)
10. One-upmanship and intellectual curiosity, especially among resident physicians
11. The opinion that a certain number of laboratory studies are necessary to maintain and improve clinical skills (Handler, 1979)
12. Defensive medicine being blamed for the increasing number of laboratory studies and its frequent citation as one of the least desirable effects of the current rise in medical litigation (Tancredi and Barondess, 1978)

whole new avenue of laboratory testing that is clearly necessary.

HIGH COST OF LABORATORY TESTS

Between 1969 and 1976, the total annual expenditure for health care in the United States increased from $64 billion to $139 billion. During 1975, approximately 10 per cent of the total health care budget, $12 billion, was spent for laboratory studies. If the current annual growth rate continues at 15 per cent, four times this amount ($48 billion) will be spent on laboratory tests in 1985 (Conn, 1978).

There is increasing concern about the cost of laboratory studies, as well as the cost of health care in general (Lyle, 1979). A number of cost controls have been suggested. Holding physicians responsible for the cost of unnecessary medical services has been advocated (Eisenberg, 1978). Blue Cross and Blue Shield have recently urged their member plans to stop paying for routine laboratory tests required by hospitals and to pay only when a physician personally orders these studies (McNerney, 1979). Reimbursement for obsolete tests, such as the protein-bound iodine (PBI) and liver flocculation tests, has been discontinued. Holland (1974) and Balint (1978) have emphasized that new procedures should be carefully evaluated in terms of cost-effective improvements in patient care before being implemented.

NEED TO ASSESS RELIABILITY OF TEST RESULTS

Physicians encounter many difficulties in obtaining reliable laboratory test results. There are many processes that occur from the time a physician requests a test until the result is returned for interpretation (see Chapter 6). It is important to remember that all of these processes require time and that all of them are subject to errors. Yet, to be clinically useful, test results must be accurate, precise, timely, and interpretable. We find it useful to group the errors that can occur in the production of laboratory data in this way:

1. *Prelaboratory errors* can occur with test requests, patient preparation, and the collection and handling of specimens. Such errors would include misinterpretation of orders by the nurse, ordering the wrong kinds of tests, mistaken identification of the patient, improper preparation of the patient, and poor preservation of the specimen.

2. *Intralaboratory errors* can occur with the performance of tests, for example, inaccurate and imprecise laboratory methods, calculation errors, and transcription errors.

3. *Postlaboratory errors* can occur during the communication of results. Examples would be illegible reports, lack of appropriate reference intervals, and poor report format.

The test for plasma activated partial thromboplastin time (APTT) illustrates difficulties that can occur in each of these categories. Prelaboratory errors can occur under certain conditions. For instance, if the blood specimen is not collected so that the blood tube is filled and so that the blood is completely mixed with anticoagulant, the APTT can be prolonged. Also, if the properly collected blood specimen is not preserved correctly (refrigerated) and if the test is not performed promptly, the APTT can again be prolonged.

Intralaboratory errors can also occur. When the APTT is measured, if the reagents are outdated and if the timing and temperature control mechanisms of the coagulation analyzer are not correct, the APTT can be erroneously shortened or prolonged.

A postlaboratory error can occur when the results of the APTT are communicated to the clinician. If the partial thromboplastin reagent has been changed since the reference interval was obtained, the APTT can be misinterpreted as shortened or prolonged by the clinician. This is because different sources of partial thromboplastin can have different sensitivities to various coagulation factor deficiencies and can therefore change the reference interval as well as test result decision levels (see Chapter 3).

THE PROBLEM-SOLVING APPROACH AS A SOLUTION

This book proposes an approach to improve the effectiveness of laboratory testing in solving clinical subproblems. This involves strategies for clinical problem solving as well as ways of organizing and presenting information about laboratory test results. Our approach is problem oriented, but we prefer the term "problem solving." Our methods are not only compatible with problem solving; they are also specifically designed to aid problem solving.

The organ panels of Henry and Arras (1970) constitute a problem-solving approach, which we decided to develop further. Our belief is that, in addition to organ panels, the laboratory ought to solve other discrete clinical problems. However, the list of presenting clinical illnesses that are amenable to clinical laboratory solutions (e.g., coma) is not very long. Lundberg (1975) was able to develop a master list of 45 problems in which there is extensive involvement of the laboratory. He presented problem-solving approaches to the solution of these problems in a continuing series in the *Journal of the American Medical Association.* (See JAMA citations in Chapter 5 references for examples.) It occurred to us that although relatively few presenting clinical illnesses have clinical laboratory solutions, many of the subproblems encountered in diagnosing and managing these illnesses do.

Our concept of subproblems requires explanation. All of us know that complex problems can often be solved by dividing them into the smaller problems of which they are composed (i.e., "divide and conquer"). The complex decisions, in turn, are broken up into a number of smaller, easier decisions (Williams, 1981). So it is with clinical decision problems. These complex problems are composed of subproblems in diagnosis and management that are easier to formulate and solve than the original problem. Many of these subproblems are largely or entirely dependent on laboratory data for their solution. For example, the clinical problem of septicemia can be divided into several subproblems, for example, identification of the infectious agent, determination of the antibiotic sensitivity of the infectious agent, and choice of treatment.

Clinical subproblems can be viewed as being general or particular in scope or of being on different levels (Table 1–2). We believe that the ability to make more confident diagnostic and management decisions based on laboratory studies increases as the level of the subproblem becomes more particular. The particular subproblem of confirming or excluding a diagnosis of acute myocardial infarction by using serial creatine phosphokinase (CPK) and lactic dehydrogenase (LDH) isoenzyme measurements can frequently be solved with confidence approaching 100 per cent—a high predictive value (see Chapter 10 for a discussion of acute myocardial infarction).

We organized our presentation of subproblems and strategies for their solution according to organ systems except for screening subproblems (Chapter 8) and the subproblem of the unexpected test result (Chapter 9). Collectively, these chapters on clinical subproblems and their strategies appear in Part 2 of this book. In Part 3, we include information necessary for the in-depth evaluation of individual test results whether high or low, for 22 different common tests. In addition this information permits construction of test result patterns for a wide variety of diseases and disorders.

Each clinical subproblem is presented in the following manner:
1. Definition and significance.
2. Pathophysiology.
3. Clinical contexts.
4. Strategy.
5. Interpretation.
6. Test requests and reports.

The subproblems have been organized this way because effective clinical problem solving using strategies in unique situations requires certain kinds of knowledge about laboratory studies and their pathophysiologic relationship to disease. This knowledge is important for sound interpretations. The content and further rationale for these sections follow.

DEFINITION AND SIGNIFICANCE

Each clinical subproblem is defined in order to provide a clear concept of what is to be solved. Particular subproblems were chosen either because they are common, e.g., pleural effusion (see Chapter 11); or because even though they are relatively uncommon, they are important (i.e., effective therapy is potentially available, as in pheochromocytoma [see Chapter 16] and Wilson's disease [see Chapter 17]).

PATHOPHYSIOLOGY

Each clinical subproblem includes a discussion of basic pathophysiology to help the reader understand the rationale for laboratory testing. We believe that, when possible, strategies should be designed to discover pathophysiologic derangements in the patient, not simply patterns of test results for specific diseases. Taken with the history and physical examination, this leads to sound interpretations. This book presupposes some understanding of the fundamental principles of anatomy, chemistry, pathology, and physiology. However, an at-

Table 1–2. GENERAL AND PARTICULAR CLINICAL SUBPROBLEMS

Example	Subproblem	Problem Level
Multiphasic screening	Is the patient healthy or ill? (entire body)	1
Complete blood count	Is there a hematologic problem? (organ system)	2
Hepatic panel	Is there a liver problem? (specific organ)	3
Acute myocardial infarction	Is there a myocardial infarct? (specific disease)	4

tempt has been made to clarify and expand on the relationship between these fundamental concepts and laboratory studies.

CLINICAL CONTEXTS

A discussion of each strategy should perhaps begin with the clinical situation in which that particular strategy applies. There are a number of reasons for this.

Interpretation of Data. One reason is that the interpretation of the laboratory and other data varies, depending on the clinical decision that is being made. For example, the interpretation will vary if the diagnosis is being ruled in (confirmed) compared with its being ruled out (excluded). Consider the subproblem of acute myocardial infarction (see Chapter 10).

Confirming a diagnosis of acute myocardial infarction by laboratory studies requires the combined performance of serum CPK and LDH isoenzymes (performed in parallel) every 12 hours for 48 hours (performed in series) — a strategy that is sensitive and specific. The performance of CPK isoenzymes provides a sensitive index of acute myocardial infarction through the detection of CPK-MB (the CPK isoenzyme of heart origin). However, the detection of CPK-MB does not reliably confirm acute myocardial infarction. This is because CPK-MB is found in diseases and disorders other than acute myocardial infarction; that is, it is not specific for this condition. The performance of LDH isoenzymes is required to exclude the presence of these other diseases and disorders through the detection of an LDH "flip" (increase of LDH-1 and LDH-2 isoenzymes with the amount of LDH-1 equal to or greater than LDH-2). This LDH "flip" is not present in these other diseases and disorders. (See Chapter 10 for further discussion of CPK and LDH isoenzymes in the diagnosis of acute myocardial infarction.)

Excluding a diagnosis of acute myocardial infarction can be accomplished by the performance of sequential serum CPK isoenzymes without the performance of serum LDH isoenzymes — a strategy that is sensitive but not specific. Because sequential CPK measurements are nearly 100 per cent sensitive for acute myocardial infarction, the absence of CPK-MB effectively excludes a diagnosis of acute myocardial infarction. It is of no consequence that CPK-MB is not specific for acute myocardial infarction and that it is found in a variety of other diseases and disorders. The measurement of LDH isoenzymes is superfluous.

Reference Values. Another reason for discussing the clinical contexts in which a particular strategy applies concerns reference values and reference intervals. *Reference values* refer to a set of values of a measured quantity obtained from a group of individuals (or a single individual) in a defined state of health (Dybkaer and Gräsbeck, 1973; Winkel and Statland, 1979). The term replaces the obsolescent term *normal values. Reference interval* refers to all reference values that lie between a lower limit and an upper limit and usually includes 95 per cent of the reference population (see Chapter 3).

Sunderman (1975) proposed that reference values include the following specifications:

1. The reference population and the way in which it was chosen.

2. The environmental and physiologic conditions under which the specimens were obtained.

3. The technique and timing of specimen collection, transport, preparation, and storage.

4. The analytic method that was used, with data regarding its accuracy, precision, and quality control.

5. The data set that was observed and the reference intervals that were derived.

One can appreciate that reference intervals for serum CPK and LDH isoenzymes may differ, depending on the reference population from which they were derived. Consider the differences in reference populations of patients in a cardiac-care unit compared with all patients visiting the emergency department. The cardiac-care unit reference population is defined as being susceptible to acute myocardial infarction as interpreted by clinical history, physical examination, and electrocardiogram. The emergency department reference population is defined by having any of a wide variety of diseases and disorders that prompted the visit to the emergency department. Therefore, the reference values for the emergency department are appropriate for a select group of patients, whereas the reference values for the cardiac care unit are appropriate for other patients.

Predictive Values. Still another reason for emphasizing the clinical situation in which a particular strategy applies has to do with the variation of the predictive value of laboratory studies, depending on the clinical situation. The *predictive value* of a test refers to the probability that an individual has a given disease when the particular test in question has a certain value (i.e., positive or negative). It is important to know the clinical situation in which each strategy applies because the predictive value of the test under consideration varies with the diagnostic sensitivity and diagnostic specificity of the test, and the prevalence of the disease in the population being examined. *Prevalence* or prior probability refers to that percentage of individuals who have the disease in the population being considered. *Diagnostic sensitivity* refers to the probability that an individual suffering from the disease will have a positive test result; *diagnostic specificity* refers to the probability that a healthy individual will have a negative test result.

Given a CPK-MB of a certain diagnostic sensitivity and diagnostic specificity, the predictive value of a positive test for CPK-MB for acute myocardial infarction will be higher in the coronary-care unit than in the emergency department because the prevalence of acute myocardial infarction is higher in the coronary-care unit than in the emergency department (see Chapter 4).

Why Physicians Order Tests. We agree with Johnson (1973) that clinical contexts can be grouped into three broad categories: diagnosis, management, and screening. Henry and Howanitz (1979) stated that physicians select and evaluate clinical laboratory tests in the course of patient care for at least one of the following reasons:

1. To confirm a clinical impression.
2. To rule out a possible diagnosis or disease.
3. To use as a therapeutic or management guide.
4. To use as a prognostic guide.
5. To detect disease (screen).

Young (1979) listed the reasons for ordering laboratory tests in a similar but slightly different manner:

1. To diagnose disease.
2. To screen for disease.
3. To determine the severity of disease.
4. To determine appropriate management of the patient.
5. To monitor progress of the disease and to monitor therapy.
6. To monitor drug toxicity.
7. To predict response to treatment.

These alternate groupings can be related to our three broad categories:

1. Diagnosis: Reasons 1. and 2. of Henry and Howanitz (1979) and reason 1. of Young (1979).
2. Management: Reasons 3. and 4. of Henry and Howanitz and reasons 3. through 7. of Young.
3. Screening: Reason 5. of Henry and Howanitz and reason 2. of Young. We have included a section for each of these three categories in every subproblem.

Diagnosis

Diagnosis involves more than just the type of logic that is needed for ruling in and out. Burke (1978) has reviewed the physician's logic in making a decision, particularly with respect to the use of laboratory studies in medical diagnosis. Chapter 2 is devoted to the relationship between clinical problem solving and laboratory studies.

Burke (1978) has pointed out that *diagnostic reasoning* proceeds from effect to cause, that is, from symptoms, signs, and laboratory data to etiology. On the other hand, *pathogenetic reasoning* (the method by which medical students have usually been taught) proceeds from cause to effect, that is, from etiology to symptoms, signs, and laboratory findings. Burke's outline of the sequence of diagnostic reasoning is shown in Figure 1–2. He observed that medical students and physicians in training tend to adopt an exhaustive approach to medical diagnosis, relying heavily on the laboratory rather than on clinical testing. In contrast, experienced physicians favor a more pointed and abbreviated approach; they use a minimum number of tests, often clinical, and are parsimonious in requesting laboratory studies. In the words of Moser (1979), for clinical laboratory testing, "a rifle, not a shotgun, approach should be used." It is possible that because experienced physicians have developed a better intuitive sense of the probability of a given diagnosis with a smaller number of data, they are able to function using fewer laboratory measurements.

Management

Tests are used to make management decisions more often than is commonly realized. Murphy and Henry (1978) have said that the

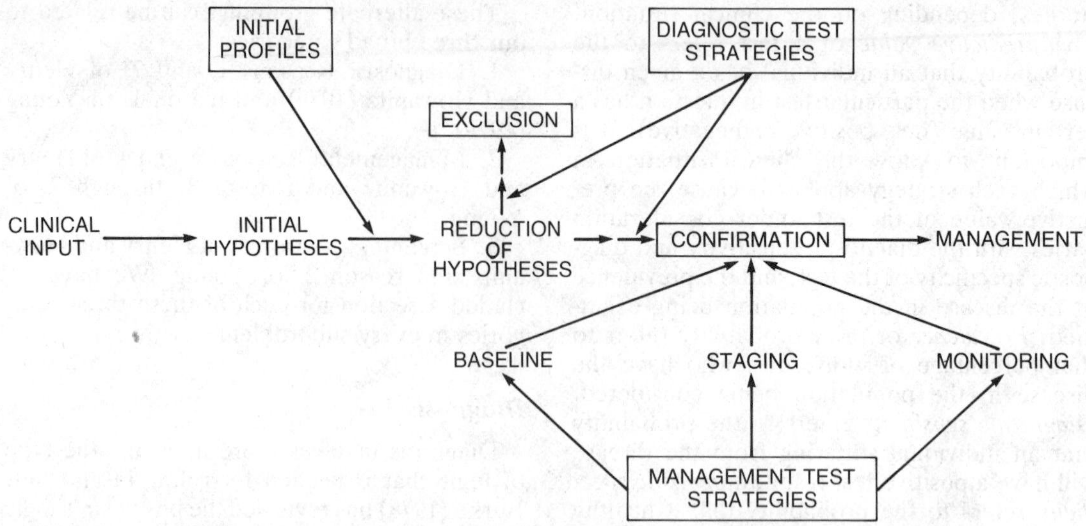

Figure 1–2. The sequence of diagnostic reasoning. (From Benson ES, Rubin M (eds): Logic and Economics of Clinical Laboratory Use. New York and Amsterdam, Elsevier North-Holland, Inc, 1978, p. 61.)

majority of laboratory tests (60 per cent) performed at the Upstate Medical Center in Syracuse, New York, are carried out to monitor therapy (i.e., to manage a condition). Brecher (1978) concurred, finding that in many settings 60 to 80 per cent of the most common laboratory tests are performed to monitor therapy rather than to make an initial diagnosis. Primary-care hospitals may differ from tertiary-care hospitals and may tend to have tests performed more often for diagnostic than management purposes. According to Burke (1978), it is in the area of management strategies that data—even qualitative and crude—are probably lacking.

In our discussions of clinical subproblems in Chapters 8 through 17, management is one of the broad categories of clinical reasons for initiating strategies. The reader will notice, however, that management strategies are less well defined than diagnostic strategies.

Management reasons for initiating strategies include the following:

1. To assess the severity of disease for prognosis.
2. To determine the extent of disease for staging.
3. To predict the response to medical therapy.
4. To predict the response to surgical therapy.
5. To monitor progress of a disease without therapy.

6. To monitor progress of a disease with therapy.
7. To monitor drug therapy.

Screening

Tests are also done for screening purposes. Employing tests for screening affects the choice of strategy to be used. Screening is the performance of studies that are not predicated on clinical features of disease.

Screening comprises the following categories:

1. Targeted screening.
2. Multiphasic screening.
   a. Hospital admission screening (profiling).
   b. Outpatient screening.

Targeted screening is designed to confirm or exclude the presence of a specific disease in a particular population by using one or a small number of tests. For example, the serum VDRL is used to exclude the presence of syphilis in sexually active persons.

Multiphasic screening uses a battery of laboratory tests to discover unexpected complications of disease, to confirm or document previously suspected disease, to exclude disease, or to provide baseline values against which the evolution of disease processes or the effects of therapy can be gauged.

Screening is the term for the testing of healthy volunteers from the general population for the purpose of separating them into groups with high and low probabilities for a given disorder. The screening encounter is initiated by the screener, and the volunteer is not a patient. The term for the testing of patients who seek health care for disorders that may be unrelated to their chief complaints is *case finding*. The testing of patients by using combinations of tests performed on automated equipment is termed *profiling*. Because the term is applied to patients, profiling is not the same as screening healthy volunteers (Burke, 1981; Sackett and Holland, 1975).

The cost-effectiveness of multiphasic screening has been under debate. It is difficult to document the concept that multiphasic screening is truly effective. On the other hand, the concept that multiphasic screening produces economic loss is at best unproved (Werner and Altshuler, 1979) (see Chapter 8).

STRATEGY

In this book, we discuss strategies for various clinical subproblems as well as the reasons for the strategies. The discussion of each strategy includes which studies to order as well as when and how often to order them. Details of patient preparation are included. Test methodologies and methods of specimen collection and handling are discussed. After all, good test methods give reliable results only when the patient is properly prepared and the specimens are properly collected and preserved. Communication of test results to physicians is also addressed. The difference between communication of data (values and units) and information (data plus reference intervals, graphs, diagnostic/management lists, and interpretive comments) is stressed. It is sometimes useful to depict strategies in flow charts or decision tables; Chapter 5 discusses how to do this.

Conventional textbooks of medicine usually discuss diseases through pathogenetic reasoning. Laboratory findings thus are usually listed as data that are interpreted as high, "normal," or low. In many cases, there is no information concerning the significance of how high or how low the test result can be, whether it is necessary to do some tests or all tests, or how often it is necessary to repeat the studies. The influence of test methodologies, specimen collection and handling, and details of patient preparation is often ignored. Statland and Winkel

(1981) reviewed the effects of selected physical, dietary, and smoking activities on chemistry test results.

It is likely that some investigators will propose alternative strategies to ours. Skendzel (1978) showed that physicians' criteria for interpreting laboratory data vary, depending on their training or area of particular interest, and often differ from the criteria of the pathologist. West (1975) concluded: "Under certain common circumstances some diabetologists would classify as 'normal' more than half of the one- and two-hour (glucose) values considered to be 'abnormal' by other well-qualified diabetologists." In this book, however, by providing both strategies and the reasons for them, we hope to give the reader the necessary information required to modify them.

INTERPRETATION

Our discussions of interpretations of laboratory test results include reference intervals, decision levels, and diagnostic sensitivity and diagnostic specificity of measurements whenever this information is available.

It must be determined not only whether test results are outside the reference intervals but also how far outside they are. Various levels of deviation from the reference intervals differ in significance. The different kinds of significance attached to various levels of deviation of a particular result have been called *decision levels* (Statland, 1979), *referent values* (Galen, 1977; Galen and Gambino, 1975), *discrimination values, cutoff points, operating positions* or *points of operation* (Sunderman, 1975), *panic values* and *critical values* (Lundberg, 1977).

Knowledge of the diagnostic sensitivity and diagnostic specificity of a test or test sequence is important. One way in which this knowledge is used is in the ability to calculate the predictive value of a measurement for a given level of disease prevalence. The predictive value of a test sequence is assessed with assumptions on the prevalence or prior probability of the disease under consideration (see Chapter 3).

According to Kassirer and Pauker (1978), "The principles relevant to the proper use of laboratory studies are not well understood by the medical community and [that] physicians would make better decisions regarding the use of diagnostic tests if they were more facile with these concepts." Casscells (1978) suggested that misunderstanding of laboratory data can contribute to the overuse of the laboratory.

Almost two decades ago, Zieve (1966) formulated reasons for the tendency of clinicians to misinterpret laboratory test results or to request laboratory tests they neither need nor really use:

1. Technical error.
2. Physiologic variation.
3. Overinterpretation of test values.
4. Unfamiliarity with procedures or with physiologic factors affecting them.
5. Unawareness of extraneous factors that influence tests.
6. Unawareness of the distributions of normal.
7. Uncritical acceptance of published opinions regarding the comparative value of tests supposedly measuring the same function.
8. Unnecessary use of tests.
9. Unnecessary repetition of tests.
10. Failure to interpret tests in relation to clinical findings.

Generally, this book should lead to improved understanding of the principles important for the effective use of laboratory tests.

TEST REQUESTS AND REPORTS

There are a number of ways in which to implement requests for laboratory tests as well as to generate reports based on the test results. For each of the clinical subproblems in this book, suggestions are made as to how to implement test requesting and interpretive reporting.

A number of ways have been suggested for implementing test request schemes; these methods differ from the traditional selection of laboratory tests by physicians. Henry and Arras (1970) developed a number of organ panels, which contain laboratory tests appropriate for such problems as metabolic disorders, hypertension, pulmonary disorders, and arthritis. These panels allow the physician to order an appropriate set of tests depending on the disease or disorder to be evaluated.

Altshuler and colleagues (1972) developed a programmed accelerated laboratory investigation (PALI), in which results outside the reference intervals on profile tests automatically cause additional tests to be performed (see Chapter 8). Cole (1980) used structured test profiles, designed to match the test ordering patterns of physicians. Such profiles have been able to reduce the number of sample collection errors as well as communication errors. Organizing laboratory services around such ordering patterns results in a more efficient laboratory system.

No less important than test requests is the actual report to the clinician after laboratory test results are in. Such interpretive reporting communicates not only data but also information on how data can be applied in terms of patient diagnosis and management. An *interpretive report* goes further than merely describing the results of the test in terms of data attributes (value and units), e.g., a glucose level of 90 mg/100 ml. Included are such items as reference intervals and decision levels that aid the clinician in applying a particular result to patient-care decisions. Interpretive reports can also add graphics to help the significance of the data to be understood. Lists of diagnostic and management possibilities or, occasionally, the actual confirmation or exclusion of a diagnosis is also possible (Speicher and Smith, 1980).

Interpretive reports are a natural way of presenting the results and interpretations of problem-solving strategies. Such reports can be generated through a variety of media, from simple paper and manual systems to more sophisticated computer-assisted systems.

Test request schemes and interpretive reports can help to improve patient care and laboratory efficiency. As an alternative to a conventional menu of individual measurements, a laboratory director can offer problem-solving test sequences. The ordering of these sequences can initiate an effective group of tests designed to solve a particular clinical subproblem. Once the test sequence has been completed, pathologists can follow through with well-designed interpretive reports based on the results of the laboratory measurements (see Chapter 7).

POTENTIAL BENEFITS OF THE PROBLEM-SOLVING APPROACH

As stated earlier there is a need to improve the use of laboratory tests by making them easier to use and more relevant to patient care. A way to accomplish this is to adopt a problem-solving approach to laboratory testing. Educational and research benefits can follow.

The concept of a problem-solving method is not new. Weed (1970) originally proposed that medical records should be restructured along problem-oriented lines. Later, Weed and Henry (1977) and Weed (1979) proposed a similar restructuring of the laboratory. Henry, along with other clinical specialists, developed organ panels that are indeed problem oriented (Henry and Howanitz, 1979). Henry believes that these organ panels are compatible with the problem-oriented record of Weed and that they can be ordered by attending physicians by means of a suitable request form (Fig. 1–3).

We have endorsed the concept of the problem-oriented medical record and agree that a problem-oriented laboratory is the natural extension of this approach into the arena of laboratory studies. To this end, we have developed the problem-solving strategies in this book.

IMPROVED PROCEDURES IN CLINICAL PRACTICE

Our problem-solving approach provides the reader with strategies rather than merely lists of tests useful for diagnosing and managing patients' illnesses. These strategies can be offered as problem-solving test sequences as an alternative to conventional menus of laboratory studies. The test results can be returned to attending physicians in the form of interpretive reports. We believe that this approach will provide information germane to patient diagnosis and management and will be more relevant to patient care. The problem-solving approach encourages the efficient use of laboratory studies.

Griner (1979) suggested that the combined efforts of a house staff, faculty, and hospital administration can bring about improved use of the laboratory. His group was able to halt proliferating laboratory studies without adversely affecting patient care or teaching programs (Table 1–3).

Eisenberg (1977) cautioned that educational programs should be long term; indeed, 18 months after an educational program had decreased admission prothrombin time determinations from 87 to 55 per cent, the rate returned to preadmission levels. Martin and coworkers (1980) demonstrated that although a financial incentive was of no value, an educational program consisting of chart reviews produced a 47 per cent decrease in use of laboratory tests by medical residents.

One must be careful in efforts of this kind. The goal is not simply to reduce laboratory testing but rather to ensure that enough, but not too many, tests are performed to effect optimal patient care. Again, it is difficult to define an optimal level of testing.

EDUCATIONAL BENEFITS

Ward and colleagues (1976) improved the competence of medical students in the use of

STATE UNIVERSITY HOSPITAL SYRACUSE, N.Y.

DATE

PAT # X REF #

PAT. NAME

AGE

X THE APPROPRIATE ☐ BOXES

CLINICAL PATHOLOGY	DEPT #	SEQ #	ROOM #
ORGAN PANEL STUDIES	**31**		

SEND ONE REQUISITION TO INITIATE PANEL STUDY AND ANOTHER REQUISITION WITH EACH SPECIMEN.

DIAGNOSIS	ORDERED BY	REQUISITIONED BY
	M.D.	R.N.

COLLECTED BY	TIME	AM / PM

PATIENT CONTAGIOUS ☐ YES ☐ NO

ARTHRITIS	**3486**	METABOLIC	**3643**
BLOOD GAS PANEL (ART. AND VEN. SPECIMENS)	**3510**	MUSCLE	**3676**
		RENAL	**3791**
CARDIAC INJURY	**3494**	WATER ACID BASE	**3858**
CARDIAC EVALUATION	**3528**		
CARDIOVASCULAR (HYPERTENSION)	**3619**		
CVA	**3551**		
GENERAL HEALTH	**3569**	TYPE OF SPECIMEN	
		SERUM	
HEPATIC	**3577**	URINE	

Figure 1–3. Request form for organ panel studies. (Information courtesy of Bettina G. Martin, MS, HT (ASCP), Syracuse, New York.)

Table 1–3. FACTORS CONTRIBUTING TO
EXCESSIVE USE OF LABORATORY TESTS
IN THE TEACHING HOSPITAL*

Institution
   High proportion of tertiary care patients
   Multiplicity of physicians involved in the care of
      individual patients
   Lack of individualization of preadmission or admission
      testing according to patient risk or prior information
   Application of test "routines" in high-intensity care
      areas (for example, intensive care unit)
   Peer pressure (from teachers or fellow students)
   Desire for new knowledge
   Isolation of clinical pathologist from clinician

Physician
   Inadequate knowledge of test characteristics
   "Blanket" testing (e.g., simultaneous ordering of
      secondary, diagnostic tests in addition to primary,
      screening tests)
   Erroneous inferences from test results leading to
      additional tests
   Diagnostic "overkill" (e.g., using two or more
      confirmatory tests when one will suffice)
   Inappropriate test (wrong test, or right test at wrong
      time)
   Medicolegal considerations

Laboratory
   Logistical conveniences (e.g., phlebotomy teams;
      comprehensive laboratory test requisition form)
   Laboratory inefficiencies (e.g., long turn-around time)

Patient
   Need for reassurance
   Patient expectations

*Adapted from Griner PF, Medical House Staff, Strong
Memorial Hospital, Rochester, NY: Use of laboratory
tests in a teaching hospital: Long-term trends. Ann Intern
Med 90:248, 1979.

the laboratory through a course in the interpretive aspects of laboratory medicine. In a similar manner, Murphy and Henry (1978) emphasized the opportunities for educating medical students and house officers about the proper use of the laboratory during rounds and conferences. Burke and Connelly (1981) concluded that systematic instruction aimed at improving laboratory utilization is capable of evaluation and, in a simulated format, leads to improved clinical problem solving.

Our experience indicates that problem-solving strategies can serve as a systematic method for teaching medical students and house officers how to use the laboratory in patient care. We believe that medical students should be thoroughly instructed in the use of the laboratory. This instruction is every bit as impor-

tant as that given in medicine, surgery, pediatrics, obstetrics, and gynecology. Educational programs for residents and physicians in practice are also important (Connelly and Steele, 1980).

The number of different laboratory tests available is well over five hundred. Pathologists, let alone medical students and physicians in practice, find it impossible to keep up with all of them. The problem-solving approach can be used to teach students how to make appropriate use of the laboratory most of the time, e.g., for acute myocardial infarction, acute hepatitis, and peptic ulcer disease. Perhaps a hundred subproblems would suffice. For specialists, additional problem-solving strategies, which are more commonly encountered in their particular specialty practice, could be developed and taught. For instance, in the case of surgeons, a strategy might be developed to exclude a bleeding diathesis in patients scheduled for surgery; for gastroenterologists, a strategy might be developed for diagnosing the malabsorption syndrome. By using Boolean factor analysis, Werner and Altshuler (1981) determined that the greater part of laboratory work requested by physicians falls into a restricted number of typical panels, certainly less than a hundred. Is this a reflection of a limited number of clinical subproblems having laboratory solutions?

OPPORTUNITIES FOR RESEARCH

The problem-solving view provides an opportunity for scientific inquiry about the use of laboratory studies for diagnosis and management in a number of ways:

1. How can decision-making aids for interpreting laboratory test results be designed and implemented? For example, Altshuler and associates (1972, 1975) provide references to a microfiche source of information on all laboratory test results. The microfiche gives further information about the significance and possible interpretation of test results. Research in the use of computer aids for reporting and interpretation systems would likewise fall in this area.

The design and implementation of problem-solving strategies allow more insight into the role of laboratory tests in diagnosis, management, and screening. This is particularly true of such quantitative tools as the predictive value model of Galen and Gambino (1975). This model emphasizes the relationship between the diagnostic sensitivity and diagnostic specificity of laboratory measurements, the prevalence of disease, and the predictive value of a test or test sequence. Such a model is useful in determining appropriate design and interpretation of strategies, and refinement of the model is aided by the design of such interpretative schemes.

These strategies must be clinically evaluated and must be proved to be more effective than alternate approaches before widespread acceptance can be expected. Beck and colleagues' (1981) investigations using the "iron screen" for diagnosing iron deficiency anemia is an example of such an evaluation.

2. How to understand physician problem solving in regard to laboratory test requesting and interpretation? Skendzel (1978) showed that, contrary to what has been written in textbooks (Copeland, 1974), physicians do not use a change of three times the analytic standard deviation of successive laboratory measurements to indicate a real change in the patient. Skendzel (1978) noted that physicians developed their own estimates of what constitutes a clinically important change. For example, some physicians felt that a serum glucose had to change 35 mg/100 ml between successive measurements to be interpreted as a real change (see Chapter 6).

3. How can both intralaboratory and extralaboratory test request and report systems be designed and implemented? The structured test profiles used by Cole (1980) illustrate the way in which such request mechanisms can be oriented not only toward more effective use of laboratory services but also toward improved problem-solving ability of the physicians who request and use the tests. Studies in these various areas, which are motivated by the problem-solving view of the laboratory, have only just begun.

REFERENCES

Achord JL: Abuse of the data-gathering process. South Med J 70:1262–1264, 1977.

Altshuler CH, Bareta J, Cafaro AF, et al: The PALI and SLIC systems. CRC Crit Rev Clin Lab Sci 3:379–402, 1972.

Altshuler CH, Bareta J, Cafaro AF, et al.: AIDE (Accessible information for diagnosis and evaluation): An information retrieval system. In Stefanini M, Isenberg HD (eds): Progress in Clinical Pathology.

Vol VI. New York, Grune & Stratton, Inc, 1975, pp 307–323.

Balint JA: When is a new test a valid test?, editorial. Dig Dis 23:291–292, 1978.

Barnard F: Growth of medical laboratory work during 1920–2000. Br Med J 1:383–384, 1976.

Barnett RN, McIver DD, Gorton WL: The medical usefulness of Stat tests. Am J Clin Pathol 69:520–524, 1978.

Beck JR, Cornwell GG, French EE, et al: The "iron screen": Modification of standard laboratory practice with data analysis. Hum Pathol 12:118–126, 1981.

Benson ES: Strategies for improved use of the clinical laboratory in patient care. In Benson ES, Rubin M (eds): Logic and Economics of Clinical Laboratory Use. New York, Elsevier North-Holland, Inc, 1978, pp 245–256.

Brecher G: Laboratory medicine 1953–1978 and the next 10 years. Hum Pathol 9:615–618, 1978.

Burke MD: Clinical decision-making: The role of the laboratory. In Benson ES, Rubin M (eds): Logic and Economics of Clinical Laboratory Use. New York, Elsevier North-Holland, Inc, 1978, pp 59–64.

Burke MD: Clinical problem solving and laboratory investigation: Contributions to laboratory medicine. In Stefanini M, Benson ES (eds): Progress in Clinical Pathology. Vol VIII. New York, Grune & Stratton, Inc, 1981, pp 1–24.

Burke MD, Connelly DP: Systematic instruction in laboratory medicine: Effects on the clinical problem solving performance of medical students. Hum Pathol 12:134–144, 1981.

Casscells W, Schoenberger A, Graboys TB: Interpretation by physicians of clinical laboratory results. N Engl J Med 299:999–1001, 1978.

Cole GW: Biochemical test profiles and laboratory system design. Hum Pathol 11:424–434, 1980.

Conn RB: Clinical laboratories. Profit center, production industry or patient-care resource? N Engl J Med 298:422–427, 1978.

Connelly DP, Steele B: Laboratory utilization. Problems and solutions, editorial. Arch Pathol Lab Med 104:59–62, 1980.

Copeland BE: Statistical tools in clinical pathology. In Davidsohn I, Henry JB (eds): Clinical Diagnosis by Laboratory Methods, ed 15. Philadelphia, WB Saunders Company. 1974, pp 1–14.

Dybkaer R, Gräsbeck R: Theory of reference values, editorial. Scand J Lab Invest 32:1–7, 1973.

Eisenberg JM: An educational program to modify laboratory use by house staff. J Med Educ 52:578–581, 1977.

Eisenberg JM, Rosoff AJ: Physician responsibility for the cost of unnecessary medical services. N Engl J Med 299:76–80, 1978.

Finkelstein SN: Technological change and laboratory test volume. In Benson ES, Rubin M (eds): Logic and Economics of Clinical Laboratory Use. New York, Elsevier North-Holland, Inc, 1978, pp 225–234.

Galen RS: The normal range. A concept in transition. Arch Pathol Lab Med 101:561–565, 1977.

Galen RS, Gambino SR: Beyond Normality: The Predictive Value and Efficiency of Medical Diagnosis. New York, John Wiley & Sons, Inc, 1975.

Gorry GH, Pauker SG, Schwartz WB: The diagnostic importance of the normal finding. N Engl J Med 298:486–489, 1978.

Griner PF, Medical House Staff, Strong Memorial Hospital, Rochester, NY: Use of laboratory tests in a teaching hospital: Long-term trends. Ann Intern Med 90:243–248, 1979.

Handler RP: Diagnostic tests necessary to maintain clinical skills, letter. N Engl J Med 300:507, 1979.

Henry JB, Arras MJ: An innovation in health care delivery: Organ panels. South Med J 63:907–916, 1970.

Henry JB, Howanitz PJ: Organ panels and the relationship of the laboratory to the physician. In Young DS, Nipper H, Uddin D, et al (eds): Clinician and Chemist. The Relationship of the Laboratory to the Physician. Washington DC, American Association for Clinical Chemistry, Inc, 1979, pp 157–174.

Holland WW, Whitehead TP: Value of new laboratory tests in diagnosis and treatment. Lancet 2:391–394, 1974.

Johnson EA: Some basic considerations of the needs for improved clinical laboratory data analyses. Hum Pathol 4:5–8, 1973.

Kassirer JP, Pauker SG: Should diagnostic testing be regulated?, editorial. N Engl J Med 299:947–949, 1978.

Kosowsky DI: The clinical laboratory industry: Future outlook. Med Mktg Media 11:46–55, 1976.

Lundberg GD: The modern clinical laboratory: Justification, scope, and directions. JAMA 232:528–529, 1975.

Lundberg GD: Panic values—five years later. Med Lab Observer 9:27–34, 1977.

Lyle CB: Economic irony and cost containment, editorial Ann Int Med 90:267–268, 1979.

Martin AR, Wolf MA, Thibodeau LA, et al: A trial of two strategies to modify the test-ordering behavior of medical residents. N Engl J Med 303:1330–1336, 1980.

McNerney WJ: Blues frown on routine hospital diagnostic tests. Med World News, February 19, 1979, p. 25.

Moser R: No more "battered" patients: Blue Cross urges curb on hospital tests. Time, February 19, 1979, p. 80.

Murphy J, Henry JB: Effective utilization of clinical laboratories. Hum Pathol 9:625–633, 1978.

Russe HP: The use and abuse of laboratory tests. Med Clin North Am 53:223–231, 1969.

Sackett DL, Holland WW: Controversy in the detection of disease. Lancet 2:357–359, 1975.

Skendzel LP: How physicians use laboratory tests. JAMA 239:1077–1080, 1978.

Speicher CE, Smith JW: Interpretive reporting in clinical pathology. JAMA 243:1556–1560, 1980.

Statland BE: Interpretive Clinical Chemistry. Fullerton, Calif, Beckman Instruments Company, April 1979.

Statland BE, Winkel P: Response of clinical chemistry quantity values to selected physical, dietary, and smoking activities. In Stefanini M, Benson ES (eds): Progress in Clinical Pathology. Volume VIII. New York, Grune & Stratton, Inc, 1981, pp 25–44.

Sunderman FW: Current concepts of "normal values," "reference values," and "discrimination values" in clinical chemistry, editorial. Clin Chem 21:1873–1877, 1975.

Tancredi LR, Barondess JA: The problem of defensive medicine. Science 200:879–882, 1978.

Ward PCJ, Harris IB, Burke MD, et al: Systematic instruction in interpretive aspects of laboratory medicine. J Med Educ 51:648–656, 1976.

Weed LI: Medical Records, Medical Education, and Patient Care: The Problem-Oriented Record as a Basic Tool. Cleveland, The Press of Case Western Reserve University, 1970.

Weed LI: Problem-oriented laboratory testing. In Young DS, Nipper H, Uddin D, et al (eds): Clinician and Chemist: The Relationship of the Laboratory to the Physician. Washington, DC, American Association for Clinical Chemistry, Inc, 1979, pp 31–55.

Weed LI, Henry JB: Problem-oriented lab acts to correlate medical data. Int Medicine News, Vol 10, December 15, 1977, p 5.

Werner M, Altshuler CH: Utility of multiphasic biochemical screening and systematic laboratory investigation. Clin Chem 25:509–511, 1979.

Werner M, Altshuler CH: Cost effectiveness of multiphasic screening: Old controversies and a new rationale. Hum Pathol 12:111–117, 1981.

West KM: Substantial differences in the diagnostic criteria used by diabetes experts. Diabetes 24:641–644, 1975.

Williams BT: Perspectives on clinical decisions. Hum Pathol 12:106–110, 1981.

Winkel P, Statland BE: Reference values. In Henry JB (ed): Clinical Diagnosis and Management by Laboratory Methods, ed 16. Philadelphia, WB Saunders Company, 1979, pp 29–52.

Young DS: Why there is a laboratory. In Young DS, Nipper H, Uddin D, et al (eds): Clinician and Chemist: The Relationship of the Laboratory to the Physician. Washington DC, American Association for Clinical Chemistry, Inc, 1979, pp 3–22.

Zieve L: Misinterpretation and abuse of laboratory tests by clinicians. Ann NY Acad Sci 134:563–572, 1966.

STRATEGIES AND CLINICAL PROBLEM SOLVING

In this chapter, two phases of clinical problem solving — diagnosis and management — are discussed. Diagnosis is discussed from a traditional viewpoint and as an example of hypotheticodeductive reasoning. The implications of the hypotheticodeductive model of clinical reasoning for developing systems to support clinical problem solving are summarized. Ways of organizing the selection of laboratory tests are presented, and methods of interpreting laboratory test results in order to facilitate clinical problem solving are suggested.

Throughout this book, we stress the problem-solving nature of clinical reasoning and the importance of decisions, not as an end in themselves, but as a requirement for clinical problem solving. The goal of clinical problem solving is to resolve the patient's problem by correct diagnosis and effective therapy (Connelly and Johnson, 1980). The problem-solving process involves decisions of both low and high orders. *Low-order decisions* involve such issues as selection of questions to ask, clinical laboratory tests to order, form of therapy to choose, and determination of the reliability of data obtained (see Chapter 6). *High-order decisions* involve interpreting previously obtained data and deciding to consider a particular working diagnosis.

DIAGNOSIS AND THE HYPOTHETICODEDUCTIVE MODEL: AN OVERVIEW

TRADITIONAL VIEW

Traditional viewpoints of the diagnostic process imply that one stage of clinical problem solving involves the generation and testing of

17

hypotheses. For example, Isselbacher and colleagues (1980) discuss this stage by drawing a similarity between generating and testing diagnoses in clinical problem solving and generating and testing hypotheses in the scientific method. In both clinical problem solving and the scientific method, observational data suggest a series of hypotheses. These hypotheses are tested for correctness by further observation, and a conclusion is reached. In the medical context, observational data are signs, symptoms, and laboratory test values. Conclusions reached during diagnosis are *working diagnoses*.

Degowin and Degowin (1969) see diagnosis as the art or act of recognizing the presence of a diagnosis from its symptoms, signs, and laboratory findings. Four steps, which physicians repeat, are needed, in order to arrive at a diagnosis.

1. Accumulating facts.
2. Evaluating facts.
3. Preparing hypotheses.
4. Choosing among hypotheses (differential diagnosis).

Similarly, Johns (1980) reiterates the analogy between clinical reasoning and the scientific method. His group considers the distinction between facts (a group of data) and information an important one. In addition to facts, information implies both meaning and knowledge; information is what prompts physicians to take certain actions, such as seeking further knowledge. According to the view of John's group, experienced physicians direct the interview according to preliminary hypotheses and weigh clinical data in the context of previous information. Observations (facts) can support, refute, or help distinguish among diagnoses under consideration.

Campbell (1978) agrees with Johns that experienced physicians do not approach a diagnostic problem in a passive manner. In his view, physicians generate hypotheses and continuously weigh facts until the diagnosis is revealed by gathering information to support or refute these hypotheses. Campbell believes that experienced physicians think of these possibilities (hypotheses) from the very first moment in which they encounter a patient.

Murphy (1976) discusses the strategy of the diagnostic process and the tactics physicians use to select appropriate data for consideration. He emphasizes that in this selection process, an important consideration is to balance the description of the patient, as completely detailed and individualized as possible, against the goal of categorizing the patient as belonging to a number of diagnostically meaningful groups.

A more categorical description of the diagnostic process is given by Feinstein (1973*a*). He describes diagnosis as a sequence of conclusions, which transform evidence obtained from the patient into names of diseases. He separates this sequence of conclusions into intermediate conclusions (stations) and the strategies that determine what the next conclusion in the sequence will be. In diagnosis an explanation is sought for the patient's manifestations. Manifestations cause physicians to consider abnormalities in gross structural or functional portions of the body, such as organs, body regions (e.g., pelvis, head, chest), channels in the body (e.g., biliary tract, digestive tract, respiratory tract) or systems (e.g., cardiopulmonary, hematopoietic, immunologic). Subdivisions of these gross structural or functional body parts, such as cardiac muscle in the cardiopulmonary system, can also be considered.

COGNITIVE VIEW

The traditional views of the diagnostic process, espoused by the investigators mentioned in the previous paragraphs, are consistent with the description of the diagnostic process described by cognitive psychologists, as an example of hypotheticodeductive reasoning. In the traditional view, hypotheses include diseases, syndromes, abnormalities of organs, and pathologic mechanisms. Also, a number of strategies and operations are traditionally performed by physicians during diagnosis, such as determining the "closeness of fit" of clinical data to hypotheses, the "spiraling pursuit" of the diagnosis, and the differential diagnosis (Cutler, 1979). In information-processing terms, the diagnostic process, strategy, and other operations are performed by physicians in order to evaluate hypotheses or search for more information to include or exclude hypotheses.

In the information-processing view, diagnosis is a hypothesis-driven process. Thus, according to Elstein and associates (1978), a discussion of diagnosis should include the following:

1. How hypotheses are formed.

2. How hypotheses under consideration are excluded.

3. How hypotheses under consideration are included for further consideration or accepted as true.

4. How hypotheses guide the search for more information.

The medical problem solver is viewed as converting an open-ended problem into a series of closed ones by setting up diagnostic hypotheses as trial goals. Very early in the problem-solving process, hypotheses are generated. Additional data are searched for with these initial hypotheses in mind. Hypotheses direct and limit the search for additional data. This problem-solving approach constitutes the hypotheticodeductive method of problem solving.

In the information-processing view, hypotheses have several fates: consideration and rejection, replacement by a better alternative, or confirmation as a tentative or final diagnosis. Hypotheses can be "a fairly specific diagnostic label" (such as infectious mononucleosis) or a "multilevel formulation" (such as acute infection, probably viral in origin, possibly infectious mononucleosis). These hypotheses are used to formulate possible diagnostic problem solutions, which are used to cluster (or group) cues. Cues include all pertinent findings—chief complaint, routine history, physical data, and laboratory test results. Therefore, the information-processing model characterizes cue acquisition and the interpretation of cues, as well as generation and evaluation of hypotheses.

PROBLEM SOLVING AND OUR APPROACH

The information-processing view of diagnostic reasoning will be useful for our purposes in this book in a number of ways. This view allows for a more precise description of the diagnostic process. It allows us to use the experimental findings from the study of physicians' problem solving, in designing methods to facilitate clinical problem solving. In addition, this view of diagnosis facilitates the use of representation techniques, such as decision tables and flow charts, for describing and implementing diagnostic problem solving for manual or computerized systems (see Chapter 5).

A number of research efforts on medical diagnostic reasoning have described the diagnostic process in information-processing terms. Elstein and colleagues (1978) have summarized their research efforts. A broad range of methods and settings was used. In a core study, actors were taught to play the role of patients. Physicians interviewed the "patient" in a videotape-equipped "physician's office" and were encouraged to think aloud during the interview. The videotaped encounter was later used in a "simulated recall" session. During this session, physicians were encouraged to reflect aloud about their thinking in the original interview. Other methods and settings used included viewing films of patients, paper-and-pencil patient management problems, and the recording of verbal responses to clinical information written on cards.

The methods and settings used in these experiments are typical of those used by cognitive psychologists to describe diagnostic reasoning in terms of the information-processing view. The findings of Elstein's group (1978) and of other researchers, which are incorporated into our discussion of diagnosis that follows, support our intuitions about how to facilitate problem solving by physicians using strategies and how to present information about laboratory test results to physicians.

We believe that a problem-solving approach to the ordering and interpretation of laboratory tests is used by experienced physicians during diagnosis. Furthermore, insight into the diagnostic problem solving of experienced physicians, provided by both a traditional view and the information-processing view of diagnosis, may prove useful when applying laboratory studies to clinical problems, systematizing laboratory approaches to clinical problems, and presenting information about the interpretation of laboratory studies in more powerful ways.

The remainder of this chapter continues the discussion of diagnosis from both traditional and information-processing viewpoints, with application of these views to clinical problem solving by the use of strategies.

DATA COLLECTION AND AUTHENTICATION

Clinical problem solving depends on gathering data about a patient's condition. One class of low-order decisions during diagnosis is data authentication. Medical data have great variability and potential inaccuracy (Koran, 1975). The methods and data of clinical medicine are not perfectly reliable or accurate.

Typically, in the early stages of the diagnostic process, signs and symptoms are the primary input. A number of subjective variables affect the correctness of this type of data (Connelly and Johnson, 1980), such as the physician's assessment of the reliability and understanding of the patient and the physician's perception of his or her own skills.

In the later stages of the diagnostic process, it is typical for data to come from other physicians, laboratory and other studies (clinical laboratory, radiology), and written medical records. The validity of data in this stage will be explored if the results are unusual or unexpected in the context of working hypotheses (Kassirer and Gorry, 1978). One fact may contradict another. Such checking for validity is common when unexpectedly "abnormal" laboratory measurement values lead to repeat orders or to inquiries to the laboratory by the physician. In Chapter 9, a general procedure for determining the validity of the unexpectedly "abnormal" test result will be discussed with application to two concrete examples: The unexpected elevation of serum alkaline phosphatase and the unexpected elevation of serum calcium levels. In Part 3, Unexpected Test Results, there is information that permits the reader to determine the validity of test results for 22 different common tests. Laboratories attempt to ensure the authenticity of the data they produce through quality control programs. This is one way in which the clinical laboratory supports the medical problem solver (see Chapter 6).

Authenticated data can be interpreted as to its significance and probable meaning (Connelly and Johnson, 1980). For example, a range of "normal" laboratory values can be used by the medical problem solver to determine whether a particular laboratory value is beyond the reference interval for a healthy population and is therefore more likely to be significant. The assessment of the meaning and significance of such a deviation in a laboratory value depends on knowledge relating to the datum as well as other facts in the case. For example, in a patient with prolonged diarrhea and decreased skin turgor, a serum sodium value above the upper reference limit would more likely be considered significant than if

this test result was found in a patient without symptoms or physical findings.

HYPOTHESIS FORMATION

Kassirer and Gorry (1978) used protocol analysis to study the strategies of physicians' "taking the history of the present illness." In their experimental design, a physician was given clinical information about a patient in response to questions by the physician being studied. They concluded that hypotheses were activated by relatively few facts, in some instances after only the age, sex, and presenting complaint of the patient were known. Triggers of a hypothesis included individual symptoms, causes of a disease, complications of the disease, another hypothesis, or a discrepancy between new information and already existing hypotheses. Nonspecific evidence, like nausea, did not generate hypotheses. More specific evidence could generate both general hypotheses (fever and chills trigger infection) or specific hypotheses (dysuria triggers urinary tract infection).

Elstein and co-workers (1978) concluded that hypothesis generation frequently took place quite early before data collection was far advanced and that hypotheses generated early in diagnosis are frequently general. These general hypotheses imply additional steps the problem solver must take in order to arrive at more specific hypotheses. In some cases, however, a specific disease hypothesis is generated right away.

Frequently, diagnosis in the early stage is heavily "data driven," in the sense that certain data "suggest" hypotheses (diseases). In some cases, more than one datum is needed to suggest a disease. In this case, a "pattern" of data is associated with a disease (Price, 1971). This type of knowledge permits the generation or triggering of hypotheses early in the diagnostic process. If a particular pattern of data is observed, certain hypotheses are triggered. This type of knowledge is referred to as *symptom centered* (Rubin, 1975) and can be represented by if . . ., then . . . statements.

It is important to remember that triggered hypotheses can be general disease processes or specific disease entities. Usually, the implication is that certain gross structural or functional units of the body are affected or that certain pathophysiologic processes are active. For ex-

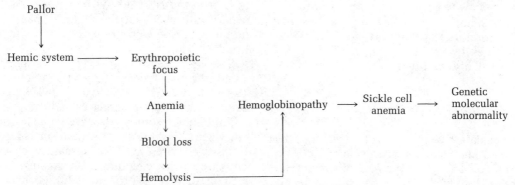

Figure 2–1. Sequential stations in diagnostic reasoning for a patient with the manifestation of pallor. (Adapted from Feinstein AR: An analysis of diagnostic reasoning: I. The domains and disorders of clinical macrobiology. Yale J Biol Med 46:225, 1973.)

ample, Feinstein (1973a) gave the following sequential stations for a patient who presented with pallor as the chief finding (Fig. 2–1). The manifestation of pallor first implies a functional abnormality at a body site or "domain." In this case, the implied domain is the hemic system. A particular "focus" in the hemic system is also implied (the erythropoietic focus). In this example, the patient's first finding gives an initial direction for diagnostic reasoning. It can be inferred that causes relating to the erythropoietic focus should be pursued further.

Just as signs and symptoms can trigger such a process, so can certain laboratory studies. Some test results can imply that certain organs or systems are affected and that significant pathophysiologic processes are active. In our previous example, a laboratory test result (such as a low hematocrit or low hemoglobin reading) could raise the possibility of similar hypotheses to that of pallor if the clinician has not yet considered anemia (see Part 3: Blood hemoglobin, low). A 12-channel chemistry profile could also be used to trigger certain "suggested" diagnostic hypotheses (Galen, 1975a). Indeed, in this regard, computer programs have been used to generate diagnostic suggestions (Hobbie and Reese, 1981). (See Chapter 8 concerning profiling.)

Campbell (1978) further illustrates this point (Fig. 2–2). A woman who presents with a lump in her breast causes the generation of these hypotheses: cancer, not cancer, or some other disorder. In a similar fashion, a patient presenting with crushing anterior chest pain can raise these hypotheses: Acute myocardial infarction, not acute myocardial infarction, or some other disorder.

Hypothesis generation is not the only function of symptom-centered knowledge in diagnosis; it also guards against errors of omission by providing a checklist for collecting information (Connelly and Johnson, 1980). Recall of data and communication of data to others are facilitated by the organization of information in a context-dependent way.

In summary, hypothesis generation appears to be an important process. Vague or common findings are not as helpful as a recognized pattern of findings. Hypothesis generation frequently takes place before much information is collected. Laboratory-test-to-disease knowledge can be of as much use as symptom-to-disease knowledge in certain situations, for example, low serum thyroxine (T_4) and high thyroid-stimulating hormone (TSH) associated with hypothyroidism. We attempt to provide laboratory-test-to-disease knowledge in Chapters 8 through 17 and in Part 3 as a way of

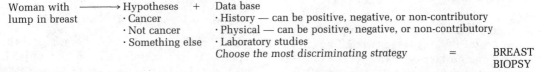

Figure 2–2. Sequence of diagnostic reasoning. (Adapted from Campbell EJ: Symposium on the Pathologist and the Diagnostic Process. St. Louis, Mo., Fall Meeting of the College of American Pathologists, September 19, 1978.)

teaching how to generate hypotheses from test results. Manual and computer systems that take laboratory test results as input and trigger hypotheses by producing diagnostic "suggestions" will also be discussed.

HYPOTHESIS EVALUATION

After data have been used to generate hypotheses, the physician must employ a reasoning process to explain the patient's manifestations. The final diagnosis needs to be sufficiently specific in order for appropriate therapy to be selected (Connelly and Johnson, 1980).

Several types of knowledge are required for this stage of diagnosis. The physician must know the ways in which the possible causes of the patient's problem manifest themselves and must also be able to compare the findings obtained so far with those exhibited by the diseases under consideration. Finally, the physician must be able to verify the adequacy of the current explanations for the patient's symptoms.

The knowledge used by the physician to determine the way in which possible causes manifest themselves has been referred to as *disease-centered knowledge* (Rubin, 1975). This knowledge provides expectations about what a patient with a certain disease "looks like" (Connelly and Johnson, 1980). In this respect, a hypothesis implies a list of clinical findings that may be observed if the hypothesis is true (Elstein et al., 1978). These lists allow data to be collected with a view toward their usefulness in testing hypotheses. As we discuss later, this list is also useful in interpreting the value of a particular clinical finding or laboratory test result to a hypothesis.

Concrete examples of such lists of clinical findings are summarized in the cue-hypothesis matrix of Table 2–1 (Elstein et al, 1978). The matrix is composed of cues (clinical manifestations) and hypotheses. This particular case involves a 19-year-old female college student who presented with fatigue, excessive sleeping, and severe headaches. An expert was asked to assign a value for each hypothesis, which was often entertained by physicians when diagnosing this case, by assigning a value to each cue (clinical manifestation). Each clinical manifestation was rated as to whether it tended to confirm (+), disconfirm (−), or not contribute

to a hypothesis. Table 2–1 shows what the expert who filled out the matrix expected to find in a person who has each of the diseases listed.

Disease-centered knowledge is further divided into two types (Connelly and Johnson, 1980; Rubin, 1975). *Prototype knowledge* concerns diseases (their variances and categories) and the manifestations that are typically present when the disease, its variant, or category of disease is present. These diseases, variants, and categories are hierarchically organized (Elstein et al, 1978; Wortman, 1972). (A hypothesized prototype-knowledge structure for a kidney disease is given in Figure 5–4.) The organization of such knowledge provides the physician with a picture of what a typical patient with the disease "looks like."

System knowledge (Connelly and Johnson, 1980) allows the physician to predict and explain the relationship between disease and its symptoms and signs to various pathophysiologic entities. Armed with such knowledge, the physician can deduce the way in which disease combinations or new diseases would present in terms of their manifestations. This type of knowledge would also "back up" the recall of prototype knowledge and provide a way to justify and explain diagnostic decisions in terms of the underlying pathophysiology of the disease. System knowledge, then, can be used in a number of ways in order to diagnose a case, particularly a new one.

Chapters 8 though 17 discuss the relationship between the pathophysiology of a disease and changes in laboratory test results. We believe this kind of system knowledge about laboratory test results is as important for accurate diagnosis as knowledge about the relationship between clinical signs and symptoms to the underlying pathophysiology of a particular disease. Likewise, for a "typical" patient, we have included values for certain laboratory test results to provide prototype knowledge in terms of laboratory measurements. (See Chapter 15, which discusses prototype as well as system knowledge for liver function tests.)

Excluding Hypotheses

Besides the hypothesized diseases and their typical clinical manifestations, the physician must also know how to choose among them. This knowledge allows the physician to ask a

Table 2–1. CUE-HYPOTHESIS MATRIX*

Finding	Hypotheses Often Entertained													
	INFEC	STREP	CNS	MONO	FLU	HEPAT	LEUK	LYM	ANEM	MEA	IPA	HA	CSA	ASA
Given at start of problem 19-year-old woman														
Chief complaint: fatigue, poor appetite													+	
Temperature 102°F oral†	+	+	+	+	+	+		+	+	+	+	+		+
Ambulatory, alert														
Present illness														
Excessive sleeping†	+	+	+	+	+	+	+	+	+	+				
Anorexia — 3 days	+	+	+	+	+	+	+	+						
Severe throbbing frontal headache†	+	+	+	+	+	+			+	+				
No visual disturbances			−											
Generalized weakness	+	+	+	+	+	+	+	+	+	+				
Mild chills and fever†	+	+	+	+	+	+	+	+			+			
General achiness, 5 days' duration†	+	+	+	+	+	+	+	+						
No cold or runny nose	−	−			−	−	−	−						
Probable exposure to influenza†	+	−	+	+	+		−				+			

Key:
INFEC	= Infection	IPA	= Inflammation-produced anemia
STREP	= Strep infection	HA	= Hemolytic anemia
CNS	= CNS infection	CSA	= Congenital spherocytic anemia
MONO	= Infectious mononucleosis	ASA	= Autoimmune spherocytic anemia
FLU	= Influenza	+	= Confirms hypothesis
HEPAT	= Infectious hepatitis	−	= Disconfirms hypothesis
LEUK	= Leukemia	Blank space	= Does not contribute to hypothesis
LYM	= Lymphoma		
ANEM	= Anemia		
MEA	= Mixed etiology anemia		

*Adapted from Elstein AS, Shulman LS, Sprafka SA, et al.: Medical Problem Solving: An Analysis of Clinical Reasoning. Cambridge, Mass, Harvard University Press, 1978, p 55.

†Signifies a critical finding, as defined in text.

sequence of questions of the form: "Does the patient have disease X?" (Connelly and Johnson, 1980). The manifestations of the patient must be compared with the typical manifestations of the hypothesized disease. If the patient's manifestations are sufficiently "consistent" with those of the hypothesized disease, that disease is the diagnosis. Otherwise, a different disease will have to be chosen or more data will have to be evaluated.

One way in which the list of hypothesized diseases can be reduced is to exclude those that have a "poor fit." For example, the physician can use the knowledge that a finding is often present when a given disease is present to help eliminate the hypothesis. The hypothesis can be eliminated when the patient does not exhibit the manifestation that is typically present when the given disease is present. Using the absence of a finding that is typically present—when a given disease is present—to weigh heavily against that hypothesis is commonly referred to as "ruling out" that disease. In Chapter 4 we shall see that sensitive tests are useful in ruling out certain diseases.

A system used by some physicians that relies heavily on the elimination strategy is called the *method of exhaustion* (Murphy, 1976). This process consists of eliciting all possible facts about a patient and arriving at a "most probable diagnosis" by exclusion of all other possible diagnoses.

Experimental findings from psychological experiments suggest that physicians do not take full advantage of negative data in order to limit the number of hypotheses they are considering (Wortman, 1966). Wortman believed that his subjects (physicians) tended to define individual diseases by positive instances of particular pathologic findings rather than by taking advantage of negative information. Elstein and colleagues (1978), however, found that a hypothesis might be excluded by a physician using a rule such as this: "If feature A is absent, it cannot be diagnosis X." These investigations tried to model the physician's hypothesis evaluation using a simple linear combination of +, −, or non-contributory values of a clinical manifestation from a cue-hypothesis matrix, as shown in Table 2–1. They found that linear combinations emphasizing positive data modeled the physicians' behavior closer than balanced (positive and negative) combinations. This result is consistent with the belief that negative information is used suboptimally by physicians (Gorry et al, 1978).

Including Hypotheses for Further Consideration

Similar to the elimination strategy, physicians usually attempt to prove that a hypothesis is true by matching the typical characteristics of that hypothesis against patient manifestations (Elstein et al, 1978; Kassirer and Gorry, 1978; Kleinmuntz, 1965, 1968). A physician might use a rule to help confirm that a particular hypothesis is true; "If three out of the following five features are present, then the diagnosis is X."

However, even though a patient might manifest all the typical findings of a hypothesis, it does not necessarily mean that a particular hypothesis is correct. Frequently, the same set of manifestations can be present in a number of diseases because many combinations of findings are not specific for a single disease. Just as signs and symptoms can be nonspecific, laboratory test results can also be nonspecific. We discuss laboratory test specificity in Chapter 4 as a statistical concept and apply it in the sections on test interpretation in Part 2 of this book.

The ability to distinguish the likelihood of one hypothesis over another is important. This discrimination strategy is sometimes referred to as *differential diagnosis*. Kleinmuntz (1965, 1968) exemplifies this strategy in his "20 questions" experiments involving neurologic disease. A neurologist thought of a disease while another physician tried to diagnose the disease by asking questions. Inquiries were made about the presence or absence of signs, symptoms, biographic data, or laboratory test results until the physician reached a diagnosis. Because the questions asked could be answered only yes or no, the entire diagnostic session could be transformed into a treelike graph, as in Figure 2–3. The questions are the "nodes" in the tree and are always connected to two paths. The first question asked becomes the top node ("root" of the tree). A path connecting the root of the tree to a terminal "node" (diagnosis) schematically represents the questions, answers, and conclusions during a session. In a separate study, physicians were requested to state their reasons for asking each of the questions about the set of initial problems.

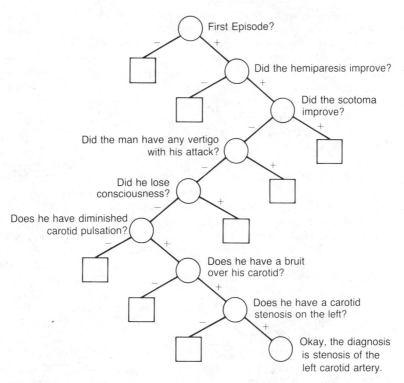

Figure 2–3. Tree-like graph in medical diagnosis. (Adapted from Kleinmuntz, B: Diagnostic problem solving by computer. Jpn Psychol Res 7:192, 1965.)

These experiments emphasize the physician's selection of an item that has one value for some diseases and a different value for the rest. The set of candidate diseases being considered is reduced on the basis of the item's value in the patient being considered. The new reduced set of hypothesized diseases is further reduced by choosing another differential expectation and checking whether or not it is true.

In evaluating the correctness of the hypothesis, the physician relies on more than the presence or absence of expected findings. Kassirer and Gorry (1978) observed that cause-and-effect relationships between hypotheses and the number of findings accounted for by hypotheses are also important. In this regard, Elstein and co-workers (1978) believed that not only were there simple rules for combining data pertinent to a particular hypothesis but also that physicians appeared to be striving for a parsimonious solution.

How Hypotheses Guide the Search for More Information

We discussed the "closeness of fit" of the patient's manifestations to each of the hypoth-

esized diseases. Our model of the hypothesis evaluation stage of medical diagnosis (Elstein et al, 1978) assumes that a hypothesis implies a list of clinical findings, which may be observed if the hypothesis is true. These lists allow data to be collected with a view toward their usefulness in testing hypotheses. This list is useful, therefore, in interpreting the value of a particular manifestation to a hypothesis and is one of the factors involved in hypothesis evaluation. Each manifestation, in the context of a particular hypothesis, tends to be viewed by the physician as either confirming (having a positive weight), disconfirming (having a negative weight), or not contributing (having a zero weight) to a hypothesis. (Such was the situation for the case summarized in a cue-hypothesis matrix of Table 2–1.) It is also suggested that the same general evaluation rule need not be applied to all hypotheses. One hypothesis might use a rule: "At least three out of five features must be present to make a diagnosis X." Another hypothesis might use the rule: "If the following three features are present, then it must be diagnosed as X."

However, "closeness of fit" is not the only consideration in choosing the best hypothesis. *Clustering* is also an intricate part of the judgments involved at this stage of diagnosis. Clustering refers to the manner in which findings are attributed to certain hypotheses. Certain hypotheses compete, in the sense that they provide alternative explanations for some groups of manifestations. Improper clustering can lead to erroneous conclusions.

For example, in a patient presenting with polyuria, tachypnea, and furuncles (Feinstein, 1973b), a monopathic explanation for the patient's manifestations would be diabetes mellitus. It could be, however, that a renal disease is causing the polyuria; a cardiac disease, the tachypnea; and solvents used in the patient's occupation, the furuncles. Conventional wisdom (i.e., the principle of parsimony, or "Ockham's razor"*) tells us that simple (monopathic) explanations are preferred to ones that are complex (polypathic). This is fine if the simple explanation turns out to be the true one. According to the principle of parsimony, the smallest number of diagnoses, which accounts for all findings, is preferred; however, using this principle can lead to errors in patients with coincidental diseases.

In striving for a parsimonious problem solution, the physician may use knowledge concerning the cause-and-effect relationships between hypotheses, as well as consider the number of findings accounted for by a hypothesis. Hypotheses are associated with functional relationships that are known to exist or are hypothesized to exist. For example, the physician may functionally attribute anemia to a gastrointestinal disorder (like bleeding), in order to explain in parsimonious terms the presence of anemia in a patient who has blood in the stool. Likewise, knowledge of the hierarchical disease classification, which pertains to a particular disease category, can similarly affect the evaluation of hypotheses by unifying a number of elementary hypotheses. It is important to remember that disease categorization can be performed not only on the basis of common signs and symptoms or laboratory test results but also on the similarity of effect on particular organs or because of a similar disease mechanism.

Another factor that affects the hypothesis evaluation process is the number of manifes-

tations encompassed by the present disease set. A diagnosis will be considered adequate only when it encompasses all elementary hypotheses and accounts for both normal and abnormal findings in a particular patient (Kassirer and Gorry, 1978). In this regard, by checking for complications, related conditions, or unrelated disorders, a physician can refine a hypothesis in order to encompass all of a patient's manifestations.

Even though each physician has an idiosyncratic way of approaching a particular diagnosis, there seem to be patterns to the order in which categories of hypotheses are considered. Kassirer and Gorry (1978) believe that, generally speaking, the initially activated general hypotheses are evaluated by comparing data from the patient with more specific categories of the hypothesized disorders. Some initial hypotheses are rejected, and more specific hypotheses are substituted for these more general ones. A few particular hypotheses are then tested further for confirmation.

In general, then, clinical diagnosis proceeds from symptoms and signs, to syndromes, to diseases, to specific etiologies. For example, in the case of the 19-year-old college student we discussed earlier (Table 2–1), a list of frequently considered hypotheses is given in Table 2–2, along with the times at which these hypotheses occurred during the diagnostic process. These hypotheses can be represented in a hierarchical disease classification, as in Figure 2–4. In this case, there are two functionally unrelated problems, anemia and infection. As the diagnoses progressed in this particular experiment, the physicians started from general hypotheses and arrived at more particular hypotheses by asking for pertinent data. Because each hypothesis, according to our model, implies a list of findings that will probably be true if the disease is present, it is easy to see how this is done.

Often a clinician can ascertain which organ is involved before the cause or mechanism of disease is determined. This is accomplished with a grouping of symptoms, signs, and laboratory test results related to anatomy, physiology, or biochemistry (see the discussion on organ panels in Chapter 1). Certain manifestations, symptoms, or signs imply affected organs, channels, and systems in the body. This implication is an associational one in the sense that it requires no reasoning, just recall (e.g., dysuria points to the bladder, ocular pain to

---

*From William of Ockham, a medieval cleric, who espoused the scientific and philosophic rule that simple explanations using a single cause are preferred over complex explanations using multiple causes.

Table 2–2. NUMBER OF SUBJECTS (PHYSICIANS) WHO CONSIDERED MAJOR HYPOTHESES AT SELECTED POINTS IN THE WORKUP OF A SIMULATION*

Hypothesis†	Total at any Point	As First Hypothesis	At Quarter Mark	At Halfway Mark	At Conclusion
Infection‡	21	14	15	19	5
Infectious mononucleosis	20	2	9	15	20
Infectious hepatitis	18	5	9	11	5
Hemolytic anemia	17	—	—	—	—
Hereditary spherocytic anemia	10	—	—	—	8
Viral illness or viral respiratory infection	8	—	4	6	1
Meningitis	7	—	5	4	0
Anemia	6	—	—	3	—
Influenza	4	—	3	1	0
Encephalitis	4	—	2	3	0
Leukemia	4	—	—	1	0
Lymphoma	4	—	0	0	1

*Adapted from Elstein AS, Shulman LS, Sprafka SA, et al.: Medical Problem Solving: An Analysis of Clinical Reasoning. Cambridge, Mass., Harvard University Press, 1978, p. 69.

†Twelve hypotheses in addition to those listed were each considered by one or two subjects at some point in the problem.

‡Includes acute febrile illness, viral illness, bacterial infection, and viral respiratory infection.

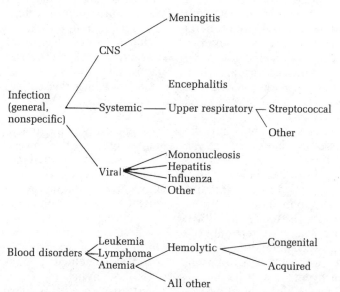

Figure 2–4. Cognitive organization of a simulation (as given in Table 2–2). (Adapted from Elstein AS, Shulman LS, Sprafka SA, et al.: Medical Problem Solving: An Analysis of Clinical Reasoning. Cambridge, Mass., Harvard University Press, 1978, p 72.)

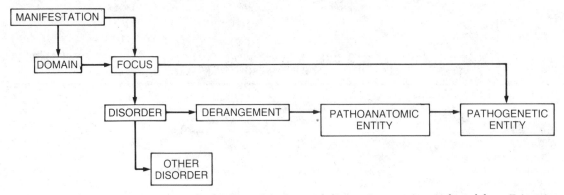

Figure 2–5. Sequential stations in the intellectual pathway of diagnostic reasoning. (Adapted from Feinstein AR: An analysis of diagnostic reasoning: I. The domains and disorders of clinical macrobiology. Yale J Biol Med 46:224, 1973.)

the eye, or diarrhea to the gastrointestinal tract).

Our example of a patient presenting with pallor (Fig. 2–1), which we discussed earlier, is a particular instance of a general "sequence of stations" in diagnostic reasoning (Feinstein, 1973a) and is graphically demonstrated in Figure 2–5.

Disorders are associated with categorized underlying causes— "derangements" (general pathologic processes), "pathoanatomic entities" (specific typographic and morphologic abnormalities), or "pathogenetic entities" (etiologic). In our example (Fig. 2–1), the general pathologic process or derangement giving rise to the disorder of anemia is hemoglobinopathy. The hemoglobinopathy is attributed to a specific morphologic abnormality, sickle cell anemia, whose etiology is a genetically induced molecular abnormality.

There are other factors that enter into the order in which diseases are considered and the decision as to the "best" diagnosis. For example, the ordering of diseases being considered appears to be a function of their relative probability, seriousness, population base rate, treatability, and novelty (Elstein et al, 1972). Physicians are more likely to remember a disease that they have seen quite often or have recently diagnosed (Connelly and Johnson, 1980). The order of hypotheses to be considered is also affected by the hierarchy of disease hypotheses that a physician is considering (Fig. 2–4). One of the functions of the data gathered by the physician is to refine more general hypotheses (syndromes, pathologic processes) into more particular hypotheses (etiologies).

In the gestalt explanation of some diagnoses (Murphy, 1976), diagnosis takes place by the association of certain patterns or pictures of patients with various diseases. The diagnosis is made when the pattern of a particular disease matches the pattern built up for a patient. The classic visual diagnosis of Parkinson's disease is an example of such a diagnosis.

Degowin and Degowin (1969) also distinguish between diagnosis at a glance from the more stepwise diagnosis discussed in this section. In making a diagnosis at a glance, physicians are unaware that they are logically pursuing a solution. However, with more difficult diagnoses, each fact obtained during an examination prompts a sequence of reasoning steps. The physician performs a "spiraling pursuit," in which revised lists of hypotheses are created based upon a review of preceding findings.

Apparently, after some experience with certain diagnoses, the physician begins to recognize a sequence of patient data that efficiently diagnoses a certain set of candidate diseases. Once such a sequence is developed and remembered, it can be reapplied to any case as a standard procedure (the gestalt). In fact, such standard procedures represented in the form of a "decision tree" or flow chart have been documented (Connelly and Johnson, 1980). A physician who is a novice at diagnosis must dynamically build such decision trees. But with experience, previously built decision trees can be retrieved from memory and used without elaborate reasoning. It is such stored procedures that allow the "effortless" diagnosis, or diagnosis at a glance.

COGNITIVE LIMITATIONS DURING DIAGNOSIS AND HOW TO OVERCOME THEM

The hypotheticodeductive model presents the problem solver as having some characteristics common to all problem solvers regardless of the decision problem. These common characteristics are inherent limitations that determine the approach to be used in solving common or unique problems (Connelly and Johnson, 1980). During medical problem solving, therefore, the physician has the same limitations as any decision maker in a similar situation. Of course, because of the particular content of the physician's problem, there are limitations and strategies unique to the medical task. In this section, we discuss problem-solving limitations and the strategies that can be used to overcome them.

Problem solvers can be identified according to how successful they are in comparison with their colleagues. Likewise, the "expert" physician can be distinguished from less successful colleagues in terms of problem-solving abilities. The comparison of the expert physician with the "non-expert" is a useful method to ascertain those cognitive skills the expert has developed in order to outperform a colleague. We discuss some differences between experts and non-experts in this section.

Memory Limitations

Many cognitive psychologists describe the human problem solver as a very adaptable limited information processor. The elementary processes of the mind limit problem-solving capabilities and the ability to process information. These limits can be usefully related to psychologic concepts of memory and problem solving.

An analogy can be drawn between the problem-solving processes of the human and the computer. In this analogy, physicians are viewed as having inputs (patient manifestations), outputs (diagnoses), memory (disease classifications, associations), and programs (matching strategies, discrimination functions). In these terms, a particular problem solver has resource limitations that limit the amount of information that can be considered at one time, such as short-term memory capacity. There are limitations in the clarity and accessibility of data, internal or external to the problem solver (Connelly and Johnson, 1980). A laboratory report that is smudged and hard to read limits the problem-solving ability of the physician using it, just as a poorly performed x-ray procedure of the chest would limit the problem solver's ability to make use of the radiograph.

One of the major results of the short-term memory resource limitations of problem solvers is the restriction on the number of active hypotheses that can be under consideration at any one time. The expert problem solver comes up with a lower number of hypotheses in comparison with the non-expert. This is an example of the expert's skill in limiting the amount of information considered or produced in such a way as to avoid degrading overall performance (Connelly and Johnson, 1980). Considering a small number of hypotheses is more efficient than considering a large number.

The concept of there being a limit to the number of active hypotheses under consideration is consistent with the view that human memory can be short term or long term. Short-term memory is characterized by a limited time span for retaining information, as well as a finite amount of room (or "chunk" capacity). An example is forgetting an unfamiliar telephone number some seconds after looking it up in the directory.

The chunk limit of short-term memory can be clearly demonstrated in certain verbal learning experiments. One such is an experiment in which a subject is presented with a list of unrelated English words one at a time and asked to recall the entire list. Recall will be more successful for the words in the last part of the list. The number of recalled words tends to increase if they are related in a conceptual way. For example, if some words are types of furniture or kinds of animals, they can be more easily remembered. This phenomenon is explained by the encoding of several words into a chunk. With unrelated words, a chunk would be equal to one word. The chunk limit of short-term memory in various experiments is generally found to be seven plus or minus two (7 ± 2) chunks. Interestingly, 7 ± 2 is the same order of magnitude as the number of active hypotheses of physicians in the studies by Kassirer and Gorry (1978).

Long-term memory is not encumbered by either of these limitations. It is practically infinite in size and retains information for a long time. Such knowledge as associations, disease classifications, and diagnostic strategies is believed to be retained in a physician's long-term memory. See Figures 5–6 and 5–7, for an artist's conception of short-term and long-term memories.

In clinical problem solving, there are a number of heuristics that are helpful in limiting the number of hypotheses under consideration without degrading the overall problem-solving performance. One such heuristic is to avoid hypothesizing the disease until it is suggested by some clinical findings. A hypothesis may be "triggered" if a certain combination of findings is present that makes a hypothesis likely to be true; if the findings occur with diseases that are too serious to ignore; or if the findings are associated with rare diseases that will be diagnosed only if they are suspected early.

The expert diagnostician can limit the number of triggered hypotheses by considering the frequency of their occurrence in the population. This information can either help eliminate rare diseases from further consideration or help order the likelihood of active hypotheses.

Finally, a differential test can be used to distinguish among active hypotheses. In later chapters, we suggest combinations of laboratory findings that are useful for triggering certain hypotheses as well as for differential diagnosis.

The physician can restrict the number of hypotheses by using disease classification schemes. More elementary hypotheses and diseases can be grouped together by virtue of their common characteristics. Such a disease grouping can be treated as a more specific hypothesis in the sense that it can be triggered by combinations of clinical findings, discriminated with a differential test, or rejected by elimination strategies. The hypothesis groupings can then be dealt with as a single hypothesis, eliminating or confirming the presence of many other hypotheses. In Figure 2–4, the cognitive organization used to solve the particular simulation of the case in Table 2–2 is represented as such a hierarchy of groups.

In later chapters, we will discuss such hierarchies in terms of their laboratory findings. It is important to realize that strategies can aid clinical problem solving by confirming or rejecting specific diseases and by confirming or rejecting classes of diseases or pathologic processes. In this regard, we will discuss combinations of laboratory tests that can trigger, discriminate, reject, or confirm such disease groupings, such as inflammation of various organs (see Chapter 8).

Disease, time-course, and severity must be kept in mind during clinical problem solving. The expert copes with problems by using discrete categories of diseases, indexed by time-course and severity factors. For example, the physician may categorize extrahepatic obstructive disease as either complete or incomplete, depending on the degree of blockage (Connelly and Johnson, 1980). By indexing the disease categories by severity, age, or time-course, the physician is better able to reject or confirm hypotheses because disease categories are more distinct. We discuss discrete disease categories in later chapters in terms of their time course and severity as well as their expected laboratory test results. Table 11–1 shows how the operating characteristics of conventional spirometric tests differ for young, minimally symptomatic smokers versus middle-aged, moderately symptomatic smokers.

An expert often appears to solve certain medical problems in a way that seems largely effortless and automatic. For the novice, these problems require deliberate and conscious mental effort (Connelly and Johnson, 1980). The expert is able to determine what "works" in certain tasks and to deal with such situations in a deterministic manner by recalling this knowledge. This is particularly true of familiar or recurring tasks. Many common medical problems can be dealt with in this manner.

In the following chapters, we attempt to map out deterministic strategies for common medical problems that can be resolved largely through the use of laboratory tests and to define the task situations for which these strategies are applicable, to aid the physician in determining their usefulness for a particular case. When predetermined procedures are not appropriate, we shall provide information to help resolve the problems.

Cost and Time Limitations

The physician must consciously decide when to halt the cycle of data collection, authentication, interpretation, development of potential explanations, selection of expectations, comparison of expectations with manifestations, and identification of additional data required. This cycle is repeated until an explanation can account for the patient's signs enough to allow for the selection of an appropriate therapy.

The diagnostic process is limited by cognitive and practical factors. It is impractical to elicit all facts about a patient before coming to a decision, just as it is impractical to order all laboratory tests available. Diagnosis cannot go on indefinitely because it is constrained by cost and time. These additional constraints are significant because presenting symptoms, signs, or laboratory test results may not be associated with the proper diagnosis. In fact, the proper diagnosis may be contradicted by the initially gathered data.

A way to view the expert selection of data during the diagnostic process is to draw an analogy involving the following dilemma (Winston, 1977). Imagine climbing to the top of a hill. One third of the way to the top, a thick blinding fog settles over the hill. How do you proceed? One strategy would be to take a single step forward and then a single step backward to your original position in each of four perpendicular directions. The direction of the steepest slope would be the direction in which to proceed (Fig. 2–6). Eventually you would achieve the "top of the hill" if certain restrictions on the shape of the hill and surrounding area are satisfied.

The "top of the hill" in diagnosis is the correct diagnosis for a particular patient's medical problem. A single step in a particular direction represents the physician's selection of a particular piece of data to aid in determining the diagnosis. One expert strategy for determining which piece of data to ask for next is to consider the effect of the possible values of a piece of data on the current hypotheses concerning the patient's problem. This process would be analogous to taking a single step forward and then backward to the original position in the four perpendicular directions. Eventually the physician should achieve the proper diagnosis if the problem "terrain" has a certain shape (Fig. 2–6).

A "hill-climbing" strategy performs poorly in certain kinds of "terrain." Foothills, ridges, and broad planes can be traps (Fig. 2–7). In such problem terrains, we are not guaranteed to achieve the correct diagnosis by asking for a piece of data that has the greatest potential positive effect on the probability of the diagnosis. If there are other plausible but incorrect diagnoses (Fig. 2–7A), the physician may be led to pursue an erroneous but plausible diagnosis. Perhaps the correct diagnosis is quite similar to other plausible diagnoses, and this "ridge" of plausible diagnoses steers us away (Fig. 2–7B). In the event that only a narrow amount of information is required to achieve a certain diagnosis, the physician may stumble aimlessly through a "broad plain," never beginning an ascent towards the correct diagnosis (Fig. 2–7C).

In our discussions of clinical subproblems and problem-solving methods, we suggest ways to avoid such pitfalls when using laboratory studies. We have attempted to incorporate cost and time considerations as well in our clinical

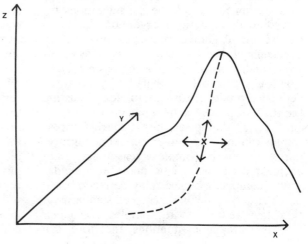

Figure 2–6. Method of steepest ascent. (Adapted from Winston PH: Artificial Intelligence. © 1977. Addison-Wesley, Reading, Mass., p 93. Reprinted with permission.)

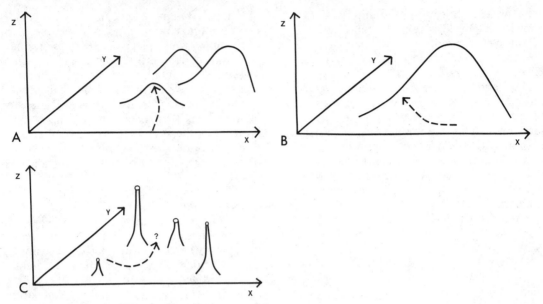

Figure 2–7. Traps encountered in the method of steepest ascent. (Adapted from Winston PH: Artificial Intelligence. © 1977. Addison-Wesley, p 94. Reprinted with permission.)

problem-solving strategies and to provide guidelines for doing so when designing such strategies.

MANAGEMENT DECISIONS

The objective of diagnostic problem solving is more than reaching a correct diagnosis. The overall goal is providing effective therapy, which lessens the negative effects of an unalterable problem or eliminates the cause (Connelly and Johnson, 1980). The previous sections of this chapter have focused on the diagnostic phase of clinical problem solving. This section addresses the considerations involved in therapeutic intervention. Unfortunately, the cognitive processes involved in management decisions have not been as intensively studied as has diagnostic reasoning.

However, we believe that the hypothetico-deductive model is also useful for discussing the thought processes of clinicians when managing patients' illnesses. Just as diagnostic reasoning can rely on either predefined procedures or more complex reasoning, management decisions can be made in a similar way. Therapeutic choices may be made based on clear and predefined accepted standards or they may require more complex reasoning. Certain therapeutic situations, therefore, can

be represented by "algorithmic" procedures, just as some diagnostic situations can be. Factors can influence a certain therapeutic situation enough to make algorithmic procedures useless. Such factors as the patient's clinical condition, concurrent disease, and disease complications can affect therapeutic decisions. Therapy availability, cost, and the physician's prior experience with the treatment can also affect decisions. In contrast to the diagnostic phase, the patient's own views regarding the possible outcomes of certain therapeutic procedures are important.

Monitoring the effects of therapy on diseases is a particularly important form of laboratory activity constituting 60 to 80 per cent of the volume of laboratory work, especially in tertiary-care facilities (Brecher, 1978; Murphy and Henry, 1978). Broadly speaking, monitoring is done by repeatedly sampling particular groups of data about which the physician has certain expectations. Data are expected to follow certain trends if the therapy is an adequate one. The physician may choose to adjust the therapy or change it entirely, depending on the trend or stability of the data. The physician may also decide to change the diagnosis or retain it, based on monitoring data.

The physician's resource limitations are an important determinant of therapeutic outcome. The physician depends heavily on memory of recent patient data as well as medical knowledge. Of particular importance is that knowledge relating the effects of certain therapeutic maneuvers to aspects of the patient's hypothesized disease or disease state.

In some of the following chapters, therapeutic selection and monitoring using laboratory test results will be discussed. These therapeutic decision situations have been chosen based on how frequently they occur, their seriousness, and dependence of the decision on laboratory studies.

APPROACH TO CLINICAL PROBLEM SOLVING BY STRATEGIES

The hypotheticodeductive model of clinical problem solving serves as a guide in the organization and content of this book. The diagnostic process can be viewed as a procedure in which the clinician solves a problem by solving a series of subproblems. Thus, strategies (procedures) are presented for resolving particular diagnostic and management subproblems with the use of laboratory studies. The hypotheticodeductive model elucidates the limitations of the medical problem solver. These insights have led us to include information that relates disease and laboratory findings.

Because incomplete knowledge about a disease and its symptoms and signs can lead to inappropriate laboratory test selection, we will be emphasizing the relationship between laboratory tests and clinical contexts or pathophysiologic states. Likewise, our recognition of the effects of low-order decisions on data verification and authentication motivated us to describe the process of producing laboratory results (see Chapter 6). Problem-solving approaches similar to those used in diagnostic situations are presented. The approach to evaluating an unexpectedly elevated serum alkaline phosphatase or calcium level is an example of such a data verification procedure (Chapter 9). We also discuss a model of laboratory operation, which can be helpful in understanding a general approach to authenticating laboratory test results (Chapter 7).

Because therapeutic selection and monitoring constitute an important phase of medical problem solving and are often highly dependent on laboratory studies, we have included approaches to these management decision sit-uations. Besides presenting strategies for effectively dealing with clinical subproblems, we discuss methods for representing and implementing these strategies. Methods useful in representing clinical problem-solving strategies include decision tables and flow charts. Implementation methods include both manual and computerized systems.

SUBPROBLEMS AND CLINICAL PROBLEM SOLVING

During diagnosis, the clinician progresses through a consideration of a series of hypotheses to explain the patient's problem. Usually, the kinds of hypotheses considered early in the process are relatively general, such as: "Inflammation is causing a sore throat." Later in the process, more specific hypotheses are involved, such as: "β-hemolytic streptococcal pharyngitis is causing a sore throat." In considering each of these hypotheses, the clinician must resolve a number of subproblems, such as: "Confirm inflammation present," or "Eliminate inflammation as possibility" (see Chapter 8).

Consider a complex problem, e.g.: "Determine the cause of fatigue." A number of subproblems may need to be solved in order to arrive at a solution. These may include somewhat more specific subproblems, such as: "Is anemia present"? Or even more specifically: "Confirm that autoimmune hemolytic anemia is present." The resolution of many of these subproblems depends almost entirely on the intelligent ordering and interpretation of laboratory studies. One reason for the growth in numbers of laboratory studies is their ability to rule in (determine the presence of) or rule out (determine the absence of) certain pathologic states or diseases in given clinical contexts.

As an example of such use of laboratory studies, consider the problem of determining the presence or absence of hemolysis and its specific cause. Table 2–3 illustrates a hemolytic anemia profile. Notice that the results of certain studies are useful in ascertaining the presence of hemolysis; other studies are useful in determining its cause, if present. This is reflected in the profile subdivisions. Screen I contains laboratory studies, principally to help determine whether or not hemolytic anemia exists; Screen II contains laboratory studies that can be used to determine specific causes.

Table 2–3. HEMOLYTIC ANEMIA PROFILE

	Patient	Normal Adult Range	
		Males	*Females*
Hemolytic Anemia Screen I			
1. Coulter S blood counts			
Red blood cells	_____	4.7– 6.1	4.2– 5.4 × 10^6 μl
Hemoglobin	_____	14.0–17.0	12.0–16.0 g/dl
Hematocrit	_____	42.0–52.0	35.0–47.0 %
Mean corpuscular volume	_____	80–100	fl
2. Red blood cell morphology	_____	Normal	
3. Reticulocytes	_____	0.5– 1.5	%
4. Haptoglobin	_____	50.0–150.0	mg/dl
5. Bilirubin: Total	_____	0.1– 1.0	mg/dl
Indirect	_____	0.1– 0.8	mg/dl
Hemolytic Anemia Screen II			
1. Direct Coombs' test	_____	Negative	
2. G6PD Screening test	_____	Negative	
3. Glycerol lysis time: Immediate	_____	26–73	Seconds
(GLT$_{50}$): Incubated	_____	17–36	Seconds
4. Hemoglobin electrophoresis	_____	Hgb A; Hgb A$_2$ < 4.5%, F < 2%	
5. Hemoglobin instability test	_____	Negative	
6. Urinary hemosiderin	_____	Negative	

*Information courtesy of Eugene L. Gottfried, M.D., New York, NY.

Physicians use laboratory tests to aid in discriminating between rival hypotheses. Strategies to resolve discrimination subproblems can be designed especially in situations where very specific tests are available. For example, in discriminating between benign or malignant breast tumors, the breast biopsy is a very specific test around which a decision strategy should be designed. The discrimination between "acute myocardial infarction or not for patients presenting to the emergency department with chest pain" can also be reduced to a laboratory-based decision strategy. The strategy in this case would involve the study of serial CPK and LDH isoenzymes (see Chapter 10). In a middle-aged alcoholic adult who presents with severe abdominal pain, the physician may have initial hypotheses of "acute pancreatitis," "not acute pancreatitis," or "some other disorder." In this situation, a strategy that offers a powerful discrimination in solving the subproblem of acute pancreatitis would be required (see Chapter 14).

Just as individual laboratory tests can be thought of as being confirmatory, exclusionary, or discriminating, decision strategies that are based on these laboratory studies can have the same characteristics. Related to these ideas are the concepts of specificity, sensitivity, prevalence, and predictive value (see Chapters 3 and 4).

Our problem-solving strategies, therefore, are simply decision strategies to solve subproblems arising during clinical problem solving. Although a strategy can depend on a single laboratory measurement, it is more common to use groups of studies that are performed in parallel (simultaneously), in series (sequentially), or both (i.e., a test sequence). A liver profile, or panel, is an example of a group of laboratory measurements performed in parallel. A glucose tolerance test is an example of a group of studies performed in series. Measurement of CPK and LDH isoenzymes is a strategy useful in the subproblem of confirming acute myocardial infarction, which consists of a group of tests that are performed both in parallel and in series. Galen and Gambino (1975) stress that parallel testing increases sensitivity and decreases specificity, whereas series testing decreases sensitivity and increases specificity (see Chapter 14).

One way to categorize various problem-solving strategies is by problem level (Table 1–2). Multiphasic screening strategies, for example, are concerned with the general problem of health versus illness (a level 1 subproblem). The results of a complete blood count (CBC) can be directed at the question of diseases within the hematologic system (a level 2 subproblem). Many strategies are directed at the solution of more particular subproblems, such as the presence or absence of abnormal function in a particular organ (a level 3 subproblem), or at one specific disease (a level 4 subproblem). (See Chapter 1 for additional discussion of the concept of problem level.)

When decisions on specific diseases are being addressed, problem-solving strategies can achieve a high degree of certainty. Galen (1975b) demonstrated this through the high predictive value of the use of serial and parallel CPK and LDH isoenzymes in the diagnosis of acute myocardial infarction. We believe that problem-solving strategies ought to be used in as categorical a manner as possible. That is, whenever possible, the strategy ought to be directed at the presence or absence of a particular disease or the presence or absence of pathologic function in one particular organ.

One of the difficulties physicians encounter is the lack of information on how to design and evaluate problem-solving strategies. Unfortunately, it is not always possible to distinguish good strategies from bad ones. Without information on the sensitivity, specificity, and predictive value of each problem-solving strategy, comparisons cannot be made. These issues are discussed in detail in Chapter 4.

PROVIDING INFORMATION AND IMPLEMENTING STRATEGIES

The usefulness of laboratory tests resides within the context of the problem-solving process. Inappropriate and incomplete laboratory test selection can result from misunderstandings about the relationship of a symptom or sign to laboratory data. Because physicians direct their attention to data in the context of what they believe to be important, other disease-characteristic data may be ignored (Altshuler, 1980; Wheeler, 1977). (See Chapter 8 for a discussion of how unexpected, but significant, data may be ignored.) To effectively design, use, or evaluate strategies for confirming, eliminating, or refining hypotheses, the diagnostic characteristics of laboratory studies must be understood, including reference intervals, sources of variability, sensitivity, specific-

ity, and predictive value. A general discussion of these characteristics is presented in Chapter 4, and these characteristics of laboratory studies are described in our treatment of individual problems.

The hypotheticodeductive model of clinical problem solving suggests not only the effective information and educational experience necessary but also the methods of support that can aid the medical problem solver. We need to develop not only more sensitive and specific laboratory tests in order to clearly confirm or exclude hypotheses but also strategies that will result in more efficient problem solving, with these more sensitive and specific laboratory tests used as inputs.

One way to implement effective strategies for problem solving is to use a laboratory-based consultant. By taking advantage of the specific nature of a consultation request, the consultant can deal with a subproblem that is focused and can use knowledge specific to that subproblem (Connelly and Johnson, 1980). The laboratory consultant should know how to deal effectively with the complex subproblems of data authentication and interpretation within specified contexts. Thus, a laboratory-based consultant provides a method of designing and implementing strategies and providing information on the use of data resulting from these strategies (Speicher, 1977).

Likewise, systems that provide this information can be devised. Interpretive reports are now commonly provided with certain test results by the laboratory (Speicher and Smith, 1980). Computers have also been used in medical decision support by the laboratory (Elevitch, 1982; Hobbie and Reese, 1981; Warner, 1979; Williams, 1982). These systems can provide reminders or additional information at the time a decision is being formulated. They can augment the physician's memory and associative skills as well as partially direct the problem-solving process itself. Manual and computer methods of implementing strategies will be discussed in later chapters.

REFERENCES

Altshuler CH: The problem: Assuring appropriate transfer and utilization of laboratory information. In Werner M: Consultation in Laboratory Medicine by Pathologists (workshop). Chicago, American Society of Clinical Pathologists, 1980, pp 49–55.

Brecher G: Laboratory medicine 1953–1978 and the next 10 years. Hum Pathol 9:615–618, 1978.

Campbell EJM: Symposium on the Pathologist and the Diagnostic Process. St. Louis, Mo, Fall Meeting of the College of American Pathologists, September 19, 1978.

Connelly DP, Johnson PE: The medical problem solving process. Hum Pathol 11:412–419, 1980.

Cutler P (ed): Problem Solving in Clinical Medicine: From Data to Diagnoses. Baltimore, The Williams & Wilkins Company, 1979.

Degowin EL, Degowin RL: Bedside Diagnostic Examination, ed 2. New York, The Macmillan Company, 1969.

Elevitch FR: Computer-assisted clinical laboratory interpretive reports. Laboratory Medicine 13:45–47, 1982.

Elstein AS, Kagan N, Shulman LS, et al: Methods and theory in the study of medical inquiry. J Med Educ 47:85–92, 1972.

Elstein AS, Shulman LS, Sprafka SA et al: Medical Problem Solving: An Analysis of Clinical Reasoning. Cambridge, Mass, Harvard University Press, 1978.

Feinstein AR: An analysis of diagnostic reasoning: I. The domains and disorders of clinical macrobiology. Yale J Biol Med 46:212–232, 1973a.

Feinstein AR: An analysis of diagnostic reasoning: II. The strategy of intermediate decisions. Yale J Biol Med 46:264–283, 1973b.

Galen RS: Multiphasic screening and biochemical profiles: State of the art. In Stefanini M, Isenberg HD (eds): Progress in Clinical Pathology. Vol VI. New York, Grune & Stratton, Inc, 1975a, pp 83–110.

Galen RS: The enzyme diagnosis of myocardial infarction. Hum Pathol 6:141–155, 1975b.

Galen RS, Gambino SR: Beyond Normality: The Predictive Value and Efficiency of Medical Diagnosis. New York, John Wiley & Sons, Inc, 1975.

Gorry GA, Pauker SG, Schwartz WB: The diagnostic importance of the normal finding. N Engl J Med 298:486–489, 1978.

Hobbie RK, Reece RL: Interpretive reporting by computer. Hum Pathol 12:127–134, 1981.

Isselbacher KJ, Adams RD, Braunwald E, et al (eds): The practice of medicine. In Harrison's Principles of Internal Medicine, ed 9. New York, McGraw-Hill Book Company, 1980, pp 1–7.

Johns RJ: Clinical information and clinical problem solving. In Harvey AM, Johns RJ, McKusick VA, et al (eds): The Principles and Practice of Medicine, ed 20. New York, Appleton-Century-Crofts, 1980, pp 1–5.

Kassirer JP, Gorry GA: Clinical problem solving: A behavioral analysis. Ann Intern Med 89:245–255, 1978.

Kleinmuntz B: Diagnostic problem solving by computer. Jpn Psychol Res 7:189–194, 1965.

Kleinmuntz B (ed): Formal Representation of Human Judgment. New York, John Wiley & Sons, 1968, pp 149–186.

Koran LM: The reliability of clinical methods, data and judgments. Part 1 and 2. N Engl J Med 293:642–646, 695–701, 1975.

Murphy EA: The Logic of Medicine. Baltimore, The Johns Hopkins University Press, 1976.

Murphy J, Henry JB: Effective utilization of clinical laboratories. Hum Pathol 9:625–633, 1978.

Price RB, Vlahcevic ZR: Logical principles in differential diagnosis. Ann Intern Med 75:89–95, 1971.

Rubin AD: Hypothesis Formation and Evaluation in Medical Diagnosis. MIT-AI Technical Report 316. Cambridge, Mass, Massachusetts Institute of Technology, 1975.

Speicher CE: Trends in clinical pathology and the emerging role of the clinical pathologist. Pathologist April 1977, pp 85–89.

Speicher CE, Smith JW: Interpretive reporting in clinical pathology. JAMA 243:1556–1560, 1980.

Warner HR: Computer-Assisted Medical Decision-Making. New York, Academic Press, Inc, 1979.

Weinstein MC, Fineberg HV, et al: Clinical Decision Analysis. Philadelphia, WB Saunders Company, 1980.

Wheeler LA, Brecher G, Sheiner LB: Clinical laboratory use in the evaluation of anemia. JAMA 238:2709–2714, 1977.

Williams BT: Computer Aids to Clinical Decisions. Volumes I and II. Boca Raton, Fla, CRC Press, 1982.

Winston PH: Artificial Intelligence. Reading, Mass, Addison-Wesley Publishing Company, 1977.

Wortman PM: Representation and strategy in diagnostic problem solving. Hum Factors 8:48–53, 1966.

Wortman PM: Medical diagnosis: An information-processing approach. Comput Biomed Res 5:315–328, 1972.

INTERPRETATION OF STRATEGIES

Interpretation of strategies is the process by which laboratory and other data are applied to the diagnosis and management of patients' clinical problems in a meaningful manner. Optimal interpretation of laboratory test results requires a knowledge of concepts of "normality," accuracy, precision, sensitivity, specificity, incidence, prevalence, predictive value, reference interval, and decision level.

THE LANGUAGE OF LABORATORY STUDIES

Laboratory data are the product of the laboratory. The studies themselves are sometimes called determinations, measurements, estimates, procedures, tests, or examinations. To be clinically useful, data need to be expressed and interpreted in terms that are understood by physicians. Unfortunately, different terms may express the same concept about laboratory data, and similar terms may have subtly different meanings. To avoid incorrect interpretations, it is important that we understand these terms.

The data resulting from laboratory studies can be of several classifications. A *qualitative* measurement of urinary glucose, for example, indicates whether glucose is present or absent. A *semiquantitative* measurement of urinary glucose states not only whether glucose is present or absent but also the approximate amount of glucose present. The statement, "Urinary glucose is present $2+$," is semiquantitative because the term $2+$ implies an approximate glucose concentration (Table 3–1). The plus ($+$) system for reporting test results should be abolished and replaced with approximate numerical results, since the plus ($+$) designation can have a different meaning for different reagent products. A *quantitative* measurement of urinary glucose states exactly how much glucose is present (e.g., the urinary glucose concentration is 100 mg/100 ml).

Laboratory data can be referred to as *variates*. A variate is simply a variable that can take on a limited set of values. There are two types of variates, continuous and discrete. Quantitative laboratory data (e.g., values of serum glucose concentration) constitute a *continuous* variate because the values of glucose

Table 3–1. CONCENTRATIONS OF URINARY GLUCOSE BY SEMIQUANTITATIVE METHODS*

	Approximate Glucose Concentration (mg/100 ml)		
Report	**BMC† Dipstick**	**Ames‡ Dipstick**	**Clinitest‡ Tablets**
Trace	40 or more	100 or more	250 or more
1 +	100	250	500
2 +	250	500	750
3 +	1000	1000	1000
4 +	—	2000 or more	2000 or more

*The concentration of a given report (e.g., 2 +) can vary according to the method used.
†Bio-Dynamics/bmc, Division of Boehringer Mannheim Gmbh, Indianapolis, Indiana.
‡Ames Division, Miles Laboratories, Inc., Elkhart, Indiana.

that can occur in the serum are continuous. Qualitative laboratory data (e.g., a measurement of urinary glucose stating whether glucose is present or absent) constitute a *discrete* and *binary* variate because there are only two possible values.

We can transform a continuous variate into a discrete variate by deciding that all values less than a cut-off value are negative and all values equal to or greater than a cut-off value are positive. For example, we can decide that any patient with a fasting serum glucose less than 140 mg/100 ml does not have diabetes mellitus and that any patient with a fasting serum glucose equal to or greater than 140 mg/100 ml does have diabetes mellitus (see Chapter 16). This cut-off value may also be referred to as a *decision level* (Statland, 1980). (Decision levels are discussed in more detail later in this chapter.)

Decision levels can be helpful in differential diagnosis; for instance, if the patient's serum calcium level is greater than 15 mg/100 ml, the diagnosis is more likely to be metastatic malignancy than primary hyperparathyroidism. Decision levels can also be helpful in determining whether a given laboratory test result is consistent with the patient's clinical picture; that is, the patient's serum calcium level should be greater than 13 to 14 mg/100 ml to explain the symptoms of anorexia, lethargy, and constipation, due to hypercalcemia (see Chapter 9). In each of these decision situations the serum calcium level is well above the usual reference interval of 9.2–11.0 mg/100 ml.

Statland (1980) described three decision levels for each of 25 common laboratory tests. His decision levels for three of these tests are given in Table 3–2.

UNITS

Each value of quantitative laboratory data contains a number and a unit of concentration. For example, a quantitative measurement of serum glucose is 100 mg/100 ml. The value 100 mg/100 ml includes a number, 100, and a unit, mg/100 ml. Units are often a source of confusion and require special attention to avoid misinterpretations.

For example, mg/100 ml is synonymous with milligrams per deciliter, mg/dl, milligrams per cent, and mg%; mg/100 ml is not synonymous with millimoles per liter (mmol/liter) or mEq/liter. Actually, for serum glucose, 100 mg/100 ml equals only 5.5 mmol/liter. We can readily imagine the adverse consequence of misinterpreting a serum glucose level of 5.5 mmol/liter as 5.5 mg/100 ml. Serum calcium is commonly reported as either mg/100 ml or mEq/liter. The units of the former are twice the latter, and serious misinterpretation can result if the units are not clearly specified. FitzSimons (1979) related the case of a patient who died because of the administration of saline, 54 gm/liter. A surgeon asked for "normal saline," which the pharmacist understood to be one normal solution of sodium chloride—the chemist's interpretation of the word "normal" being one equivalent/liter (i.e., 54 gm/liter).

Mmol/liter is the unit of expression of glucose concentration used by the International System of Units (Le Système Internationale d'Unités, or SI units). SI units were proposed during a series of General Conferences on Weights and Measures and suggested for adoption by the World Health Organization Council on Scientific Affairs of the American Medical Association (AMA), 1978.

Table 3–2. EXAMPLES OF DECISION LEVELS*

Analyte (Reference Interval)	Level 1	Level 2	Level 3
Magnesium	*0.8 mEq/liter*	*1.8 mEq/liter*	*5.0 mEq/liter*
(1.2–2.4 mEq/liter)	Values of *0.8 mEq/liter* or below are associated with weakness, irritability, tetany, and convulsions.		
	A value of *1.8 mEq/liter,* however, in conjunction with these symptoms, rules out hypomagnesemia as the cause of the patient's clinical problem. Other causes such as alcoholism, malnutrition, malabsorption, and severe diarrhea should be evaluated.		
	A value of *5.0 mEq/liter* or above is above the upper reference limit and is usually due to renal insufficiency or excess magnesium sulfate given as an anticonvulsant.		
Phosphorus	*1.5 mg/100 ml*	*2.5 mg/100 ml*	*5.0 mg/100 ml*
(2.5–5.0 mg/100 ml)	A value of *1.5 mg/100 ml* or lower may be caused by hyperparathyroidism (primary), vitamin D deficiency, malabsorption, administration of glucose (hyperalimentation), hyperinsulinism, and loss of phosphate in urine (Fanconi's syndrome). Hemolytic anemia often occurs concomitant with low phosphorus levels.		
	A value below *2.5 mg/100 ml* associated with elevated serum calcium chloride suggests primary hyperparathyroidism.		
	A value of *5.0 mg/100 ml* is the upper reference limit for adults and may indicate renal insufficiency, hypoparathyroidism, and excessive vitamin D intake. Children, however, have higher reference values.		
Potassium	*3.0 mEq/liter*	*5.8 mEq/liter*	*7.5 mEq/liter*
(3.7–5.3 mEq/liter)	Causes of low potassium include renal tubular disease, hyperaldosteronism, malnutrition, treatment of diabetic ketoacidosis, hyperinsulinism, metabolic alkalosis, diuretic therapy, and gastrointestinal loss. Values below *3.0 mEq/liter* may be associated with weakness, digoxin toxicity, and cardiac arrhythmia.		
	A value of *5.8 mEq/liter* requires diagnostic measures to classify the patient correctly. Causes of hyperkalemia include renal glomerular disease, adrenal-cortical insufficiency, diabetic ketoacidosis, excessive intravenous potassium therapy, and sepsis.		
	A value above *7.5 mEq/liter* may be associated with cardiac arrhythmias, which may need therapeutic measures. Serum sodium and urine electrolyte values should be ordered to help classify the patient.		

*Adapted from Statland BE: Turning lab values into action. Diagnostic Medicine 3:65, 67, 69, Sept-Oct, 1980.

There has been much interest in the area of converting traditional units to SI units. Linke and colleagues (1979) have compiled a brief review of the mathematics and chemical calculations that are useful in understanding laboratory data units and conversions.

Young (1978) has given theoretical justification for the use of SI units. An advantage cited includes standardization of the terminology of laboratory data among different clinical laboratories and between clinicians and research scientists and improved understanding of the interrelationship of biochemical constituents of body fluids through molar and metric terminology.

As an example, Young (1978) explained that changing a serum albumin of 4.0 gm/100 ml and a serum bilirubin of 0.4 mg/100 ml into SI units would equal a serum albumin of 620 μmol/liter and a serum bilirubin of 6.9 μmol/liter. In mass terms, there is 10,000-fold more albumin than bilirubin; in molar terms, however, the amount is only 100-fold more. Molar terminology gives us a better intuitive understanding of how an increase in molar concentration of other compounds that bind to albumin can result in displacement of bilirubin from binding sites on the albumin molecule.

Other countries appear to have accepted SI units more readily than the United States (Ta-

Table 3–3.   INTRODUCTION OF SI UNITS*

Year of Introduction	Countries
1970	Netherlands
1971	Denmark, Finland
1974	Australia
1975	United Kingdom
1976	New Zealand, South Africa, Sweden
1977	Norway
1978	Federal Republic of Germany
1979	Czechoslovakia, Democratic Republic of Germany
1980	Hungary, Italy
1981	Japan, Switzerland, Yugoslavia
1982	Ecuador

SI = International System of Units.

*Young DS: SI units for clinical laboratory data. JAMA 240:1618, 1978. Copyright 1978, American Medical Association.

ble 3–3). American physicians and laboratory scientists have been actively debating the merits and disadvantages of SI units (Bromage, 1978; Novack, 1978; Rose, 1978; Wilkinson, 1978). The American Association for Clinical Chemistry has endorsed the use of SI units. The Council on Scientific Affairs of the AMA (1978) made the following recommendations regarding the use of SI units in clinical chemistry:

1. That the use of mass concentration units (weight/volume) be retained by medical laboratories until it is shown that a change to molar concentrations will improve patient care (diagnosis, treatment, followup) or prove a considerable advantage with respect to laboratory technique.

2. That no abrupt changes in the current use of mass concentrations or in milliequivalent units for certain electrolytes be undertaken until an overall plan and schedule have been agreed on by representative medically oriented groups and appropriate councils of the AMA.

Young (1975) constructed tables of all clinical laboratory measurements of the Massachusetts General Hospital. The tables give "normal" laboratory values in traditional and equivalent SI units and include multiplication factors for converting traditional units to SI units. Henry (1979), Conn (1980), and Halsted (1981) have constructed similar tables. (See the Appendix for tables of "normal" values in traditional and SI units.) Marsters (1978) has compiled an English language bibliography of SI units in laboratory medicine. A book by Lippert and Lehmann (1978) includes an intro-duction to SI units as well as conversion tables and "normal ranges" (reference intervals).

The College of American Pathologists (CAP) faces the issue of SI units in the arena of its laboratory surveys program. Because laboratories in both Canada and the United States participate in the surveys, it appears that adoption of SI units by Canada will necessitate the CAP's implementation of a dual-unit reporting system.

LABORATORY STUDIES IN DISEASE

GENERAL CONSIDERATIONS

In the diagnostic process, the physician uses his or her senses to obtain a patient's medical history and to perform the physical examination. In order to obtain more objective information, the physician may order a number of laboratory and radiologic tests. The relative contribution of these three pieces of data (history, physical examination, and laboratory/x-ray studies) to the diagnostic process has changed markedly with time.

In 1900, for instance, the laboratory contributed a small portion of the clinical data base. From 1900 until approximately the 1950s, this amount steadily grew and then came automation with an explosive increase in laboratory testing. At present, the laboratory contributes much more of the data on which a diagnosis is made. Some diagnoses are based solely on laboratory studies. Patient management may rely on laboratory studies more heavily than diagnosis does. By "laboratory," we mean all data generated in all divisions of the clinical laboratory—chemistry, clinical microscopy, cytology, hematology, immunology, immunohematology, microbiology, nuclear medicine, and surgical pathology.

New laboratory tests are constantly being introduced, often with exaggerated claims about their usefulness. Consider the following (Schwartz, 1973). Assume that you have available to you a test for the diagnosis of cancer; it is a common form of cancer (e.g., cancer of the lung, gastrointestinal tract, or cervix). The test has the following characteristics:

1. It is positive in 95 of 100 patients who have the disease, i.e., cancer.

2. It is negative in 95 of 100 patients who do not have cancer.

Now assume that you are going to apply this test to a population that you know from past experience will contain five people with this particular form of cancer per thousand. In other words, in a group of 1,000 people, five will have the cancer you are interested in detecting. At the time you see these people, they have no objective signs or symptoms of cancer, and the previously described test—with its unique characteristics—is going to be performed on them.

The problem is as follows: On the third day of testing, the technologist walks into your office and says: "We have found our first patient with cancer." Now you realize that you have found a patient with a positive test. What is the probability that the patient actually has cancer? Ten per cent? Twenty per cent? Greater than 50 per cent?

This actual problem was given to a total of 290 physicians, medical students, house officers, and practicing physicians. The great majority of the participants stated the probability incorrectly. More than half the physicians gave a value of 50 per cent or greater. The correct answer is 9 per cent. That is, a test even this good (positive in 95 of 100 patients with cancer, negative in 95 of 100 patients without cancer) has only an approximate 10 per cent probability of diagnosing cancer when it is positive in a group of people where the prevalence of cancer is five in 1000 people.

To help the reader understand the poor overall performance of the test, we shall discuss the rationale for laboratory testing and shall introduce some new definitions. Although the words will not seem new, we must be very careful about their meanings. You may have used the terms "accurate," "precise," "sensitive," "specific," "incidence" and "prevalence" before, perhaps at times synonymously. We shall see in later chapters that these are not synonymous terms and that a clear understanding of their definitions allows physicians to communicate intelligently with one another when considering the result of a laboratory test (see Chapter 4).

WHY DO PHYSICIANS ORDER TESTS?

As we mentioned in Chapter 1, physicians use the laboratory (and any other testing modality, for that matter) for a number of reasons

(Galen and Gambino, 1975; Henry, 1979; Johnson, 1973; Young, 1979):

1. Diagnosis—to obtain a correct diagnosis in a patient known to be ill. *Example:* A person complaining of weakness visits the physician. A simple hematocrit is found to be low for that patient's age and sex. The physician may order additional tests, such as red blood cell indices or serum iron concentration and vitamin B_{12} concentration in order to determine the specific etiology of the known anemia. (See Part 3: Blood hematocrit, low.)

2. Management—to provide information concerning disease prognosis in a patient who has a known diagnosis. *Example:* A patient is known to have leukemia and an extremely high blood leukocyte count. A bone marrow examination is found to be consistent with acute leukemia. After initial chemotherapy, another bone marrow examination may be done. If a marked reduction in leukemic cells is not found, this may indicate a poor prognosis; on the other hand, evidence of a normally regenerating marrow would be consistent with a good prognosis. (See Part 3: Blood leukocyte count, high or low.)

3. Management—to provide data to assist in monitoring complicated or protracted treatment. *Example:* The patient may have a diagnosis of Hodgkin's disease. The chemotherapeutic approach may involve the use of drugs that severely depress the blood leukocyte and platelet counts. Measurements of total leukocyte and platelet counts may be done during the course of therapy to avoid the complications of a low leukocyte count (e.g., infection) and those of a low platelet count (e.g., hemorrhage). (See Part 3: Blood leukocyte and platelet counts, low.)

4. Screening—to detect so-called subclinical disease in an apparently healthy population. *Example:* The measurements of urinary glucose in all college freshmen are taken in hopes of determining clinically undetected diabetics. The attempt here is to find disease in patients who are apparently healthy but whose laboratory values indicate disease that has not made itself clinically apparent (subclinical disease). This is what is meant by screening healthy populations for "abnormal" laboratory values. This screening of healthy populations should be distinguished from what some have called "profiling." Profiling usually means performing a number of selected tests on patients who are already symptomatic or who show a high

likelihood of having disease—often these are patients being admitted to the hospital. An example might be the performance of 12-channel serum chemistry tests on adults with chest pain who are being admitted to the hospital. We shall subsequently show that screening is not always a productive way of finding disease (see Chapter 8 for further discussion of screening).

5. Screening—to delineate risk factors. *Example:* The measurement of serum cholesterol, high-density lipoprotein (HDL), and triglyceride levels determines the likelihood that a given patient will suffer the complications of atherosclerosis (heart attack, stroke, peripheral vascular disease). This testing is meant to indicate whether illness is more likely to develop in certain individuals with given laboratory values. (See Chapter 10 for the use of serum lipids to quantify risk for atherosclerosis).

WHAT CONSTITUTES "NORMAL"?

Physicians use laboratory studies to answer a number of questions. The answers to these questions (correct diagnosis, subclinical illness, therapeutic monitoring) would be vastly simplified if we could clearly distinguish "disease" from "non-disease." Although initially this may seem an easy distinction, anyone who has had experience in clinical medicine knows that it is not always a simple matter. Of course, in some diagnostic situations, it may be relatively easy to distinguish disease from non-disease. Obviously, a patient with a depressed skull fracture or a draining cutaneous wound has disease. Likewise, an extremely high or extremely low laboratory value is often associated with a clear-cut clinical disease. An example is serum glucose value of 300 mg/100 ml or greater in a patient with obvious diabetic ketoacidosis, or, on the other hand, an extremely low serum glucose value (under 20 mg/100 ml) in a patient with hypoglycemia secondary to an insulin overdose.

In modern medical practice, the situation is often much less clear-cut than in these examples. Patients with suspected clinical disease may not have extreme laboratory values. The question, then, is: Do they have disease?

For many laboratory tests, age, sex, metabolites, and drugs all can seriously affect blood levels of various *analytes*. (An analyte is simply something that can be measured.) It is not reasonable—even though it is often done—to measure the blood level of a particular analyte in a group of medical students or nurses, to find its frequency distribution about a mean, and to label any value outside that distribution indicative of disease.

The values of a particular analyte for non-diseased and diseased patients usually overlap. The question for values lying in this overlap area is always: "Does the value indicate the patient has disease, or not?" Often, when the blood level of a particular analyte is extremely high or low, the patient has clear-cut clinical evidence of a disease and a laboratory test is not needed for diagnosis. The real problem is early, or subclinical, disease. It is in this situation that laboratory determinations can be the most useful. We will discuss how overlap areas for serum glucose and serum ceruloplasmin between healthy and ill patients are handled in the subproblems of diabetes mellitus (Chapter 16) and Wilson's disease (Chapter 17).

Part of the problem is the confusion about what we mean by "normal" and "abnormal" in the laboratory setting. Murphy (1976) has outlined a number of meanings for the word "normal." From the list of words given in column 1 in Table 3–4, let's use serum urea nitrogen (SUN) as an example. We see that

Table 3–4.   MEANINGS OF THE WORD "NORMAL" IN MEDICINE*

Paraphrase	Where Used	Preferable Term
Probability function (bell-shaped curve)	Statistics	Gaussian
Most representative of its class	Descriptive sciences	Averge, median, modal
Commonly encountered in its class	Descriptive sciences	Habitual
Most suited to survival	Genetics, operations research	Optimal, "fittest"
Carrying no penalty	Clinical medicine	Innocuous, harmless
Commonly aspired to	Politics, sociology	Conventional
Most perfect of its class	Metaphysics, esthetics, morals	Ideal

*Adapted from Murphy EA: The Logic of Medicine. Baltimore, The Johns Hopkins University Press, 1976, p. 125.

"normal" values for SUN can be given a number of meanings (Galen and Gambino, 1975):

1. Within normal probability distribution: This is frequently given as the "normal laboratory range" and is often quoted on laboratory report forms. This is not true for SUN because its distribution is skewed to the right in a healthy reference population.

2. Most representative of its class: This would be the value as defined by a median, or average. It would depend upon the population tested.

3. Commonly encountered in its class: These are the values of SUN that commonly occur in a healthy population.

4. Most suited to survival: We simply do not have enough information on many analytes to discuss them in this fashion. For SUN, this would be the values for a person who is most suited for survival.

5. Carrying no penalty: Many times in clinical medicine, when we speak of normal values, this is what is meant. Normal values in this sense are laboratory values that do not indicate that the patient has disease.

6, 7. Commonly aspired to, and the most perfect of its class: These have essentially no meaning in the context of using the laboratory for patient care.

The normal range is ordinarily determined by measuring a given analyte, let's say, SUN, in a population of people who appear to be free of disease. Often this population is young (e.g., medical students, nurses, or medical technologists). The SUN test results are then statistically analyzed. A standard deviation is determined, and a range is calculated that includes those values, which are two standard deviations on either side of the mean value. This range accounts for 95 per cent of the test results within the population and defines the high "normal" value and the low "normal" value. More sophisticated analyses can be made for old people, young people, men, women, different races, patients on various diets, and so forth. Elveback (1970, 1972, 1973) has written extensively about the pitfalls of defining "normal" values (i.e., parametric statistics, inappropriate reference populations, and related issues). She prefers to use the percentile method for calculating the reference interval.

These range determinations are sometimes useful; however, they may not address the clinician's major problem, which is: "How far above or below the mean should the value be before I consider disease in a patient? And if I consider disease, which disease?" Oftentimes, a particular test is proposed as useful in a given disease after the following kind of study is done.

1. The test, as developed in the investigator's laboratory, is applied to a known, previously healthy sample population, and 95 per cent confidence limits are determined. This then constitutes "normal," "high normal," and "low normal."

2. This same test is then applied to a population of diseased patients. If the test has been developed by an investigator with a particular interest in a certain disease, the new test will be applied to the clinic or in-hospital patient population, many of whom are known to have the disease because of previous clinical or laboratory tests. In this patient population, the test proves positive in most of the people known to have this disease.

Here then, we have a test that is clearly negative in known healthy people and clearly positive in those known to have the specific disease. In essence, we have a test that is both highly specific and highly sensitive. The question, however, is this: "Do we have a clinically useful test?" Perhaps, but not necessarily so. Here is the reason: The diagnostic procedure was not given its most severe test, i.e.: "What will be the results of the test when it is applied to a population of patients who are clearly not well and do not clearly have the disease in question?" In other words: "How will the test perform in patients who are sick from other diseases that may clinically resemble the disease we are trying to diagnose?"

For example, most patients who have an acute myocardial infarction have left-sided chest pain and, in addition, an elevated serum LDH. On the other hand, most healthy people have serum levels of LDH in the 95 per cent confidence range. We can say then that the serum LDH is in the "normal range" in most healthy people and that it is elevated in most patients with heart attacks who have chest pain. "Does this mean that every patient with chest pain and an elevated serum LDH has had a heart attack?" No, because LDH is an ubiquitous enzyme and is elevated in the serum in a wide variety of degenerative, neoplastic, and inflammatory conditions, many of which can produce chest pain. (See Part 3: Lactic dehydrogenase, high.) The dilemma is: How certain can we be that the elevated serum

LDH in this adult male patient confirms the clinical impression that the patient has had a heart attack?" (See Chapter 10 for the use of serum enzymes and isoenzymes to diagnose acute myocardial infarction.)

CLARIFYING LANGUAGE

In order to further understand this type of problem, we need to develop a vocabulary to enable us to talk to one another in words that mean the same thing to all of us. Laboratory data are often described in the language of statistics and the descriptive sciences (e.g., bell-shaped curves, averages, medians, or modes). However, clinical problems concern a single patient; statistical language refers to populations, not individuals. Medical decisions usually concern patients. "Does the patient have diabetes mellitus? Has the patient had an acute myocardial infarction? Is the patient responding to therapy? Is the patient likely to have cardiovascular disease if this serum level of HDL cholesterol is maintained?" It is these questions that most of us are concerned with when we order laboratory tests.

As we have mentioned, the term *reference interval* is replacing *"normal" values ("normal" range)* in the clinical laboratory literature. Although the terms *reference values* and *referent values* subtly differ from the term reference interval, they are sometimes used synonymously. We shall discuss these differences later. The terms *"normal" range* and *reference range* should probably be avoided because "range" implies a difference between two limits rather than all values that lie between two limits (Dybkaer and Grasbeck, 1973).

"Normal" is a subjective word that implies different meanings to different persons. "Normal values," as used in laboratory medicine, can apply to any number of reference populations. The spectrum of these groups can vary from those individuals who are in a state of complete physical, mental, and social well-being, absolute health—as outlined in the World Health Organization Constitution (1973)—through subjectively healthy people, screened ambulant persons, non-ill individuals confined to bed, or hospitalized persons. As we can see, the term "normal" is ambiguous and difficult to define; therefore, we shall be very careful when we use it.

Reference values can be defined as a set of values of a measured quantity obtained from a group of individuals (or a single individual) in a defined state of health (Dybkaer and Gräsbeck, 1973; Winkel and Statland, 1979). Sunderman (1975) listed the following major categories of specifications to accompany reference values in clinical chemistry (see Chapter 1):

1. The reference population (clinical class) and the way in which it was chosen (considered in our clinical contexts for each subproblem in Part 2, Clinical Subproblems).
2. The environmental and physiologic conditions under which the specimens were obtained (considered in our strategy for each subproblem).
3. The techniques and timing of specimen collection, transport, preparation, and storage (considered in our strategy for each subproblem in Part 2).
4. The analytic method that was used with data regarding its accuracy, precision, and quality control (considered where possible in our strategy for each subproblem in Part 2).
5. The data set that was observed and the reference intervals that were derived (considered where possible in our strategy for each subproblem in Part 2).

The term *reference interval* refers to all the quantitative reference values for a given measurement that lie between two reference value limits, a lower limit and an upper limit. By convention, the reference interval refers to all reference values between the reference value limits found in 95 per cent of the reference population chosen. Unless otherwise specified, we shall use the term reference interval according to this definition.

Galen and Gambino (1975) (Galen, 1977) coined the term *referent value*. They pointed out that even though "reference interval" is semantically better than "normal values," it still refers basically to a healthy population or a reference population (clinical class). It tells us nothing about disease. They use the term referent value as an empirical value, which enables us to distinguish a diseased patient from the reference population (clinical class) with a definite predictive value. We agree that the "referent value" concept has a useful place in laboratory medicine; however, we prefer the synonym *decision level* (Statland, 1980) because it more explicitly embodies the use of the value in the process of deciding between health and disease and is less likely to be confused with "reference values" and "reference interval."

Harris (1981) reviewed the statistical aspects of reference values. His discussion includes additional important topics, such as univariate versus multivariate reference ranges, subject-specific reference values, and reference values for a serial change. See Gräsbeck and colleagues (1981) for further discussion of these concepts.

DECISION LEVELS

Decision levels (referent values) are values of a measured quantity, which enable us to distinguish an individual with a disorder or disease from a reference population (clinical class) of similar individuals without the disorder or disease. If the diagnostic sensitivity and specificity of the decision level for the disorder or disease are known and if the prevalence of the disease or disorder in the reference population (clinical class) is known, the predictive value of the decision level for the disorder or disease can be calculated. The predictive value of a decision level of a measurement can be determined experimentally by defining the presence or absence of a given disorder or disease in a reference population by analysis of outcome. (All criteria—clinical history, physical examination, ancillary studies and procedures—are used to define the presence or absence of the disorder or disease.) The predictive value of the measurement decision level is then determined retrospectively by correlating the diagnostic sensitivity and specificity of the measurement decision level with outcome (Galen, Reiffel and Gambino, 1975).

Cole (1979) suggested that the following test result ranges be defined for each laboratory test:
1. Physiologic range.
2. Problem detection range.
3. Problem confirmation range.
4. Problem exclusion range.
5. Specific or toxic range.
6. Therapeutic range.
   a. Significant deviation between results.
   b. Significant trend between results.

ACCURACY AND PRECISION

Until recently, laboratory professionals had been primarily concerned with accuracy and precision; as we shall see, these goals are not enough. It is still important, however, to ensure that laboratory determinations are as accurate and precise as possible. Good laboratories can provide information about the accuracy and precision of their tests.

Accuracy means closeness to the true value. It is more or less a "gold standard" phenomenon. The closer a determination is to some accepted standard, the more accurate you are said to be. In laboratories, this is ordinarily gauged by comparing the value measured with what was obtained by a very standard technique in a reference laboratory.

There are real problems with ensuring accuracy in anything one measures in a biologic fluid. Often, the true values are not known. There is the problem of interference of protein with the measurement of many analytes, and, in many instances, the definition of what is measured depends upon how it is measured. For example, the value for a colorimetric measurement of protein concentration can differ from the value for an immunologic measurement, and the value for a measurement in weight (for instance, in nanograms per 100 ml) of a substance can be considerably different from a value for a measurement based on the activity of that same substance. In other words, we can measure the actual weight of immunoglobulin in a solution or its activity as antibody. The values for the two measurements will differ. Accuracy, then, is the closeness to a true value obtained in some standard way. (Chapter 17 illustrates how the accuracy of serum ceruloplasmin measurements affects the decision levels for confirming or excluding a diagnosis of Wilson's disease.)

Although accuracy is difficult to attain in a clinical laboratory, as a rule precision is not. *Precision* means the nearness of replicate measurements on the same sample to one another. Some methods by which we can measure precision are the determination of mean or average, standard deviation, and coefficient of variation. (Chapter 6 describes how the precision of serum creatinine measurements can influence the renal transplant surgeon's management decision of whether or not to administer intravenous azathioprine and corticosteroids.)

Other investigators have provided further information on these topics. Barnett (1979) addresses in greater detail the statistical concepts in this chapter, and Galen and Gambino (1975) present the concepts of sensitivity, specificity, prevalence, predictive value, and efficiency.

REFERENCES

Barnett RN: Clinical Laboratory Statistics, ed 2. Boston, Little, Brown & Company, 1979.

Bromage PR: SI units: kilo-everything, letter. N Engl J Med 299:557–558, 1978.

Cole GW: The clinical usefulness of multiple result ranges for a laboratory test, as exemplified by serum urea nitrogen. In Young DS, Nipper H, Uddin D, et al (eds): Clinician and Chemist: The Relationship of the Laboratory to the Physician. Washington, DC, American Association for Clinical Chemistry, Inc, 1979, pp. 265–272.

Conn RB: Laboratory reference values of clinical importance. In Conn HF, Conn RB (eds): Current Diagnosis. Philadelphia, WB Saunders Company, 1980, pp 1153–1172.

Council on Scientific Affairs (AMA): Adoption of International System of Units for clinical chemistry. JAMA 240:2664, 1978.

Dybkaer R, Gräsbeck R: Theory of reference values, editorial. Scand J Lab Invest 32:1–7, 1973.

Elveback LR: How high is high? A proposed alternative to the normal range. Mayo Clin Proc 47:93–97, 1972.

Elveback LR: The population of healthy persons as a source of reference information. Hum Pathol 4:9–16, 1973.

Elveback LR, Guillier CL, Keating FR Jr: Health, normality, and the ghost of Gauss. JAMA 211:69–75, 1970.

FitzSimons DW: SI units, letter, JAMA 242:710, 1979.

Galen RS: The normal range. A concept in transition. Arch Pathol Lab Med 101:561–565, 1977.

Galen RS, Gambino SR: Beyond Normality: The Predictive Value and Efficiency of Medical Diagnosis. New York, John Wiley & Sons, 1975.

Galen RS, Reiffel JA, Gambino SR: Diagnosis of acute myocardial infarction. Relative efficiency of serum enzyme and isoenzyme measurements. JAMA 232:145–147, 1975.

Gräsbeck R, Alström T, Solberg HE (eds): Reference Values in Clinical Medicine: The Current State of the Art. New York, John Wiley and Sons, Ltd, 1981.

Halsted JA, Halsted CH (eds): The Laboratory in Clinical Medicine. Interpretation and Application. Philadelphia, WB Saunders Company, 1981.

Harris EK: Statistical aspects of reference values in clinical pathology. In Stefanini M, Benson ES (eds): Progress in Clinical Pathology. Volume VIII. New York, Grune & Stratton, Inc., 1981, pp. 45–66.

Henry JB, Howanitz, PJ: Organ panels and the relationship of the laboratory to the physician. In Young DS, Nipper H, Uddin D et al (eds): Clinician and Chemist: The Relationship of the Laboratory to the Clinician. Washington, DC, American Association for Clinical Chemistry, Inc, 1979, pp 157–174.

Henry JB (ed): Clinical Diagnosis and Management by Laboratory Methods, ed 16. Philadelphia, WB Saunders Company, 1979.

Johnson, EA: Some basic considerations of the needs for improved clinical laboratory data analyses. Hum Pathol 4:5–8, 1973.

Linke EG, Henry JB, Statland BE: Theory and practice of laboratory technique. In Henry JB (ed): Clinical Diagnosis and Management by Laboratory Methods, ed 16. Philadelphia, WB Saunders Company, 1979, pp. 53–76.

Lippert H, Lehmann HP: SI Units in Medicine. Baltimore, Urban and Schwarzenberg, 1978.

Marsters RW: SI units in laboratory medicine. Clinical Chemistry News, November 29, 1978, pp. 9–10.

Murphy EA: The Logic of Medicine. Baltimore, The Johns Hopkins University Press, 1976, p 125.

Novack GD: SI units: Kilo-everything, letter. N Engl J Med 299:558, 1978.

Rose JC: Sounding board: Pressures on the millimeter of mercury. N Engl J Med 298:1361–1364, 1978.

Schwartz WB, Gorry GA, Kassirer JP, et al: Decision analysis and clinical judgment. Am J Med 55:459–472, 1973.

Statland BE: Turning lab values into action. Diagnostic Medicine 3:56–75, Sept–Oct, 1980.

Sunderman FW: Current concepts of "normal values," "reference values," and "discrimination values" in clinical chemistry, editorial. Clin Chem 21:1873–1877, 1975.

Wilkinson RS: SI units: Kilo-everything, letter. N Engl J Med 299:557, 1978.

Winkel P, Statland BE: Reference values. In Henry JB (ed): Clinical Diagnosis and Management by Laboratory Methods, ed 16. Philadelphia, WB Saunders Company, 1979, pp. 29–52.

World Health Organization: Basic Documents, 23rd ed, WHO, Geneva, 1973, p. 1.

Young DS: "Normal laboratory values" (case records of the Massachusetts General Hospital) in SI units. N Engl J Med 292:795–802, 1975.

Young DS: SI units for clinical laboratory data. JAMA 240:1618–1621, 1978.

Young DS: Why there is a laboratory. In Young DS, Nipper H, Uddin D, et al (eds): Clinician and Chemist: The Relationship of the Laboratory to the Physician. Washington, DC, American Association for Clinical Chemistry, Inc, 1979, pp 3–22.

CHAPTER 4

STATISTICAL CONCEPTS USEFUL IN THE PROBLEM-SOLVING APPROACH

PREDICTIVE VALUE
  Predictive Value of a Laboratory
    Measurement
  Predictive Value and Bayes'
    Theorem
OTHER STATISTICAL
  APPLICATIONS

In a study by Berwick and colleagues (1981), physicians showed a frequent lack of consensus on the meaning of common terms in use (e.g., "false-positive rate") and often seemed willing to draw conclusions unsupported by available data. Performance was inversely correlated with length of time since graduation from medical school, and practicing physicians tended to err more frequently than medical students, interns, and residents. This lack of understanding of probabilistic reasoning has been noticed by others (Casscells et al., 1978).

In this chapter, we discuss the predictive value model of laboratory measurements; the associated concepts of sensitivity, specificity, and prevalence; and Bayes' theorem (Archer, 1978; Galen and Gambino, 1975; McNeil et al., 1975; Vecchio, 1966). The predictive value model allows us to characterize the behavior of laboratory measurements needed for confirming the presence of disease, excluding disease, and screening for disease. The predictive value of a test estimates the chances that a test result indicates the presence or the absence of disease. The first section of the chapter discusses how this estimate is made. The predictive value concept is no more than an easily digestible version of Bayes' theorem (Burke, 1981).

PREDICTIVE VALUE

PREDICTIVE VALUE OF A LABORATORY MEASUREMENT

The predictive value of a laboratory measurement depends on three quantities:

1. Prevalence—the frequency of patients with a certain disease in the group we are examining with the measurement.

2. Sensitivity—the percentage of true-positive results in patients with the disease.

3. Specificity—the percentage of true-negative results in healthy patients.

We shall illustrate in more detail the meaning of these three terms by using an example, pregnancy testing (see Chapter 8).

47

Table 4–1. PREVALENCE OF PREGNANCY

	No. With Positive Result	No. With Negative Result	Total
No. pregnant			100
No. not pregnant			900
Total			1000
Prevalence: ———————— 10% ————————
Sensitivity: ————————————————————
Specificity: ————————————————————
Predictive Value of a Positive: ————————

Imagine an evaluation of a pregnancy test performed on a urine sample. The group of women in the evaluation of this test have previously been examined by other means in order to determine which individuals are pregnant. For our example, 10 per cent of the women in our evaluation group are pregnant (the prevalence of pregnancy) out of a total of 1,000 women (see Table 4–1). The pregnancy test is performed on the urine specimen from each individual who is known to be pregnant, and it is determined if the result is positive or negative. The results of this stage of the evaluation are shown in Table 4–2.

Of the 100 pregnant women, 90 had a positive test result (a true-positive) and 10 had a negative test result (a false-negative). The percentage of positive results obtained when the urine test was performed on pregnant women is 90 per cent. This percentage represents the true-positive results and is referred to as the sensitivity of the test. Sensitivity of a test is an expression of the positivity of the test in disease.

Table 4–2. PREVALENCE OF PREGNANCY AND SENSITIVITY OF PREGNANCY TEST

	No. With Positive Result	No. With Negative Result	Total
No. pregnant	90	10	100
No. not pregnant			900
Total			1000
Prevalence: ———————— 10% ————————
Sensitivity: ———————— 90% ————————
Specificity: ————————————————————
Predictive Value of a Positive: ————————

Another step in our evaluation of the urine test is to test the urine of women who are known not to be pregnant. The results of this stage of the evaluation are shown in Table 4–3. The same test, applied to the group of non-pregnant women, was truly negative in 720 out of 900 women (80 per cent). The 80 per cent figure represents the true-negative results and is the specificity of the test. In general, specificity is obtained by performing the test on individuals who are free of disease, and it represents the negativity of the test in health.

Based on this data obtained from our evaluation of the pregnancy test, how good would our test be in confirming or ruling out pregnancy? A measure of use in deciding these questions is the percentage of positive results of the test that are true positives (TP) when the test is applied to a population like the one we have selected.

From Table 4–4, there are 90 out of 270 positive results that are true-positive results, or 33 per cent (a positive test result in an individual who was pregnant). This percentage of true-positive results of all the positive results is referred to as the *predictive value* of a test. In the evaluation of this test, only 33 per cent of the positive test results occurred in women who were pregnant. A predictive value of 33 per cent indicates that this test would not be of use in confirming whether a woman were pregnant in a population like the one in the test evaluation because roughly 67 per cent of the positive test results would be in women who were not pregnant.

Does it seem surprising that the predictive value of the test is 33 per cent when the evaluation showed that the test was 90 per cent sensitive and 80 per cent specific? In Table 4–4, the explanation for the low predictive value of the test is apparent when we consider the total number of women in the evaluation who were pregnant (100) versus the total number of women in the study who were not pregnant (900).

If we assume that sensitivity is an intrinsic property of the test and its relationship to pregnancy or non-pregnancy, the percentage of true positives will remain the same regardless of the total number of pregnant women tested. Also, the percentage of pregnant women with a false-negative result will remain the same (FN). The sensitivity, multiplied by the total number of pregnant women, will then give us the number of women who have a true-positive result.

Table 4–3. PREVALENCE OF PREGNANCY, SENSITIVITY OF PREGNANCY TEST, AND SPECIFICITY OF PREGNANCY TEST

	No. With Positive Result	No. With Negative Result	Total
No. pregnant	90	10	100
No. not pregnant	180	720	900
Total			1000

Prevalence: _____ 10%

Sensitivity: _____ 90%

Specificity: _____ 80%

Predictive Value of a Positive: _____

Likewise, if we assume that specificity is an intrinsic property of the test, the percentage of true negatives (TN) will remain about 80 per cent regardless of the actual number of non-pregnant women tested. The number of non-pregnant women who have a negative test result, subtracted from the total of non-pregnant women, gives us the number of women who are not pregnant but have a positive test result, the false positives (FP). As the total number of non-pregnant women in the study increases, the number of non-pregnant women with a positive test result also increases at a fixed rate. This rate is determined by the specificity of the test.

In the calculation of the percentage of positive results that are true-positive results (the predictive value), the number of pregnant women with a positive result depends on the total number of pregnant women and the sensitivity of the test. However, the total number of positive results is a combination of this previous value (the true-positive results) and also of the false positives. The predictive value of a positive test is therefore heavily dependent on the total number of women in our evaluation who are not pregnant as well as the sensitivity and specificity of the test, i.e., the TP divided by the sum of the TP plus the FP × 100.

If, in another evaluation, we increase the total number of non-pregnant women used in the study relative to the number of pregnant women that were used in the previous study, the predictive value would decrease dramatically. In this case, the total number of non-pregnant women who have a positive test result would increase dramatically. It is this increase in false-positive results relative to the total number of true-positive results that causes the decrease in the predictive value of the test.

In summary, if we are going to use a test to confirm the presence of a disease, we need a test that, when positive, is frequently associated with the disease. However, the percentage of true-positive results (the predictive value) of a test is dramatically affected by the prevalence rate of the disease in the population that we are testing. This is illustrated in Table 4–5 for two tests, one of which is 95 per cent sensitive and specific, whereas the other is 99 per cent sensitive and specific. At very low prevalence rates, even highly sensitive and specific tests have a very low percentage of true-positive results.

A negative test result also has usefulness in decision making. A negative result on a test associated with disease increases our confidence that the disease is not present, and if the association is strong, allows us to reject the disease as a possibility. It is natural to want to know the predictive value of a negative test result: It is the percentage of all negative test results that are truly negative. The true-negative results occur when the test result is negative in individuals who do not have disease. In our evaluation example (Table 4–4), of 730 negative test results, 720 were truly negative—which gives the negative test result a predictive value of 98.6 per cent (720/730 × 100), i.e., the TN divided by the sum of the TN plus the FN × 100. If a particular woman's urine specimen has a negative test result, it is highly probable that the woman is not pregnant. Thus, even though a positive test result is not of much help in confirming that a woman

Table 4–4. PREVALENCE OF PREGNANCY, SENSITIVITY OF PREGNANCY TEST, AND SPECIFICITY OF PREGNANCY TEST PLUS PREDICTIVE VALUE OF A POSITIVE PREGNANCY TEST RESULT

	No. With Positive Result	No. With Negative Result	Total
No. pregnant	90	10	100
No. not pregnant	180	720	900
Total	270	730	1000

Prevalence: _____ 10%

Sensitivity: _____ 90%

Specificity: _____ 80%

Predictive Value of a Positive: _____ 33%

Table 4–5. EFFECT OF PREVALENCE ON PREDICTIVE VALUE*

Effect of Prevalence†		Effect of Prevalence‡	
Prevalence (%)	Predictive Value of a Positive Test (%)	Prevalence (%)	Predictive Value of a Positive Test (%)
0.1	1.9	0.1	9.0
1.0	16.1	1.0	50.0
2.0	27.9	2.0	66.9
5.0	50.0	5.0	83.9
50.0	95.0	50.0	99.0

*Adapted from Galen RS, Gambino SR: Beyond Normality: The Predictive Value and Efficiency of Medical Diagnoses. New York, John Wiley & Sons, Inc., 1975, p. 16. Used with permission.
†Sensitivity = 95%; specificity = 95%.
‡Sensitivity = 99%; specificity = 99%.

is pregnant, a negative test result is very helpful in confirming that the woman is not pregnant.

Of course, the predictive value of a negative test result is also highly dependent on the prevalence of the disease-free state. As the prevalence of pregnancy in the test population increases, the predictive value of a negative test result to rule out pregnancy decreases because a proportionately greater number of negative test results occurs in pregnant women. As the prevalence of pregnancy increases in our tested population, the predictive value of

a positive test result in confirming pregnancy increases.

The relationships and definitions that we have discussed are summarized in Tables 4–6 and 4–7. Note that sensitivity is the percentage of true-positive results in those individuals having the disease. The total number of individuals having the disease is the sum of those individuals with a true-positive test result added to the number of individuals with a false-negative test result. Specificity is the percentage of true-negative test results in those people who are in a state of health and are

Table 4–6. PREDICTIVE VALUE TABLE*

	Number With Positive Test Result	Number With Negative Test Result	Totals
Number with disease	TP	FN	TP + FN
Number without disease	FP	TN	FP + TN
Totals	TP + FP	FN + TN	TP + FP + TN + FN

TP = True positives; the number of sick subjects correctly classified by the test.
FP = False positives; the number of subjects free of the disease who are misclassified by the test.
TN = True negatives; the number of subjects free of the disease who are correctly classified by the test.
FN = False negatives; the number of sick subjects misclassified by the test.
Prevalence = Percent of total subjects examined who are diseased.

$$\text{Sensitivity} = \text{positivity in disease} = \frac{TP}{TP + FN} \times 100 = \frac{TP}{\text{no. diseased}} \times 100$$

$$\text{Specificity} = \text{negativity in health} = \frac{TN}{TN + FP} \times 100 = \frac{TN}{\text{no. without disease}} \times 100$$

$$\text{Predictive value of a positive test} = \frac{TP}{TP + FP} \times 100 = \frac{TP}{\text{no. positive}} \times 100$$

$$\text{Predictive value of a negative test} = \frac{TN}{TN + FN} \times 100 = \frac{TN}{\text{no. negative}} \times 100$$

*From Galen RS, Gambino SR: Beyond Normality: The Predictive Value and Efficiency of Medical Diagnoses. New York, John Wiley & Sons, Inc., p. 124. Used with permission.

Table 4–7. PREDICTIVE VALUE TABLE*

	Number With Positive Test Result	Number With Negative Test Result	Totals
Number with disease	pa	p(1 − a)	p
Number without disease	(1 − p)(1 − b)	(1 − p)b	(1 − p)
Totals	pa + (1 − p)(1 − b)	p(1 − a) + (1 − p)b	1

Sensitivity = a
Specificity = b

$$\text{Predictive value of positive} = \frac{pa}{[pa + (1 - p)(1 - b)]}$$

$$\text{Predictive value of negative} = \frac{(1 - p)b}{p(1 - a) + (1 - p)b}$$

*From Galen RS, Gambino SR: Beyond Normality: The Predictive Value and Efficiency of Medical Diagnoses. New York, John Wiley & Sons, Inc., p. 124. Used with permission.

thus free of the disease. The total number of individuals without disease is the sum of those people with a true-negative test result and those with a false-positive test result.

On the other hand, the predictive value of a positive result is the percentage of individuals with true-positive test results. All those individuals with positive test results includes those with true-positive test results and those with false-positive test results. Likewise, the predictive value of a negative test result is the percentage of true-negative test results in all individuals who had a negative test result. The group of individuals who have a negative test result is composed of those with true-negative test results and those with false-negative test results.

To confirm whether a patient has a disease, we would like the predictive value of a positive test result to be high. To reject a disease, we would like to have a test whose predictive value of a negative test result is quite high.

There is no test that would ever be free of any false-positive or false-negative results. In fact, as we shall see later, sensitivity and specificity are coupled in an inverse way. The higher the sensitivity of the test (positivity in disease), the lower the specificity of the test (negativity in health). We shall illustrate why this is so by using a quantitative test in which it is possible to define the positivity of the test results at a variety of test values. By changing the value above which we consider the test positive (decision level of the test), we can vary the sensitivity and specificity in a predictable way. The example used later in this chapter is the fasting serum glucose test for determining diabetes mellitus. For certain quali-

tative tests, however, sensitivity and specificity are inherent in the test system in such a way that we cannot vary them in the laboratory. Different test systems (or strategies) can also have various degrees of sensitivity and specificity.

So far in this chapter, we have not adhered strictly to the epidemiologic definition of the word *prevalence* (Galen and Gambino, 1975). Epidemiologists refer to prevalence as the number of people who have a given disease at a particular time per 100,000 individuals. We have used the word prevalence as the percentage of people who have a given disease. The two definitions, however, are conceptually the same in terms of their effect on predictive value. It is important to realize the distinction between prevalence and *incidence*. The prevalence of disease can vary over time because it is determined by the number of individuals who have a disease at the time a measurement is made. During epidemics, the prevalence of disease will be high at the height of the epidemic and low at the beginning or end of the epidemic. The incidence rate refers to the percentage of a population who contracts a disease over a given period of time or the number of individuals per 100,000 population who develop a disease in a given year. The formulas for the incidence rate and prevalence rate are as follows (Friedman, 1976):

Incidence rate =

$$\frac{\text{number of new cases of a disease}}{\text{total population at risk}} \text{ per unit of time}$$

$$\text{Prevalence rate} = \frac{\text{number of existing cases}}{\text{total population}}$$

The distinction between incidence and prevalence is an important one in the attempt to calculate predictive values. Clearly, the two are not always equal. For example, in June the prevalence of upper respiratory tract infections may be 70/100,000 for a given group of people. If we were to do a study to detect upper respiratory tract infections in January, the prevalence could be 500/100,000, which is a higher figure. This means that although incidence rates take into consideration the number of people who have developed a disease over an entire year, the prevalence rate indicates that most people develop an upper respiratory tract infection during the winter months. If you are diagnosing upper respiratory tract infections based on a laboratory test, a positive test result in January is more likely to be a true-positive result than a positive test result in June. There are simply more cases of upper respiratory tract infection in January.

Most diseases that we are concerned with are not very prevalent in the population. We are a remarkably healthy people. Diabetes mellitus, including all age groups under 80, has a prevalence of about 3 per cent. That is fairly high for any disease. Certainly, it is much higher than the prevalence for most other endocrine or metabolic diseases and for almost any cancer you can name.

Previously, we discussed the sensitivity, specificity, and predictive value of a test result. Any test or diagnostic maneuver that you choose to employ will have a certain degree of sensitivity (positivity in disease) and specificity (negativity in health). No test is simultaneously very sensitive and very specific; the more sensitive a test is, the less specific it is, and vice versa.

It is important to remember that most tests are neither very sensitive nor specific and that the prevalence of most diseases in our population is not very high. As a matter of fact, a number of authors have shown that getting good information on the sensitivities and specificities of common tests is difficult and that we simply do not know the prevalence of many diseases in the general population (Harris, 1981).

Prevalence, or prior probability considerations, prompt the following observations:

1. If most tests are not highly sensitive and specific and if disease prevalences in the general population are not very high, using laboratory tests to screen for disease in asymptomatic people is probably going to be very unproductive. Most of our positive results will be false positives, and there will be too many false-negative results. With very few exceptions, this has been the experience of most investigators who have tried to use laboratory tests or x-ray procedures to screen for disease in clinically asymptomatic, healthy, large populations. Obviously, the cost considerations can be enormous. (See Chapter 8 on screening subproblems, and see Chapter 17 concerning cystic fibrosis.)

2. The key to using tests in a way that will help instead of confuse us, then, has to do with increasing the prevalence or prior probability of disease. If, before the laboratory test is done, we take a good history, particularly a family history, and do a thorough physical examination, we can begin to rule out patients in whom further laboratory testing will undoubtedly be unproductive and can begin to group patients into cohorts in which further testing is likely to be productive. (In this way, we are increasing the prevalence of disease.) The signs, symptoms, and historical features we look for should have high sensitivity for the disease we are considering, e.g., predisposing factors, tachypnea, and dyspnea for pulmonary embolism (see Tables 11–4 and 11–5).

In other words, we do not have to use statistical calculations constantly in order to apply the concepts of predictive value theory (i.e., Bayes' rule). If we have an intuitive appreciation of how the model works, we can use this knowledge to make laboratory studies work more powerfully. A good workup, history, and physical examination will increase the prior probability of the disease that we are attempting to diagnose; then we apply the most effective test or strategy known (Appelgate, 1981).

Other variables associated with disease can have an effect on predictive value calculations. We already mentioned that disease prevalence can vary over time and can affect these calculations. Variations in sensitivity, specificity, and predictive value can also occur in different stages or after different durations of a disease (see Table 11–1). Population variables like age, sex, and the presence of other diseases can also potentially affect these indexes. Determining specificity of a test using healthy subjects is in a sense an estimate of "ideal" specificity. In many decision situations, the specificity that we need to know is the specificity of a test for a particular disease when that test is applied to patients who have similar diseases. The difficulty is frequently not in differentiating disease from perfect health but in differentiating a disease from a variety of other similar diseases.

Another useful measure of a test is efficiency or effectiveness. The efficiency of a test is represented by the percentage of all results that are true results, whether positive or negative (Burke, 1981; Galen and Gambino, 1975).

PREDICTIVE VALUE AND BAYES' THEOREM

This section discusses the relationship between Bayes' theorem and predictive value concepts. Bayes' theorem is the predictive value model cast in the terminology of probability. The formula for calculating predictive value is Bayes' rule. The use of Bayes' rule to aid medical decision making for diagnosis has been suggested in a variety of medical contexts: acute myocardial infarction (Bloomberg, 1975; Galen and Gambino, 1975; Galen, Reiffel, and Gambino, 1975), pheochromocytoma (Galen and Gambino, 1975), application of tumor markers (Galen, 1974; Galen and Gambino, 1975) hepatic metastases (Baden, 1971; Kim, 1977), thyroid function testing (Homburger and Hewan-Lowe, 1979), and neonatal screening for genetic disease (Galen and Gambino, 1975; Whitby, 1974).

In our discussion of Bayes' theorem, when we talk about the probability of an event A, we shall use *probability* to mean the frequency of occurrence of event A. We denote the probability of an event A by $P(A)$. $P(A)$ will be referred to as an unconditional probability, prior probability, or the a priori probability of event A. Calling $P(A)$ an a priori or unconditional probability indicates that the frequency of occurrence of event A is not dependent on any other events. However, the occurrence of some events varies, depending on the occurrence or non-occurrence of related events (Mendenhall and Shaeffer, 1973). Such situations will be described using conditional probabilities or a posteriori probabilities, which we shall discuss later.

Simple Form of Bayes' Rule

The simple form of Bayes' rule is directly related to the predictive value model. Bayes'

rule allows us to calculate the probability of an event based on the knowledge of other mutually exclusive events, which we know have occurred. The predictive value formula for a positive test result that was presented earlier allows us to calculate the frequency (probability) of a person's having a disease, given that we know the occurrence of a test result. The predictive value formula—Bayes' rule—is just a special way of viewing Bayes' theorem in regard to tests. Bayes' rule can be applied to calculate the probability that a patient has a particular disease, given that we know that the patient has certain signs, symptoms, or laboratory test results in the same way the predictive value formula can be used. Up to now, our discussion of the predictive value model has been somewhat restricted to laboratory measurements. Because a large body of literature on the use of Bayes' theorem and medical decision making already exists, it is useful to know Bayes' rule.

What good is knowing the probability that a medical diagnosis is true? We could argue that in diagnostic decision making, we are trying to decide the merit of one disease hypothesis over another, not probabilities. One way of viewing the use of probabilities in this situation is to consider the possible diagnostic classes for a patient (the hypotheses) as being associated with a probability of being true. This probability would be calculated from the evidence we have accumulated using Bayes' rule. An "optimal way" of deciding which diagnostic class is the best to choose for a particular patient would then be to choose the disease that has the highest conditional probability (predictive value).

Our next example will deal with the data given for the pregnancy test in our discussion on predictive value, as modified from Duda and Hart (1973). Rather than evaluating the test in our previous example, let's pose a different situation. An obstetrician wishes to decide whether a woman is pregnant or not and to use the data from our urine test evaluation to come up with a decision rule whereby the percentage of time a patient is correctly classified as pregnant or non-pregnant is maximized. In other words, the obstetrician is seeking a decision rule whereby a wrong decision will be made a minimal percentage of the time.

Several probabilities are at the physician's disposal and will be assumed to be true. The obstetrician knows that the probability of seeing a pregnant woman in practice is 0.3. In other words, the prior probability or prevalence of pregnancy in this practice population is 30 per cent. If we denote pregnancy by the letter "p," the probability of pregnancy is P(p) = 0.3. This probability is an unconditional (a priori) probability because it reflects our prior knowledge of how frequently we expect to see a pregnant woman. This a priori probability of a disease in a population is an estimate of the prevalence of the disease. The prevalence in the obstetrician's practice of non-pregnancy would be 70 per cent. The probability of a woman's not being pregnant P(p̄) would be equal to 0.7. This probability is an estimate of the prevalence of non-pregnancy in the practice population.

Note that 0.7 + 0.3 = 1.0. Some of the requirements of event probabilities for use in the simple Bayes rule are that:

1. They must be greater than or equal to zero (0).

2. The sum of the probability of all possible events we are considering must equal one (1.0).

Pregnancy and non-pregnancy are also mutually exclusive events in the sense that each woman that we see must be in one state or the other, not in both simultaneously.

It is also important to realize that the physician finds it hard to predict whether the next woman seen will be pregnant or not, based on the previous sequence of women already seen. In this sense, the sequence of women is random because the sequence of pregnant or non-pregnant women is unpredictable.

Would it be possible to decide, based just on these a priori probabilities, whether the next woman seen will be pregnant or not? If the only information we use are these a priori probabilities, we could follow the following decision rule: Decide that a woman is pregnant if P(p) is much greater than P(p̄); otherwise, decide she is not pregnant. The percentage of times we will be correct using this decision rule, of course, is dependent on the value of the a priori probabilities. If the prior probability that a woman is pregnant is much greater than the probability that she is not, deciding pregnancy will make us right most of the time. We shall always decide that a woman is pregnant. Take the probability (prevalence) that a woman is pregnant = 0.3 and follow this decision rule (always deciding that a woman is

not pregnant); we will be in error 30 per cent of the time in the "long run" (on the average). It can be shown that the probability of error (percentage of time that we are wrong) using this decision rule is the smallest probability of error that is possible using any other decision rule we can imagine (Duda and Hart, 1973).

This situation is, of course, highly unrealistic because a physician would make such a decision based on additional evidence related to whether a woman was pregnant or not. Let's add such evidence for pregnancy to our example. Refer back to our simple test that measures some quantity of chemical in the urine in such a way that most pregnant women have a positive test and most non-pregnant women have a negative test. In our first example in this chapter, we arrived at this conclusion by taking a sample of women known by other means to be pregnant or not pregnant. These two groups were given the test, thus allowing us to approximate P(+/p) and P(+/p̄). P(+/p) = the probability of a positive test result, given that a patient was pregnant (sensitivity). P(+/p̄) = probability of a positive test result, given that a patient is not pregnant. Let's say, P(+/p) = 0.9 and P(+/p̄) = 0.2. These are the conditional probabilities of the test's being positive, given that a woman is pregnant or not pregnant.

How can we combine this new information with our previous a priori probabilities to arrive at the decision of pregnancy or non-pregnancy? In other words: How does the laboratory test result influence our belief concerning the state of women whose test result we have? The answer in this case is obtained by using Bayes' rule.

The formula for predictive value is that which we used previously for our test calculation in the pregnancy test evaluation. The pregnancy decision has been stated in such a way as to approximate the basic assumptions of Bayes' rule. We are dealing with true probabilities. The hypotheses that we are considering are mutually exclusive and exhaustive. A woman cannot be pregnant and not pregnant at the same time; and therefore, pregnancy and non-pregnancy are mutually exclusive. A woman can only be either pregnant or not pregnant; therefore, the hypotheses are exhaustive.

Bayes' and the predictive value formulas for a woman whose pregnancy test is positive would be:

$$\text{P.V.} = P(p/+) = \frac{P(p) \, P(+/p)}{P(p) \, P(+/p) + P(\bar{p}) \, P(+/\bar{p})}$$

$$= \frac{\text{prevalence (sensitivity)}}{[(\text{prevalence})(\text{sensitivity}) + (1 - \text{prevalence})(1 - \text{specificity})]}$$

$$= \frac{\text{TP}}{\text{TP} + \text{FP}}$$

$P(p) \, P(+/p)$, the term in the numerator and the first term in the denominator of Bayes' rule, is the fraction pregnant times the fraction pregnant with a positive test [(prevalence) (sensitivity)]. This would be the fraction of positive tests in pregnant women (TP). $P(\bar{p}) \, P(+/\bar{p})$, the second term in the denominator, is the fraction of non-pregnant women with a positive test [FP = (1 − prevalence) (1 − specificity) = (non-pregnant) (false-positive rate)]. This is the fraction of non-pregnant women with positive tests. The fraction of true-positive tests $P(p/+)$ (predictive value of a positive test result) is the true positives divided by all positives (true positives and false positives). The terms of the predictive value equation are synonymous with the corresponding probabilities.

For the moment, disregard the denominator of this formula. The denominator merely acts as a scaling factor for the conditional probabilities calculated. This scaling is done so that the conditional probability of pregnancy given a positive test result and the conditional probability of non-pregnancy given a positive test will add up to one (i.e., $P(p/+) + P(\bar{p}/+) =$ 1). This is a requirement for the conditional probabilities to be considered true probabilities by definition. Note that this denominator will be the same for $P(p/+)$ and $P(\bar{p}/+)$.

The calculation that makes a difference as to the merit of a hypothesis is in the numerator of the equation. What is the numerator saying? In this case, we are taking the unconditional probability of pregnancy and multiplying it by the conditional probability of a woman who is pregnant having a positive test. We can view this calculation as a revision of the unconditional probability of pregnancy based on our knowledge of the conditional probability of a positive test, given that a woman is pregnant. We are revising our belief in a hypothesis from the belief we had knowing the frequency of occurrence of pregnancy. We are revising our belief by the conditional probability of a related event. This is in accordance with common sense. Bayes' rule is no more than a formali-

zation of this common-sense reasoning strategy. As in our previous example, when we assume the actual numbers for this example, we have:

$$P(p/+) = \frac{P(p) \, P(+/p)}{P(p) \, P(+/p) + P(\bar{p}) \, P(+/\bar{p})}$$

$$= \frac{0.3(0.9)}{0.3(0.9) + 0.7(0.2)}$$

$$= \frac{0.27}{0.27 + 0.14} = 0.66$$

The fact that the test was positive has increased the probability of the hypothesis—pregnancy—from 0.3 to 0.66. Just as our belief in a woman's being pregnant would increase given a positive result, the probability calculation has also resulted in an increased probability of pregnancy.

How can this calculation of conditional probability be used in a decision rule similar to the one we used, given only a prior probability? If in the "long run" we wish to minimize the percentage of errors we make in classifying patients as either pregnant or not pregnant, we would write our decision as: Decide pregnancy if $P(p/+)$ is greater than $P(\bar{p}/+)$; otherwise, decide non-pregnancy.

Using Bayes' rule to calculate the latter probability, we have:

$$P(\bar{p}/+) = \frac{P(\bar{p}) \, P(+/\bar{p})}{P(p) \, P(+/p) + P(\bar{p}) \, P(+/\bar{p})}$$

$$= \frac{0.7(0.2)}{0.3(0.9) + 0.7(0.2)}$$

$$= \frac{0.14}{0.27 + 0.14} = 0.34$$

Note in our example, $P(p/+) + P(\bar{p}/+) = 1$; i.e., $0.66 + 0.34 = 1$.

We would decide that a woman with a positive test would be pregnant because 0.66 is greater than 0.34. Note that, following this decision rule for the fixed fraction of pregnant women given in our example, we would decide that a woman was pregnant, given a positive test result in all cases. We know from our previous results, however, that some women have positive tests even though they are not pregnant. The decision rule we are using minimizes the percentage of time we shall be in error. In fact, it guarantees that the percentage of error we make is lower than any other decision rule that we can imagine based on probability arguments. We are guaranteed this minimum error rate in the long run (on the average).

Some have objected to this method of making decisions because we are guaranteed correct decisions only on the average. The ones who might object argue that they are interested in making the correct decision for an individual patient, not the correct decisions in the long run. It is unclear to us what is meant by "correct" in this objection. In a probability sense, we can be correct only on the average. Perhaps those individuals objecting to this average guarantee believe there is a better way of making decisions that guarantees more than a minimum percentage error rate in the long run. The clinical utility of making decisions this way is under debate (Brett, 1981; Ingelfinger, 1975; Schwartz, 1979).

Because the denominator in Bayes' rule is a scaling factor, it can be omitted in our decision rule. If we eliminate this scaling factor, we can equivalently write our decision as: Decide p if $P(p) \, P(+/p)$ is greater than $P(\bar{p}) \, P(+/\bar{p})$; otherwise, decide $\bar{p}$.

Assume for the moment that $P(+/p) = P(+/\bar{p})$, that a positive result on the chemical test is equally likely to be associated with pregnancy or non-pregnancy. In this case, our decision rule is totally dependent on the a priori probabilities. The observation of a positive test result would have no effect on our decision. Let's now assume that $P(p) = P(\bar{p})$; it is equally likely that a woman is either pregnant or not pregnant. Using our decision rule, we would be basing our opinion on only the conditional probabilities of pregnancy, given a positive test result. For intermediate situations between these two extremes, we can view Bayes' rule as weighing the a priori and conditional probabilities to produce an overall probability of the hypothesis being true.

This ends our discussion of the simple case of using Bayes' rule with discrete test results. This is the same as using predictive value to decide between two competing hypotheses based on the conditional probability of one test result related to the hypotheses. The test results we have been considering are discrete in the sense that the result of the urine test could take only two possible values (+ or −).

Bayes' Rule and Continuous Values

Now look at an application of Bayes' rule and the predictive value model when the test results can have an infinite number of values, as modified from Duda and Hart (1973). Because the test results are continuous, we shall have to deal with a distribution of probabilities rather than a probability for each discrete event. Our example will be the decision to classify a patient as having diabetes mellitus or not having diabetes mellitus based on the result of a fasting serum glucose measurement.

In order to use Bayes' rule or the predictive value model to compare these two hypotheses, we need to know several probabilities. We need the a priori probabilities of a person's being diabetic or not being diabetic (prevalence) as well as the conditional probabilities relating the fasting serum glucose, given that the person is diabetic or non-diabetic (sensitivity and specificity).

To arrive at these hypothetical, class-conditional probabilities, let's imagine taking one group of people who are known to be diabetic by some independent means and measuring their fasting serum glucose. We shall refer to this group as D and refer to the values of their fasting serum glucose as x. From this sample of all possible diabetics, we might infer an approximation of the actual probability distribution of glucose values for all diabetics. This distribution might follow one of the common continuous distribution of values (like the gaussian distribution). Assume that the true distribution is as shown in Figure 4–1 by the curve marked P(x/D). Remember that this curve tells us the distribution of probabilities of glucose levels, given the fact that we are dealing with people who are diabetic.

Likewise, taking another group of people who are known by independent means not to be diabetic, we might discover a distribution of probabilities relating their fasting serum glucose levels to the fact they are non-diabetic. Assume that this distribution corresponds to

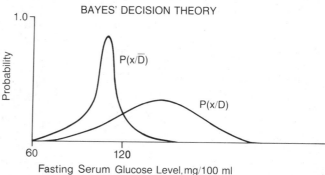

Figure 4–1. Hypothetical class-conditional probabilities for diabetes mellitus (D) and non-diabetes mellitus ($\overline{D}$) for given values of fasting serum glucose (x). (Adapted from Duda RO, Hart PE: Pattern Classification and Scene Analysis. New York, John Wiley & Sons, Inc, 1973, p 12. Used by permission.)

the curve labeled $P(x/\overline{D})$ in Figure 4–1. This curve would allow us to find the probability, given that a person is non-diabetic, of a certain value, x, of fasting serum glucose.

Let's assume, for this example, that the a priori probability of a person being diabetic (prevalence) is $P(D) = 2/3$ and the a priori probability of a person being non-diabetic (prevalence) is $P(\overline{D}) = 1/3$. Such a situation might arise when patients are referred by another physician who has screened out most of the non-diabetic patients.

The decisions we are asked to make are the following: Given a patient's fasting serum glucose level, is it more probable that this patient is a diabetic or a non-diabetic? Furthermore, what decision rule can we use to minimize the percentage of error that we make in classifying patients as either diabetic or non-diabetic?

For this particular decision, we can use a formula analogous to the one we used when the probabilities were discrete. We would write:

$$P(D/x) = \frac{P(D)\ P(x/D)}{P(x)}, \quad \text{or}$$

$$= \frac{\text{prevalence (sensitivity)}}{\text{total positive}}$$

where

$$P(x) = P(D)\ P(x/D) + P(\overline{D})\ P(x/\overline{D})$$

or

$$P(x) = [(\text{prevalence})\ (\text{sensitivity}) + (1-\text{prevalence})\ (1 - \text{specificity})].$$

Given a particular fasting serum glucose level (e.g., x = 120 mg/100 ml), we could use the conditional probability distribution to calculate the probability that a person is diabetic,

given that the serum glucose level is 120 mg/100 ml. Likewise, we can use the formula

$$P(\overline{D}/x) = \frac{P(\overline{D})P(x/\overline{D})}{P(x)}$$

to calculate the conditional probability that a person was not diabetic, given a certain serum glucose level.

The results of such calculations are given in Figure 4–2. The reader should note several things about these probabilities. For a given value of serum glucose, the conditional probability of being a diabetic, added to the conditional probability of not being a diabetic, always adds up to one in agreement with the definition of a probability. For example, look at the conditional probabilities wherein the serum glucose level is 60 mg/100 ml. From Figure 4–2, we can see that, given a fasting serum glucose level of 60 mg/100 ml, the probability of not being a diabetic is equal to one (1) and the probability of being a diabetic is zero (0). These two probabilities, of course, add up to one (1). The same is true for any level of fasting serum glucose.

If we follow the decision rule analogous to the one we used in the discrete probability case, we would assign patients whose serum glucose level was 120 mg/100 ml or less to the class called non-diabetic. This is because at 120 mg/100 ml fasting blood glucose, the conditional probability curves for diabetic and non-diabetic classes are equal. This area is referred to as R_1 in Figure 4–2. Likewise, for values of fasting serum glucose above 120 mg/100 ml, we would assign these patients to be in the diabetic class. This is referred to as R_2 in Figure 4–2. This decision rule allows us to define decision regions R_1 and R_2, because it

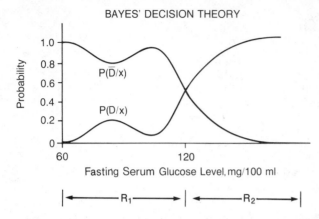

Figure 4–2. A posteriori probabilities for diabetes mellitus (D) and non-diabetes mellitus ($\overline{D}$) for given values of fasting serum glucose (x) when $P(D) = 2/3$ and $P(\overline{D}) = 1/3$. (Adapted from Duda RO, Hart PE: Pattern Classification and Scene Analysis. New York, John Wiley & Sons, Inc, 1973, p 12. Used by permission.)

assigns a patient to the class that has the highest conditional probability, given a certain value on a laboratory test.

In this particular example, R_2 corresponds to the decision region in which patients are classified as diabetic. As in the discrete case, following this decision rule guarantees us that the percentage of errors we make is minimized over any other decision rule that we can imagine using probability concepts. Using this decision rule, we can assign with increasing probability, patients, whose serum glucose levels are 130 mg/100 ml, 140 mg/100 ml, or 150 mg/100 ml, respectively, to the class called diabetic. In other words, each of the values for serum glucose can indicate diabetes mellitus with a certain probability. In this sense, they are referent values or decision levels for the diagnosis of diabetes mellitus (Chapter 3). By changing the value above, which we consider the fasting serum glucose positive for determining diabetes mellitus, we can vary the sensitivity and specificity in a predictable way. However, as sensitivity increases, specificity decreases and as sensitivity decreases, specificity increases—they are coupled in an inverse way. (See Chapter 16 for diagnosing diabetes mellitus.)

OTHER STATISTICAL APPLICATIONS

Decision models based on statistical concepts such as Bayes' theorem have been one of the most popular forms of models used in computer-assisted diagnostic systems. A large body of literature has evolved regarding the use of Bayes' theorem and similar techniques in medical decision making (Miller et al.,

1977). More details about the application of these techniques have been documented by Ledley and Lusted (1959), Lusted (1968), Ross (1972); and Wardle and Wardle (1978). These techniques have been used in the diagnosis of a variety of types of medical problems, including the acute abdomen (deDombal et al., 1975; Scheinok and Renaldo, 1967), hematologic diseases (Engle et al., 1976), pleuritic chest pain (McNeil and Sherman, 1978), and thyroid disease (Cobelli and Salvan, 1975).

In association with Bayesian techniques, other researchers have attempted to design computer approaches to diagnosis and treatment by structuring clinical problems using the formal techniques of decision analysis (Barnoon and Wolfe, 1972; McNeil and Sherman, 1978; Pauker, 1977; Schwartz et al., 1973; Weinstein and Fineberg, 1980). In this technique, relative likelihood or probability is assigned to each possible event that could occur in a particular decision context. The relative worth, or utility, of each potential consequence of a decision is assigned. From the utility and probability of each event, it is possible to calculate an expected utility for each important course of action. The basic decision rule used selects the action that has the highest expected value.

Decision analysis has been suggested as a way to make laboratory tests more diagnostically useful as well as economical (Benson, 1978). In this regard, a number of investigators have attempted to discover statistical relationships that would be useful for clinical problem solving using various forms of statistical analysis, such as multivariate analysis, numerical taxonomy, and discriminate functions (Beck et al., 1978; Lahniser et al., 1980; Sher, 1980; Statland et al., 1979; Winkel, 1973).

REFERENCES

Appelgate WB: Decision theory for clinicians: Uses and misuses of clinical tests. South Med J 74:468–473, 1981.

Archer PG: The predictive value of clinical laboratory test results. Am J Clin Pathol 69:32–35, 1978.

Baden H, Anderson B, Augustenborg G, et al: Diagnostic value of gamma-glutamyl transpeptidase and alkaline phosphatase in liver metastases. Surg Gynecol Obstet 133:769–773, 1971.

Barnoon S, Wolfe H: Measuring the Effectiveness of Medical Decisions. Springfield, Ill, Charles C Thomas, Publisher, 1972.

Beck JR, Cornwell GG, Rawnsley HM: Multivariate approach to predictive diagnosis of bone marrow iron stores. Am J Clin Pathol 70:665–670, 1978.

Benson ES, Rubin M (eds): Logic and Economics of Clinical Laboratory Use. New York, Elsevier North-Holland, Inc, 1978.

Berwick DM, Fineberg HV, Weinstein MC: When doctors meet numbers. Am J Med 71:991–998, 1981.

Blomberg DJ, Kimber WD, Burke MD: Creatine Kinase isoenzymes: Predictive value in the early diagnosis of acute myocardial infarction. Am J Med 59:464–469, 1975.

Brett AS: Hidden ethical issues in clinical decision analysis. N Engl J Med 305:1150–1152, 1981.

Burke MD: Clinical problem solving and laboratory investigation: Contributions to laboratory medicine. In Stefanini M, Benson ES (eds): Progress in Clinical Pathology, vol VIII. New York, Grune & Stratton, Inc, 1981, pp 1–24.

Casscells W, Schoenberger A, Graboys TB: Interpretation by physicians of clinical laboratory results. N Engl J Med 299:999–1001, 1978.

Cobelli C, Salvan A: A medical record and a computer program for diagnosis of thyroid diseases. Methods Inf Med 14:126–132, 1975.

deDombal FT, Horrocks JC, Walmsley G, et al: Computer-aided diagnosis and decision-making in the acute abdomen. J R Coll Physicians Lond 9:211–218, 1975.

Duda RO, Hart PE: Pattern Classification and Scene Analysis. New York, John Wiley & Sons, Inc., 1973.

Engle RL, Flehinger BJ, Allen S, et al: HEME: A computer aid to diagnosis of hematologic disease. Bull NY Acad Med 52:584–600, 1976.

Friedman GD: Medical usage and abusage: "Prevalence" and "incidence." Ann Intern Med 84:502–504, 1976.

Galen RS: False positives. Lancet 2:1081, 1974.

Galen RS, Gambino SR: Beyond Normality: The Predictive Value and Efficiency of Medical Diagnoses. New York, John Wiley & Sons, Inc, 1975.

Galen RS, Reiffel JA, Gambino SR: Diagnosis of acute myocardial infarction: Relative efficiency of serum enzyme and isoenzyme measurements. JAMA 232:145–147, 1975.

Harris JM: The hazards of bedside Bayes. JAMA 246:2602–2605, 1981.

Homburger HA, Hewan-Lowe K: Predictive values of thyroxine, thyrotropin, and triiodothyronine concentrations in serum. Clin Chem 25:669–674, 1979.

Ingelfinger FJ: Decision in medicine, editorial. N Engl J Med 293:254–255, 1975.

Kim NK, Yasmineh WG, Freier EF, et al: Value of alkaline phosphatase, 5'-nucleotidase, γ'glutamyl-transferase, and glutamate dehydrogenase activity measurements (single and combined) in serum in diagnosis of metastases to the liver. Clin Chem 23:2034–2038, 1977.

Lahniser DJ, Oud PS, Raaijamkers MCT, et al: Decision tree optimization in a prescreening system for cervical smears. In Gelsenia ES, Kanal LN (eds): Pattern Recognition in Practice. Amsterdam, North-Holland Publishing Company, 1980, pp 453–462.

Ledley RS, Lusted LB: Reasoning foundations of medical diagnosis. Science 130:9–21, 1959.

Lusted LB: Introduction to Medical Decision Making. Springfield, Ill, Charles C Thomas, Publisher, 1968.

McNeil BJ, Keeler E, Adelstein SJ: Primer on certain elements of medical decision making. N Engl J Med 293:211–215, 1975.

McNeil BJ, Sherman H: Example: Bayesian calculations for the determination of the etiology of pleuritic chest pain in young adults in a teaching hospital. Part B. Comput Biomed Res 11:187–194, 1978.

Mendenhall W, Schaeffer RL: Mathematical Statistics with Applications. Belmont, Cal, Wadsworth Publishing Company, Inc, 1973.

Miller MC, Westphal MC, Reigart JR, et al: Medical Diagnostic Models. A Bibliography. Ann Arbor, MI, University Microfilms International, 1977.

Pauker SG: The practical use of decision analysis in patient care. In First Annual Symposium on Computer Applications in Medical Care. Boston, Tufts University School of Medicine, Oct 1977.

Ross P: Computers in medical diagnosis. CRC Crit Rev Clin Radiol Sci 3:197–243, 1972.

Scheinok PA, Rinaldo JA: Symptom diagnosis: Optimal subsets for upper abdominal pain. Comput Biomed Res 1:221–236, 1967.

Schwartz WB: Decision analysis. A look at the chief complaints. N Engl J Med 300:556–559, 1979.

Schwartz WB, Gorry GA, Kassirer JP, et al: Decision analysis and clinical judgement. Am J Med 55:459–472, 1973.

Sher PP: Mathematical and computer-assisted procedures in clinical decision making. Hum Pathol 11:420–423, 1980.

Statland BE, Winkel P, Burke MD, et al: Quantitative approaches used in evaluating laboratory measurements and other clinical data. In Henry JB (ed): Clinical Diagnosis and Management by Laboratory Methods, ed 16. Philadelphia, WB Saunders Co, 1979, pp 525–555.

Vecchio TJ: Predictive value of a single diagnostic test in unselected populations. N Engl J Med 274:1171–1173, 1966.

Wardle A, Wardle L: Computer aided diagnosis—A review of research. Methods Inf Med 17:15–28, 1978.

Whitby LG: Screening for disease: Definitions and criteria. Lancet 2:819–822, 1974.

Weinstein MC, Fineberg HV, Elstein AS, et al: Clinical Decision Analysis. Philadelphia, WB Saunders Co, 1980.

Winkel P: Patterns and clusters—Multivariate approach for interpreting clinical chemistry results. Clin Chem 19:1329–1338, 1973.

CHAPTER 5

REPRESENTATION TECHNIQUES USEFUL IN THE PROBLEM-SOLVING APPROACH

In this chapter, we discuss some techniques for representing clinical problem solving that are not based on statistical concepts. We will present two diagrammatic methods that can be used to represent decisions dependent on the value of conditions—decision tables and flow charts. In addition, we discuss some techniques of knowledge representation from the field of artificial intelligence. All these techniques are useful in describing symbolically the problem-solving approaches discussed later in this book. These techniques can help us to communicate and execute clinical problem-solving approaches using strategies.

DECISION TABLES

Decision tables show what actions should be taken for different combinations of conditions. Use of a decision table implies that a decision is composed of conditions, actions, and the relationship between the conditions and the associated actions (London, 1972). *Conditions* are defined as events or facts that influence the action to be taken. Conditions have possible values, such as Yes/No, True/False, 120 mg/100 ml, or less than 20 U/ml. *Actions* are any process to be carried out, such as ordering an SGOT determination, diagnosing a myocardial infarction, or treating with a diuretic. A decision is defined as choosing the appropriate action under present conditions.

Some knowledge for ordering laboratory tests or interpreting test results can be cast in decision tables, e.g., the knowledge that for certain test values further laboratory tests, calculations, or interpretations are appropriate. In this situation, it is possible to take the narrative description of the procedure to be followed and to write a decision table from it. In order to write such a table, we must do the following:

1. Isolate the conditions.
2. Isolate the actions.
3. State the condition combinations calling for different actions.

AN EXAMPLE

For an example, let's use the following narrative description for ordering thyroid tests and evaluating the results, as modified from Kasanof (1974):

A clinical impression of suspected hyperthyroidism is important, but not sufficient for the diagnosis; such impressions should be confirmed by laboratory tests. The serum T_3 [triiodothyronine] uptake, serum T_4 [thyroxine], and calculated free thyroxine index [FTI] are tests of choice for suspected hyperthyroidism. In the young adult with suspected hyperthyroidism, if laboratory test results are equivocal, the tests may be repeated in a few months. In older patients with suspected hyperthyroidism and cardiac arrhythmia, a full workup should be ordered immediately in the face of equivocal laboratory test results.

This narrative contains the statement of various conditions under which to order various thyroid tests. The first step in writing a decision table for this narrative is to isolate these conditions and actions. Reviewing the narrative, we can form a list of the conditions:

1. Young adult.
2. Older patient.
3. Clinically suspect hyperthyroidism.
4. Equivocal laboratory test results.
5. Cardiac arrhythmia.

In the narrative, several actions should be taken if we clinically suspect hyperthyroidism. We can list these actions:

1. Order the serum T_3 uptake.
2. Order the serum T_4 test.
3. Calculate the FTI.
4. Repeat the laboratory tests.
5. Order a full workup immediately.

In these lists of conditions and actions, the relationship between the conditions and actions is not expressed. Conditions and actions are listed separately; the relationship between

them is expressed in terms of rules. Rules are merely a statement of the combination of conditions for a particular action(s). Rules are often written in the form *if . . . then. . . .*

In our example, a number of rules are described. The text, "A clinical impression of suspected hyperthyroidism is important but not sufficient for the diagnosis; such impressions should be confirmed by laboratory tests. The serum T_3 uptake, serum T_4, and calculated free thyroxine index are tests of choice for suspected hyperthyroidism" expresses the first rule.

Rule A   *If:*   Clinically suspect hyperthyroidism,
          Then: 1. Order serum T_3 uptake,
          and   2. Order serum T_4,
          and   3. Calculate FTI.

The text, "In the young adult with suspected hyperthyroidism, if laboratory test results are equivocal, the tests may be repeated in a few months" expresses the second rule.

Rule B   *If:*   1. Clinically suspect hyperthyroidism,
          and   2. Young adult,
          and   3. Equivocal laboratory test results,
          Then: Repeat laboratory tests in a few months.

The text, "In older patients with suspected hyperthyroidism and cardiac arrhythmia, a full workup should be ordered immediately in the face of equivocal laboratory test results" expresses the third rule.

Rule C   *If:*   1. Clinically suspect hyperthyroidism,
          and   2. Older patient,
          and   3. Cardiac arrhythmia present,
          and   4. Equivocal laboratory test results,
          Then: Order a full workup immediately.

This extraction of the rules, which express the relationship between the conditions and actions, is another step in writing a decision table.

Table 5–1 shows the rules of the narrative in the form of a decision table. Conditions and actions are separated by a double horizontal line. The upper left quadrant of the table contains a list of all the conditions. This quadrant of possible conditions is above the quadrant containing the list of possible actions.

Table 5–1. DECISION TABLE FOR ORDERING THYROID TESTS AND EVALUATING THE RESULTS

Conditions/Actions		Rules			
C1	Clinically suspect hyperthyroidism	T	T	T	T
C2	Young adult	T	F	T	F
C3	Older patient	F	T	F	T
C4	Cardiac arrhythmia	–	–	F	T
C5	Lab tests are equivocal	U	U	T	T
A1	Order serum T_3 uptake	X	X		
A2	Order serum T_4	X	X		
A3	Calculate FTI	X	X		
A4	Repeat tests in few months			X	
A5	Do a full workup immediately				X

Key:
T = True or yes; F = false or no; U = unknown; – = indifference; C = condition; X = take action; A = action; blank space = do not take action.

Horizontally, across from the conditions, is a series of symbols. T represents True or Yes, and F represents False or No. U represents unknown, and (—) represents indifference to a value. The quadrant in which the conditions are listed is often called the *condition stub.* The quadrant in which the actions are listed is often referred to as the *action stub.* Horizontally, opposite the list of actions, there are either a series of spaces or Xs. By convention, a space means: "Do not take action," and an X means: "Take action."

In such a table, each vertical column represents a rule (in this case there are four). Rule C in our example is in column 4 in the table; Rule B is in column 3. Rule A has become columns 1 and 2 because the rule implies that we order the serum T_3 uptake, order the serum T_4, and calculate the FTI regardless of whether the patient is old or young when we clinically suspect hyperthyroidism.

The decision table sets forth the same procedures as does the narrative description. However, the fact that the decision table is more explicit than the corresponding sentences in the narrative is one of several advantages of using a decision table (Gildersleeve, 1970). Other advantages include more immediate comprehensibility, amenability to standardization, and ease of organizing the procedures into relatively independent modules.

To summarize, the decision table consists of three basic elements: conditions, actions, and a series of rules. The part of the table that lists the conditions and actions is referred to as the *stub;* the part that contains the rules is referred to as the *entry.* The four quadrants of the table may be identified as the condition stub, action stub, condition entry, and action entry. Since our table is divided into vertical columns, each vertical column is one rule. This format constitutes the most common method of drawing a decision table.

PRINCIPLES OF DECISION TABLES

Tables can use different sorts of values in the entry part. *Limited-entry* refers to the situation in which the permissible values in the entry part of the table are either T (true), F (false), – (Indifference), and X (Take action). *Extended-entry* refers to the situation in which other values are associated with conditions other than T, F, or –. For example, a condition could have the three values: greater than, less than, or equal to represented by >, <, or =. *Mixed-entry* tables contain both the limited and extended-entry conditions.

Other extensions of the basic decision table form are also possible. For instance, more than the inclusion or exclusion of an action can be indicated in the action entry quadrant. The X for action can be replaced by numbers indicating not only the actions to be taken but also the order in which the actions are to be taken.

Several principles for designing tables are important to keep in mind:

1. A condition is entered in such a table only if it has an effect on the actions. If a certain condition does not affect the action being taken, we would not test for the value of that condition.

2. There must be a value in the condition entry of each rule in a table. The indifference symbol (–) does not mean that the condition has no value; it merely means the condition may have any one of the set of legal values. It does not mean that the condition does not arise; it means that the value of the condition will not affect the action being taken.

Table 5–2 illustrates this point. We see four conditions and two possible actions (London,

Table 5–4. DECISION TABLE ILLUSTRATING LOGICAL CONTRADICTIONS BETWEEN RULES 1 AND 2 AND BETWEEN RULES 3 AND 4

	1	2	3	4
C1	F	F	F	F
C2	T	T	F	F
C3	T	T	F	F
C4	T	F	T	F
A1	X	X		
A2			X	X

Key:
T = True; F = false; C = condition; X = take action; A = action; blank space = do not take action.

Table 5–4. DECISION TABLE ILLUSTRATING LOGICAL CONTRADICTIONS BETWEEN RULES 1 AND 2 AND BETWEEN RULES 3 AND 4

	1	2	3	4
C1	T	T	F	F
C2	T	T	F	F
C3	–	T	–	T
A1	X		X	X
A2		X		

Key:
T = True; F = false; C = condition; X = take action; – = indifferent; A = action; blank space = do not take action.

1972). Scanning this table from left to right, we see that the first two rules have both a true and a false shown for condition C4. We also note that the first two rules do not differ in any of the first three conditions, C1, C2, and C3. Thus, whether Condition 4 is T or F does not affect the decision. The same situation arises in Rule 3 and Rule 4. It is an indifferent situation for which the indifference symbol is intended. We could then rewrite this table as in Table 5–3.

3. When using indifference symbols, we

must be careful not to introduce logical contradictions or redundancies into the table (London, 1972). Consider Rule 1 and Rule 2 of Table 5–4; they may be a logical contradiction. Rule 1 says: If C1 and C2 and C3 are true, take action A1. Rule 2 says: If C1 and C2 and C3 are true, take action A2. The same sort of problem arises with Rule 3 and Rule 4. In this case, Rule 4 is included in Rule 3. If two or more rules have the same condition entries but the actions specified are different, a contradiction may exist in the table.

4. Redundancies occur in tables when two or more rules have the same condition entries and the actions are the same. This is shown in Rules 1 and 2; and in Rules 3 and 4, Table 5–5.

5. In cases of decisions wherein conditions

Table 5–3. DECISION TABLE ILLUSTRATING THE USE OF THE INDIFFERENCE SYMBOL (—) TO ELIMINATE THE INDIFFERENT CONDITION IN TABLE 5–2

	1	2
C1	F	F
C2	T	F
C3	T	F
C4	–	–
A1	X	
A2		X

Key:
T = True; F = false; C = condition; X = take action; – = indifferent; A = action; blank space = do not take action.
*Rules 1 and 2 of Table 5–2 are consolidated into Rule 1, and Rules 3 and 4 of Table 5–2 are consolidated into Rule 2.

Table 5–5. DECISION TABLE ILLUSTRATING REDUNDANCIES BETWEEN RULES 1 AND 2 AND BETWEEN RULES 3 AND 4

	1	2	3	4
C1	T	T	T	T
C2	T	T	F	F
C3	F	F	T	T
A1	X	X		
A2			X	X

Key:
T = True; F = false; C = condition; X = take action; – = indifferent; A = action; blank space = do not take action.

can have more than two values, the restriction of having only two values (T or F) for conditions forces us to use extended entry. As we mentioned earlier, such extended-entry conditions can have more than two values. For example, condition entries might be SGOT* = 50 U/ml, SGOT greater than SGPT,† SGOT less than SGPT. The entry condition in the tables can take on any value as long as the values are specified beforehand. Mixed-entry tables use both extended- and limited-entry conditions. If both logical comparisons and multiple value conditions are needed for the decision, these can be freely mixed in the condition stub. Such a table is shown in Table 5–6.

DESIGN GUIDELINES

It is important that the final table depend upon the use to which it is being put. Decision tables used in interpreting laboratory test results will generally be used to review a decision-making procedure for a typical user of such tables, i.e., a physician. In this situation, a good table is one that shows the decision to be simple, complete, and easily understood.

To design a table, observe the following procedures:

Step 1

Study the problem under consideration and isolate all relevant conditions; list them in the condition stub of the table. Conditions should be stated as clear and concise questions. Abbreviations should be explained at the bottom of the table or in a cross reference. Positive statements rather than negative expressions of a condition are generally preferred in order to avoid the use of double negatives for a positive case. At this point, examining the conditions should show which of them are better treated as T, F, or − and which are better treated as more complex items (SGOT = 30 U/ml, SGOT = 20 U/ml).

Condition sequence does not affect the validity of the table but does affect its ease of being conceptualized. In general, it is a good idea to have major conditions, which are most discriminating, at the head of the table. We can start by listing the conditions in the se-

---

*Serum glutamic-oxaloacetic transaminase.
†Serum glutamic-pyruvic transaminase.

Table 5–6. DECISION TABLE ILLUSTRATING EXTENDED-ENTRY CONDITIONS

	1	2	3
C1	T	F	SGOT = 30 U/ml
C2	SGOT = 100 U/ml	T	F
C3	F	T	−
A1		X	
A2	X		X

Key:
T = True; F = false; C = condition; X = take action; − = indifferent; A = action; blank space = do not take action.

quence by which they are identified in the narrative and later revising this sequence for communication purposes.

Following these guidelines should result in the listing of all conditions necessary for the problem or process that is being studied. If the number of conditions listed is large, it may be necessary to divide the list and produce a number of linked decision tables. At this step, it is important to identify all conditions to avoid difficulty later in the development of the table.

Step 2

Actions should be isolated from the narrative description of the procedure. The list of actions should be sequenced for clarity. As mentioned before, if actions are to be taken in a logical sequence that is different from the listed sequence, numbers rather than Xs can be used in the action entry area to represent the sequence.

Step 3

Fill in the condition and action entries. There are two standard techniques for filling in this part of the table (London, 1972).

Classic Technique. With this method, all possible combinations of conditions are placed in the condition entry quadrant producing a table representing all possible rules. Each of these rules is examined one by one, and the condition entry is considered. All condition entries are completed for each rule. At the conclusion of this step, a complete table is produced.

A variety of techniques can now be used to consolidate this complete table into a simpler table. For example, we have seen that complex rules (rules containing −) can be formed from simple rules (contain no −). This occurs when an unconsolidated table has a condition that can be viewed as an indifferent one for the decision. Rules are consolidated whose action is identical and whose condition values are the same except for one pair of conditions.

The classic technique has major disadvantages. It is time consuming in that each step must be carefully performed and checked. Shortcuts in the technique often lead to errors in the table. If errors do occur, the later they are discovered, the harder it is to correct them. The refinement of the table is somewhat mechanical, but the overall purpose of the decision can be lost in the process of simplifying the table. The time required to go through all the steps may not be worthwhile. The larger the table, the more difficult it is to use the classic technique because as the number of conditions increases, the number of entries required increases exponentially. For example, in a limited-entry table with seven conditions, a matrix of 2^7 (128 rules) would be required. Being confronted with all these rules may cause all sequential logic to be lost as the table is constructed.

In contrast, the classic technique can be useful when the logic of the problem appears very involved and not well understood by the designer of the table. In those cases, when the decision-making procedure is well understood for normal conditions, if not for exceptional conditions, this technique assures that these exceptional conditions will be specified. Finally, the classic technique is also amenable to mechanization, using an appropriate computer language.

Progressive Rule Development Method. This is an alternative technique for preparing the condition and action entries of a decision table. This method does not require that all possible combinations of conditions be defined. Instead, it requires that conditions be written in the table as they are identified. Condition entries and action entries for each rule are written down as the problem is analyzed. Problem logic is thus in sight at all times, and sequencing becomes a part of the table development. As combinations of the conditions are considered, it may be obvious that particular combinations are not important for the action specified by a rule. Indifference

should be specified opposite the indifferent condition in the rule. Indifference symbols are thus entered onto the table as they are needed.

This technique has some advantages over the classic method in that the logic of the decision is continually under review by the table designer. Ambiguities in the table are more likely to be apparent. In addition, more conditions are able to be handled in a single table than with the classic technique.

A COMPLEX EXAMPLE

We shall now apply these new ideas to a concrete example with another narrative on the evaluation of thyroid tests, as modified from Kasanof (1974).

If you suspect hyperthyroidism in your patient because of one or more clinical symptoms, e.g., tremor, anxiety, tachycardia, atrial fibrillation, or a palpably enlarged gland, order a serum T_4, a T_3 uptake, and determine the free thyroxine index (FTI). A patient clinically suspected of having hyperthyroidism with a markedly elevated FTI should be treated for hyperthyroidism. In such a patient, if the FTI is not markedly elevated, further testing is indicated.

Appropriate further testing is a radioiodine uptake, before and after suppression by hormone, or a serum T_3 determination. If the T_3 is markedly elevated or the uptake high, the patient should be treated for hyperthyroidism. In case the serum T_3 is not high and hyperthyroidism is still clinically suspected, order an iodine uptake suppression test. If the uptake suppression test is pathologic, the patient is hyperthyroid, and if it is "normal," hyperthyroidism is not indicated. A pathologic test is one in which the uptake after suppression is equal to or greater than 50 per cent. If all test results are within the reference intervals for a healthy population, the evidence is against hyperthyroidism. However, if hyperthyroidism is still clinically suspected, wait a few months and retest.

We can now compile the following condition list and condition values:

1. Clinically suspect hyperthyroidism? True, False.
2. FTI markedly elevated? True, False.
3. Serum T_3 markedly elevated? True, False.
4. Radioiodine uptake suppression test? Less than 50 per cent, Greater than 50 per cent, Equal to 50 per cent.

Likewise, we can list the actions:

1. Order a serum T_3 determination.

Table 5–7. DECISION TABLE, USING BOTH EXTENDED- AND LIMITED-ENTRY CONDITIONS (MIXED-ENTRY TABLE), FOR ORDERING THYROID TESTS AND EVALUATING THE RESULTS

Conditions/Actions	Rules								
Clinically suspect hyperthyroidism?	T	T	T	T	T	T	T	T	F
FTI elevated?	U	T	F	F	F	F	F	F	F
Serum T_3 elevated?	U	U	U	U	T	F	–	F/U	F/U
Radioiodine uptake suppression test?	U	U	U	U	U	U	≥50%	<50%	<50%
Order a serum T_4	X								
Order a serum T_3 uptake	X								
Order a serum T_3			X						
Determine the FTI	X								
Order a radioiodine uptake suppression test				X		X			
Treat for hyperthyroidism		X			X		X		
Wait a few months to retest								X	
Hyperthyroidism not indicated								X	X

Key:
T = True or yes; F = false or no; U = unknown; – = indifferent; X = take action; blank space = do not take action.

2. Order a serum T_4 determination.
3. Order a serum T_3 uptake.
4. Determine the FTI.
5. Order a radioiodine uptake with suppression by hormone.
6. Treat for hyperthyroidism.
7. Hyperthyroidism not indicated.
8. Wait a few months to retest.

The relationship between the conditions and actions can be placed in a table, as shown in Table 5–7. Note that extended-entry symbols have been used.

ENHANCEMENTS

In the previous sections, we discussed some of the standard terminology and techniques applicable to decision tables. A number of enhancements can be added to these basic structures, including techniques that enable us to use the tables more flexibly, such as table linkage, table initialization, and the ELSE clause (explained in the section on MYCIN later in this chapter). All these techniques may be applied to all types of tables and are simple modifications of the basic structures discussed previously.

In many complex decision procedures, clarity can be insured only by splitting the problem into smaller subproblems. Problem splitting is represented even in narrative descriptions of decisions. For example, in the previous narrative, a small subproblem was the decision to suspect hyperthyroidism "because of one or more clinical symptoms, e.g., tremor, anxiety, tachycardia, atrial fibrillation, or palpably enlarged gland."

The major parts of the problem are often described in a paragraph or subsection corresponding to each decision. Parts of the problem are then related by using summaries and cross-references within a paragraph or subsection. It is useful to view this splitting as a division of the decision into a number of major blocks, each block describing a separate subdecision. The relationship between the decision blocks is shown by appropriate linkages between the blocks. If a decision problem is examined, it may be found that it can be split logically into several subtables of a few conditions each. However, with multiple tables a system of cross-references is needed to link one table to another.

FLOW CHARTS

We have seen how narrative descriptions can be formalized in a decision table by isolating conditions, actions, and their relationships. Another diagrammatic representation technique is a substitute for the decision table. Flow charting uses symbols as a special notation for the processes and decision. These standard symbols are connected by arrows to indicate the direction of decision flow. They are an equivalent way of representing conditional logic of the if . . . then . . . form.

SYMBOLS USED

Commonly, a diamond is used to replace the *if . . . then . . .* statement. A square/rectangle is used to symbolize a process or action. Arrows connecting these symbols indicate the beginning and the end of the statement. The connector symbol is used when direct lines cannot be drawn between other symbols because of space restriction, such as page continuations or crossing lines. In data processing, refinements of the symbols have been used to indicate more specific actions. These special symbols include start and termination symbols as well as symbols to indicate what type of device is being used for input/output (Grams, 1972). However, flow charts can be drawn with only these three basic symbols shown (Fig. 5–1).

FLOW CHARTS AND DECISION TABLES

The relationship between decision tables and flow charts is shown in Figure 5–2, which represents the logic in the decision table of Table 5–7. The relationship between conditions and actions in a decision table is represented in a flow chart by the linking of the exits from a decision diamond to other decision diamonds or action symbols.

Note that the sequence of conditions in the decision table is represented as the linear sequence of the decision diamonds in the flow chart. The two-valued conditions are represented not as T/F but by labeled arrows leaving

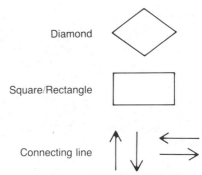

Figure 5–1.   Symbols for flow charts.

the decision diamonds. Lists of actions in the decision table are transformed into rectangular action boxes in the flow chart (Grams, 1972).

Some investigators believe that flow charts are superior to narrative when the logic of a problem is complex. However, flow charts have serious drawbacks compared with decision tables:

1. They force sequential thinking even when sequence of flow may not be the key factor in a particular decision.

2. By spreading the logic of the decision over a considerable area, flow charts may destroy the visualization of the relationships between the various conditions. This relationship may not be apparent until one traces the path of each diamond to establish the logic.

3. The actual drawing of such diagrams requires considerable planning in the placing of symbols, connections, and so on. Decision tables do not suffer from these problems. (Decision tables, of course, have their own special problems.)

Flow charts represent the sequence of logic, with graphic symbols for each decision and action. Flow charts for clinical decisions have been appearing in the literature for some time. The flow chart in Figure 5–2 represents the decisions narrated in an article on evaluation of the thyroid gland by laboratory tests. Our narrative used earlier was a modification of the text presented in this article.

Decisions cast in flow charts imply that the results of an early decision have a high discrimination ability. Once flow has passed through a decision diamond, we inevitably eliminate a portion of the flow chart from further consideration. For example, in the flow chart on evaluation of the thyroid gland by laboratory tests (Fig. 5–2), a marked elevation in the FTI would result in ignoring a large section of the flow chart. Thus, this type of representation is

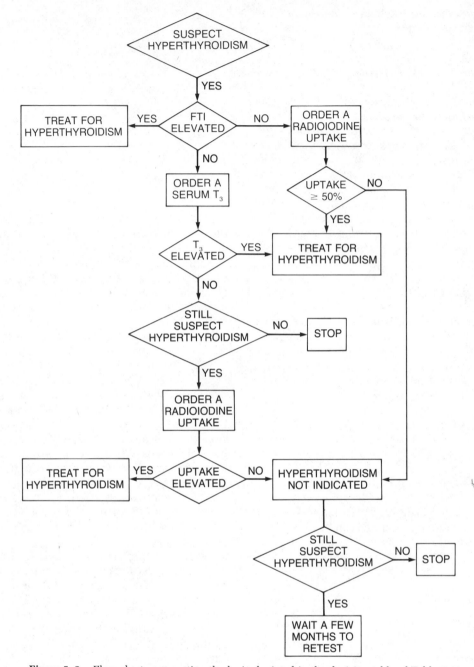

Figure 5–2. Flow chart representing the logic depicted in the decision table of Table 5–7.

not adequate for problems where such high discrimination conditions are not present.

SUMMARY

We have discussed two equivalent techniques for diagrammatically representing de-

cisions based on conditions. The terminology of decision tables and a typical decision table format have been shown. These ideas were applied to both a simple decision and a more complex one. The flow chart representation of decisions was also briefly discussed.

Flow charts are logically equivalent to decision tables. The relationship between a simple decision table and a flow chart was given. Flow charts have the inherent disadvantage of requiring the sequencing of decisions. Holland (1975) has taken Kunin's (1975) flow charts for the detection of urinary tract infections and depicted them in a series of decision tables.*

We have started to view medical knowledge for the interpretation of laboratory test results as "recipes," or strategies for solving a clinical problem. The sequence of logic in a recipe can be illustrated with a flow chart formed from graphic symbols for each act or decision (*Lancet* editorial, 1982). Likewise, the logic of a decision problem in medicine can be represented in the form of a decision table.

These techniques may be adequate for some decisions we wish to represent but not flexible enough for more complex decisions. In the next section, we shall discuss contemporary representations for more complex decisions. These representations can be tied in closely with our earlier discussion of medical diagnosis.

TECHNIQUES FOR MEDICAL KNOWLEDGE REPRESENTATIONS IN THE FUTURE

PRODUCTION RULES

In our discussion of decision tables, we called each of the vertical columns in the table a rule. Rules can also be written in the form:

If: (followed by a set of conditions),
Then: (followed by a set of actions).

Rules written in this form are referred to as *production rules.* Rules can be thought of as

---

*Other flow charts include: the diagnostic workup and treatment of the hypertensive patient (Maronde, 1975*a, b*), jaundice in older children and adults (Ostrow, 1975), joint pain or arthritis (Fries, 1976), evaluation of the obese patient (Bray, 1976*a, b*), postpartum assessment of maternal-fetal incompatibility (Lupovitch and Centeno, 1976), anemia (Wallerstein, 1976), chest pain (Hurst, 1976), acute diarrhea (Satterwhite, 1976), jaundice in the newborn (Thaler, 1977), fever of unknown origin (Vickery, 1977), sore throat (Komaroff, 1978), lymphadenopathy (Greenfield, 1978), syphilis (Lee, 1979), gonococcal infection (Riccardi, 1979), cholestatic jaundice in adults (Fisher, 1981), hematuria (Brewer, 1981*a, b*), splenomegaly (Eichner and Whitfield, 1981), hypercalcemia (Wong and Freir, 1982), and evaluation of the male partner of an infertile couple (Swerdloff, and Boyers, 1982). These are available in the literature as part of Lundberg's (1975) series of articles, Towards Optimal Laboratory Use in the *Journal of the American Medical Association.*

packets of knowledge. The If part of the rule represents a list of things to look for; the Then part of the rule represents a list of things to do (Winston, 1977). In this section, we shall discuss the representation of knowledge using production rules.

In our previous examples, we used rules as an intermediate stage in transforming knowledge in narrative form to knowledge in decision table form. Why not just use the rules as our final representation?

Using production rules would be equivalent to either a decision table or a flow chart, and we could use these production rules to make decisions in a way analogous to the way in which we use a decision table. For example, if all of our production rules for a particular decision were in a long list, we could scan down the If part of all the decision rules and take the action specified in the Then part of rules, the conditions of which are satisfied.

Representing Deduction by Production Systems

This section discusses the representation of deductive reasoning, the special form of reasoning in which conclusions follow from certain premises. We deduce a fact to be true by drawing an inference from other facts that are believed to be true. A chain of facts and deduced facts can be generated to conclude further facts. Productions can be used to create new facts from known facts. This is using a production system to represent deductive reasoning.

When productions are used to represent deductive reasoning, we speak of the productions as being triggered by a certain combination of facts (found in the If portion). Additionally, we restrict the action part of each production rule to the single action of asserting new facts. This special type of production rule is a deduction. Such restrictive production rules may also be called premise-conclusion pairs rather than condition-action pairs (Winston, 1977).

Assume that we are given the following production rule as a piece of knowledge:

If: A patient has an elevated serum T_4 level,
Then: Conclude that the patient has hyperthyroidism.

Knowing that a patient has an elevated serum T_4 level provides the fact that matches the condition for triggering the production rule. We can conclude by deduction that the patient has hyperthyroidism.

Typically, many productions are used in a deduction system. Basic facts known to be true at the beginning of the reasoning process are gradually added to as productions are triggered and the system concludes further facts. The combination of known facts that were given at the beginning—plus the facts we are concluding—can match the conditions of production rules not previously fired to form a chain of reasoning. This is an example of using intermediate facts to generate new facts.

Chaining

You can see how production rules allow us to create chains of reasoning. We can work from known facts to deduced facts. This is referred to as *forward chaining.*

In *backward chaining,* we work our way from the conclusion part of production rules to find out what facts would support a particular conclusion. By backward chaining through the production rules, we are able to work backward from a conclusion or a hypothesis to premises trying to find the conditions needed to satisfy the premises either by observation or deduction from other rules. This causes a backward-moving chain to be formed, which ends in success if we are able to verify our original hypothesis. We shall be unsuccessful at verifying our original hypothesis if the required premise facts are shown to be false, are unable to be observed, or are unable to be deduced from productions.

Each type of chaining has its own advantages and disadvantages. If we are backward chaining, we shall avoid collecting facts that are irrelevant to the conclusion we are hypothesizing. If we are forward chaining, we shall set off all the productions which can be satisfied at any one time. This will allow us to discover all the facts that can be deduced. Which method is better for a particular type of decision is dependent on what type of decision we want to make. If we are creating a system that would discover all the facts that can be deduced from a set of facts, forward chaining would be our choice. However, if irrelevant facts or irrelevant conclusions are not to be collected, backward chaining would be our choice.

An Example of a Production Rule System

This section describes MYCIN, a computer program that has been designed to choose an appropriate antimicrobial drug for patients with septicemia. In this program, all knowledge is stored as production rules. From these rules, it is able to determine whether a patient's infection is significant, the offending organism's identity, useful drugs for a given clinical condition, and what drug would be best for a particular patient. The last decision considers the patient's age, sex, drug allergies, kidney and liver function, as well as the route of administration.

Knowledge is expressed principally in production rules. A typical production would be constructed as follows:

If:
1. The site of the culture is blood, and
2. The identity of the organism is not known with certainty, and
3. The stain of the organism is gram-negative, and
4. The morphology of the organism is a rod, and
5. The patient has been seriously burned,

Then: There is weakly suggested evidence (0.4) that the identity of the organism is Pseudomonas.

As in our previous rules for hyperthyroidism, the rules in MYCIN have premises in the If clause with actions stated in the Then clause. In addition to these two types of clauses, the rules can also have the ELSE clause. When a rule has the ELSE clause, the action stated in the ELSE clause is executed if the conditions of the rule are not met. This is similar to the action of an ELSE clause column in a decision table. The If clause of a MYCIN rule is composed of the ANDing of a number of conditions. Therefore, each condition must be true for the action clause to be executed. When a rule is found to have a false condition, the action to be taken is indicated by the ELSE clause, if it is present. In addition to this technique of triggering actions, the computer system ignores all rules in which the truth of the premise cannot be ascertained or in which a premise is known to be false and the rule contains no ELSE clause.

In order to diagnose a case of bacteremia, MYCIN has access to a computerized data base of patient information. This data base contains facts known about the patient input by a physician, or deduced by the system from the interaction of the data base and the production rules. In order for new facts to be ascertained about the patient, all applicable rules are used. The backward chaining technique is used to deduce new facts. The program hypothesizes that the conclusion of each rule is true and tries to search back through the If clause of each production to reach this conclusion. If in the process of backward chaining the system cannot deduce a particular premise condition, it will ask the user for that result in some cases.

The backward reasoning of the system can be represented by a reasoning network (Fig. 5–3). In this diagram, the underlined words are the names of the conditions the system is trying to discern. For example, TREATFOR stands for the organisms the system concludes that the patient needs to be treated for.

Immediately under each of these underlined words are the numbers of the production rules that have a conclusion about this particular parameter. Rules that have multiple conditions in an If clause have a number associated with

each of the conditions to specify the position of that condition in the If clause. For example, looking at Rule #044, we see that there are three conditions in the If clause involving SITE, NUMCULS, and NUMPOS. Each of these conditions would have to be ascertained as true in order for the system to reach a conclusion using Rule #044, which concerns SIGNIFICANCE. In some cases, these conditions cannot be deduced by the system and it asks the user for the value of a condition. This is shown in our figure by ASK, followed by a number.

The task that MYCIN was designed to perform is actually represented in the system by a production rule. This rule is known as the *goal-rule* for the system. In order to diagnose a patient, the program simply attempts to apply the goal-rule to the patient's data. The goal-rule is:

Rule #092

> *If:*   1. There is an organism that is causing illness that requires therapy, and
>
>   2. Consideration has been given to the possible existence of addi-

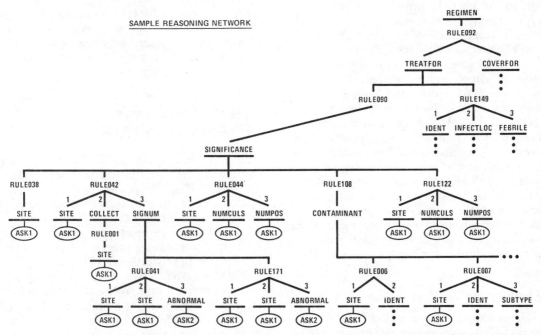

Figure 5–3. An example of the kind of reasoning network generated by the MYCIN mechanisms. Names of clinical parameters are underlined. When rules have multiple conditions in their If clause, a number has been included to specify the position of the associated clinical parameter within the clause. (From Shortliffe EH: Computer-Based Medical Consultations: MYCIN. Copyright 1976 by Elsevier Science Publishing Co., Inc, New York. Reprinted with permission.)

tional organisms causing conditions that require therapy, even though they have not actually been recovered from any current cultures,

Then: Do the following:
1. Compile the list of possible therapies that, based upon sensitivity data, may be effective against the organism, and
2. Determine the best therapy recommendations from the compiled list.

Otherwise: Indicate that the patient does not require therapy.

Because MYCIN uses backward chaining, the first step it performs in the consultation is to try to evaluate the premise of the goal-rule. From Figure 5–3, the conclusion we would like to arrive at is REGIMEN, so indicated as the top node on the sample reasoning network. In order to arrive at this conclusion, we use Rule #092, the goal-rule indicated below REGIMEN. As we have seen, Rule #092 has two conditions. The first is concerned with whether an organism is causing an illness that requires therapy and is represented by TREATFOR on our sample reasoning network. The second condition is concerned with giving consideration to the possible existence of other organisms causing illnesses that require therapy, which is represented by COVERFOR.

MYCIN would now look for all rules that could reach conclusions about TREATFOR. From the sample reasoning network, two rules can be used, Rule #090 and Rule #149. Rule #090 has one premise condition referred to as SIGNIFICANCE. A number of rules are applicable for making conclusions about this condition. The premise conditions for these additional rules can sometimes be deduced by the system. In this case, the reasoning network is expanded to more levels in the diagram. In other cases, the system is not able to use any knowledge rule to arrive at the value of the condition and the user of the system is asked to provide this input directly.

Weighing the Truth of a Rule

The reader may have noticed that the rules in MYCIN have a significant difference from the rules we discussed in our decision tables. The difference is the inclusion of a certainty factor (CF), which is associated with the action part of a rule. The CF in this program is a number between 1 and −1, which represents belief or disbelief in the truth of the conclusion that a rule reaches if its conditions are satisfied. In our decision table examples, we concluded facts as being simply true or not true. MYCIN associates a number representing the degree of belief or disbelief in the truth of the conclusions.

We point out that the CF associated with deduced facts is not a probability. It is based on a theory of inexact reasoning (judgment) developed by the designers of the system. In simple terms, each fact deduced by the system is associated with a measure of belief that the particular hypothesis based on evidence to date is true. Each fact deduced by the system is also associated with a measure of disbelief that a particular hypothesis is true based on the present evidence. These measures are represented by numbers from 0 to 1 in the case of measure of belief, and −1 to 0 in the case of disbelief. The CF is calculated from these belief measures in a way analogous to the calculation of probabilities in Bayes' theorem. As such, the CF suffers from some of the same difficulties as does Bayes' theorem.

CFs are assigned to the various rules by infectious disease specialists working on MYCIN. Because of this, the CFs suffer from errors introduced by asking individuals to assign numbers for degrees of belief in certain hypotheses. The interested reader may consult additional references for the details of calculating CFs (Shortliffe, 1976).

MEDICAL KNOWLEDGE REPRESENTED IN FRAMES

In this section, we shall discuss another method of representing medical knowledge. The central ideas of this approach can be easily related to our previous discussion on the cognitive view of medical diagnosis (see Chapter 2). This knowledge representation has heavily influenced a computer program, referred to as the Present Illness Program (PIP).

PIP was designed to take the present illness of a patient presenting with edema. Its behavior closely resembles the problem solving of the clinicians who participated in the project. That is to say, when the program is given a series of findings from typical cases of patients presenting with edema, the computer program outputs conclusions similar to those made by clinicians presented with the same findings.

The knowledge used by the program to reach these conclusions is organized in both a short- and long-term memory. We shall expound on the details of this program in our discussion.

Cognitive Concepts Review

But first, we shall review the central cognitive concepts about medical diagnosis. The physician is a hypothesis generator and evaluator. Hypotheses that explain the patient's signs are activated by certain combinations of manifestations. When hypotheses are activated, they are brought into short-term memory. A hypothesis in short-term memory can help guide further information gathering or provide a list of typical findings for the hypothesis.

The hypotheses are said to provide a basis for expectation because they identify the relevant clinical features that should be true if the hypothesis is true. To evaluate the truth or falsity of a particular hypothesis after it is activated, the cognitive view espouses that the physician "matches" the relevant clinical features of the hypothesis with the manifestations of the patient. The closer the "fit" of the relevant clinical features to the manifestations of the patient, the more belief the physician places in a particular hypothesis. If the "fit" is not very good, the physician decreases belief in that particular hypothesis or excludes it altogether from further consideration.

The list of relevant clinical features associated with a hypothesis does more, however, than just provide a means of evaluating whether or not the hypothesis is true. This list of relevant clinical features also provides the means to guide further information gathering. The cognitive view of diagnosis espouses that diagnosis is "hypothesis driven." One of the ways in which the hypothesis drives the process is by providing a list of relevant features to ask for in order to confirm or disconfirm a hypothesis. Such features would be the most likely ones for a physician to ask when considering a particular hypothesis.

Another characteristic of diagnosis, from a cognitive viewpoint, is that hypotheses activated early in the diagnosis tend to be rather broad and nonspecific. As the diagnosis proceeds, these are replaced with more specific hypotheses (i.e., refined). The relationship between the nonspecific and specific hypotheses were represented in Chapter 2 by a hierarchical tree of disease classes. Disease classes at the top of the tree are broad, elementary hypotheses, whereas disease classes at the lower parts of the tree are more specific, refined hypotheses.

A final idea about the cognitive view of diagnosis regards the point at which diagnosis stops. Presumably, there are a number of factors that cause a physician to accept certain diagnoses for the present time. One of these factors is felt to be related to how well clinical features associated with the final diagnosis help explain all the manifestations known to be present in the patient. A hypothesis that best encompasses all the positive and negative findings about a patient is an adequate one. A second factor is the physician's preference for a parsimonious explanation for findings in a patient.

Hypothesis Representation in PIP

We shall see that the knowledge representation techniques used in PIP are closely related to the cognitive view of diagnosis. Just as a hypothesis in the cognitive model of diagnosis is associated with a list of typical findings, so are the hypotheses in PIP.

Hypotheses used in PIP are represented by frames. Each disease, clinical state, or physiologic state known about by the system is represented by individual frames. A frame for the nephrotic syndrome is shown in Figure 5–4. By reading the frame, we can get a good idea of typical manifestations present in and causes or complications of the nephrotic syndrome. Underlined words in the frame (such as Name:) are referred to as the *slot names* of the frame. Following each slot name is a list of values filling that slot. For example, in the Name: slot, we have the value Nephrotic Syndrome. As another example, in the May-Be-Caused-By: slot is a list of conditions that can cause the nephrotic syndrome, such as acute glomerulonephritis, chronic glomerulonephritis, or nephrotoxic drugs. The frame for Nephrotic Syndrome explicitly gives us a list of characteristics of the nephrotic syndrome, which we would expect to be present in a patient manifesting this syndrome.

To confirm that a hypothesis is true, PIP matches the characteristics of that activated hypothesis against the manifestations known about the patient. The Finding: slots tell what the typical findings are for a particular hypothesis. In a particular patient, it is quite likely that some, but not all, of these findings would

```
NAME:    NEPHROTIC SYNDROME

IS-A-TYPE-OF:    CLINICAL STATE
FINDING:   LOW SERUM ALBUMIN CONCENTRATION
FINDING:   HEAVY PROTEINURIA
FINDING:   >5GRAMS/24HRS PROTEINURIA
FINDING:   MASSIVE, SYMMETRICAL EDEMA
FINDING:   EITHER FACIAL OR PERI-ORBITAL,
              AND SYMMETRICAL EDEMA
FINDING:   HIGH SERUM CHOLESTEROL CONCENTRATION
FINDING:   URINE LIPIDS PRESENT
MUST-NOT-HAVE:
           PROTEINURIA ABSENT
IS-SUFFICIENT:
           BOTH MASSIVE EDEMA AND >5GRAMS/24HRS PROTEINURIA
MAJOR-SCORING:
           SERUM ALBUMIN CONCENTRATION
              LOW: 1.0
              HIGH: -1.0
           PROTEINURIA:
              >5GRAMS/24HRS: 1.0
              HEAVY: 0.5
              EITHER ABSENT OR LIGHT: -1.0
           EDEMA:
              MASSIVE AND SYMMETRICAL: 1.0
              NOT MASSIVE BUT SYMMETRICAL: 0.3
              ERYTHEMATOUS: -0.2
              ASYMMETRICAL: -0.5
              ABSENT: -1.0
MINOR-SCORING:
           SERUM CHOLESTEROL CONCENTRATION:
              HIGH: 1.0
              NOT HIGH: -1.0
           URINE LIPIDS:
              PRESENT: 1.0
              ABSENT -0.5
MAY-BE-CAUSED-BY:
           ACUTE GLOMERULONEPHRITIS,
           CHRONIC GLOMERULONEPHRITIS,
           NEPHROTOXIC DRUGS,
           INSECT BITE,
           IDIOPATHIC NEPHROTIC SYNDROME,
           SYSTEMIC LUPUS ERYTHEMATOSUS, OR
           DIABETES MELLITUS
MAY-BE-COMPLICATED-BY:
           HYPOVOLEMIA
           CELLULITIS
MAY-BE-CAUSE-OF:
           SODIUM RETENTION
DIFFERENTIAL-DIAGNOSIS:
           IF NECK VEINS ELEVATED,
              CONSIDER: CONSTRICTIVE PERICARDITIS
           IF ASCITES PRESENT,
              CONSIDER: CIRRHOSIS
           IF PULMONARY EMBOLI PRESENT,
              CONSIDER: RENAL VEIN THROMBOSIS
```

Figure 5–4. A typical "frame." Information about a disease, a physiologic state, and so on, is stored in the form of a frame within the long-term memory. Included in the typical frame, as shown here for nephrotic syndrome, are descriptions of typical findings, numerical factors to be used in scoring, and links to other frames (e.g., May-Be-Caused-By; May-Be-Complicated-By). There are also rules for excluding (Must-Not-Have) and satisfying (Is-Sufficient) the fit of the frame to the case at hand. (From Pauker SG, Gorry, GA, Kassirer JP, Schwartz, WB: Towards the simulation of clinical cognition: Taking a present illness by computer. Am J Med 60:988, 1976.)

a hypothesis with the frame of that hypothesis. A positive number represents belief, and a negative number represents disbelief in a hypothesis. Positive numbers represent a belief that the hypothesis is true. These numbers are arrived at by combining numbers in the Major-Scoring: and Minor-Scoring: slots of the hypothesis frame. Look in the Nephrotic Syndrome frame Major-Scoring: slot. If the serum albumin concentration is low, this gives a $+1$ weight to the nephrotic syndrome hypothesis; in the same slot, if proteinuria is either absent or light, this counts as a -1 weight against the hypothesis.

Weight combinations determine whether a hypothesis is true or false. After the findings of the frame are matched against the patient's manifestations, the appropriate weights are combined for matching manifestations. If the combined number is greater than a certain threshold, PIP accepts the hypothesis as true. If the conditions in the Is-Sufficient: slot are met, this is all that is necessary for the hypothesis to be accepted as true. In the case of the nephrotic syndrome, you can see that if the conditions Massive Edema and >5 Grams/24 Hrs Proteinuria are met, PIP would accept the value, Nephrotic Syndrome, as true. If the combined weights of a hypothesis are above a negative numbered threshold, this hypothesis would be rejected. A hypothesis would also be rejected if one of the conditions in the Must-Not-Have: slot were met. In the case of the nephrotic syndrome, we see that with Proteinuria absent, Nephrotic Syndrome would be eliminated from further consideration.

The matching and weighing mechanisms for hypotheses are representations of the association of findings and disease and the weighing (judgment) of the degree of truth or falsity of a particular hypothesis. Hypotheses represent the program's conjecture about what is wrong with the patient in a fashion analogous to how we view a physician as considering certain hypotheses. A frame in the program explicitly states sets of prototypical findings that can either support or refute a particular hypothesis. This is analogous to speaking of the physician as associating sets of manifestations that can either support or refute the presence of a certain disease. PIP matches prototypical findings and manifestations known about the patient. This is analogous to speaking of a physician matching findings associated with a particular disease against those known about a patient.

be present. Only with certain combinations of these findings would it be reasonable to conclude that a hypothesis was true. Indeed, it is rarely the case that we are absolutely convinced of the truth of a hypothesis. Often, we believe or do not believe to a certain degree in a particular hypothesis. PIP associates a number for the degree of belief or disbelief in

Table 5–8. COMPARISON OF HYPOTHESIS STATES IN PIP AND IN THE COGNITIVE MODEL

PIP Hypothesis State	Physician Hypothesis State
Active	Short-term memory; conscious thinking
Inactive	In long-term memory; no findings to suggest it
Semiactive	"In the back of your mind"

Hypothesis States in PIP

In our cognitive model of diagnosis (Chapter 2), we spoke of certain combinations of findings triggering hypotheses in the physician's memory. How do we represent this idea? In PIP, each hypothesis has a set of associated triggers. If the combination of reported findings about a particular patient matches any one of these triggers, that hypothesis is immediately activated. It is only after activation that non-trigger findings of relevance to a particular hypothesis are noticed. This is analogous to the concept of short- and long-term memory in our cognitive model of diagnosis. Remember that in the cognitive view, a hypothesis can be further considered by the physician only if it is brought into short-term memory. Likewise, PIP only considers the hypothesis further if it is activated.

There are three states that hypotheses can have in PIP—active, inactive, and semiactive. We can relate the states of PIP's hypotheses to those in our cognitive model (Table 5–8).

The semiactive state of hypotheses in PIP corresponds to the observation that a physician is more likely to pay attention to the minor symptoms of a particular disease if that disease is somehow related to the present diagnosis than to the minor symptoms of unrelated disorders. A semiactive hypothesis will be triggered by combinations of more minor symptoms than if it were in an inactive state.

PIP Organization

Before we discuss PIP further, it will be useful to overview the program's organization. Figure 5–5 shows an overview of the PIP program. There is a data base in which clinical data are stored for the patient being diagnosed. The supervisor program is presented with this clinical data, which it uses to generate hypotheses by moving frames from long-term memory (associated memory) to short-term

memory (processing memory). The supervisor program also oversees the evaluation (matching and weighing) of each hypothesis to determine whether it should be accepted, rejected, or considered further.

Memory is organized into two types. The program's short-term memory is where activated hypotheses are processed. Short-term memory contains only the activated hypotheses and deductions associated with them. Long-term memory contains all the frames of the system. The frames are linked together in a network (Fig. 5–6). In this diagram, links between frames represent various relationships between diseases, clinical states, and physiologic states. Looking back at Figure 5–4, notice that this frame contains several slots that we did not discuss earlier. These are the slots named May-Be-Caused-By:, May-Be-Complicated-By: and May-Be-Cause-Of:. These are the names of the relationships represented by the links in our diagram.

Links are used in addition to triggers as

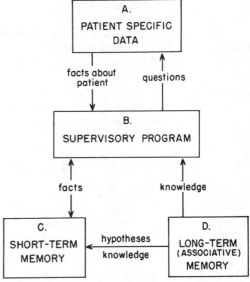

Figure 5–5. Overview of computer program organization. Clinical data (A) are presented to the supervisory program (B), which places them in short-term memory (C). The supervisory program, after consulting both short-term (C) and long-term memories (D), generates hypotheses and moves the information associated with these hypotheses from long-term to short-term memory. The supervisory program then asks for additional patient-specific data relevant to its hypotheses. At every stage, each hypothesis is evaluated (scored) by the program to determine whether it should be rejected, accepted, or considered further. (From Pauker SG, Gorry GA, Kassirer JP, Schwartz WB: Towards the simulation of clinical cognition:Taking a present illness by computer. Am J Med 60:987, 1976.)

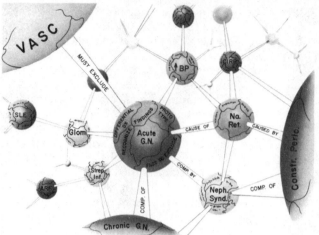

Figure 5–6. The associative (long-term) memory. The associative memory consists of a rich collection of knowledge about diseases, signs, symptoms, pathologic states, "real-world" situations, and so forth. Each point of entry into the memory allows access to many related concepts through a variety of associative links shown as rods. Each rod is labeled to indicate the kind of association it represents: disease status, clinical states (e.g., nephrotic syndrome), and physiologic states (e.g., sodium retention). Acute G.N. = acute glomerulonephritis; Chronic G.N. = chronic glomerulonephritis; VASC = vasculitis; CIRR = cirrhosis; Constr. Peric. = constrictive pericarditis; ARF = acute rheumatic fever; Na Ret. = sodium retention; SLE = systemic lupus erythematosus; ↑ BP = acute hypertension; GLOM. = glomerulitis; Strep. inf. = streptococcal infection; Neph. Synd. = nephrotic syndrome. (From Pauker SG, Gorry GA, Kassirer JP, Schwartz WB: Towards the simulation of clinical cognition: Taking a present illness by computer. Am J Med 60:989, 1976.)

sources of active hypotheses. Links represent other disorders (complementary hypotheses) that might be necessary in addition to a given hypothesis to account for the manifestations of a patient. In our cognitive model, these links would be described as associations the physician has between certain hypotheses. These associations could be based on physiologic knowledge (causal), knowledge that one disease often complicates another, or knowledge that one hypothesis is often associated with another but the reason for it is not understood.

We also did not refer to the Differential-Diagnosis: slot earlier. This contains rules that identify conditions that are often confused with a particular hypothesis. If these conditions are met while PIP is considering a particular hypothesis, the action part of the rules will be processed. This is analogous to when a physician checks out certain diseases known to be confused merely because one of these diseases is being considered.

PIP Activity Summary

The overall activity of PIP can be characterized as shown in Figure 5–7. Initially, PIP has all its knowledge stored in long-term memory with no hypotheses in short-term memory. Some of the frames in long-term memory will be brought into short-term memory if certain combinations of manifestations are known about the patient.

Frames are shown extending "tentacles" (daemons) into short-term memory, where each tentacle constantly searches for matching conditions. Figure 5–7 shows what happens if in fact there is a match to one of these daemons causing the movement of a frame (in this case, acute glomerulonephritis) into short-term memory. We see that the frame (acute glomerulonephritis) has moved into short-term memory and as a side-effect, frames that were linked to it by various relationships have now moved closer to short-term memory. Some of these frames had not previously had their tentacles dangling in short-term memory and would not have been brought into short-term memory with any combinations of facts. However, it is now possible that their matching conditions will be met and they too will be brought into short-term memory. This corresponds to a transition of the frame from inactive to semiactive.

After hypotheses have been brought into short-term memory, they guide the search for more information. We will not discuss this mechanism fully here. Basically, the program tries to fully characterize findings in terms of location, severity, temporal pattern, and so forth, according to specific rules written previously. All hypotheses are then re-evaluated to appraise the effect of these findings on the likelihood of a particular hypothesis. PIP then identifies the highest-scoring active hypothesis and asks about an expected finding associated with this hypothesis that has not already been investigated. PIP then pursues expected findings of complementary hypotheses to the leading active hypothesis. This search for new information corresponds to the cognitive view that medical diagnosis is "hypothesis driven."

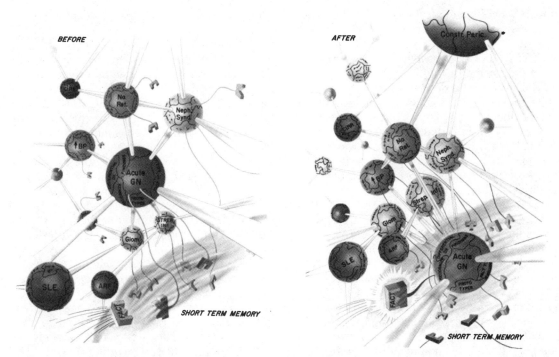

Figure 5–7. Hypothesis generation. *Before:* In the nascent condition (when there are no hypotheses in short-term memory), tentacles (daemons) from some frames in long-term memory extend into the short-term memory where each constantly searches for a matching fact. *After:* The matching of fact and daemons causes the movement of the full frame (in this case, acute glomerulonephritis) into short-term memory. As a secondary effect, frames immediately adjacent to the activated frame move closer to short-term memory and are able to place additional daemons therein. Note that, to avoid complexity, the daemons on many of the frames are not shown. (From Pauker, SG, Gorry GA, Kassirer JP, Schwartz WB: Towards the simulation of clinical cognition: Taking a present illness by computer. Am J Med 60:990, 1976.)

In regard to the weight that PIP assigns to a hypothesis, calculating this score is somewhat complicated. Our previous discussion mentioned only the "local" score part of the total score for a particular hypothesis. This local score reflected the degree to which the facts found about the patient supported the hypothesis directly. This is basically arrived at by summing up the values found in the frame for each of these facts and normalizing this number by the maximum possible score. Another component of a matching score is the "propagation" score, which includes effects of related hypotheses.

Finally, PIP also takes into account the ratio of the number of findings, which are accounted for by a particular hypothesis, to the total number of reported findings to arrive at a final weight that a hypothesis is true. This rather complicated way of assigning a hypothesis a weight is just a reflection of the observation that a physician increases or decreases belief in a hypothesis because:

1. The patient presents with certain manifestations commonly associated with that hypothesis (local score).

2. Related hypotheses help explain a patient's condition (propagated score).

3. The particular hypothesis accounts for many of the manifestations recorded about the patient (findings accounted for/total number of findings). Pauker and associates (1976), and Kassirer and Gorry (1978) provide additional details related to this subject area.

SYSTEMS BASED ON ARTIFICIAL INTELLIGENCE TECHNIQUES

A number of investigators have constructed computer-based consultation systems using an artificial intelligence representation technique like PIP. The earlier and better known of these systems are CASNET, INTERNIST, MYCIN, and PIP (Kulikowski, 1980; Shortliffe, 1976; Szolovitz and Pauker, 1978).

CASNET represents knowledge about the pathogenesis of disease in a *Causal Associa-*

tional *Net*work and deals with the diagnosis and treatment of glaucoma (Weiss et al., 1978).

INTERNIST's knowledge base covers a large proportion of the field of internal medicine. This system is designed to use this knowledge base in a way similar to that used by an expert clinician. The knowledge is represented as a variety of links that represent the evoking strengths of findings for specific diseases, the relationship of typical findings to specific forms of a disease, the causal connections between diseases, and a hierarchy of diseases (Barnett, 1982; Miller et al., 1982; Pople et al., 1975).

MYCIN was designed to select appropriate antibiotics for patients with infections and represents infectious disease knowledge as production rules (Shortliffe, 1976). It uses backward chaining of these rules in order to select antibiotics and determine the most likely organisms causing the patient's disease. A frame scheme like PIP's, wherein frames stand for prototypical descriptions of a disease or physiologic state, has been applied to digitalis therapy and acid-base problems (Patil, 1979; Pauker, 1976; Silverman, 1975).

These earlier systems have been succeeded by a number of consultation programs in other medical problem domains that use a variety of representation schemes. For example, mixtures of frames, semantic nets, and production rules have been used in CENTAUR (Atkins, 1979), NEUREX (Reggia, 1978), NEUROLOGIST (Catanzarite, 1979), and the RX project (Blum and Wiederhold, 1979).

The authors have been involved in a knowledge-based medical diagnosis project, MDX, which imposes an order on production rules based on the notion of conceptual structures (Chandrasekaran et al., 1979; 1980). It is an ongoing project to experiment with representing ideas using diagnostic medicine as a domain and has been dealing with the domain of liver disease. It is based on the view that knowledge should be organized around the deep conceptual structures of the domain. The conceptual structure can be viewed as an organization of "specialists" in which the interspecialist communication enables problem solving to be focused and purposeful. Some of the MDX specialists correspond to bodies of knowledge that are not directly involved in the clinical problem-solving process of diagnosis. Rather, they act as auxiliary experts to be called upon to render advice in their area of expertise. RADEX, which is the radiology auxiliary specialist, is an example (Chandrasekaran et al., 1980).

Systems that generalize the representation techniques of earlier systems have come into use. The CASNET representation can be included in both IRIS (Trigoboff et al., 1977) and EXPERT (Weiss and Kulikowski, 1979). IRIS is a general software system for experimenting with different reasoning and control strategies. EXPERT provides a general consultation software system with routines to implement knowledge bases in a variety of domains. MYCIN has given rise to EMYCIN (VanMelle and Scott, 1980), which uses the MYCIN control structure for chaining production rules and routines to create the knowledge base needed.

There has been some preliminary use of these generalized knowledge-engineering systems for consultation programs oriented more specifically toward laboratory measurement consultation. EXPERT is being used to construct a series of decision-making models for endocrinology and serum protein electrophoresis consultation (Kulikowski, 1980). CLOT (Nii, 1980), a project to implement a consultation system for coagulation disorders, is in the preliminary stages. Fragments of the knowledge base of MYCIN that relate to culture and antibiotic sensitivity testing also relate to laboratory consultation.

REFERENCES

Algorithms for the clinician, editorial. Lancet 2:528–529, 1982.

Atkins JS: Prototype and production rules: An approach to knowledge representation for hypothesis formation. Proc 6th Int Joint Conf Artif Intell, Tokyo, Japan, 1979, pp 1–3.

Barnett GO: The computer and clinical judgment, editorial. N Engl J Med 307:493–494, 1982.

Blum, RL, Wiederhold G: Inferring knowledge from clinical data banks utilizing techniques from the computer and artificial intelligence. Proc 3rd Ann Symp Comput Appl in Med Care, Washington, 1979, pp. 303–307.

Bray GA, Jordan, HA, Sims, EAH: Evaluation of the obese patient: 1. An algorithm. JAMA 235:1487–1491, 1976a.

Bray GA, Dahms WT, Greenway F, et al: Evaluation of the obese patient. 2. Clinical Findings. JAMA 235:2008–2010, 1976b.

Brewer ED, Benson GS: Hematuria: Algorithms for diagnosis: I. Hematuria in the child. JAMA 246:877–880, 1981a.

Brewer ED, Benson GS: Hematuria: Algorithms for diagnosis: II. Hematuria in the adult and hematuria secondary to trauma. JAMA 246:993–995, 1981b.

Catanzarite VA, Greenburg AG: Neurologist: A computer program for diagnosis in neurology. Proc 3rd Ann Symp Comput Appl in Med Care, Washington, 1979, pp. 64–71.

Chandrasekaran B, Gomez F, Mittal S et al.: An approach to medical diagnosis based on conceptual structures. Proc Int Joint Conf Artif Intell, Tokyo, Japan, 1979, pp. 1–9.

Chandrasekaran B, Mittal S, Smith JW: RADEX—Towards a computer-based radiology consultant. In Gelsema ES, Kanal LN (eds): Pattern Recognition in Practice. New York, Elsevier North-Holland Publishing Co, 1980, pp. 463–474.

Eichner ER, Whitfield CL: Splenomegaly. An algorithmic approach to diagnosis. JAMA 246:2858–2861, 1981.

Fisher MG: Cholestatic jaundice in adults. JAMA 245:1945–1948, 1981.

Fries JF, Mitchell, D.: Joint pain or arthritis. JAMA 235:199–204, 1976.

Gildersleeve, TR: Decision Tables and Their Practical Value in Data Processing. Englewood Cliffs, NJ, Prentice-Hall, 1970.

Grams RR: Problem Solving, Systems Analysis and Medicine. Springfield, Ill, Charles C Thomas, Publisher, 1972.

Greenfield S, Jordan MD: The clinical investigation of lymphadenopathy in primary care practice. JAMA 240:1388–1393, 1978.

Holland RR: Decision tables: Their use for the presentation of clinical algorithms. JAMA 233:455–457, 1975.

Hurst JW, King SB, III: The problem of chest pain. Emphasis on the workup of myocardial ischemia. JAMA 236:2100–2103, 1976.

Kasanof D (ed): Solving thyroid problems by deduction. Patient Care, February 1, 1974, pp. 28–51.

Kassirer JP, Gorry GA: Clinical problem solving: A behavioral analysis. Ann Intern Med 89:245–255, 1978.

Komaroff AL: A management strategy for sore throat. JAMA 239:1429–1432, 1978.

Kulikowski CA: Artificial intelligence methods and systems for medical consultation. IEEE Transactions on Pattern Analysis and Machine Intelligence 2:464–476, 1980.

Kunin CM: Urinary tract infections: Flow charts (algorithms) for detection and treatment. JAMA 233:458–462, 1975.

Lee TJ, Sparling PF: Syphilis, an algorithm. JAMA 242:1187–1189, 1979.

London KR: Decision Tables. New York, Auerbach Publishers, Inc, 1972.

Lundberg GD: The modern clinical laboratory. Justification, scope and directions. JAMA 232:528–529, 1975.

Lupovitch A, Centeno O: Postpartum assessment of maternal-fetal incompatibility: Use of a programmable calculator for interpretive reporting of laboratory data. JAMA 235:2530–2534, 1976.

Maronde RF: The hypertensive patient. An algorithm for treatment. JAMA 233:990–992, 1975*a*.

Maronde RF: The hypertensive patient: An algorithm for diagnostic work-up. JAMA 233:997–1000, 1975*b*.

Miller RA, Pople HE, Myers JD: INTERNEST-I; An experimental computer-based diagnostic consultant for general internal medicine. N Engl J Med 307:468–476, 1982.

Nii PH (ed): AGE in Heuristic Programming Project 1980. Stanford, Cal, Stanford University, 1980, p 56.

Ostrow DJ: Jaundice in older children and adults. Algorithms for diagnosis. JAMA 234:522–526, 1975.

Patil RS: Design of a program for expert diagnosis of acid base and electrolyte disturbances. AIM Workshop, May 1979.

Pauker, SG, Gorry GA, Kassirer JP et al: Towards the simulation of clinical cognition: Taking a present illness by computer. Am J Med 60:981–996, 1976.

Pople HE, Myers JD, Miller RA: DIALOG: A model of diagnostic logic for internal medicine. Proc 4th Int Joint Conf Art Intell, Tbilisi, 1975, pp. 848–855.

Reggia JA: A production rule system for neurological localization. Proc 2nd Ann Symp Comput Appl in Med Care, Washington, 1978, pp. 254–260.

Riccardi NB, Felman YM: Laboratory diagnosis in the problem of suspected gonococcal infection. JAMA 242:2703–2705, 1979.

Satterwhite TK, DuPont HL: The patient with acute diarrhea. An algorithm for diagnosis. JAMA 236:2662–2664, 1976.

Shortliffe EH: Computer-Based Medical Consultations: MYCIN. New York, American Elsevier Publishing Company, Inc, 1976.

Silverman H: A digitalis therapy advisor. Cambridge, Mass, Massachusetts Institute of Technology, Rep MAC-TR 143, 1975.

Swerdloff RS, Boyers SP: Evaluation of the male partner of an infertile couple: An algorithmic approach. JAMA 247:2418–2422, 1982.

Szolovits P, Pauker SG: Categorical and probabilistic reasoing in medical diagnosis. Artificial Intelligence 11:115–144, 1978.

Thaler MM: Jaundice in the newborn. Algorithmic diagnosis of conjugated and unconjugated hyperbilirubinemia. JAMA 237:58–62, 1977.

Trigoboff M, Kulikowski CA: IRIS: A system for propagation of inferences in a semantic net. Proc 5th Int Joint Conf Art Intell, 1977, p. 274.

VanMelle W, Scott C: Demo-based session: EMYCIN: A knowledge-based system to aid in constructing knowledge-based consultation programs. 6th AIM Workshop, Aug, 1980.

Vickery DM, Quinnell RK: Fever of unknown origin: An algorithmic approach. JAMA 238:2183–2188, 1977.

Wallerstein RO: Role of the laboratory in the diagnosis of anemia. JAMA 235:490–493, 1976.

Weiss S, Kulikowski CA, Amarel S, et al: A model-based method for computer-aided medical decision-making. Artificial Intelligence 11:145–172, 1978.

Weiss S, Kulikowski CA: EXPERT: A system for developing consultation models. Proc 6th Int Joint Conf Art Intell, Tokyo, Japan, 1979, pp. 942–950.

Winston PH: Artificial Intelligence. Reading, Mass, Addison-Wesley Publishing Co, 1977.

Wong ET, Freier EF: The differential diagnosis of hypercalcemia. An algorithm for more effective use of the laboratory tests. JAMA 247:75–80, 1982.

Chapter 6

STRATEGIES AND THEIR LIMITATIONS

Physicians use strategies to confirm a clinical impression, to exclude less likely diagnoses, and to manage a patient's illness once the diagnosis has been made. In addition, they use strategies to screen for occult disease. In the process of designing or executing a strategy, a knowledge of the workings of the laboratory service is necessary. This chapter describes this knowledge in the context of a discussion of the laboratory information loop (Connelly, 1978).

80

THE LABORATORY INFORMATION LOOP

DESCRIPTION

The laboratory information loop represents an enlarged concept of the clinical laboratory. Instead of viewing the laboratory as the physical place where studies are performed (responsibility starting when a specimen is admitted to the laboratory and ending when the report is sent out), we might think of the laboratory information loop as embracing all that happens from the time a physician orders a study until the results of that study are placed in the physician's hands. There are three limbs:

1. *The prelaboratory limb*—all steps that occur from the time the physician orders the study until the specimen is brought into the laboratory.

2. *The intralaboratory limb*—all steps that occur from the time the specimen is admitted to the laboratory until the report is released from the laboratory.

3. *The postlaboratory limb*—all steps that occur from the time the report is released from the laboratory until the results are placed in the hands of the ordering physician.

Lundberg (1981) further enlarged the concept of the laboratory information loop to what he called the "brain-to-brain turn-around time loop" (Fig. 6–1).

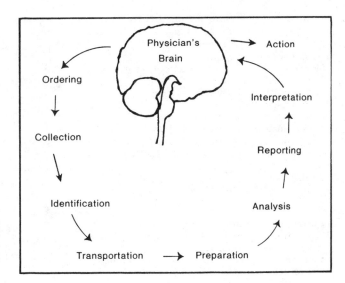

Figure 6–1. The nine steps in the performance of any laboratory test. The brain-to-brain turn-around time loop. (From Lundberg GD: Acting on significant laboratory results, editorial. JAMA 245:1763, 1981. Copyright 1981, American Medical Association.)

CHARACTERISTICS OF LABORATORY DATA

The quality of data produced by the laboratory through the laboratory information loop can be measured by four criteria:

1. *Accuracy*—how closely the data conform to the true values.

2. *Precision*—how well the data can be reproduced.

3. *Turn-around time*—the timeliness of the data (i.e., the total elapsed time from the moment the physician requests a test until the results are placed in the physician's hands).

4. *Interpretability*—relevance to patient care (i.e., the ease with which the data can be applied to patient diagnosis and management).

Accuracy

Accuracy refers to how closely the data conform to the true values. All of us realize that laboratory data are not always accurate and that a certain number of mistakes are inevitable. Intuitively, we realize that good laboratories will make fewer mistakes than poor laboratories. However, no one knows the true magnitude of mistakes for either good or poor laboratories. Estimates of the frequency of mistakes have ranged from 1 to 5 per cent.

What is surprising is this: If mistakes in laboratory data are this common, why doesn't the laboratory hear more complaints from physicians? We suspect that physicians have simply learned to ignore data that do not fit with their clinical impressions. The danger with this behavior is that they may ignore accurate data because the data do not make sense to them when in reality the data may be providing them with clues to diagnoses they never considered. This tendency to ignore unexpected abnormalities in laboratory test results has been well documented (Kelley and Mamlin, 1974; Schneiderman et al., 1972; Wheeler et al., 1977; Wigton et al., 1981; Williamson et al., 1967). Chapter 8 discusses the overlooking of important test results by physicians in more detail.

Grannis and co-workers (1972) studied types and frequency of laboratory mistakes (Tables 6–1 and 6–2). Their study, however, dealt only with mistakes occurring in the intralaboratory limb. We are unaware of any study that addresses the total frequency of mistakes in all limbs of the laboratory information loop. (See Chapter 3 for additional discussion of accuracy.)

Precision

Precision refers to the reproducibility of data. It is commonly quantified in terms of the coefficient of variation (CV). Barnett (1979) states that the CV is simply another way of expressing the standard deviation (SD) of a series of measurements on the same sample.

Table 6–1. TYPES OF LABORATORY MISTAKES*

Specimen mix-up
Specimens labeled with wrong accession numbers in the clerical area.
Sera transferred to mislabeled tubes in the specimen preparation area.
When a specimen was removed from the AutoAnalyzer sampler wheel to insert an emergency specimen, an improper cup number was recorded and all specimens on the wheel were assigned false values.
Analytical tubes interchanged during pipetting of specimens, or by misplacing cuvets in the Gilford spectrophotometer 4-position cuvet holders.

Incorrect chart readings
Incorrect reading of AutoAnalyzer peak.
Incorrect read-off from standard curve.
Read-off from standard curve assigned to wrong specimen.
Read-off from wrong standard curve (e.g., reading LDH values from SGOT or SGPT chart, or reading sodium from the potassium peak, or vice versa).

Dilution and calculation errors
Analyst forgot to correct results for dilution.
Samples diluted by first-shift technologist were analyzed by a second-shift technologist, who was not informed of the prior dilution.
A newly employed analyst thought a "1 to 2" dilution meant one volume of serum and two volumes of diluent, rather than one volume of each.

Reagent and standard solutions
Distilled water, rather than buffer, was used to prepare a reagent.
pH meter standardized with wrong buffer.
Reagent contaminated.
New reagent used without checking against old reagent; baseline correction changed and all specimens had elevated values.
Outdated substrate or standard solutions used.

Instrument problems
Slow clock used for a timed reaction.
Recorder not properly warmed up; blank reading unstable.
Broken balance was used to weigh out standards.
AutoAnalyzer: dirty membrane; clot in line; manifold lines worn; manifold lines improperly installed.

Other
Specimens left at room temperature by first-shift technologist to be analyzed by second-shift technologist; second-shift technologist did not report for work and specimens were not analyzed until the next day.
Analyst calculated results mentally, rather than drawing a standard curve or calculating a factor; the results were grossly incorrect.
Initial computer printout was incorrect, and a subsequent corrected printout was ignored.

*From Grannis GF, Grümer H-D, Lott JA, et al: Proficiency evaluation of clinical chemistry laboratories. Clin Chem 18:232, 1972.

It is defined as 100 times the SD divided by the mean, and it is expressed as a percentage. Its chief value is that it relates the SD to the level at which the measurements are made. It is important, therefore, when we are critically using the CV, to be certain that it was determined at the level at which it is being used. For example, if one SD for the measurement of serum SGOT is 5 U/ml, this would represent a CV of 12.5 per cent at a serum SGOT level of 40 U/ml (the approximate upper limit of the reference interval) but a CV of only 2.5 per cent at a serum SGOT level of 200 U/ml. The CV for the measurement of any single analyte is expressed in terms of either within-day CV or day-to-day CV. Usually, the day-to-day CV is larger than the within-day CV.

It is commonly accepted by statistical argument that a change of three times the day-to-day CV for any given analyte is required to indicate a real day-to-day change in the concentration of that analyte in the body fluids or tissues of a patient (Copeland and Hoyt, 1980). For example, if the day-to-day CV for serum glucose is 6 per cent at a level of 100 mg/100 ml, a change of 18 mg/100 ml in day-to-day concentration of serum glucose would have to occur in order to represent a real change in the serum glucose of a patient. We shall see later in this chapter, however, that physicians

Table 6–2. FREQUENCY OF LABORATORY MISTAKES*

Type of Mistake	Rate of Occurrence (Mistakes per 100 Specimens) 1/1/69–12/31/70		
Specimen mixup	0.89		
Clerical area		(0.35)	
Specimen preparation area		(0.12)	
Analytical areas		(0.42)	
Manual area			(0.13)
AutoAnalyzer area			(0.13)
Enzyme area			(0.16)
Incorrect chart readings	0.66		
Dilution and calculation	0.60		
Poor reagent or standard solutions	0.75		
Other, or unexplained	0.56		
Mistakes in proficiency laboratory	0.19		
Total	3.65		

*From Grannis GF, Grümer H-D, Lott JA, et al.: Proficiency evaluation of clinical chemistry laboratories. Clin Chem 18:232, 1972.

Table 6–3. EXAMPLE OF A LABORATORY WITH A TURN-AROUND TIME OF 1 HOUR OR LESS*

Laboratory A

This is a laboratory with a turn-around time of 1 hour or less. All procedures are performed manually, and no stats are honored. Only one or two tests are performed per request slip and per specimen to control volume and to ensure maximum speed. There is no splitting of specimens to other laboratories. This is a 7-day-a-week, 24-hour-a-day operation. Results are transmitted by television terminal display, by telephone, or by manual entry hard copy or photocopy. Tests offered include:

Amylase, fluids	Magnesium, serum
Amylase, serum	pCO_2, blood
Amylase, urine	pH, blood
Bicarbonate, serum	pO_2, blood
Bilirubin, direct, serum	Potassium, serum
Bilirubin, total, serum	Prothrombin, plasma
Fibrinogen, plasma	Sodium, serum
Glucose, cerebrospinal	Sodium, urine (random)
fluid	Urea nitrogen, serum
Glucose, serum	Urea nitrogen, urine
Glucose, urine (random)	(random)

*Adapted from Lundberg, GD: Managing the Patient-Focused Laboratory. Oradell, NJ, Medical Economics Company, 1975, p 18.

tend not to use this statistical rule. (See Chapter 3 for additional discussion of precision.)

Turn-Around Time

Turn-around time is the total elapsed time from the point at which the physician orders a laboratory study until the results have been received. In Chapter 1, we noted not only that the volume of laboratory studies is increasing but also that physicians are requesting test results in shorter turn-around times. Requirements for different kinds of turn-around times are reflected in the following terms. (The times listed are based on our perceptions of a physician's usual need.)

1. *Stat*—as soon as possible, usually less than 1 hour.

2. *Expedite*—as soon as possible after stat, usually less than 3 hours.

3. *Today*—as soon as possible after expedite, usually less than 8 hours.

4. *Routine*—varies from less than 8 hours, to days, to weeks.

It is our perception that the intensity of medical practice, especially at tertiary-care hospitals, is increasing in that physicians need certain test results in ever-decreasing turn-around time (e.g., arterial blood gases and

serum potassium in critically ill patients or patients in surgery). Fallon (1981) states that "the cause of the lack of oxygen" (i.e., arterial blood gases) "should be assessed in less than 5 minutes by a good laboratory." He suggested that there is a need to resolve what constitute emergency-type tests for life-threatening situations and to determine methods for handling these efficiently and quickly in the institution. He added that because stat tests are viewed by the laboratory as a source of annoyance and an interruption of normal routine—stat tests are less efficient and more costly (Barnett et al., 1978)—it is easy to understand that dependency on regular laboratory service for the acute management of unstable patients can be risky.

Gambino (1977) proposed the convenience of dividing laboratory testing into four classes on the basis of turn-around times as follows:

1. Immediate feedback is essential (e.g., for blood gases, electrolytes, and coagulation studies).

2. Less than 1 hour is often essential and 15

Table 6–4. EXAMPLE OF A LABORATORY WITH A TURN-AROUND TIME OF 4 HOURS OR LESS*

Laboratory B

This is a laboratory with a turn-around time of 4 hours or less. Nearly all tests are automated. There is no specimen splitting. No stats are honored. One test or one panel is performed per request slip and per specimen. All urine specimens are random. This is a 7-day-a-week, 24-hour-a-day operation with mass volume. Results are transmitted by television terminal display, telephone, automated or manual entry hard copy. Tests offered include:

Alkaline phosphatase,	Osmolality, serum
serum†	Osmolaity, urine
Amylase, fluids	Phosphate, inorganic,
Amylase, serum	serum†
Amylase, urine	Porphobilinogen, urine
Bicarbonate, serum†	Potassium, serum†
Calcium, serum†	Potassium, urine
Chloride, serum†	Protein, cerebrospinal
Creatinine, serum†	fluid
Fibrinogen, plasma	Prothrombin, plasma
Glucose, cerebrospinal	Sodium, serum†
fluid	Sodium, urine
Glucose, serum†	Urea nitrogen, serum†
Lactic acid, blood	Urea nitrogen, urine
Magnesium, serum	Uric acid, serum†

*Adapted from Lundberg GD: Managing the Patient-Focused Laboratory. Oradell, NJ, Medical Economics Company, 1975, p 19.

†SMA 11—Bone, kidney, and electrolyte panel. (SMA = sequential multiple analyses and is a trademark of the Technicon Corp, Tarrytown, N.Y.)

minutes is preferable (e.g., for glucose, electrolytes, coagulation studies, spinal fluid studies, hematology studies).

3. Same-shift turn-around time is highly desirable (e.g., for cardiac enzymes, isoenzymes, admission profiles, hematology studies, microbiology studies, and levels of therapeutic drug studies).

4. Several days is acceptable, (e.g. for many hormone assays, some trace element testing, and general screening tests).

Gambino (1977) explained that these turn-around times may require different types of laboratory service. Immediate feedback is best achieved in a "stat" laboratory; same-shift turn-around time, in a central laboratory within walking or short running distance; and several-day turn-around time, he believed, permits regional centralization.

Lundberg (1975) organized the response of the chemistry laboratories of the Los Angeles County–University of Southern California Medical Center into laboratories A, B, and C on the basis of turn-around times (Tables 6–3, 6–4, and 6–5).

Table 6–5. EXAMPLE OF A LABORATORY WITH A TURN-AROUND TIME OF 24 HOURS OR LESS*

Laboratory C

This is a laboratory with a turn-around time of 24 hours or less. Nearly all tests are automated. There is no specimen splitting. No stats are honored. One test or one panel is performed per request slip and per specimen. This is a 7-day-a-week, 8-hour-a-day (any shift) laboratory with mass volume. Results are reported by automated or manual entry hard copy. Tests offered include:

Acid phosphatase, serum	Glutamic pyruvate
Albumin, serum†	transaminase, serum†
Alkaline phosphatase,	Hemoglobin, serum
serum†	Hemoglobin, urine
Bilirubin, direct, serum†	Lactate dehydrogenase,
Bilirubin, total, serum†	serum†
Bromsulphalein	Lipase, serum
Calcium, urine, 24-hour	Lipase, urine (random)
Creatinine, urine, 24-hour	Phosphate, urine, 24-hour
Creatine phosphokinase,	Potassium, urine, 24-hour
serum†	Sodium, urine, 24-hour
Estriol, placenta, urine	Sweat chloride test
Globulin, serum†	Urea nitrogen, urine, 24-
Glutamic oxaloacetic	hour
transaminase, serum†	Uric acid, urine, 24-hour

*Adapted from Lundberg GD: Managing the Patient-Focused Laboratory. Oradell, NJ, Medical Economics Company, 1975, p 19.

†SMA 9—Liver, heart, and enzyme panel.

Barnett and associates (1978) listed the frequency of stat tests from 53 hospitals (Table 6–6). Table 6–7 lists the turn-around times of these stat tests and demonstrates that larger hospitals have longer turn-around times. Dove and co-workers (1980) monitored laboratory and x-ray studies performed on 148 outpatients

Table 6–6. FREQUENCY OF PERFORMANCE OF STAT TESTS*

Tests performed by more than 90% of laboratories
Serum acetone
Serum amylase
Serum electrolytes
Glucose
Microbilirubin
Salicylates
Urea nitrogen
Urinalysis†
Calcium
Complete blood count
Prothrombin time
Partial thromboplastin time
Platelet count
Type and cross-match†
Inoculate media†
Gram stain†
Spinal fluid
    Sugar
    Protein
    Cell count
    Culture
    India ink†
Draw blood only†

Tests available in 75–89% of laboratories
Blood alcohol
Blood gases
Fibrinogen
Direct Coombs' test
Transfusion reaction investigation
Inoculate media†

Tests available in 50–74% of laboratories
Ammonia
Barbiturates
Serum glutamic oxaloacetic transaminase (SGOT)
Creatine phosphokinase (CPK)
Osmolality
Sedimentation rate
Bleeding time
Fibrin split products
Thrombin time
Cord ABO
Cord Rh
Cord direct Coombs' test
Pregnancy test
Fecal occult blood

Tests available in fewer than 50% of laboratories
Digoxin
Alkaline phosphatase
Phenothiazines

Table continued on opposite page

Table 6–6. FREQUENCY OF
PERFORMANCE OF STAT TESTS
(Continued)

Plasma, hemoglobin
Acid-fast smear
Quellung—*Haemophilus influenzae,* type B
Prepare cytology fluid
Prepare cell block
Examine cytology fluid
Prepare bone marrow

*Adapted from Barnett RN, McIver DD, Gorton WL: The medical usefulness of stat tests. Am J Clin Pathol 69:521, 1978.

†Less than 90 per cent of the large hospitals indicated that these services were available on a stat basis. It is our feeling, however, that it is likely that the house staff rather than the laboratory takes responsibility for performing these tests, and that this is not an indication of test unavailability.

to determine how long it took to obtain, review, and insert reports in the medical record in a Veterans Administration Medical Center. An average of 27 days was required for all of these tasks.

We believe that the majority of stat test requests are for other than life-threatening situations. For example, Cole (1980) reduced the number of daytime stat test requests in an 820-bed university tertiary-care hospital from an average of 114 to 16 (an 86 per cent decrease) by scheduling venipuncture rounds every 2 hours from 8:00 A.M. to 4:00 P.M. and making the test results available through faster turn-around times. We have had a similar experience in a 100-bed community hospital.

We perceive an increasing requirement for special laboratories to handle studies for life-threatening situations, especially in large acute-care hospitals. By consensus (Fallon, 1981), the most common tests needed in emergency situations include blood gases, oxygen saturation, hemoglobin, and hematocrit, and determinations of serum sodium, potassium, glucose, osmolality, and colloidal osmotic pressure. Others would also include basic tests for blood clotting and for measurements of serum amylase and urea nitrogen. Another group, Weil and colleagues (1981), reported the most useful tests as blood gases, hematocrit, hemoglobin, oxygen saturation, methemoglobin, carboxyhemoglobin, with serum lactate, electrolytes, osmolality, colloid osmotic pressure, and total protein.

In addition to the staffing, equipment, and design of special laboratories, limitations on turn-around time depend on how quickly the sample can be delivered to the laboratory and how quickly the test results can be delivered to the physician. Because the reporting of results can be accomplished electronically, the limitation that remains is the speed with which the specimens can be delivered to the laboratory. In spite of dedicated specimen couriers and mechanical specimen-delivery systems (discussed later in this chapter), distance of the special laboratories from the patient remain a major impediment to very rapid turn-around times (i.e., less than 5 minutes). For this reason, special acute-care laboratories should be located as close as possible to the patients who require their services.

Gabel (1978) stated that for tests to be useful in an acute-patient monitoring situation, they must be understood in depth (including potential sources of error) and repeated frequently so that trends may be noted and defensive action taken. (See Chapter 7 for a discussion of problem-solving acute-care laboratories.)

Interpretability

Even accurate and precise data produced within an acceptable turn-around time may not be interpretable. For example, laboratory data are usually expressed in terms of values consisting of numbers and units (e.g., a creatinine value of 1.2 mg/100 ml). These data are useless unless we know the appropriate reference intervals (i.e., 0.6 to 1.2 mg/100 ml for males and 0.5 to 1.0/100 ml for females) for specific creatinine methods (true creatinine). Total chromogen methods are about 0.3 mg/100 ml higher (Woo et al., 1979). Decision levels that correlate the data with other laboratory data or clinical signs and symptoms can be helpful. For instance, a creatinine of 4.0 mg/100 ml correlates approximately with a creatinine clearance that is 25 per cent of the healthy value and is also the level above which serum electrolyte changes (an increased anion gap) secondary to renal failure occur (Emmett and Narrins, 1977).

Other kinds of inputs can make laboratory data even more relevant and useful for patient care. These inputs include graphic-analogue displays, diagnostic-management lists, and interpretive comments. Along with reference intervals-decision levels, these inputs constitute the features of interpretive reports (Speicher and Smith, 1980). Chapter 7 discusses the contribution of interpretive reports to interpretability.

Table 6–7. TURN-AROUND TIMES OF STAT TESTS IN 38 HOSPITALS*

Test	Turn-around Time in Small Laboratories (n = 9)		Turn-around Time in Medium Laboratories (n = 16)		Turn-around Time in Large Laboratories (n = 13)	
	Range (Minutes)	*Median (Minutes)*	*Range (Minutes)*	*Median (Minutes)*	*Range (Minutes)*	*Median (Minutes)*
Chemistry						
Acetone	5–60	12	10–60	15	10–90	25
Alcohol	15–120	30	20–120	45	20–120	60
Ammonia	30–70	45	20–90	45	45–120	60
Amylase	15–60	25	15–60	32	20–120	45
Blood gases	5–25	15	5–45	15	10–120	15
Barbiturates	15–120	60	30–240	90	20–240	60
Calcium	15–60	20	10–60	28	20–120	35
Digoxin	10–180	45	45–180	90	120–120	120
Electrolytes	15–60	20	15–60	22	10–120	30
Serum glutamic oxaloacetic transaminase (SGOT)	15–60	20	10–45	20	20–60	30
Creatine phosphokinase (CPK)	15–60	15	10–30	20	20–60	30
Alkaline phosphatase	20–60	45	10–60	20	20–60	60
Glucose	10–60	15	10–30	20	15–120	30
Microbilirubin	10–60	20	10–60	22	20–60	45
Osmolality	10–15	15	10–60	20	20–120	30
Phenothiazines	60–60	60	20–150	120	15–120	60
Salicylates	15–60	30	10–120	28	20–120	30
Urea nitrogen	15–60	20	10–60	20	20–120	35
Draw blood only	7–15	10	5–15	10	10–15	15
Urinalysis, hematology, blood bank						
Urinalysis	5–60	15	8–30	15	15–60	30
Complete blood count	5–60	15	15–60	20	8–60	20
Plasma hemoglobin	15–60	22	10–120	60	5–90	38
Sedimentation rate	60–75	62	10–120	70	20–90	65
Prothrombin time	15–60	20	15–60	25	20–60	30
Partial thromboplastin time	15–60	20	15–60	30	20–60	30
Platelet count	7–60	30	17–45	30	20–90	30
Bleeding time	5–60	10	5–30	15	7–60	60
Fibrin split products	20–60	45	20–180	40	20–120	60
Fibrinogen	15–60	20	15–60	30	15–120	30
Thrombin time	20–60	42	15–45	28	25–60	30
Type and cross match	30–60	60	15–60	60	25–60	45
Direct Coombs' test	15–60	15	5–30	18	5–60	20
Cord ABO	10–60	10	5–45	18	10–60	10
Cord Rh	10–60	10	5–130	20	10–60	10
Cord direct Coombs' test	10–60	15	5–30	15	5–60	15
Transfusion reaction	30–150	60	20–150	75	10–120	60
Bacteriology, cytology, miscellaneous						
Inoculate media	5–15	10	1–30	8	1–15	5
Gram stain	5–60	10	5–20	15	5–60	20
India ink	10–60	10	5–60	15	5–60	15
Acid-fast smear	10–60	25	15–60	20	20–60	30
Quellung—*Haemophilus influenzae*, type B	30	30	—	—	—	—
Pregnancy test	5–130	12	5–120	12	3–60	12
Cerebrospinal fluid sugar	10–60	15	6–60	20	10–90	30
Cerebrospinal fluid protein	10–60	30	10–60	20	10–90	30
Cerebrospinal fluid cell count	5–60	10	5–60	18	15–60	25
Cerebrospinal fluid culture	10–60	10	5–60	10	5–60	16
Fecal occult blood	3–60	5	2–16	10	2–60	15
Prepare cytology fluid	10–60	12	5–60	15	5–90	20
Examine cytology fluid	15–60	15	15–60	18	60–60	60
Prepare bone marrow	35–60	60	35–60	60	60–120	60
Prepare cell block	15–60	15	15–50	15	20–30	20

*From Barnett RN, McIver DD, Gorton WL: The medical usefulness of stat tests. Am J Clin Pathol 69:522, 1978.

THE PRELABORATORY LIMB

SIGNIFICANCE

Problems in the prelaboratory limb can seriously affect the accuracy, precision, and turn-around time of laboratory data. Adverse effects on longer turn-around time include delays in executing the physician's order, in collecting the specimen, and in transporting the specimen to the laboratory. Most of us are familiar with the deterioration of accuracy secondary to poor specimen collection and handling, such as decreased serum glucose levels in specimens not refrigerated or not collected in fluoride tubes, increased serum potassium levels in specimens allowed to stand for hours on a desk or bench top at room temperature, and prolonged plasma prothrombin times or activated partial thromboplastin times in specimens not properly collected or preserved (see Chapter 1). Many of us, however, are not aware of the manner in which problems in the prelaboratory limb can cause deterioration of precision.

"STATE-OF-THE-ART" PRECISION CAPABILITY IN CLINICAL CHEMISTRY MEASUREMENTS

In reviewing the "state-of-the art" precision capability in clinical chemistry measurements, Copeland and Hoyt (1980) concluded that with the exception of serum calcium, medical decision needs are being fulfilled. They recommended that performing repeated analyses of serum calcium is a practical way to increase the precision of serum calcium measurements. For example, repeating a calcium measurement four times improves the precision twice as much as that of a single measurement, according to this formula:

$$\text{average SD} = \frac{\text{individual SD}}{\sqrt{\text{number of measurements}}}$$

Copeland and Hoyt (1980) summarized the studies of Barnett (1977), Elion-Gerritzen (1978), and Skendzel (1978) concerning the

Table 6–8.   STUDIES OF THE PRECISION NEEDED BY PHYSICIANS FOR MEDICAL DECISION MAKING*

	Elion-Gerritzen (1978) and Senior Internists Chiefs of Medicine 1 SD (concentration)	1 SD Estimate Barnett (1977) General Practitioners, Internists 1 SD (concentration)	Skendzel (1978) Internists 1 SD (concentration)	1 SD Actual Average 1 SD Day to Day (Ross & Fraser)
Glucose mg/dl	9.0 (125)† 18.0 (250)	12.6 (110)	17.0 (110)	3.7
BUN mg/dl	1.9 (20)† 3.7 (40)	3.5 (21)	3.0 (21)	0.8
Sodium mEq/L	2.6 (119)	2.0 (130) 3.8 (140)	2.0 (130) 3.0 (140)	1.6
Potassium mEq/L	0.19 (2.4)	0.20 (3.6) 0.25 (5.0)	0.2 (3.6) 0.3 (5.0)	0.11
Creatinine mg/dl	0.05 (0.8)† 0.17 (2.6)	0.25 (0.8)	0.2 (0.8)	0.09
Calcium mg/dl	0.26 (11.4)	0.31 (10.3)	0.2 (8.5) 0.2 (10.3)	0.28
Triglyceride mg/dl	—	13.6 (160)	10.0 (160)	8.6
Cholesterol mg/dl	18.0 (250)† 25.0 (350)	16.0 (240)	10.0 (250)	9.2
Uric Acid mg/dl	—	—	0.4 (7.2)	0.19

Note: We have chosen to convert the relative standard deviation (RSD) values to concentration one standard deviation (1 SD) values. The concentration level is given in parentheses.

*Adapted from Copeland BE, Hoyt LH: Clinical chemistry. In Jones RJ, Palulonis RM (eds): Laboratory Tests in Medical Practice. Chicago, American Medical Association, 1980, p 82.

†Coefficient of variation from the elevated level assumed to apply proportionally in normal range.

precision needed by physicians for medical decision-making (Table 6–8).

POOR PRECISION ATTRIBUTABLE TO THE PRELABORATORY LIMB

According to Copeland and Hoyt (1980), a change of three times the quality control SD must occur before a given analyte in a patient's blood can be considered to have changed significantly. As can be seen by the following example, this decision rule does not always work.

Maher (1974) recommended that when following a patient in whom a successful renal transplant was performed (serum creatinine below 2 mg/100 ml), any day-to-day increase at least 25 per cent above baseline should be considered as presumptive evidence of rejection. Maher believed that a 25 per cent increase would be greater than the sum of physiologic plus methodologic variation.

Williams and co-workers (1975) tested Maher's hypothesis because the renal transplant surgeons noted that a 25 per cent increase was occurring in transplant patients who were not experiencing a rejection. Three serum pools, in which the mean creatinine levels were approximately 1.3 mg/100 ml, 1.8 mg/100 ml, and 2.9 mg/100 ml, were made up. These pools were distributed to areas in the hospital where renal transplant patients were housed. Aliquots of the serum pools were kept frozen and thawed on the days of analysis. Samples from each of these pools were sent to the laboratory on 20 successive days. The samples were sent through the usual channels of specimen collection and processing. The results of the Technicon AutoAnalyzer creatinine analyses on these samples are given in Tables 6–9 and 6–10 (AutoAnalyzer technic N–11B, Technicon Corp., Tarrytown, N.Y.). The intralaboratory quality control data for the Technicon AutoAnalyzer measurement of creatinine showed a day-to-day CV of 5 to 6 per cent at a level of 0.9 to 1.0 mg/100 ml serum creatinine.

Pool I showed an increase at least 25 per cent above baseline between day 1 and day 2 and between day 15 and day 16. Pool II showed an increase greater than 25 per cent of baseline between day 3 and day 4. This was not surprising because the CVs of Pools I and II were 11 and 10 per cent, respectively. On three

Table 6–9. RESULTS OF CREATININE ANALYSES

Day	Pool I	Pool II	Pool III
1	1.2*	1.7	2.9
2	1.5	2.1	3.4
3	1.4	1.3	3.0
4	1.2	1.7	2.8
5	1.2	1.8	2.8
6	1.4	1.8	3.0
7	1.3	1.9	3.0
8	1.4	2.0	3.3
9	1.2	1.8	2.9
10	1.4	2.0	3.0
11	1.3	1.8	2.8
12	1.3	1.7	2.5
13	1.1	1.6	2.5
14	1.1	1.6	2.6
15	1.1	1.8	3.2
16	1.5	1.9	3.0
17	1.3	1.9	3.1
18	1.4	1.8	2.9
19	1.1	1.9	2.8
20	1.1	1.9	2.5

*Units are in mg/100 ml.

occasions, increases at least 25 per cent above baseline occurred, which, if these samples had come from patients, would have been interpreted as presumptive evidence of transplant rejection.

The increased CVs of the pools could have been due to a variety of causes—evaporation of water, chemical changes, or analytical bias. Although there is no certain explanation for the CVs of the pools in the patient areas being twice the intralaboratory CVs, the message is clear. If we critically use changes in serum creatinine on successive days as evidence of transplant rejection, the patient's sample should be immediately hand-carried to the laboratory, where a serum creatinine determination should be rapidly performed. This may help to reduce prelaboratory artifacts that can increase the patient's CV. On the other hand, it may not remove the analytical bias

Table 6–10. RESULTS OF CREATININE ANALYSES

	Pool I	Pool II	Pool III
Mean	1.28*	1.80	2.90
Standard deviation	0.14	0.17	0.25
Coefficient of variation	11%	10%	9%

*Units are in mg/100 ml.

associated with "blind" controls. Allen and associates (1969) reported that "blind" control specimens tend to have higher CVs than "known" control specimens.

When Williams and colleagues (1975) had the transplant patients' samples quickly taken to the laboratory and rapidly analyzed for creatinine, the problem of false-positive rejection data disappeared.

IMPROVING THE PRELABORATORY LIMB

Ideally, specimen collection and handling should be the responsibility of the laboratory and under its control. Proper identification, collection, preservation, and transportation of specimens are as important to generating accurate and precise data as are well-performed, well-controlled technical procedures (Lundbery, 1981). As mentioned, the CV for serum creatinine can be as large for the prelaboratory limb as for the intralaboratory limb.

The importance of proper identification of specimens has been recognized by many hospital transfusion services, where only trained laboratory personnel are allowed to collect blood specimens to be used for cross-matching. This policy has markedly decreased the incidence of transfusion reactions caused by giving the wrong blood to transfusion recipients.

Long physical distances between the sites of specimen collection and the laboratory can cause specimen deterioration and increased turn-around times. Of course, the larger and more spread out the institution, the greater are the problems. Yet, there are a number of ways of overcoming the problems of long physical distances:

1. Improve methods of specimen preservation, such as by adding fluoride to blood specimens for glucose analysis or using ice to preserve specimens for lactate analysis. These methods decrease specimen deterioration but do nothing to decrease turn-around time.

2. Improve transportation of specimens to the laboratory. New developments, such as special vertical lifts (dumbwaiters) for specimens and automated mechanical and pneumatic transportation systems, are essential. Nosanchuk (1977) showed that most specimens for routine laboratory studies could be safely transported by pneumatic tube if the system had the right engineering characteristics. Lapidus (1982) coupled a slow-speed pneumatic tube with a gravity transport system for transporting specimens to the laboratory simply and economically.

3. Decentralize the laboratory and create satellite laboratories. This is an expensive solution and causes the additional problem of controlling the quality of data in multiple locations. Nevertheless, this solution is being increasingly applied in operating room suites, outpatient clinics, and emergency departments. Henry and colleagues (1975) addressed the issues that must be considered when contemplating a satellite laboratory for ambulatory and emergency patient care.

4. Expedite test requests through electronic communication devices and improved test request forms.

Table 6–11. METHODS OF COMMUNICATING LABORATORY TEST RESULTS

Direct oral communication
Remote telephone communication
Remote hard copy generated by electromechanical device
Hard copy report handed to physician
Hard copy report delivered by courier
Television transmission of hard copy report
Computer-generated report transmitted electronically
    Hard copy generated by remote printer
    Soft copy displayed on remote cathode-ray tube

Table 6–12. HOW STATS ARE REPORTED*

	Laboratories			
	Small *(n = 9)*	*Medium* *(n = 16)*	*Large* *(n = 13)*	*Total* *(n = 38)*
Telephone physician	5	5	7	17
Telephone floor	8	13	11	32
Carry to floor	6	3	2	11

*From Barnett RN, McIver DD, Gorton WL: The medical usefulness of stat tests. Am J Clin Pathol 69:523, May 1978.

Table 6–13.   TABLE OF CRITICAL VALUES*

The system of critical laboratory values, also called panic values, was originated by George D. Lundberg, M.D. and first published in MLO in 1972. Such a system is now required of all laboratories by both the JCAH and the CAP. Dr. Lundberg developed his original critical values at the Los Angeles County/USC Medical Center, but this revised table is based on his more recent experience at the University of California, Davis, Medical Center in Sacramento, where he has been professor and chairman of the department of pathology.

Test	Low	Possible Effect	High	Possible Effect
Packed cell volume	<15 vol. %	Heart failure and anoxemia	None	
Blood hemoglobin	<5 gm %	Heart failure and anoxemia	None	
Blood platelets	<30,000 cu mm	Hemorrhage	None	
Blood platelets (newborn and pediatrics)	<20,000 cu mm	Hemorrhage	None	
Prothrombin time	None		>40 seconds	Hemorrhage
Serum bilirubin, total (newborn)	None		>18 mg/dl	Brain damage
Serum calcium	<6 mg/dl	Tetany and convulsions	>13 mg/dl	Coma
Serum calcium (newborn)	<6 mg/dl	Tetany and convulsions	>13 mg/dl	Coma
Serum glucose	<40 mg/dl	Brain damage	>700 mg/dl	Diabetic coma
Serum glucose (newborn)	<30 mg/dl	Brain damage	>300 mg/dl	Diabetic coma
Serum phosphate	<1 mg/dl	Seizures and coma	None	
Serum potassium	<2.5 mEq/L	Muscle weakness, paralysis, cardiac arrhythmias	>6.5 mEq/L	Cardiotoxicity with arrhythmias
Serum potassium (hemolyzed)	<2.5 mEq/L	Muscle weakness, paralysis, cardiac arrhythmias	>8.0 mEq/L	Cardiotoxicity with arrhythmias
Serum potassium (newborn)	<2.5 mEq/L	Muscle weakness, paralysis, cardiac arrhythmias	>8.0 mEq/L	Cardiotoxicity with arrhythmias
Serum salicylate	None		>700 µg/ml	Continuing untreated toxicity
Serum sodium	<120 mEq/L	Extremes of dehydration, vascular collapse, or edema, hypervolemia, heart failure	>160 mEq/L	Extremes of dehydration, vascular collapse, or edema, hypervolemia, heart failure
Serum bicarbonate	<10 mEq/L	Complex interwoven patterns of acidosis, alkalosis, and anoxemia	>40 mEq/L	Complex interwoven patterns of acidosis, alkalosis, and anoxemia
Arterial or capillary blood pCO_2	<20 mmHg	Complex interwoven patterns of acidosis, alkalosis, and anoxemia	>70 mmHg	Complex interwoven patterns of acidosis, alkalosis, and anoxemia
Arterial or capillary blood pH	<7.2 units	Complex interwoven patterns of acidosis, alkalosis, and anoxemia	>7.6 units	Complex interwoven patterns of acidosis, alkalosis, and anoxemia
Arterial or capillary blood pO_2	<40 mmHg	Complex interwoven patterns of acidosis, alkalosis, and anoxemia	None	
Positive blood culture		Worsening sepsis		
Positive CSF Gram stain		Untreated bacterial meningitis		
Positive CSF culture		Untreated bacterial meningitis		

A critical laboratory value is a value at such variance with normal as to represent a pathophysiologic state which is life threatening unless some action is taken in a very short time and for which an appropriate action is possible. It is a laboratory responsibility to communicate these values immediately and flawlessly to the responsible clinicians.

*From Clinical Laboratory Reference. Oradell, NJ, Medical Economics Company, Inc, 1981, p 7.

5. Give physicians the opportunity to choose between a conventional menu of individual tests and a list of strategies designed to solve particular subproblems with the greatest discrimination, in the shortest time, and at the lowest compatible cost. Once a particular strategy has been requested, the clinical laboratory could be responsible for the proper collection and handling of all sequential or parallel specimens, together with the appropriate analytic measurements. The resulting data could be most effectively communicated to the physician in a coherent interpretive report instead of by a scattered piecemeal array of individual data (see Chapter 7).

INTRALABORATORY LIMB

The intralaboratory limb includes all steps that occur from the time the specimen is brought into the laboratory until the time the report is released from the laboratory. The manner in which the accuracy of data is adversely affected by problems in the laboratory is shown in Table 6–1.

POSTLABORATORY LIMB

The postlaboratory limb includes all steps that occur from the time the report is released from the laboratory until the results are placed in the hands of the ordering physician. The laboratory information loop is not closed until the results of the studies are communicated to the ordering physician. In addition, for these results to impact on patient care in a meaningful way, they must be communicated in the appropriate time frame.

There are a variety of methods available for communicating laboratory test results (Table 6–11). Barnett and co-workers (1978) studied the methods of communication of stat test results in small versus large hospitals (Table 6–12). The method of communication should be appropriate for the required turn-around time. Because the results of certain laboratory studies have life-saving implications for patient care, policies have been devised in most laboratories for the immediate communication of this critical information (see Table 6–13).

The reporting of the results of therapeutic drug monitoring measurements is another example of the necessity for appropriate turn-around times in closing the laboratory information loop. If the results of blood levels for any given drug are not received in time to adjust the next dosage level, the results of that blood level are worthless, a waste of money, and should not have been done (see Chapter 7).

Interpretive reporting may be used to communicate the results of laboratory tests. Instead of merely communicating data, i.e., numbers and units, interpretive reports communicate information. (See Chapter 2 for the distinction between data and information.) This information can then be assimilated by the physician into the diagnostic and management processes.

REFERENCES

Allen JR, Earp R, Farrell EC, et al: Analytical bias in a quality control scheme. Clin Chem 15:1039–1044, 1969.

Barnett RN: Analytical goals in clinical chemistry. Pathologist 31:319–322, 1977.

Barnett RN: Clinical Laboratory Statistics, ed 2. Boston, Little, Brown & Company, 1979.

Barnett RN, McIver DD, Gorton WL: The medical usefulness of stat tests. Am J Clin Pathol 69:520–524, 1978.

Cole GW: Biochemical test profiles and laboratory system design. Hum Pathol 11:424–434, 1980.

Connelly DP: The role of reporting and interpretation in effective laboratory utilization. In Benson ES, Rubin M (eds.): Logic and Economics of Clinical Laboratory Use. New York, Elsevier North-Holland, Inc, 1978, pp. 157–162.

Copeland BE, Hoyt LH: Clinical chemistry. In Jones RJ, Palulonis RM (eds.): Laboratory Tests in Medical Practice. Chicago, American Medical Association, 1980, pp. 77–94.

Dove HG, Gifford R, Schneider KC: The trip of slips. Time delays in laboratory and X-ray data for outpatients in a teaching hospital. JAMA 243:537–539, 1980.

Elion-Gerritzen WE: Medical Significance of Laboratory Results in Relation to Analytical Performance, thesis. Eramus University, Rotterdam, 1978.

Emmett M, Narins RG: Clinical use of the anion gap. Medicine 56:38–54, 1977.

Fallon KD: Monitoring of metabolism, acid-base balance, and relevant laboratory considerations. In Shoemaker WC, Thompson WL (eds.): Critical Care, State of the Art, Vol 2. Fullerton, Cal, Society of Critical Care Medicine, 1981.

Gabel JC: Monitoring of body chemistry during anesthesia. In Saidman LJ, Smith NT (eds): Monitoring in Anesthesia. New York, John Wiley & Sons, 1978, pp. 15–29.

Gambino SR: Laboratory services for intensive care units. In Kinney JM, Bendixen HH, Powers SR (eds): Manual of Surgical Intensive Care. Philadelphia, WB Saunders Company, 1977, pp. 143–149.

Grannis GF, Grümer H-D, Lott JA, et al: Proficiency evaluation of clinical chemistry laboratories. Clin Chem 18:222–236, 1972.

Henry JB, Martin BG, Pusch AL: Organization and response of clinical pathology to ambulatory and emergency patient care. Laboratory Medicine 6:41–45, 1975.

Kelley CR, Mamlin JJ: Ambulatory care quality. Determination by diagnostic outcome. JAMA 227:1155–1157, 1974.

Lapidus BM: Slow-speed pneumatic and gravity transport of laboratory specimens: System design. Journal of Clinical Laboratory Automation 2:23–28, 1982.

Lundberg GD: Managing the patient-focused laboratory. Oradell, NJ, Medical Economics Company, 1975.

Lundberg GD: Acting on significant laboratory results editorial. JAMA 245:1762–1763, 1981.

Maher JF: A logical approach to the diagnosis of renal transplant rejection. Immunologic, ischemic and inflammatory impairment of renal function. Am J Med 56:275–279, 1974.

Nosanchuk JS, Salvatore JD: Improved pneumatic tube system shortens stat turnaround time. Laboratory Medicine 8:21–25, 1977.

Schneiderman LJ, De Salvo L, Baylor S, et al: The "abnormal" screening laboratory results. Arch Intern Med 129:88–90, 1972.

Skendzel LP: How physicians use laboratory tests. JAMA 239:1077–1080, 1978.

Speicher CE, Smith JW: Interpretive reporting in clinical pathology. JAMA 243:1556–1560, 1980.

Weil MH, Michaels S, Puri, VK, et al: The stat laboratory: Facilitating blood gas and biochemical measurements for the critically ill and injured. Am J Clin Pathol 76:34–42, 1981.

Wheeler LA, Brecher G, Sheiner LB: Clinical laboratory use in the evaluation of anemia. JAMA 238:2709–2714, 1977.

Wigton RS, Zimmer JL, Wigton JH, et al: Chart reminders in the diagnosis of anemia. JAMA 245:1745–1747, 1981.

Williams J, Widish JR, Speicher CE: Unpublished data, 1975.

Williamson JW, Alexander M, Miller GE: Continuing education and patient care research. JAMA 201:938–942, 1967.

Woo J, Treuting JJ, Cannon DC: Creatine and creatinine. In Henry JB (ed): Clinical Diagnosis and Management by Laboratory Methods, ed 16. Philadelphia, WB Saunders Company, 1979, pp. 262–264.

CHAPTER 7

COMMUNICATION BETWEEN LABORATORY AND CLINICIAN: TEST REQUESTS AND INTERPRETIVE REPORTS

TEST REQUESTS

Physicians can order laboratory tests in a variety of ways through the completion of a laboratory request. This request is usually a piece of paper with lists of tests. Large laboratories, which offer hundreds of different tests, segregate chemistry tests on one request slip, hematology tests on another slip, and so forth.

As patterns of ordering certain groups of tests together came into being and as automated instruments became capable of performing multiple tests together, laboratory request forms were developed by which clinicians could order a whole group of tests by merely checking one block (e.g., a 12-channnel chemistry profile). Later, Henry and Arras (1970) developed the concept of organ panels whereby tests appropriate to the evaluation of a single organ could be ordered, also by checking one block (see Fig. 1–3). Cole (1980) developed a sophisticated laboratory request system in which a hierarchy of laboratory testing needs could be structured and in which smaller subsets could be combined into larger profile groups. Request slips were developed to permit physicians to order these smaller subsets and to incorporate them into larger profiles (see Figs. 8–10 and 8–11).

We believe that the pathologist needs to be more involved at "the request end of the chain" (Carter et al., 1974). The pathologist needs to find out the nature of the questions the attending physician is asking when laboratory tests are ordered, to design and implement strategies that will answer these questions, and, finally, to offer the physician the ability to request these strategies as an alternative to a menu of individual tests (see Chapter 1).

A three-step diagnostic system for iron deficiency anemia set up by Beck, Cornwell, and French, and colleagues (1981) is an excellent example of how a laboratory strategy can be used to render diagnoses of defined probability. In this system, a serum ferritin level and mean corpuscular volume are used as a screen in all patients. This is followed by a serum iron level and total iron-binding capacity in some patients and by an erythrocyte sedimentation rate in a few patients. When compared with bone marrow iron stores as a diagnostic tool for the same disease, this system was found to have 96 per cent accuracy.

INTERPRETIVE REPORTS

Interpretive reports of clinical laboratory studies contain information in addition to data. (See Chapter 2 for the distinction between data and information.) Laboratory data are simply values and units (e.g., a BUN of 60 mg/100 ml). Laboratory information consists of laboratory data plus reference intervals, decision levels, and a variety of other inputs that make the data more relevant to patient care, such as graphic and analogue displays, diagnostic and management possibilities, and interpretive comments.

We believe that interpretive reports constitute an innovative method by which the clinical laboratory can communicate and interact with clinicians. McConnell (1978) agrees that interpretive reporting is an idea whose time has come. We emphasize that we do not advocate the substitution of interpretive reports for the one-on-one personal consultations of pathologists with attending physicians. With respect to improving the quality of patient care, nothing surpasses personal consultations in laboratory medicine, particularly at the bedside. Rather, we advocate interpretive reports as a systematic approach to the communication of the results of problem-solving strategies so that millions of individual pieces of laboratory data can be more effectively applied to patient care and so that we can triage problems requiring personal consultation from the huge amount of data that every clinical laboratory deals with every day (Fig. 7–1) (Connelly, 1978).

Communicating the results of clinical laboratory studies to physicians is a part of the laboratory information loop discussed in Chapter 6, the other parts being the collection and handling of specimens and the performance of laboratory studies, respectively. In order to learn how to improve our communication of laboratory data, we decided to investigate the role of interpretive reporting in clinical pathology. We reported previously on this subject (Speicher and Smith, 1980), and much of the information in this chapter is provided by courtesy of the *Journal of the American Medical Association*.

INTERPRETIVE REPORTING IN CLINICAL PATHOLOGY

BACKGROUND

A good clinical history and physical examination have always been the basis for sound medical diagnosis and management. Modern medicine has extended this data base through

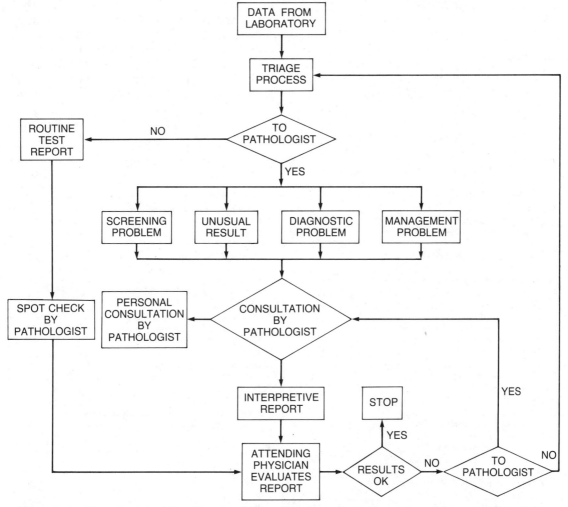

Figure 7–1. Flow chart depicting the role of the pathologist in the interpretation of laboratory data. Editing typewriters and computers can assist in these consultations.

a wide variety of techniques, of which clinical laboratory studies play a major role. These studies have grown explosively, and the accompanying paperwork has often overwhelmed the laboratory and the physician. Thick piles of charts bulging with laboratory reports hamper the ability of busy physicians to find the information they require. Computer-assisted reports have not yet solved the problem. Attempts by the laboratory to assist physicians in managing these data have included marking "abnormal" results with asterisks, printing reference intervals adjacent to test results, grouping data by system or organ (Henry, 1976), displaying data in more informative ways (Osserman et al., 1978), suggesting diagnostic possibilities (Reece and Hobbie, 1972), making

interpretive comments (Galen et al., 1975), and suggesting additional studies or performing them automatically (Altshuler et al., 1972).

In this chapter, all of these efforts to reduce laboratory data to clinically useful information are called interpretive reporting. The methods, variety, and scope of interpretive reporting have not been well documented in the medical literature. Because this approach constitutes a serious effort to improve the use of laboratory data for patient care, we undertook a survey of its frequency in the practice of pathology in the United States. Implicit in the concept of interpretive reporting should be the realization that only thoughtfully designed problem-solving strategies lend themselves to effective interpretation.

A SURVEY OF INTERPRETIVE REPORTING

Methods

The names and addresses of 3784 hospitals in the United States having more than 100 beds were obtained from the American Hospital Association *Guide to The Health Care Field* (Schecter, 1977), and a form letter was sent to the director of laboratory services of each hospital. The letter requested the directors to forward examples of each kind of interpretive report generated. The directors

Table 7–1. INTERPRETIVE REPORT*

	% Using Report		% Using Report
Screening		**Endocrinology and metabolism**	
Multiphasic screening	23	Glucose tolerance	21
Acid-base, water, and electrolytes		Thyroid function panel	20
Blood gases	18	Steroid panel	2
Serum electrolytes and osmolality	9	Hypopituitarism panel	1
Anion gap	3	Parathyroid function panel	1
Urine electrolytes and osmolality	1	Parathyroid hormone	1
Cardiovascular disease		Metabolic panel	1
Lipid panel	46	Nutritional assessment	1
Cardiac injury panel	31	**Immunology and rheumatology**	
Lactic dehydrogenase isoenzymes	28	Serum protein electrophoresis	50
Creatine phosphokinase isoenzymes	18	Immunology consultation	12
Hypertension panel	3	Immunoglobulin panel	8
Cardiac evaluation panel	1	Immunoelectrophoresis	5
Pulmonary disease		Arthritis-collagen panel	5
Cystic fibrosis	2	Febrile agglutinins	5
Pulmonary panel	1	Immune competence panel	2
α-1-Antitrypsin	1	Antinuclear antibody, antimitochondrial antibody, and antismooth muscle antibody	2
Renal and urinary tract disease		**Pediatrics, obstetrics, and gynecology**	
Renal panel	8	Fetal maturity	10
Urine protein electrophoresis	4	Placental function	5
Urine chemistry	3	Erythroblastosis panel	3
Stone analysis	2	Antibody screen	3
Prostatic panel	1	Amino acid screen	1
Gastrointestinal disease		Chromosome analysis	1
Gastric analysis	11	**Neuromuscular and bone disease**	
Duodenal analysis	1	Bone panel	1
Lactose tolerance	1	Muscle panel	1
Xylose tolerance	1	**Infectious diseases**	
Malabsorption panel	1	Antibiotic sensitivity	13
Liver, bile ducts, and pancreas		Infection by site	3
Liver panel	11	Identification and interpretation	1
Pancreatic panel	1	Viral hepatitis	1
Cholinesterase	1	Hypersensitivity pneumonitis	1
Hematology and oncology		**Blood bank**	
Coagulation screen	22	Transfusion reaction	29
Hemoglobin identification	16	Antibody identification	6
Bone marrow	12	Rhogam eligibility	1
Peripheral blood	7	Paternity test	1
Anemia study	6	**Body fluid and special topics**	
Serum iron	5	CSF proteins	8
Coagulation consultation	4	Semen analysis	7
Osmotic fragility	2	Joint fluid	5
Schilling test	1	Serous cavity fluid	3
Transition panel	1	**Therapeutic monitoring and toxicology**	
Haptoglobin	1	Therapeutic monitoring	8
		Toxicology	3

*From Speicher CE, Smith JW: Interpretive reporting in clinical pathology. JAMA 243:1556, 1980. Copyright 1980, American Medical Association.

were promised an analysis and summary of this material as well as appropriate credit in future publications. The letters were mailed through February and March 1978, with June 15, 1978, established as the cutoff date for inclusion of replies in this study.

Results

Replies were received from 183 directors of laboratory services, 146 of whom enclosed examples of their reports. At least 150 of the directors were identified as pathologists. The 37 directors who did not enclose examples replied that they were not using interpretive reports but were interested in the study. Of the 183 replies, 150 were from community hospitals, 22 were from university hospitals, and 11 were from federal hospitals. Interpretive reports were organized into 16 categories as shown in Table 7–1.

Several kinds of information were included in interpretive reports. The first was the provision of reference intervals and decision levels. Another was some type of graphic or analogue display in which graphs were used or test results outside of reference intervals were marked with asterisks or placed in different columns from test results within the reference intervals. The third was the provision of diagnostic or management possibilities that should be considered when various results occurred.

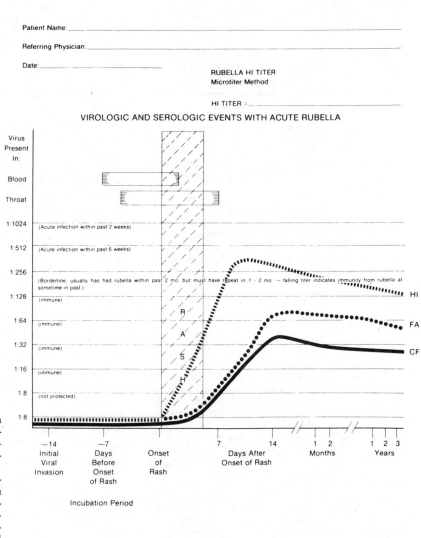

Figure 7–2. Preprinted form for interpretive reporting (Courtesy of Emma White, M. D., Bakersfield Calif.). HI = hemagglutination inhibition; CF = complement fixation; FA = fluorescent antibody. (From Speicher CE, Smith JW: Interpretive reporting in clinical pathology. JAMA 243:1557, 1980. Copyright 1980, American Medical Association.)

The fourth type of information included an interpretive comment by which the pathologist stated an opinion of the significance attributed to a given group of studies.

Interpretive reports usually included results from two or more laboratory measurements that were grouped together, e.g., an organ panel or a coagulation screen. Occasionally, these measurements were performed in a sequential manner, but most of the time they were done in parallel.

Interpretive reports were executed in a variety of ways. Most utilized preprinted forms (Fig. 7–2). Additional information was either handwritten or typed. Many reports utilized a memory typewriter (Table 7–2), and 15 per cent used a computer (Fig. 7–3).

A few respondents sent interpretive reports used in surgical pathology, cytology, and autopsy pathology. Because these reports are conventional in format, they were not included in this study. Each director who responded to the survey was sent an analysis and summary of all the interpretive reports (Speicher, 1978).

VALUE OF INTERPRETIVE REPORTS

It is our impression that many pathologists use interpretive reports. The 146 respondents who sent examples of their reports probably represent that smaller group of laboratory directors who are particularly interested in this approach, who have developed their reports more than others, and who are interested in sharing their work and seeing what others are doing.

The large number of replies from community hospitals and the small number of replies from university hospitals were not unexpected. Physicians have received these interpretive reports with mixed feelings. Although it is hazardous to generalize, physicians in community hospitals tend to welcome these reports, whereas subspecialists in university centers tend to view these reports as unnecessary because they know how to interpret their own data.

Hobbie and Reece (1978) surveyed physicians regarding computer-assisted interpretive reporting of 12-channel chemistry profiles for outpatients. It was found that 90 per cent liked this technique and 80 per cent wanted to see more follow-up suggestions. When this same system was tried in a hospital, it did not work as well and was abandoned after 6 months. Reasons for failure in the hospital were given as slow turn-around time, disinterest by hospital specialists, less interest in diagnostic than management information, and lack of commitment by laboratory staff.

Ashworth and co-workers (1978) surveyed physicians regarding computer-assisted interpretive reporting of multitest 20-channel chemistry profiles and thyroid function tests in a hospital setting; the results showed variable physician acceptance. Many internists were critical of the reports, but the majority of other physicians found them helpful. Sixty-four per cent of the internists read the interpretive remarks and found the comments helpful in 31 per cent of the cases. Other physicians read the comments 87 per cent of the time and found the comments helpful 58 per cent of the time.

Table 7–2. EXAMPLE OF INTERPRETIVE REPORTING BY CODE NUMBER USING A MEMORY TYPEWRITER*†

Serum Protein Electrophoresis

Total protein 7.6 g/100 ml. The albumin through beta regions appear unremarkable. In the mid-gamma region, a narrow zone of restriction is evident. Densitometric quantitation of this restricted zone reveals a quantity of 0.6 g/100 ml protein. The remainder of the gamma zone is unremarkable.

Immunoelectrophoresis

An IgG kappa monoclonal protein is evident. No free monoclonal light chains are noted in the serum. The normal polyclonal immunoglobulins (G, A, and M) appear normal in amount.

Laboratory impression: IgG kappa minor monoclonal protein.

Suggest:
1. Urine immunoelectrophoresis, if this has not been previously ordered.
2. Hematology consultation.
3. Such minor monoclonal proteins may be present with clinically evident lymphoproliferative disease (myeloma) and evolving lymphoproliferative disease. However, they may also coexist with a variety of nonlymphoproliferative epithelial neoplasms. Finally, in elderly individuals, they may exist as an isolated phenomenon unassociated with disease. If this is found to be the case in this patient, suggest periodic quantitation by electrophoresis.

*Courtesy of John C. Neff, M.D., Columbus, Ohio.
†Adapted from Speicher CE, Smith JW: Interpretive reporting in clinical pathology. JAMA 243:1557, 1980. Copyright 1980, American Medical Association.

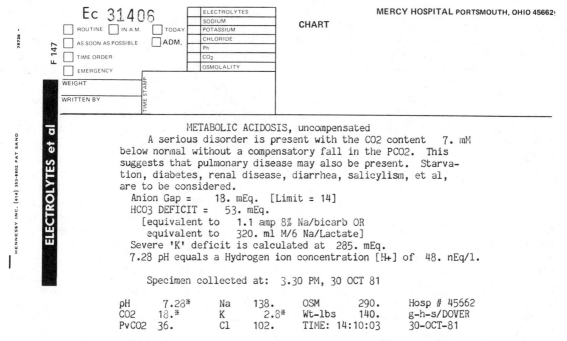

METABOLIC ACIDOSIS, uncompensated
     A serious disorder is present with the CO2 content   7. mM
below normal without a compensatory fall in the PCO2. This
suggests that pulmonary disease may also be present. Starvation, diabetes, renal disease, diarrhea, salicylism, et al,
are to be considered.
     Anion Gap =   18. mEq. [Limit = 14]
     HCO3 DEFICIT =   53. mEq.
       [equivalent to   1.1 amp 8% Na/bicarb OR
        equivalent to   320. ml M/6 Na/Lactate]
     Severe 'K' deficit is calculated at 285. mEq.
     7.28 pH equals a Hydrogen ion concentration [H+] of 48. nEq/l.

          Specimen collected at: 3.30 PM, 30 OCT 81

     pH   7.28*   Na   138.   OSM   290.   Hosp # 45662
     CO2   18.*   K   2.8*   Wt-lbs   140.   g-h-s/DOVER
     PvCO2 36.   Cl   102.   TIME: 14:10:03   30-OCT-81

Figure 7–3. Preprinted form for a computer-assisted interpretive report. (Courtesy of J. T. Gohmann, M. D., Portsmouth, Ohio.)

CONCERNS OF PHYSICIANS

Documentation in the patient's chart of diagnostic possibilities and therapeutic suggestions by the pathologist has caused some physicians to be concerned about increased medicolegal liability, especially if an appropriate suggestion was not acted on. The outpatient survey mentioned previously showed that one third of the physicians were concerned about medicolegal implications (Hobbie, 1978).

The cause of this concern is enigmatic, for the attending physician has the same prerogative of accepting or rejecting the suggestions of the pathologist as those of any other consultant. Perhaps concern stems from the fact that the pathologist's diagnostic comment is not consistently requested, or it may be that the sheer volume of laboratory reports causes an intuitive fear of overlooking something important. Whatever the reason, a problem exists and pathologists should be aware of it.

Lundberg (1980) commented: "As interpretive laboratory reporting increases, one easily can envision the day when the defense by a clinical physician for a lack of appropriate action may be that the pathologist failed to inform him or her of the true importance of the result and that the pathologist was liable."

The pathologist deals with the issue of a physician's concern about the medicolegal aspects of interpretive reports in a number of ways: One approach is to make an unequivocal diagnosis. An interpretive comment concerning myocardial infarction follows (information courtesy of Henry De Leeuw, M.D., Muskegon, Mich.):

CPK electrophoresis shows an MB band. LDH isoenzyme electrophoresis shows an elevated fast fraction with LDH-1 greater than LDH-2. This combination is virtually diagnostic of an acute myocardial infarct. No further isoenzyme determinations are necessary to document this diagnosis. (CPK indicates creatine phosphokinase; MB, creatine phosphokinase of heart origin; and LDH, lactic dehydrogenase).

Another approach is to define the meaning of diagnostic terms precisely, e.g.: "A negative cytology report does not mean that cancer is ruled out with certainty because false-negative reports may be the result of nonrepresentative material."

A third approach is to couch one's comment in terms that do not bind the physician to a certain course of action, such as: "Suggest follow-up liver panel if clinically indicated." Similarly, a disclaimer might be used to indicate that diagnoses based solely on laboratory tests should not be regarded as complete and final: "The list of diagnostic possibilities is incomplete, and the order is not necessarily significant."

Another technique was created by Ashworth and colleagues (1978). They provided a horizontal perforation line on the report to enable separation of the data section from the comment section.

BENEFITS OF INTERPRETIVE REPORTING

Interpretive reporting is thus a convenient method of communicating the results of problem-solving strategies. A review of interpretive reports encountered in our survey disclosed that many of them, if not at all, were concerned with problem solving. Multiphasic screening was concerned with the general problem of health versus illness. Other reports were directed at the solution of more particular problems, such as the presence or absence of

disordered function in a given organ or even the ruling in or out of one particular disease. When the issue of one particular disease is being addressed for those diseases that have specific laboratory findings, interpretive comments can achieve a high degree of certainty. Galen and associates (1975) demonstrated this through the high predictive values of serial CPK and LDH isoenzymes in the diagnosis of myocardial infarction (see Chapter 10 and Table 10–2).

The laboratory diagnosis of acute myocardial infarction is a good example for illustrating the manner in which reference intervals, decision levels, graphic-analogue displays, diagnostic-management lists, and interpretive comments contribute to the information content of an interpretive report. A cardiac injury panel illustrates a basic level of interpretive reporting by providing reference intervals as follows (information courtesy of John B. Henry, M.D., Washington, D.C.): "CPK 55 to 170 IU/L for men and 30 to 135 IU/L for women; and LDH, 71 to 207 IU/L for men and women." Figure 10–4 shows how the information content can be enhanced by a graphic display of serial enzyme studies. Table 7–3 shows the contribution of a diagnostic list for CPK isoenzymes.

Table 7–3. DIAGNOSTIC LIST FOR CREATINE PHOSPHOKINASE (CPK) ISOENZYMES*†

Diseases	CPK Isograms in Various Diseases‡		
	MM CPK₃	*MB CPK₂*	*BB CPK₁*
Active myocardial damage, including subendocardial infarct, infarct extension, and cardiac surgery	+ − + + + +	Trace- + + +	—
Myocardial ischemia	+ − + + +	Trace	—
Active skeletal muscle damage, including Duchenne's muscular dystrophy, extensive rhabdomyolysis, polymyositis, early dermatomyositis, myoglobinemia, and severe ischemia of extremities due to vascular disease	+ + − + + + +	0 − +	—
Rocky Mountain spotted fever	+ − + +	0 − +	—
Reye's syndrome	+ − +	0 − +	—
Normal serum	0 − + +	—	—
Brain injury	0 − + +	—	0 − +
Biliary atresia	+ − + +	—	0 − +
Malignant tumors (usually with metastases)	+ − + +	0–Trace	0 − + +
Severe shock	+ − + + +	0–Trace	0–Trace
Chronic renal failure	+ − + + +	0–Trace	0 − +

*Information courtesy of Warren B. Helwig, M.D., Newport News, Va.

†Adapted from Speicher CE, Smith JW: Interpretive reporting in clinical pathology. *JAMA* 243:1559, 1980. Copyright 1980, American Medical Association.

‡Values indicated occur at peak isoenzyme levels. MM and CPK₃ indicate slow electrophoretic CPK isoenzyme; MB and CPK₂, intermediate electrophoretic CPK isoenzyme; and BB and CPK₁, fast electrophoretic CPK isoenzyme.

The interpretive comment concerning myocardial infarction mentioned previously illustrates the most informative manner of interpretive reporting in which a diagnosis of acute myocardial infarction has been confirmed.

Interpretive reports can help busy physicians by providing the information they require to solve clinical problems. These reports can save time for the medical student, house officer, general practitioner, or specialist who has to page through lists of chemistry, hematology, microbiology, and immunology test results while trying to locate, copy, compute, and collate data germane to a particular problem. Computer-assisted interpretive reporting of 20-channel chemistry profiles and of thyroid function tests has been able to significantly reduce the number of telephone calls about "abnormal" results owing to age, sex, fasting state, age-deterioration of specimen, or hemolysis. In the same manner, laboratory staff time has been conserved by the elimination of the need for handwritten, phoned, or rubber-stamped comments that had been previously required (Ashworth et al., 1978).

It has been suggested that the insertion of problem-solving interpretive reports directly into the progress notes might save further time for clinicians. Perhaps we need a problem-oriented laboratory report that segregates significant abnormalities and prints these daily until they are resolved by the physician (Conn, 1980). It may be helpful for the pathologist to provide a summary report of significant laboratory findings in the same manner that the attending physician summarizes the important features of a hospital admission.

Interpretive reports can benefit patients by closing the gap between the mere reporting of laboratory test results and their integration into the diagnostic process. We could argue that simply stating reference intervals hardly constitutes interpretive reporting; however, without these values interpretation is impossible. Both the College of American Pathologists (CAP), through its Inspection and Accreditation Program, and the Joint Commission on Accreditation of Hospitals (JCAH) have insisted that reference intervals be provided. Furthermore, in recognition of the pitfalls of reporting raw data, these two agencies require the laboratory director or representative to review laboratory studies to ensure their relevance to patient care.

A graphic display of data, as depicted in Figure 10–4, can have far greater impact on clinical decision making than numbers alone. And why shouldn't the inclusion of appropriate "diagnostic possibilities" be useful to patient care? Don't we first have to think of a "diagnosis" to make one? Reece (1978) found that computer-assisted interpretive reports of 966 abnormal 12-channel chemistry profiles included the right diagnosis in the first five possibilities 67 per cent of the time.

These diagnostic possibilities are not really diagnoses at all. They merely represent hypotheses, which are suggested by the results of laboratory studies. This triggering of hypotheses by laboratory test results is similar to the triggering of hypotheses by the patient's signs and symptoms. It is a natural phase of the diagnostic process. The triggered hypotheses must then be evaluated by the physician. Because expert physicians intuitively tend to limit the number of hypotheses to be dealt with at one time, it is inadvisable to make the list of hypotheses too long. A page full of diagnostic possibilities will be quickly rejected by the attending physician (see Chapter 2).

We do not intend to imply that interpretive reports will enable the pathologist to make definitive diagnoses from laboratory results consistently. Rather, we mean to highlight the fact there are many ways in which the information content and clinical usefulness of laboratory data can be improved. Some of these are as simple as good form design, inclusion of better reference intervals and decision levels, and graphing or grouping of data in more comprehensible ways. Comments listing appropriate diagnostic possibilities or recognizing disease processes, such as inflammation, can also be helpful.

Two separate studies—one in which chart reminders of anemia (Wigton et al., 1981) were used and the other in which suggestions about clinical events that might need corrective action (McDonald et al., 1980) were included—were not very successful in modifying physician performance. These studies, however, differed from interpretive reports of the results of problem-solving strategies in that the reminders and suggestions were unsolicited by the physicians and probably did not address the hypotheses (i.e., differential diagnoses) they had on their minds (Burke, 1981).

Laboratory directors, particularly pathologists trained broadly in anatomic and clinical pathology, are in a unique position to contribute to patient care by interpretive reporting of data. They are aware, both as a result of individual experience and because of the volumes of data collected by the CAP, of the quantitative aspects of principles relevant to the use of diagnostic testing (Skendzel, 1978). Kassirer and Pauker (1978) believe that these principles—diagnostic sensitivity and specificity, predictive value, therapeutic significance, and cost-effectiveness, particularly in their quantitative aspects—are grasped by a small minority of physicians. Though the opinion of any consultant should not be considered absolute, that of the pathologist may be very worthwhile. Interpretive reporting should be encouraged by the pathologist, who as a rule is constantly involved in the introduction of new methods, statistical evaluation of analyses, interpretation of multiple studies, and biopsy evaluation as well as the ultimate quality control procedure in medicine—the autopsy.

THERAPEUTIC DRUG MONITORING

The information in this section is largely provided courtesy of the journal *Therapeutic Drug Monitoring* (Svirbely and Speicher, 1981).

BACKGROUND

Therapeutic drug monitoring has become possible and necessary through simultaneous advances in pharmacology, analytical chemistry, and clinical medicine. Pharmacologists have synthesized increasingly effective drugs that are potentially increasingly toxic. Analytical chemists have developed methods to measure levels of these drugs in body fluids. Physicians have applied these drug level measurements to patient care for the purpose of achieving therapeutic effects and avoiding toxic effects in both critically and chronically ill patients.

Not all drugs are candidates for monitoring. Therapeutic drug monitoring is not justified if there is no reliable method of measuring the drug, if there is no relationship between the serum drug level and the pharmacologic effect, if non-laboratory methods correlate better than the serum drug level with the pharmaco-

logic effect, or if a wide margin in dosage exists between therapeutic and toxic effects. Therefore, certain criteria are necessary before therapeutic drug monitoring is indicated (Bochner et al., 1978; Jusko, 1974; Riegelman and Sadee, 1974; Van der Kleijn et al., 1974; Wilkinson, 1974).

Furthermore, not all drug level measurements reported by clinical laboratories are acceptable for application to patient care. Acceptable drug level measurements must be accurate for the primary drug and its significant metabolites; precise, to facilitate titration of serum levels with dosage; timely, to permit changes in the next dose; and interpretable, to allow dosage in the most clinically relevant manner possible (see Chapter 6).

The attempt to achieve better assays for specific drugs in body fluids has consumed much effort in the field of therapeutic drug monitoring. Yet, accurate and precise measurements of drug levels constitute only one apect of effective therapeutic drug monitoring. This part can be conveniently considered under the category of intralaboratory considerations. Pre- and postlaboratory considerations are equally as important in obtaining a successful outcome, i.e., the prelaboratory limb and the postlaboratory limb of the laboratory information loop (see Chapter 6).

Because test request and report forms are such important components of pre- and postlaboratory considerations, respectively, their effects on the interpretation of therapeutic drug level measurements are examined in this study. Other investigators have already recognized the importance of request forms (Pippenger, 1979; Sohn, 1979).

A SURVEY OF THERAPEUTIC DRUG MONITORING

Methods

A letter was sent to 232 directors of laboratory services requesting them to forward examples of material that they use in the area of therapeutic drug monitoring and toxicology. Material requested included request forms, report forms, interpretive reports, computer applications, and newsletters or information handouts. The directors were promised an analysis and summary of this material as well as appropriate credit in future publications.

Table 7–4. THERAPEUTIC DRUG MONITORING REQUEST FORM CHARACTERISTICS*

Characteristic	% Exhibiting This Characteristic
Space for name of drug requested	100
Space for time specimen drawn	45
Space for source of specimen	9
Space for time of last dose	28
Space for amount of last dose	17
Space for route of drug administration	6
Space for urgency of request	19
Space for names of other drugs patient receiving	0
Space for clinical information, e.g., working diagnosis or evidence of hepatic, renal, or cardiac failure	0
Request form different from toxicology request form	40

*From Svirbely JR, Speicher CE: The importance of request and report forms in the interpretation of therapeutic drug monitoring data. Ther Drug Monit 2:212, 1980. By permission of Raven Press, New York.

The majority of directors were those individuals who responded to or indicated interest in the larger survey of interpretive reporting discussed earlier in this chapter. The survey was conducted from May 1, 1979, to October 31, 1979.

Results

Replies were received from 77 respondents, 53 of whom enclosed examples of their therapeutic drug monitoring request and report

Table 7–5. THERAPEUTIC DRUG MONITORING REPORT FORM CHARACTERISTICS*

Characteristic	% Exhibiting This Characteristic
Reference values	70
Decision levels	34
Graphic/analogue displays	8
Diagnostic/management lists	8
Interpretive comments	26
Computer printout	21
Computer pharmacokinetics	4
Request form used as report form	17

*From Svirbely JR, Speicher CE: The importance of request and report forms in the interpretation of therapeutic drug monitoring data. Ther Drug Monit 2:212, 1980. By permission of Raven Press, New York.

forms. The remaining 24 directors indicated interest in the survey, and some included newsletters and related material. Analysis of the 53 replies showed characteristics as given in Tables 7–4 and 7–5.

The characteristics of the request form in Table 7–4 are self-explanatory. The characteristics of the report form in Table 7–5 are common to all interpretive reports in clinical pathology and are further explained as follows. Reference intervals refer to the usual therapeutic range. Decision levels refer to levels at which toxicity is frequently encountered. Graphic-analogue displays refer to non-digital highlighting of data by asterisks, high-low columns, and so on. Diagnostic-management lists refer to additional matters the physician should consider, for example, on a serum digoxin test result report: "Renal failure, hypercalcemia, hypokalemia, alkalosis, recent myocardial infarction, myxedema, and hypomagnesemia can increase the patient's sensitivity to digoxin." Interpretive comments refer to a specific written comment, such as: "The serum level of theophylline is 40 μg/ml, which is definitely a toxic level." Computer pharmacokinetics refers to the availability of computer pharmacokinetic analysis.

The directors of laboratories who submitted therapeutic drug monitoring request and report forms were each sent an analysis and summary of all the forms (Speicher, 1980).

EFFECTIVENESS OF THERAPEUTIC DRUG MONITORING

The results of this survey indicate that request and report forms are not optimally designed to facilitate effective interpretation of therapeutic drug monitoring data. Many request forms are not designed to allow inclusion of even basic additional data; many report forms do little more than provide a drug level measurement and a therapeutic range. A minority of reports attempt to make drug level measurements more interpretable through the use of decision levels, graphic or analogue displays, diagnostic or management lists, and interpretive comments (Speicher and Smith, 1980).

Reasons to explain this poor situation in both data collection and reporting are conjectural and include the following: (1) a tradition of clinical laboratories as generators of numbers for which attending physicians provide interpretations; (2) a lack of appreciation for the requirements of effective therapeutic drug monitoring; and (3) a desire to provide drug level measurements at the lowest possible cost.

Physicians play a key role in effective therapeutic drug monitoring, yet it is a challenge for them to keep informed about drugs, especially new ones. They may be incompletely prepared to interpret bioavailability data (Schumacher, 1975; Vinson and Schumacher, 1976) and may be unaware of dangers associated with common dosing regimens (Neibergall et al., 1974). They may not appreciate that similar medications are not always bioequivalent (Martin, 1978) and that determinants of drug activity are varied and complex (Wagner, 1975).

Therefore, the simple reporting of an analytic value, while sufficient for many chemical tests, may be inappropriate for drug level measurements. Interpretive reporting of drug level measurements is necessary to ensure their relevance to patient care (Speicher and Smith, 1980).

We believe that a more aggressive approach to both the collection of data and reporting of results is required to improve the effectiveness of therapeutic drug monitoring data. Effective monitoring is a challenge of considerable magnitude that should be approached systematically. We will discuss solutions in terms of the personnel involved, the request form, and the report form.

SOLUTIONS FOR IMPROVEMENT

Adequate numbers of qualified personnel should be committed to therapeutic drug monitoring. These personnel should come from the laboratory, the pharmacy, and the clinical staff, and they should cooperate in designing a system that will work in their environment. Some should be responsible for properly collecting the specimen and the required data base (Table 7–6). It is our experience that request forms, no matter how simple and well designed, are, in practice, rarely completed, and that data collected retrospectively are often erroneous.

Concerning the request form, the amount of information required will vary with the reasons

Table 7–6. DATA BASE TO CONSIDER FOR THERAPEUTIC DRUG MONITORING REQUEST FORMS*

Patient identification
   Name, address, social security or other numbers
   Hospital number, outpatient, inpatient, room number
   Physician, service
   Personnel/locations desiring reports

Patient characteristics
   Age, sex, ethnicity, pregnancy
   Height, weight, surface area
   Personal or familial drug intolerance, reaction, allergy
   Primary disease process
   Organ involvement, especially renal, hepatobiliary, cardiac, gastrointestinal, endocrine
   Fluid balance, parenteral fluids
   Laboratory studies, especially acid-base status, serum albumin and electrolytes, creatinine clearance, urinary pH

Purpose of assay and urgency of request
   Toxicity, adequate dose, inadequate dose
   Data for calculating dose and dose interval
   Determination of reason for unexpectedly high or low serum level
   Comprehensive pharmacokinetic evaluation

Drug information
   Name of drug to be assayed, other drugs
   Time of last dose, frequency of prescribed dose, quantity of dose, route of administration

Specimen information
   Time of collection
   Nature of specimen: blood, urine, other body fluid
   Site of collection
   Order of sample, if one of a series
   Type of container, preservative
   Time of receipt by laboratory

Personnel audit trail
   Identification of phlebotomist, nurse, pharmacist, laboratory personnel

*From Svirbely JR, Speicher CE: The importance of request and report forms in the interpretation of therapeutic drug monitoring data. Ther Drug Monit 2:213, 1980. By permission of Raven Press, New York.

for which the physician is requesting the drug level determination. Oxley (1980) categorized consultative requests into four types, each with its own requirements (Table 7–7). Perhaps it may not be practical to rely on one request form to provide sufficient flexibility for all situations. Multiple types may be required. Every request form should meet the requirements of the CAP Inspection and Accreditation Program and the JCAH.

The content of the report form will vary with the type of request being answered. It

Table 7–7. TYPES OF CONSULTATIVE REQUESTS IN THERAPEUTIC DRUG MONITORING*

Type 1: To confirm
  Toxicity
  Adequate dose
  Inadequate dose
	Type 2: To provide data
	    for calculating
	  Dose
	  Dose interval

Requires:
  Single trough level
  Explanatory statement
	Requires:
	  Half-time
	  Dose history
	  Clinical history

Type 3: To determine why
  serum level is
  unexpectedly high
  or low
	Type 4: Comprehensive
	  pharmacokinetic
	  evaluation

Requires:
  Dose history
  Half-time
  Clearance
  Clinical history
  Other laboratory data
	Requires:
	  Dose history
	  Half-time
	  Clearance
	  Clinical history
	  Lab evaluation of
	  pathways for:
	  absorption, distribution,
	  metabolism, excretion

*From Svirbely JR, Speicher CE: The importance of request and report forms in the interpretation of therapeutic drug monitoring data. Ther Drug Monit 2:214, 1980. By permission of Raven Press, New York.

should be individualized as much as possible, and its content should be in keeping with good interpretive reporting (Speicher and Smith, 1980). The report form should meet the requirements of the CAP and the JCAH. It may, by necessity, be different from the request form. Listing of key references and telephone numbers for further consultation is recommended.

The achievement of effective therapeutic drug monitoring is an ambitious task. Recent advances in computers, especially those with both data-processing and word-processing capabilities, may prove helpful in collecting, storing, manipulating, and reporting the large data base involved. Computer programs have already been written that provide drug information (Frankenfeld et al., 1971; Olejar, 1971), kinetics calculations (Danek, 1978; Wagner, 1967), drug-drug interaction information (Greenlaw and Zellers, 1978; McKenney and Wasserman, 1979) and interaction with other portions of the patient data base (Gilroy et al., 1977; LaBrie, 1979). Programs have been written not only to prescribe specific drugs in given situations (Coe and Soloway, 1979; Hammond et al., 1979) but also to utilize

the principles of artificial intelligence to rival experienced clinicians in their prescribing expertise (Agarwal and Perrin, 1976; Gorry et al., 1978; Shortliffe et al., 1975). The ability to connect computers with one another affords the opportunity for communication networks providing ready access to information as well as timely and relevant solutions to patient problems.

Effective therapeutic drug monitoring requires not only that drug level measurements be accurate, precise, and timely but also that the results be interpretable and relevant to patient care. Interpretability requires that the appropriate data base be collected through the request forms and that meaningful information be disseminated through the report forms. Good request and report forms, as well as a system to ensure their proper use through adequate numbers of qualified personnel, are essential. Recent developments in computers should prove helpful in data handling and communication.

COMMUNICATING THE RESULTS OF PROBLEM-SOLVING STRATEGIES THROUGH CONSULTATIONS AND INTERPRETIVE REPORTS

PRESENT ORGANIZATION OF CLINICAL LABORATORIES

The clinical laboratory has functioned well as a generator of data. Over the last three decades, we have seen a tremendous increase in the number and variety of measurements and in the quality of the results of these measurements. Quality control has been both an intralaboratory and an extralaboratory function, and much assistance has come from such organizations as the CAP, the Center for Disease Control (CDC), and the Sunderman Institute for Clinical Science. But the laboratory has generated only individual pieces of data that have increased in number and complexity. Rather than aiding the clinician in diagnosis and management of patients, these data have often led to confusion with their long lists of numbers so that merely deciding what deserves attention and what does not is a feat in itself (see Chapter 1).

The non-physician laboratory scientist and technologist have well-defined tasks, but the role of the pathologist requires clarification.

The pathologist has management tasks, but management is only a tool to accomplish the goals of laboratory medicine. The pathologist needs to bridge the gap between laboratory technology and patient care more effectively, to design and implement problem-solving strategies, to collate and interpret laboratory measurements in order to bring their full information content to bear on patient's problems, perhaps needing to spend more time out of the laboratory to establish greater clinical relevance (Bartlett, 1974, 1982; Benson, 1978; Miller, 1975) (see Chapter 1).

The organization and orientation of the clinical laboratory have not been conducive to optimal patient care. Traditionally, laboratories have been organized into blood bank, chemistry, hematology, immunology, microbiology, surgical pathology, and cytology divisions. This kind of organization has its basis according to technology but often bears no relationship to patients' problems and their subproblems. It is not surprising that laboratories organized along these lines are not always the most readily responsive to patient care needs.

The pathologist often thinks of long lists of differential diagnoses for unusual test results, such as: "What are the causes of a high CPK?" This activity has merit, and we include lists of differential diagnoses for common chemistry and hematology test results in Part 3. In addition, the pathologist should be oriented to the clinical problems, e.g.: "Is this an acute myocardial infarction, and what is the strategy to rapidly and easily confirm or exclude this diagnosis with the greatest degree of confidence?" Through laboratory data analysis by mathematical (Beck, Meier, and Rawnsley, 1981) or nonmathematical approaches, the pathologist can help to make sense of the data by increasing the laboratory's diagnostic power.

The pathologist needs to bring the full information content of laboratory data to bear on the needs of patients. Comments and consultations should be directed toward solving patient problems.

REORGANIZATION OF LABORATORIES ALONG PROBLEM-SOLVING LINES

Reorientation of clinical laboratories along problem-solving lines can bring about greater relevance to patient care. Whenever this is physically possible, it should be done. For example, stat laboratories have emerged because of our technologic capability to perform some essential tests rapidly. Our capability has now progressed so far that it is probably possible to perform with great speed almost any test we desire. Instead of a stat laboratory, why not design a problem-solving emergency-care laboratory that is oriented toward solving the clinical subproblems that involve acutely ill patients (Wenk et al., 1980)?

Limitations of physical space, as well as of the technologist's skill and of laboratory equipment, usually restrict the ability to reorganize the laboratory physically along problem-solving lines oriented toward cardiovascular problems, renal problems, pediatric problems, and so forth. However, these limitations do not prevent reorganizing and reorienting test requests, strategies, and reports (i.e., information flow) along problem-solving lines. In other words, we can organize an information superstructure, which is problem-oriented, on top of the physical structure.

Whereas the laboratory scientist could be mainly responsible for the technical aspects of the laboratory divisions, the pathologist could be mainly responsible for a number of problem-solving areas within the laboratory that would be directly responsive to patient problems encountered by attending physicians. The pathologist could make rounds and go to conferences in areas of interests and responsibilities, and attending physicians could consult about their problems with the appropriate pathologist. In a small hospital, one or two pathologists would assume responsibility for all problem-solving areas.

The key to accomplishing this goal is in the ability to file, collate, organize, and report all laboratory information bearing on a particular patient problem. This problem-solving information would also be useful in surgical pathology and in clinical pathologic correlations at the time of autopsy.

INTERPRETIVE REPORTS, A NATURAL CONSEQUENCE OF PROBLEM-SOLVING STRATEGIES

Increasing the information content of laboratory measurements through interpretive reporting of problem-solving strategies can shorten the time required by busy clinicians to locate, collate, and interpret data about a particular patient problem. Good reference intervals, decision levels, graphic-analogue displays, diagnostic-management lists as well as interpretive comments can help clinicians to make better decisions. There would be less chance of important data being overlooked.

These measures, it is hoped, will shorten hospital stays and allow clinicians to diagnose and treat outpatients more effectively. All of these measures could reduce the cost of health care delivery. Murphy and Henry (1978) believe that the institution of organ panels at The Upstate Medical Center, Syracuse, N.Y., has been a cost-effective innovation.

REFERENCES

Agarwal RP, Perrin DD: Computer-based approach to chelation therapy: A theoretical study for some chelating agents for the selective removal of toxic metal ions from plasma. Agents Actions 6:667, 1976.

Altshuler CH, Bareta J, Cafaro AF, et al: The PALI and SLIC systems. CRC Crit Rev Clin Lab Sci 3:379–402, 1972.

Ashworth CT, McConnell TH, Ashworth RD, et al: A computer program for reporting automated chemistry (SMAC) and thyroid function tests with algorithm-derived interpretive comments. In Benson ES, Rubin M (eds): Logic and Economics of Clinical Laboratory Use. New York, Elsevier North-Holland, Inc, 1978, pp 173–186.

Bartlett RC: A plea for clinical relevance in medical microbiology. Am J Clin Pathol 61:867–872, 1974.

Bartlett RC: Making optimum use of the microbiology laboratory: 1. Use of the laboratory. 2. Urine, respiratory, wound, and cervicovaginal exudate. JAMA 247:857–859, 1336–1338, 1982.

Beck JR, Cornwell GG, French EE, et al: The "iron screen": Modification of standard laboratory practice with data analysis. Hum Pathol 12:118–126, 1981.

Beck JR, Meier FA, Rawnsley HM: Mathematical approaches to the analysis of laboratory data. In Stefanini M, Benson ES (eds): Progress in Clinical Pathology. Volume VIII. New York, Grune & Stratton, Inc, 1981, pp 67–100.

Benson ES: Strategies for improved use of the clinical laboratory in patient care. In Benson ES, Rubin M (eds): Logic and Economics of Clinical Laboratory Use. New York, Elsevier North-Holland, Inc, 1978, pp 245–258.

Bochner F, Carruthers G, Kampmann J, et al: Handbook of Clinical Pharmacology. Boston, Little, Brown & Company, 1978.

Burke MD: Clinical problem solving and laboratory investigation. Contributions to laboratory medicine. In Stefanini M, Benson ES (eds): Progress in Clinical Pathology, Volume VIII. New York, Grune & Stratton, Inc, 1981, pp 1–24.

Carter PM, Davison AJ, Wickings HI, et al: Quality and quantity in clinical pathology. Lancet 2:1555–1557, 1974.

Coe JM, Soloway HB: Computer-assisted heparin monitoring. Am J Clin Pathol 72:74–76, 1979.

Cole GW: Biochemical test profiles and laboratory system design. Hum Pathol 11:424–434, 1980.

Conn RB: Optimal utilization of the laboratory in making clinical decisions. Hum Pathol 11:407–412, 1980.

Connelly DP: The role of reporting and interpretation in effective laboratory utilization. In Benson ES, Rubin M (eds): Logic and Economics of Clinical Laboratory Use. New York, Elsevier North-Holland, Inc, 1978, pp 157–162.

Danek A: The use of computers in pharmacokinetics. Int J Clin Pharmacol 16:345–350, 1978.

Frankenfeld FM, Black HJ, Dick RW: Automated formulary printing from computerized drug information file. Am J Hosp Pharm 28:155–161, 1971.

Galen RS, Reiffel JA, Gambino R: Diagnosis of acute myocardial infarction. Relative efficiency of serum enzyme and isoenzyme measurements. JAMA 232:145–147, 1975.

Gilroy G, Ellinoy BJ, Nelson GE, et al: Integration of pharmacy into the computerized problem-oriented medical information system (PROMIS)—A demonstration project. Am J Hosp Pharm 34:155–162, 1977.

Gorry GA, Silverman H, Pauker SG: Capturing clinical expertise. Am J Med 64:452–460, 1978.

Greenlaw CW, Zellers DD: Computerized drug-drug interaction screening system. Am J Hosp Pharm 35:567–570, 1978.

Hammond JJ, Kirkendall WM, Calfee RV: Hypertensive crisis managed by computer controlled infusion of sodium nitroprusside: A model for the closed loop administration of short acting vasoactive agents. Comput Biomed Res 12:97–108, 1979.

Henry JB: Introduction to organ panels. In Henry JB, Giegel JL (eds): Quality Control in Laboratory Medicine. New York, Masson Publishing USA, Inc, 1976, pp 1–13.

Henry JB, Arras MJ: An innovation in health care delivery: Organ panels. South Med J 63:907–916, 1970.

Hobbie RK, Reece RL: A computer reporting and interpretation system: Acceptance and accuracy. In Benson ES, Rubin M (eds): Logic and Economics of Clinical Laboratory Use. New York, Elsevier North-Holland, Inc, 1978, pp 163–172.

Jusko WJ: Pharmacokinetic management of antibiotic therapy. In Levy G (ed): Clinical Pharmacokinetics—A Symposium. Washington DC, American Pharmaceutical Association, 1974, pp 111–128.

Kassirer JP, Pauker SG: Should diagnostic testing be regulated? N Engl J Med 299:947–949, 1978.

LaBrie RA: Drug intake monitoring and evaluation system (DIMES): Computerized drug monitoring. Psychopharmacol Bull 15:31–33, 1979.

Lundberg GD: The reporting of laboratory data interpretations: To omit or commit?, editorial. JAMA 243:1554–1555, 1980.

Martin EW: Hazards of Medications. Philadelphia, JB Lippincott, 1978.

McConnell TH: Interpretive reporting of laboratory data. Hum Pathol 9:129–131, 1978.

McDonald CJ, Wilson GA, McCabe GP: Physician response to computer reminders. JAMA 224:1579–1581, 1980.

McKenny JM, Wasserman AJ: Effect of advanced pharmaceutical services on the incidence of adverse drug reaction. Am J Hosp Pharm 36:1691–1697, 1979.

Miller DF: Clinical relevance: A concept whose time has

come? Laboratory Management, July 1975, pp 16–17.

Murphy J, Henry JB: Effective utilization of clinical laboratories. Hum Pathol 9:625–633, 1978.

Niebergall PJ, Sugita ET, Schnarre RL: Potential dangers of common drug dosing regimens. Am J Hosp Pharm 31:53–59, 1974.

Olejar PD (ed): Computer-Based Information Systems in the Practice of Pharmacology. University of North Carolina at Chapel Hill, 1971.

Osserman EF, Katz L, Sherman WH, et al: Computer-based case tracing (COMTRAC). JAMA 239:1772–1776, 1978.

Oxley DK: Principles of pharmacology and pharmacokinetics. In National Pathology Conference on Clinical Laboratory Pharmacochemistry and Therapeutic Drug Monitoring. Incline Village, Nevada, American Society of Clinical Pathologists, 1980.

Oxley DK, Fischer CL: Therapeutic drug monitoring. West J Med 128:47–48, 1978.

Pippenger CE: Editorial. Ther Drug Monit 1:451–452, 1979.

Reece RL, Hobbie RK: Computer evaluation of chemistry values: A reporting and diagnostic aid. Am J Clin Pathol 57:664–675, 1972.

Reece RL: Universal unified interpretive reports. Conceivable, believable, and achievable. Pathologist 32:343–350, 1978.

Riegelman S, Sadee W: Which drugs should be monitored today and tomorrow? In Levy G (ed): Clinical Pharmacokinetics—A Symposium. Washington DC, American Pharmaceutical Association, 1974, pp 169–180.

Schecter DS (ed): American Hospital Association Guide to the Health Care Field. Chicago, American Hospital Association, 1977.

Schumacher GE: Use of bioavailability data by practitioners: I. Pitfalls in interpreting the data. Am J Hosp Pharm 32:839–842, 1975.

Shortliffe EH, Davis R, Axline, SG, et al: Computer-based consultation in clinical therapeutics: Explanation and rule acquisition capabilities of the MYCIN system. Comput Biomed Res 8:303–320, 1975.

Skendzel LP: How physicians use laboratory tests. JAMA 239:1077–1080, 1978.

Sohn D: The clinician-laboratory connection, the vital link: Comments regarding the NCCLS proposed standards for clinical laboratory requisition forms. Ther Drug Monit 1:453–457, 1979.

Speicher CE: Survey of Interpretive Reporting in Clinical Pathology. Columbus, Ohio, Ohio State University, 1978.

Speicher CE: Survey of Request Forms and Report Forms in Therapeutic Drug Monitoring and Toxicology. Columbus, Ohio, Ohio State University, 1980.

Speicher CE, Smith JW: Interpretive reporting in clinical pathology. JAMA 243:1556–1560, 1980.

Svirbely JR, Speicher CE: The importance of request and report forms in the interpretation of therapeutic drug monitoring data. Ther Drug Monit 2:211–216, 1980.

Van der Kleijn E, Guelen PJM, van Wijk CGWM, et al: Clinical pharmacokinetics of benzodiazepines, barbiturates, and short chain fatty acids. In Levy G (ed): Clinical Pharmacokinetics—A Symposium. Washington DC, American Pharmaceutical Association, 1974, pp 79–102.

Vinson BE, Schumacher GE: Use of bioavailability data by practitioners. Part 2: Preliminary report of evaluation skills of pharmacists and physicians. Am J Hosp Pharm 33:1164–1166, 1976.

Wagner JG: Use of computers in pharmacokinetics. Clin Pharmacol Ther 8:201–218, 1967.

Wagner JG: Fundamentals of Clinical Pharmacokinetics. Hamilton, Ill, Drug Intelligence Publications, 1975.

Wenk RE, Weinstein W, Rudert J: Evolution of an acute care laboratory. Laboratory Medicine 11:731–737, 1980.

Wigton RS, Zimmer JL, Wigton JH, et al: Chart reminders in the diagnosis of anemia. JAMA 245:1745–1747, 1981.

Wilkinson GR: Therapeutic plasma level monitoring of anticonvulsants: From concept to practice. In Levy G (ed): Clinical Pharmacokinetics—A Symposium. Washington DC, American Pharmaceutical Association, 1974, pp 67–78.

PART **2**

CLINICAL
SUBPROBLEMS

SCREENING SUBPROBLEMS

VALUE OF SCREENING

Screening is the performance of a variety of laboratory tests on healthy or ill subjects for reasons other than diagnosing the cause of the subject's signs and symptoms. Screening, however, is actually a general term; that is, there are different kinds of screening that can intelligently be discussed only as individual activities. We can categorize these activities as *targeted screening* and *multiphasic screening*. Multiphasic screening that is performed on ill patients, such as candidates for hospital admission, is often called *profiling*. An article by Werner and Altshuler (1979) on the utility of screening forms the basis for many of our introductory comments.

Some physicians (Burke, 1981; Sackett, 1975) use the term screening to mean the testing of healthy volunteers from the general population for the purpose of separating them into groups with high and low probabilities for a given disorder. The term used for the testing of patients who seek health care for disorders that may be unrelated to their chief complaints is *case finding*. Combinations of tests performed with automated equipment are termed profiling. (See the discussion of screening in Chapter 1.)

The idea that patients can be screened by multiple laboratory tests as a method of detecting, documenting, or excluding diseases or disorders is appealing. Over the past several decades, screening for disease has been widely practiced. Multiphasic screening using automated techniques (automated multiphasic health testing) is no longer a problem for theoretical discussion. It has been predicted that by 1984, 10 million annual examinations will have been conducted in the United States (Galen, 1975). Solid proof of the effectiveness of screening, however, is still lacking. Nevertheless, the medical community appears to be divided into those favoring screening and those against it (Collen, 1979; Durbridge, 1976, 1978; Pribor, 1980, 1981). Third-party payers, in an attempt to contain escalating costs, tend to side with those who are against routine screening.

Targeted screening is designed to confirm (rule in) or exclude (rule out) the presence of a specific disease by using one or a small number of laboratory tests, such as serum T_4 and thyroid-stimulating hormone (TSH) for neonatal hypothyroidism. It is assumed that in targeted screening, the discovery of early or latent disease permits effective treatment at relatively low cost and will avert disabling

111

illness and the high costs associated with advanced and possibly incurable disease.

Certain requirements are necessary for effective targeted screening:

1. The screening test must be technically reliable.

2. There must be effective therapy for the screened condition.

3. The population at risk must be identified.

4. The screened condition must represent a significant health problem; for example, screening for cancer of the uterine cervix by examination of cervicovaginal cytologic smears satisfies all of these requirements.

Multiphasic screening (profiling) of patients by a panel of laboratory tests at the time of hospital admission is a common practice. Profiling is different from multiphasic screening of healthy outpatients in that patients being admitted to the hospital are already ill. In this group of ill patients, multiphasic data can confirm or document previously suspected disease, can discover unsuspected complications of disease, can exclude disease, or can provide baseline values against which the evolution of disease processes or against which the effects of therapy can be gauged.

Multiphasic screening of outpatients is of two kinds:

1. The first tests outpatients who are ill. In this group, the potential benefits are similar to those derived from profiling ill patients at the time of hospital admission.

2. The second tests outpatients who are healthy. The emphasis is on the detection of unsuspected disease and the provision of baseline data against which future disease processes can be evaluated.

The effectiveness of multiphasic screening by laboratory tests has been a subject for debate. It has been difficult to document the benefits of multiphasic screening of healthy outpatients, although this practice continues to have its advocates. Babb (1980) believes that executive health programs incorporating multiphasic screening are worthwhile.

On the other hand, the concept that multiphasic screening produces economic loss has remained unproved. A large and statistically well-controlled Australian study compared a group of hospital admission patients who were screened with a control group who were not screened (Durbridge, 1976). The two groups were found to be indistinguishable by any outcome measurements, including length of hospital stay. The total laboratory expense, however, was larger for the screened group than for the control group. The problem with this study is that the outcome did not distinguish a false-negative test result from a true-positive test result that had been ignored. In this study and in similar ones, the crucial but overlooked issue is that data acquired are not necessarily used. Without this obvious realization, findings such as those reported in the Australian study are to be expected a priori (Werner and Altshuler, 1979). Data generated but ignored can have no effect on decision making.

The fact that clinicians frequently overlook diagnoses in the face of disease-characteristic laboratory data has been demonstrated in a number of studies. Altshuler (1980) evaluated some 80,000 encounters between physicians and inpatients and found that the diagnosis was missed in one of four cases even when characteristic laboratory data were at hand. He illustrated the frequency of diagnostic misses by a computerized analysis of all cases with the simultaneous occurrence of a decreased free thyroxine index (FTI) decreased serum T_4 concentration, and an elevated TSH concentration encountered over a 3-year period (Table 8-1). Wheeler and co-workers (1977) analyzed 258 consecutively examined inpatients with low hemoglobin values on hospital admission. Of the patients studied, 71 per cent had an adequate follow-up and 24 per cent had no follow-up.

Because a certain number of diagnoses supported by disease-characteristic data can be overlooked, it may not be enough to provide the patient's physician with the data; it may be equally or more important to provide an interpretation of the data and suggestions for further testing. Altshuler and associates (1972) have carried the concept of interpretation one step further by devising a mechanism to follow up abnormal screening data by triggering the execution of conclusive, discriminatory tests whenever they are appropriate. His group documented the technical feasibility and the economic viability of such a sequential testing system in a large tertiary-care hospital.

Reviewing the cost-effectiveness of multiphasic screening, Werner and Altshuler (1981) developed a way of implementing the practice. They recommended that each institution develop a number of profiles best suited to it, that the bulk of tests be accommodated by a limited number of test profiles, and that appropriate mathematical analysis of the statis-

Table 8–1. CASES OF HYPOTHYROIDISM WITH A DECREASED FREE THYROXINE INDEX, A DECREASED SERUM THYROXINE LEVEL, AND AN ELEVATED THYROID STIMULATING HORMONE LEVEL

	Year		
	1975	**1976**	**1977**
Number of cases	27	30	47
Diagnosis on chart	17	15	31
Diagnosis known but not coded (chart review); includes miscoding	3	6	12
Apparent diagnostic misses	7	9	4
Types of physician involved	General practitioner Surgeon Urologist Internist Orthopedist	General practitioner Surgeon Internist Orthopedist	Obstetrician Orthopedist Surgeon Internist Urologist

*From Altshuler CH: The problem: Assuring appropriate transfer and utilization of laboratory information. In Werner M: Clinical Consultation in Laboratory Medicine by Pathologists. Chicago, American Society of Clinical Pathologists, 1980, pp 49–55.

tical data base specify optimal sets of profiles for various purposes.

TARGETED SCREENING

INFLAMMATION

Definition and Significance

Inflammation is the local reaction of vascularized tissue to injury and is often accompanied by necrosis. It is the final common pathway of practically every noxious process regardless of its etiology. However, conceptually it is useful to separate inflammation caused by infectious agents from other varieties of inflammation.

Common causes of inflammation include bacterial and viral infections as well as tumors, acute myocardial infarction, and rheumatic processes. Even if the exact etiology is unknown, confirming or excluding the presence of an inflammatory process by laboratory studies in a patient who presents with vague symptoms and signs can help determine whether to pursue further studies or to attribute the symptomatology to a psychologic origin. In patients with known inflammation, the response to therapy may have to be monitored. Therefore, a good strategy for the management of inflammation is also important.

Pathophysiology

The characteristics of an inflammatory process—swelling, heat, redness, and pain—are related to a complex series of events involving hemodynamic changes, changes in vascular permeability, leukocytic exudation, and chemical mediators (Robbins and Cotran, 1979). A good strategy for inflammation should center around the systemic effects that are manifested in the circulating blood (Gewurz et al., 1982).

The mechanisms whereby tissue injury stimulates the liver to synthesize diverse, acute-phase proteins are still unclear. C-reactive protein (CRP) is a particularly sensitive and useful acute-phase protein because the magnitude of its elevation can be more than 1000 times preinfection levels (Gambino, 1982).

Clinical Contexts

Table 8–2 summarizes the clinical indications for the use of acute-phase protein measurements in the diagnosis and management of inflammatory disease.

Diagnosis. The clinical features of inflammation include fever and tachycardia as well as vague, general symptoms of illness such as malaise and poor appetite. The patient should be examined for localized swelling, heat, redness, and pain. The characteristic presentations of various infections and rheumatic processes should be kept in mind.

Management. Laboratory studies that mirror the inflammatory response in the circulating blood can be used to monitor the course of an inflammatory process as well as its response to therapy (e.g., infections or rheumatic processes).

Table 8–2. WHEN TO USE ACUTE-PHASE PROTEIN MEASUREMENTS*

Screening for organic disease
Monitoring disease activity and response to therapy in
  inflammatory disease
  Rheumatoid arthritis, juvenile chronic arthritis,
    ankylosing spondylitis, Reiter's syndrome, psoriatic
    arthropathy
  Vasculitis syndromes
  Crohn's disease, ulcerative colitis
  Rheumatic fever
Making a differential diagnosis of inflammatory disease
  Systemic lupus erythematosus versus other arthritides
  Crohn's disease versus ulcerative colitis
Diagnosing and managing infections
  Neonatal septicemia and meningitis
  Intercurrent infection in systemic lupus erythematosus
  Intercurrent infection in leukemia
  Postoperative infection
  Infection and septicemia in burns
Seeking evidence of complications of known disease
  Hemolysis, fibrinolysis, vasculitis
  Immune complex deposition
Monitoring malignant disease
  Recurrence and response to therapy
Miscellaneous
  Assessment of myocardial infarction
  Assessment of new anti-inflammatory drugs

*From Whicher JT, Bell AM, Southall PJ: Inflammation: Measurements in clinical management. Diagnostic Medicine, July/August 1981, p 68.

Screening. Ordinarily, it is not appropriate to screen for inflammation in the absence of any clinical features of disease. However, such screening can be useful for excluding organic disease in patients with vague presentations or psychiatric disorders.

Strategy

Test Sequence. Serial and parallel performance of the following tests can be useful for diagnosing or managing an inflammatory process (Whicher, 1981; Whicher et al., 1981):

1. Leukocyte count.
2. Differential leukocyte count.
3. Erythrocyte sedimentation rate (ESR).
4. Serum protein electrophoresis (SPE).
5. Acute-phase proteins.
   a. alpha$_1$-antichymotrypsin.
   b. alpha$_1$-antitrypsin.
   c. C3 complement.
   d. C4.
   e. Ceruloplasmin.
   f. CRP.
   g. Haptoglobin.

h. Fibrinogen.
i. Orosomucoid (alpha$_1$-acid glycoprotein).

The leukocyte count, the differential leukocyte count, the ESR, SPE, and CRP are the more commonly used tests. Developments in the use of CRP have been promising.

Measurements of acute-phase proteins individually or by SPE have advantages over the ESR because they are affected by fewer variables, such as anemia. These acute-phase proteins can also be useful indicators of inflammation when the leukocyte count is depressed, for example, during chemotherapy or in overwhelming infection.

Patient Preparation. No particular preparation is required for the measurement of the ESR, SPE, and acute-phase proteins.

Specimen Collection and Handling. Sodium citrate is the anticoagulant-diluent for the Westergren ESR. A modified Westergren method has been devised that substitutes ethylenediamine tetraacetic acid (EDTA) for sodium citrate (Gambino et al., 1965). This permits the ESR to be performed on blood from the same tube used for other hematologic studies.

SPE, CRP, and all of the acute-phase reactants except fibrinogen can be measured in serum from a plain tube of clotted blood. Fibrinogen measurement requires plasma using citrate or oxalate as the anticoagulant. (See Part 3 on blood leukocyte count.)

Methodology. The physician should consult the laboratory for information on methodologies, reference intervals, accuracy and precision, and potential sources of interference. The National Committee for Clinical Laboratory Standards recommends the Westergren method as the basis for an acceptable standard ESR. However, even though anemia accelerates the ESR, there is no effective technique for correcting for anemia in the Westergren method. On the other hand, the Wintrobe method for the ESR can be corrected for anemia. The zeta sedimentation ratio (ZSR) (Coulter Diagnostics, Hialeah, Fla.) has been a satisfactory alternative to the ESR in a few clinical trials and is considerably faster than the Westergren method (Swaim, 1981).

SPE can be accomplished by a variety of methods. Cellulose acetate electrophoresis at a pH of 8.6 is satisfactory, but agarose electrophoresis is preferable because of its greater sensitivity for pathologic changes in the electrophoretic pattern.

CRP and fibrinogen are the most commonly measured acute-phase proteins. The usual methods for estimating CRP are agglutination, complement fixation, fluorescent antibody, precipitation in fluid or gel, and radioimmunoassay (Deodhar and Valenzuela, 1981). Rate nephelometry is a particularly convenient method (Gill et al., 1981). Fibrinogen can be measured by immunologic or functional techniques. The other acute-phase reactants can be measured by immunologic techniques, and some can be measured by functional techniques such as serum alpha$_1$-antitrypsin and ceruloplasmin. (See Part 3 on blood leukocyte count.)

Interpretation

Diagnosis. The presence of one or more of the following findings supports a diagnosis of inflammation:

1. Increased leukocyte count (over 11,000/mm^3).

2. Shift to the left of polymorphonuclear leukocytes (over 3 per cent bands).

3. Increased ESR, Westergren (men under 50 years > 15 mm/hr; men over 50 years > 20 mm/hr; women under 50 years > 20 mm/hr; women over 50 years > 30 mm/hr).

4. Increased CRP (approximate upper reference limit: 10 μg/ml or 0.01 g/L).

5. Increased alpha and beta globulins by SPE (approximate reference intervals: alpha$_1$, 0.1 to 0.4 gm/100 ml; alpha$_2$, 0.4 to 1.2 gm/100 ml; beta, 0.5 to 1.1 gm/100 ml). Agarose electrophoresis frequently shows a gamma migrating CRP band in the serum of subjects with inflammation.

Table 8–3 gives reference intervals and response times for clinically useful acute-phase proteins.

Leukocytosis (i.e., a white blood cell count over 11,000 per cubic millimeter) is indicative of inflammation. It can also be a false-positive measure of inflammation, since it occurs in a number of non-inflammatory states (e.g., strenuous exercise, pregnancy, acute bleeding).

A shift to the left in the differential leukocyte count is indicative of inflammation. This can sometimes be present in the absence of leukocytosis, particularly with viral infections, in which it may be accompanied by atypical lymphocytes.

The ESR can be falsely positive or negative for inflammation in the presence of macrocytosis, microcytosis, spherocytosis, hypercholesterolemia, cryoglobulinemia, polycythemia, anemia, and age.

A comparison of Figures 8–1 and 8–2 shows why the strategy for determining inflammation can be useful to diagnose a postoperative infection. Note how quickly the CRP responds. Some investigators believe that because the dynamics of liver synthesis of acute-phase reactants are different for each protein, much more information can be gained by measuring multiple rather than single acute-phase proteins (Fischer and Gill, 1975). They also believe that by using panels of acute-phase proteins it is possible to distinguish among major categories of inflammatory disease (i.e., bacterial versus viral infection). Measurement of a panel of acute-phase proteins to diagnose and manage inflammatory processes is not widely used.

Figure 8–3 shows the serum electrophoretic distribution of acute-phase proteins. Simple inspection of the electrophoretic pattern can detect elevated proteins. To determine whether a particular protein is elevated or not, it is important to remember that pregnancy and contraceptive medications elevate the lev-

Table 8–3. THE CLINICALLY USEFUL ACUTE-PHASE PROTEINS*

Protein	Normal Concentration (g/L)	Concentration in Acute Inflammation (g/L)	Response Time (hr)
C-reactive protein	0.0008–0.004	0.4	6.0–10.0
alpha-antichymotrypsin	0.3–0.6	3.0	10.0
Orosomucoid	0.5–1.4	3.0	
alpha$_1$-antitrypsin	2.0–4.0	7.0	24.0
Haptoglobin	1.0–3.0	6.0	
Fibrinogen	2.0–4.5	10.0	
C3	0.55–1.2	3.0	
C4	0.2–0.5	1.0	48.0–72.0
Ceruloplasmin	0.15–0.6	2.0	

*From Whicher JT, Bell AM, Southall PJ: Inflammation: Measurements in clinical management. Diagnostic Medicine, July/August 1981, p 64.

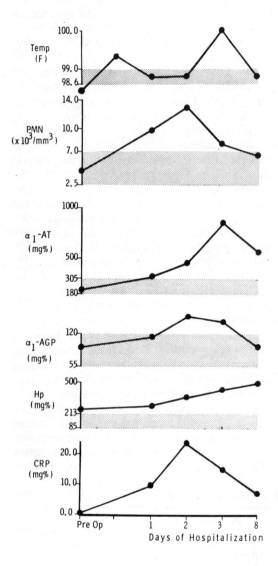

Figure 8–1. Clinical values in acute-phase reaction following an uncomplicated herniorrhaphy. Temp: temperature; PMN: polymorphonuclear leukocytes; α_1-AT: α_1-antitrypsin; α_1-AGP: α_1-acid glycoprotein; Hp: haptoglobin; CRP: C-reactive protein. (From Fischer CL, Gill CW: Acute-phase proteins. In Ritzmann SE, Daniels JC (eds): Serum Protein Abnormalities; Diagnostic and Clinical Aspects. Boston, Little, Brown & Company, 1975, p 346.)

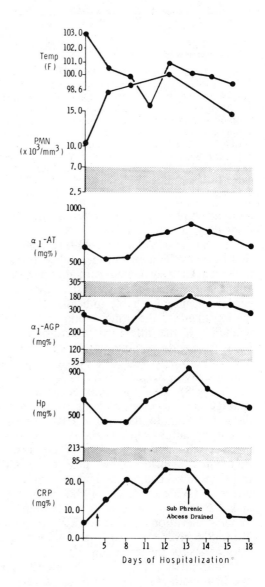

Figure 8–2. Acute-phase protein levels in surgical complication (infection). Temp: temperature; PMN: polymorphonuclear leukocytes; α_1-AT: α_1-antitrypsin; α_1-AGP: α_1-acid glycoprotein; Hp: haptoglobin; CRP: C-reactive protein. (From Fischer GL, Gill CW: Acute-phase proteins. In Ritzmann SE, Daniels JC (eds): Serum Protein Abnormalities; Diagnostic and Clinical Aspects. Boston, Little, Brown & Company, 1975, p 347.)

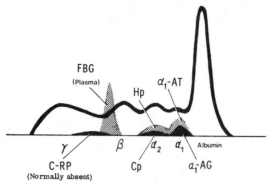

Figure 8–3. Electrophoretic distribution of the acute-phase proteins—α_1-acid glycoprotein, α_1-antitrypsin, ceruloplasmin, C-RP, haptoglobin, and fibrinogen and their relative contributions. α_1-AG: α_1-acid glycoprotein; α_1AT: α_1-antitrypsin; Hp: haptoglobin; Cp: ceruloplasmin; C-RP: C-reactive protein; FBG: fibrinogen. (From Fischer CL, Gill CW: Acute-phase proteins. In Ritzmann SE, Daniels JC (eds): Serum Protein Abnormalities: Diagnostic and Clinical Aspects. Boston, Little, Brown & Company, 1975, p 332.)

els of acute-phase proteins, whereas corticosteroids depress these levels.

Deodhar and Valenzuela (1981) point out that new developments in the ability to measure serum CRP significantly enhance its clinical applications. Studies indicate that CRP is an earlier and more reliable indicator of inflammation than are the other serum acute-phase reactants. In the differential diagnosis of bacterial from viral pneumonia, serum CRP has been reported to be useful because it rises dramatically in bacterial infections (McCarthy et al., 1978). CRP can also be a means of distinguishing ulcerative colitis from Crohn's disease, owing to the active CRP response seen in the latter (Pepys et al., 1977). Systemic lupus erythematosus (SLE), in contrast to rheumatoid arthritis, shows little or no CRP response unless complicated by an intercurrent infection (Whicher et al., 1981). Tables 8–4 and 8–5 present diseases in which high and minimal elevations of serum CRP are found. Table 8–6 gives the results of common laboratory tests for inflammation.

Management. The Westergren test is an excellent method for measuring the severity of an inflammatory process and following its response to therapy, for instance, the severity of a rheumatic process and its response to steroid therapy. Serum CRP is said to be a more reliable indicator of activity in patients with rheumatoid arthritis than the ESR is (Walsh et al., 1979).

Table 8–4. DISEASES ASSOCIATED WITH HIGH CRP LEVELS*

Active juvenile arthritis (Still's disease)
Amyloidosis, secondary
Ankylosing spondylitis
Arthritis associated with jejunoileal bypass
Bacterial infections
Crohn's disease (granulomatous colitis)
Familial Mediterranean fever
Myocardial infarction
Psoriatic arthropathy
Reiter's syndrome
Rheumatic fever
Rheumatoid arthritis
Thromboembolic complications following surgery
Vasculitis syndromes (e.g., polyarteritis)

*Adapted from Gambino SR (ed): A CRP supplement. Lab Report for Physicians 4(1):3, 1982.

The clinical course of patients with serious infections can be monitored by acute-phase protein profiles as well as by leukocyte counts, and therapy can be effectively guided by their responses (Table 8–3). Acute-phase proteins have been widely used as an adjunct to the staging and monitoring of malignancy (e.g., ceruloplasmin, often measured as serum copper) to monitor Hodgkin's disease (Whicher et al., 1981).

In myocardial infarction a sharp increase in the serum CRP level usually parallels the size of the infarct (Smith et al., 1977). In burn patients, an increase in serum CRP correlates with the severity of the burn (Daniels et al., 1974). A decrease in serum CRP levels can indicate successful therapy of acute pyelonephritis (Jodal and Hanson, 1976). A sudden increase in the serum CRP level is indicative of graft rejection in patients with renal transplants (Deodhar and Valenzuela, 1981).

Table 8–5. DISEASES ASSOCIATED WITH MINIMAL ELEVATION OF CRP*

Chronic active hepatitis
Dermatomyositis
Leukemia (not infected)
Mixed connective tissue disease
Polymyositis
Quiescent juvenile chronic arthritis
Scleroderma
Systemic lupus erythematosus (not infected)
Ulcerative colitis

*Adapted from Gambino SR (ed): A CRP supplement. Lab Report for Physicians 4(1):3, 1982.

Table 8–6. COMMON LABORATORY TEST RESULTS IN INFLAMMATION

Laboratory Test	Value	Pathophysiologic Factors
Chemistry (Serum)		
Bilirubin, total	—	
Calcium, total	—	
Carbon dioxide	—	
Chloride	—	
Cholesterol	—	
Creatine phosphokinase	↑	Related to tissue destruction, e.g., muscle, brain, thyroid, lung
Creatinine	—	
Glucose	—	
Lactic dehydrogenase	↑	Related to tissue destruction, i.e., virtually all tissues
Phosphatase, alkaline	—	
Phosphorus, inorganic	—	
Potassium	—	
Proteins, total	↑	Result of increase in acute-phase proteins and gamma globulins
Proteins, albumin	↓	Related to depressed synthesis and increased loss
Sodium	—	
Transaminase, aspartate amino	↑	Related to tissue destruction, e.g., muscle, liver, kidney, brain, pancreas, spleen, lung
Urea nitrogen	—	
Uric acid	↑	In severe tissue destruction, e.g., shock
Hematology (Blood)		
Hemoglobin	↓	Anemia associated with chronic disease
Hematocrit	↓	Anemia associated with chronic disease
Leukocyte count, total	↑	Can reach extreme elevations, a leukemoid reaction; can vary in type, e.g., neutrophilia, lymphocytosis, eosinophilia
	↓	Certain infections cause leukopenia, e.g., typhoid fever, viruses
Platelet count	↑	Slightly elevated
	↓	For example, gram-negative sepsis

Key:
— = No change; ↑ = can be increased; ↓ = can be decreased.

In pregnant women with premature rupture of the membranes, a serum CRP concentration greater than 200 μg/ml had a sensitivity of 70 per cent and a specificity of 100 per cent for infectious morbidity (Evans et al., 1980). CRP offered greater sensitivity for infectious morbidity than the leukocyte count, the differential count, and the ESR, and it was elevated at least 12 hours before any other indication of infection, including fever. Other applications of CRP include the diagnosis and management of pelvic inflammatory disease and the diagnosis and management of neonatal sepsis (Gambino, 1982).

Test Requests and Reports

A strategy for confirming, excluding, or monitoring inflammation can be offered by the laboratory, and an interpretive report may be generated, if desired.

PREGNANCY TESTING

Definition and Significance

Although most women become aware of a pregnancy 30 to 60 days after conception, some women take much longer to realize they are pregnant. There are a number of reasons why it is important to detect pregnancy before it naturally declares itself (Bish, 1979; Pelosi et al., 1981):

1. The fetus, especially in an early pregnancy, is vulnerable to damage from potentially teratogenic drugs, other substances, and ionizing radiation.

2. Knowledge of an existing pregnancy is important to medical and surgical differential diagnosis such as tubal pregnancy. In addition, pregnancy can contraindicate certain elective procedures.

3. The widespread use of steroid contraceptives gives rise to situations in which a contraceptive failure needs to be detected as early as possible to avoid possible damage to the embryo or fetus by continued administration. Pelosi and colleagues (1981) believe that all women of reproductive age admitted to hospitals should be screened for pregnancy using sensitive radioimmunoassay (RIA) or radioreceptor (RRA) tests.

4. Detection of early pregnancy is necessary in the management of infertility.

There have been important developments in immunologic pregnancy tests. Immunoassays replaced bioassays in the early 1960s. It is important to know the features of these tests, including their predictive value in given clinical situations.

Physiology

Modern pregnancy tests are based on the detection of human chorionic gonadotropin (hCG), which is synthesized by the trophoblastic tissue (syncytiotrophoblast) of the placenta. hCG is essential for maintaining the corpus luteum and supporting early pregnancy. It stimulates secretion of estrogen and progesterone by the corpus luteum and prevents menstruation. The amount of hCG secreted is directly related to the amount of trophoblastic tissue present.

hCG is a polypeptide hormone similar in structure to luteinizing hormone (LH), follicle-stimuating hormone (FSH), and TSH. All these hormones are composed of an alpha chain and a beta chain. The alpha chains are essentially identical; it is the beta chain structure that confers biologic and immunologic specificity. In practice, the distinction between hCG and LH is most important because the normal midcycle surge in LH that triggers ovulation can be mistakenly identified as hCG in non-specific pregnancy tests. This would result in a false-positive diagnosis of pregnancy.

The concentrations of hCG in maternal blood and urine peak during the first trimester (Fig. 8–4). Blood and urine assays show parallel peaks about 60 days after conception, then decrease to low levels just before term. Serum levels rise to 50 to 100 IU/ml, then decrease to 10 to 20 IU/ml at term. Values of hCG in the urine peak at 20,000 to 100,000 IU per day and decrease in later pregnancy to values of 4,000 to 11,000 IU per day (Pelosi et al., 1981). An excellent review of hCG is available by Keller (1976).

Clinical Contexts

Diagnosis. One of the common clinical settings for the diagnosis of pregnancy occurs when a woman of child-bearing age presents to a physician because she has signs or symptoms suggestive of pregnancy, such as a missed

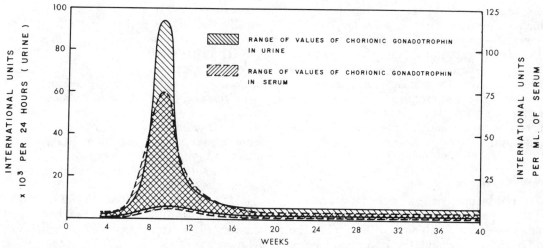

Figure 8–4. Chorionic gonadotropin levels in serum and urine. (Adapted from Greenhill JP, Friedman EA; Biological Principles and Modern Practice of Obstetrics. Philadelphia, WB Saunders Company, 1974, p 58.)

menstrual period. She may or may not be using contraceptives.

Another situation in which testing for pregnancy is indicated occurs when a woman presents with vaginal bleeding or abdominal pain, which raises the possibility of an ectopic tubal pregnancy or threatened abortion. In addition, it is important to exclude pregnancy in situations requiring management with potentially teratogenic drugs or ionizing radiation or when elective medical or surgical procedures are contemplated.

Management.   Reasons for measuring hCG include the following (Pelosi, 1981):

1. To manage infertility. Some women conceive and abort so early that neither they nor their physician are aware of the pregnancy.

2. To evaluate the quality of the pregnancy. Persistently low levels of hCG suggest spontaneous abortion, ectopic pregnancy, or an abnormal source of hCG. Elevated levels suggest multiple gestation or the presence of trophoblastic disease.

3. To monitor trophoblastic disease.

Screening.   An example of targeted screening for pregnancy is the routine screening of every woman of child-bearing age on hospital admission.

Strategy

Test Sequence.   The strategy for pregnancy testing depends on how soon after conception there is a need to confirm a diagnosis. The earlier the requirement, the more sensitive and specific the pregnancy test must be. To exclude pregnancy, a more sensitive, less specific test is adequate. Table 8–7 gives the sensitivity of

available tests for pregnancy. An important feature of the new RIA (beta-subunit hCG) in very early pregnancy is its increased specificity directed toward the beta-subunit of hCG in distinguishing hCG from LH.

Therefore, for the common situation in which a woman is curious about the possibility of pregnancy, an ordinary urine immunologic pregnancy test will suffice. When the greatest sensitivity and specificity are required for diagnosing early pregnancy (possible ectopic tubal pregnancy or exclusion of pregnancy prior to x-ray exposure), an RIA is recommended.

Patient Preparation.   To confirm pregnancy, a first-morning urine specimen is recommended because it is the most concentrated and is likely to have a high level of hCG. Blood or protein in the urine and drugs (especially methadone and phenothiazines) can interfere with urine-immunologic pregnancy tests (Horwitz, 1980).

Certain factors can interfere with serum RIA pregnancy testing (Pelosi et al., 1981):

1. Presence of other radionuclides in the patient.

2. Prior administration of hCG; this can cause a false-positive test. Wait 30 days after administration.

3. Gross lipemia; obtain specimen after the patient has fasted.

4. The occurrence of ectopic hCG, such as in trophoblastic disease or other non-placental sources of hCG (non-trophoblastic neoplasms of breast, prostate, lung, kidney, ovary, and gastrointestinal tract).

5. Presence of sarcomas and malignant melanomas.

Table 8–7.   COMPARISON OF COMMERCIALLY AVAILABLE ASSAYS*

	RIA (beta-subunit hCG)	Radioreceptor Assay	Immunoassays		
			New Tube Tests	*Tube Tests*	*Slide Tests*
Sensitivity (hCG amount detected)	0.003–0.030 IU hCG/ml of specimen	0.2 IU hCG/ml of specimen	0.2–0.25 IU hCG/ml of specimen	0.5–1.0 IU hCG/ml of specimen	1.0–4.0 IU hCG/ml of specimen
Specimen type	Serum	Serum	Urine	Urine	Urine
Time required	1–3 hours	1 hour	1.5–2.0 hours	1.5–2.0 hours	2 minutes
When 100% sensitivity can be expected (normal pregnancy)	First week of pregnancy	Day of first missed period	Day of first missed period	2 weeks after first missed period	2 weeks after first missed period
Cost	Most expensive	Expensive	Medium range	Medium range	Least expensive

*From Pelosi MA, Apuzzio J, Harrigan JT: What to expect from the new generation of pregnancy tests. Contemporary Ob/Gyn 17:236, 1981.

Specimen Collection and Handling. Clean glassware is essential for collection of urine and serum samples. Avoid hemolysis when collecting the blood sample.

Methodology. Urine immunoassays differ from serum RIA and RRA assays in their sensitivity to hCG, sample type, time required for testing, time at which greatest sensitivity can be expected, and cost (Table 8–7).

The advantages and disadvantages of the rapid latex slide immunoassays and the standard hCG tube immunoassays are given in Tables 8–8 and 8–9. Urine immunoassays for hCG cross-react with LH. This limits their specificity for early pregnancy detection. RRA for hCG can also cross-react with LH.

Urine immunoassays can be performed by inhibition of either hemagglutination or latex agglutination. Drugs and proteins in the urine interfere less with hemagglutination inhibition tests than with latex agglutination inhibition tests (Park, 1980). Serum beta-subunit hCG RIAs are more sensitive than RRAs and are therefore the test of choice for detection of pregnancy in all low-titer conditions such as ectopic pregnancy (Horwitz, 1980).

Interpretation

Diagnosis. The serum RIA test for the beta-hCG subunit is the most sensitive (0.003–0.030 IU/ml) and specific indicator of viable

Table 8–8. ADVANTAGES AND DISADVANTAGES OF THE RAPID INDIRECT LATEX SLIDE IMMUNOASSAYS*

Advantages
Convenient and rapid
Centrifugation or filtration of specimen unnecessary
Specific if urinary protein content is low (<30 mg/dl)
No drug interference with covalent hCG-latex linkage

Disadvantages
Relative insensitivity (compared with tube and RIA tests)
hCG level of 1.5–2.5 IU/ml needed for a positive test
>90% accuracy *only* after 45 days from LNMP
False-negative results on some urine specimens with specific gravity of <1.010
High technical error rate (1.5–3.0%) resulting from improper mixing technique
Occasional false-positive results caused by significant proteinuria (≥100 mg/dl)

Conclusion
Tests of choice in physicians' offices

*From Horwitz CA: Pregnancy tests 1980: Advantages and limitations. Laboratory Medicine 11:621, 1980.

Table 8–9. ADVANTAGES AND DISADVANTAGES OF THE STANDARD hCG TUBE IMMUNOASSAYS*

Advantages
Simple test procedure
Several times more sensitive than rapid slide tests
Less technical error than with rapid slide tests

Disadvantages
Relative insensitivity (compared with RIA tests)
hCG level of 0.5–1.0 IU/ml needed for a positive test
>90% accuracy *only* after 40 days from LNMP
Significant proteinuria (≥100 mg/dl) can result in serrated, atypical rings
Vibration or jarring disturbance can result in distorted, inconclusive end points

Conclusion
Tests of choice in hospitals that do not have RIA equipment for patients undergoing diagnostic curettage or elective hysterectomy

*From Horwitz CA: Pregnancy tests 1980: Advantages and limitations. Laboratory Medicine 11:622, 1980.

trophoblastic tissue available. It can confirm pregnancy within the first week. When symptomatic ectopic pregnancy or an early uterine pregnancy associated with a fertility problem is under consideration, it can confirm or exclude the diagnosis, sparing the patient unnecessary risk and expense (Bates, 1981). If the sensitivity and specificity of the beta-subunit RIA test are not required (such as in confirmation of pregnancy 2 weeks or more after the first missed menstrual period), urine immunoassays can be adequate.

The RRA for hCG is not as useful as the beta-subunit RIA for diagnosing ectopic pregnancy. The sensitivity of the RRA for hCG is approximately 0.2 IU/ml, and the test cross-reacts with LH (Bates, 1981). Milwidsky and associates (1978) found 8 of 15 (53 per cent) patients with proven ectopic pregnancy to have serum hCG levels below 0.2 IU/ml. Schwartz and DiPietro (1980) found 10 of 22 (45 per cent) patients with proven ectopic pregnancy to have serum hCG levels below the analytic sensitivity of the serum RRA test. Among 234 patients admitted to the hospital for suspected ectopic pregnancy during a 13-month period in whom the beta-subunit RIA was done, only 22 (9.4 per cent) were found to have the condition, and all 22 had positive tests. Of the 22 patients with confirmed ectopic pregnancies, 50 per cent had negative urine immunologic pregnancy tests.

Table 8–10 gives the results of common laboratory tests in pregnancy.

Table 8–10. COMMON LABORATORY TEST RESULTS IN PREGNANCY*

Laboratory Test	Value	Pathophysiologic Factors
Chemistry (Serum)		
Bilirubin, total	—	
Calcium, total	↓	Related to insufficient calcium, phosphorus, and vitamin D ingestion
Carbon dioxide	↓	Related to respiratory alkalosis caused by increasing enlargement of the uterus and the stimulatory effect on respiration by the increased hormones of pregnancy
Chloride	↑	Reciprocal relationship to bicarbonate secondary to respiratory alkalosis especially prominent during labor
Cholesterol	↑	Related to increase in cholesterol, triglycerides, and phospholipids from hepatic stimulation by increased hormones; may also be related to glucose intolerance
Creatine phosphokinase	↑	Increased during the last few weeks and remains elevated through parturition, becoming normal approximately 5 days postpartum
	↓	During 8th–20th week; minimum at 12th week
Creatinine	↓	Slightly lower in pregnant state; creatinine of 1.2 mg/100 ml represents an elevated level in pregnancy
Glucose	↑	Related to glucose intolerance secondary to ovarian and placental hormones
Lactic dehydrogenase	↑	Increases variably in normal pregnancy
Phosphatase, alkaline	↑	Placental in origin; first apparent in second trimester, increases in third trimester, and disappears 4 weeks postpartum. Higher levels in eclampsia with infarcted villi
Phosphorus, inorganic	↓	Sometimes a slight decline with no serious complications
Potassium	—	
Proteins, total	—	Alpha and beta globulins are increased but not enough to elevate total protein, especially with albumin depressed
	↓	Related to expansion of the intravascular space with a dilution of proteins
Proteins, albumin	↓	Related to expansion of the intravascular space with a dilution of albumin
Sodium	↓	Caused by dilution secondary to expansion of the intravascular space
Transaminase, aspartate amino	↓	Caused by a decrease in pyridoxine during pregnancy
Urea nitrogen	↓	Caused by dilution secondary to expansion of the intravascular space and by an increase in glomerular filtation
Uric acid	↑	Occurs with pre-eclampsia and eclampsia
	↓	Usually decreased compared with non-pregnant state
Hematology (Blood)		
Hemoglobin	↓	Related to increase in plasma volume; can be aggravated by anemia, especially from iron deficiency
Hematocrit	↓	Related to increase in plasma volume; can be aggravated by anemia, especially from iron deficiency
Leukocyte count, total	↑	During late pregnancy and labor
Platelet count	↓	Evidence of intravascular coagulation, as shown by elevated levels of fibrin degradation products and reduced platelet counts found in many women

Key:
— = No change; ↑ = can be increased; ↓ = can be decreased.

*Based on information from Friedman RB, Anderson RE, Entine SM, et al: Effects of diseases on clinical laboratory tests. Clin Chem 26:416D–419D, 1980; Wolf PL: Interpretation of Biochemical Multitest Profiles: An Analysis of 100 Important Conditions. New York, Masson Publishing USA, Inc, 1977.

Management. Serum levels of beta-subunit hCG can help to identify and follow compromised pregnancies, twin pregnancies, and trophoblastic tumors.

Test Requests and Reports

Test Requests. A strategy to confirm or exclude the diagnosis of pregnancy can be tailored to fit the needs of the requesting physician. For instance, a urine immunologic test can be done at lower cost for a woman with clinical features of normal uterine pregnancy; or a beta-subunit hCG serum RIA test can be done at higher cost to confirm early pregnancy when greater sensitivity and specificity are necessary, as in symptomatic ectopic tubal pregnancy.

Interpretive Reports. An interpretive report can be returned to the attending physician, giving the test result in IU/liter or IU/ml rather than in terms of "positive" or "negative." If the test result is positive, further comment about its specificity is appropriate, such as: Does it cross-react with LH? If the test result is negative, a comment should be made as to whether the outcome is due to the absence of a detectable level of hCG or to the possible presence of a detectable level of hCG that is below the threshold for a positive test. In the latter case, information about the analytic sensitivity of the test for hCG may be helpful.

MULTIPHASIC SCREENING

MULTIPHASIC SCREENING BY CHEMISTRY TESTS

Definition and Significance

Multiphasic screening refers to the systematic study of a patient by a panel of measurements for the purpose of detecting, documenting, or excluding disease or of providing baseline data. We have confined our attention to measurements that are performed exclusively in the clinical chemistry laboratory, i.e., the biochemical screen or profile.

Pathologists should devise innovative communicative and consultative tools to help physicians use screening tests more effectively.

Pathophysiology

Because the number of disease entities that can be detected, documented, or excluded by multiphasic screening is very large, we shall not list them as individual entities. Lufkin and associates (1969), Preston and Troxel (1971), Ward (1973), Wolf (1977), Beeler (1978), and Beeler and Catrou (1979) described a large variety of pathophysiologic mechanisms and disease entities that can be manifested in biochemical profiles.

Clinical Contexts

Diagnosis. A biochemical profile of ill patients at hospital admission or a profile of ill outpatients at a visit to a physician is often conducted with the same panel of studies regardless of the particular symptoms and signs that may be exhibited. However, some biochemical profiles can differ according to category of illness; for example, a patient admitted to a cardiovascular unit may have a different type of biochemical profile than one who is admitted to a gynecologic unit.

Management. Multiphasic screening of both ill and healthy patients provides a panel of baseline laboratory data against which the development of future disease, the course of present disease, or the response to therapy can be evaluated. These screens can be repeated to assess the severity of disease processes or to provide prognostic information.

Screening. According to the strictest definition of screening—the performance of laboratory tests in the absence of clinical features of disease—screens of healthy outpatients are the only variety of multiphasic screening that fall into this category.

Strategy

Test Sequence. There are many strategies for multiphasic screening. They differ from

Table 8–11. TEST COMPOSITION OF BIOCHEMICAL PROFILES

Profile No. 1	Profile No. 2
Sodium	Total protein
Potassium	Albumin
Carbon dioxide	Calcium
Chloride	Inorganic phosphorus
Glucose	Cholesterol
Urea nitrogen	Uric acid
	Creatinine
	Total bilirubin
	Alkaline phosphatase
	Creatine phosphokinase
	Lactic dehydrogenase
	Glutamic oxaloacetic transaminase

one another in two significant ways, namely, in the number and kinds of tests performed. Two of the more common biochemical profiles, shown in Table 8–11, are often performed together. Altshuler and co-workers (1972) developed not only an extensive multiphasic screen but also a strategy for follow-up studies that are automatically performed under supervision of the pathologist when abnormalities are discovered in the primary profile (Fig. 8–5).

Patient Preparation. Although unnecessary for most tests, a fasting blood sample can be advantageous in screening for diabetes mellitus (see Chapter 16). Part 3 presents information on common serum chemistry tests.

Specimen Collection and Handling. See Part 3 on common serum chemistry tests.

Methodology. Consult the laboratory for methodologies, reference intervals, and potential sources of interference. Methods for common serum chemistry tests are discussed in Part 3.

For the sake of economy, screens or profiles are usually generated by a single large multi-channel chemistry analyzer. In fact, the technical development of these analyzers in the 1960s has been one of the major factors fostering the growth of biochemical profiles. Performance of biochemical profiles by individual chemical methods is labor-intensive and is often prohibited because of cost.

Interpretation

Diagnosis. There are many diagnostic interpretations that can be done using biochemical profiles. Patterns for the results of a biochemical profile (18 common chemistry tests) and a hematologic profile (four common hematology tests) appear in tabular form in the discussions of each of the clinical subproblems in this book. Lufkin and associates (1969) compiled 13 different meaningful patterns of biochemical profiles; Preston and Troxel (1971), 32; Ward (1973), 26; Beeler and Catrou (1979), five; and Wolf (1977), 100. Figures 8–6 and 8–7 exemplify biochemical profiles that exhibit elevations in serum alkaline phosphatase and serum calcium, respectively. Unexplained elevations of these two analytes are discussed in Chapter 9. The tables in Part 3 can be used to construct patterns of results for 18 chemistry tests and four hematology tests in a variety of diseases and disorders.

If we use conventional 95 per cent limits for the reference intervals for each of the analytes in the screen or profile, a high number of false-positive results will be obtained (see Table 9–1). For measurements that do not bear directly on the patient's problems, it might be useful to use reference intervals with 99 per cent limits. These would be less sensitive but more specific for unexpected diseases and would tend to produce better pattern definition. Grams and co-workers (1978) established a multivariate chemical laboratory data base and were able to reduce the number of healthy patients having "abnormal" values from 53 to 9 per cent.

Management. Figure 8–8 is an example of a biochemical profile that can serve to follow the course of viral hepatitis.

Test Requests and Reports

Test Requests. Usually, a clinical laboratory's request form is designed so that a physician can order a biochemical screen or profile by checking one block. Figure 8–9 shows Henry's panel of tests for general health screening. Henry and Howanitz (1980) gave the rationale for this panel as follows:

This panel may be used to screen each patient visiting an institution for the first time and for subsequent periodic health examinations. It is designed to evaluate renal, liver, endocrine, musculoskeletal, and hematopoietic systems. If an abnormality is noted, an appropriate organ panel can be utilized. Routine screening has been criticized as having little beneficial impact on patient care despite the significant number of abnormal laboratory results generated. This panel has been designed for the early detection of those diseases where treatment is either easier or more effective when undertaken at an earlier point in time. However, the measurement of the effectiveness of screening is judged by the usefulness in altering the clinical course of a patient. Although this is subjective, our clinical colleagues believe a screening panel is of value for selected patients.

Figure 8–5 shows a report form used for the programmed accelerated laboratory investigation (PALI) of Altshuler and co-workers (1972). Figures 8–10 and 8–11 give Cole's (1980) panels of tests that can be used to tailor general or specific biochemical profiles.

Interpretive Reports. Henry, Cole, Altshuler, and many other pathologists have practiced interpretive reporting of biochemical pro-

Text continued on page 137

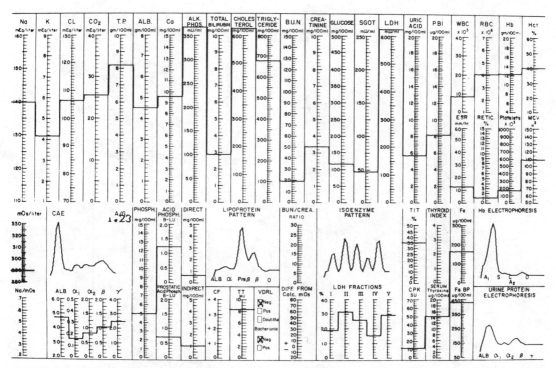

Figure 8–5. The PALI report form. The horizontal lines and the waveforms are the found values. (From Altshuler CH, Bareta J, Cafaro AF, et al: The PALI and SLIC systems. CRC Crit Rev Clin Lab Sci 3:380, 1972. Copyright by the Chemical Rubber Company, CRC Press, Inc).

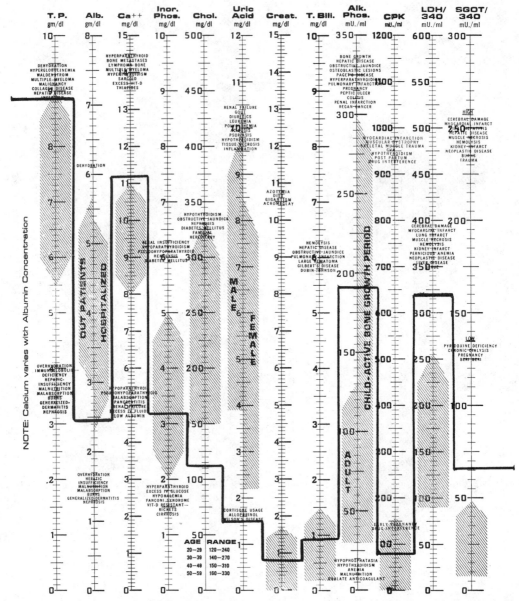

Figure 8–6. Graphic display of biochemical test results in a male with adenopathy and increased alkaline phosphatase who was found to have Hodgkin's disease. (From Wolf PL: Interpretation of Biochemical Multitest Profiles: An Analysis of 100 Important Conditions. New York, Masson Publishing, Inc, 1977, p 156).

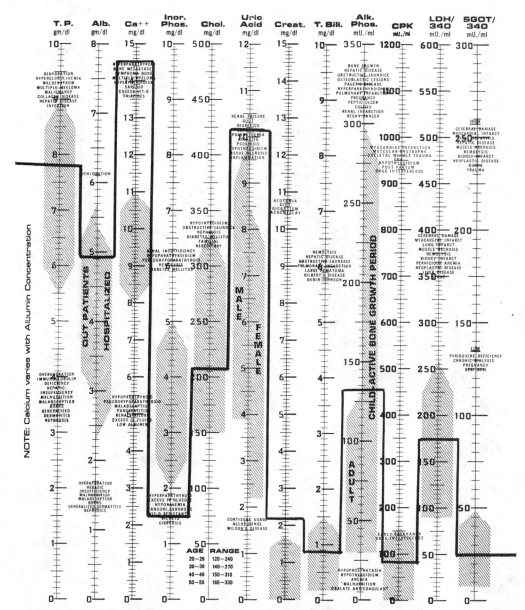

Figure 8–7. Graphic display of biochemical test results in a middle-aged male with elevated serum calcium and duodenal ulcer who was found to have hyperparathyroidism. (From Wolf PL: Interpretation of Biochemical Multitest Profiles: An Analysis of 100 Important Conditions. New York, Masson Publishing, Inc, 1977, p 29.)

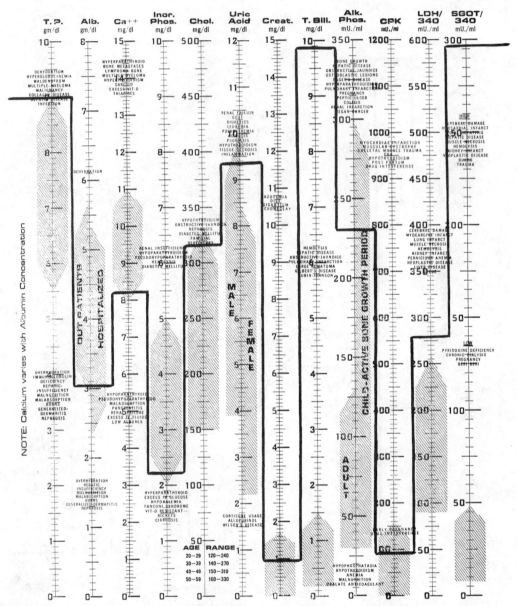

Figure 8–8. Graphic display of biochemical test results in a female drug addict who was found to have viral hepatitis. (From Wolf PL: Interpretation of Biochemical Multitest Profiles: An Analysis of 100 Important Conditions. New York, Masson Publishing, Inc, 1977, p 250.)

GENERAL HEALTH (Fasting)				
Creatinine mg/dl	0.6–1.2			
Urea Nitrogen (BUN) mg/dl	8–18			
SGO Transaminase IU/L	1–39			
Uric Acid mg/dl	Female 2.0–6.4 Male 2.1–7.8			
Chloride mEq/L	98–109			
CO_2 Content mM/L	24–30			
Sodium mEq/L	135–145			
Potassium mEq/L	4.0–4.8			
Calcium mEq/L	4.5–5.4			
Lactic Dehydrogenase IU/L	71–207			
Glucose mg/dl	65–115			
Cholesterol mg/dl	Age 20–30 130–230			
Triglyceride mg/dl	10–160			
HDL Cholesterol mg/dl	40–75			
CBC	See Hematology Report Sheet			
Urinalysis	See Microscopy Report Sheet			

Figure 8–9. Test profile for investigation of general health. (Adapted from Henry JB, Murphy J: Effective utilization of clinical laboratories. In Henry JB (ed.): Clinical Diagnosis and Management by Laboratory Methods, ed. 16. Philadelphia, WB Saunders Company, 1979, p 2042.)

CHEMISTRY

WATER/ELECTROLYTES/ACID-BASE

Test	Tube	Qty				Test	Tube	Qty			
ELECTROLYTES	(RED)	(2)	R	T	S	BONE	(RED)	(2)	R	T	
SODIUM		(1)	R	T	S	CALCIUM		(1)	R	T	S
POTASSIUM		(1)	R	T	S	PHOSPHOROUS		(1)	R	T	
CO_2 CONTENT		(1)	R	T	S	TOTAL PROTEIN		(1)	R	T	
CHLORIDE		(1)	R	T	S						
FLUID BALANCE	(RED)	(3)	R	T		RENAL	(RED)	(4)	R	T	
ELECTROLYTES		(2)	R	T	S	FLUID BALANCE		(3)	R	T	
UREA		(1)	R	T	S	BONE		(2)	R	T	
CREATININE		(1)	R	T	S	URIC ACID		(1)	R	T	
GLUCOSE		(1)	R	T	S						
PROTEINS	(RED)	(2)	R	DT		RENAL/LIVER	(RED)	(5)	R	T	
PROTEIN ELECTROPHORESIS						RENAL AND LIVER PROFILES		(4) (3)	R R	T T	
ACETONE	(RED)	(1)	R	T	S	OSMOLALITY	(RED)	(1)	R	T	S
LACTIC ACID	(GRAY/ICE)	(1)		T	S	MAGNESIUM	(RED)	(1)	R	T	S

ORGAN INJURY — ENZYMES

Test	Tube	Qty				Test	Tube	Qty			
LIVER	(RED)	(3)	R	T		CARDIAC	(RED)	(3)	R	DT	
BILIRUBIN, TOTAL		(1)	R	T		GOT		(1)	R	T	S
BILIRUBIN, DIRECT		(1)	R	T		LDH		(1)	R	T	
GOT		(1)	R	T	S	CPK ISOZYMES		(2)	R	DT	
GGT		(1)	R	T		CARDIAC #2	(RED)	(5)	R	DT	
LDH		(1)	R	T		GOT		(1)	R	T	S
ALKALINE PHOSPHATASE		(1)	R	T		LDH ISOZYMES		(2)	R	DT	
						CPK ISOZYMES		(2)	R	DT	
LIVER #2	(RED)	(4)	R	DT							
LIVER PROFILE		(3)	R	T							
LDH ISOZYMES		(2)	R	DT							
ORGAN INJURY	(RED)	(6)	R	DT		AMYLASE	(RED)	(1)	R	T	S
LIVER		(3)	R	T		ACID PHOSPHATASE		(1)	R	T	
LDH ISOZYMES		(2)	R	DT			(GREEN/ICE)				
CPK ISOZYMES		(2)	R	DT							

LIPIDS

Test	Tube	Qty				Test	Tube	Qty			
LIPID	(RED)	(2)	R	DT		LIPID #3	(REDX2)	(4)	R	DT	
CHOLESTEROL		(1)	R	DT		LIPID PROFILE #2		(3)	R	DT	
TRIGLYCERIDES		(2)	R	DT		LIPOPROTEIN ELECTROPHORESIS		(2)	R	DT	
LIPID #2	(REDX2)	(3)	R	DT							
LIPID PROFILE		(2)	R	DT							
HD LIPOPROTEIN		(2)	R	DT							

Notes:

Red, Gray, Lav., Blue = color of stoppers for blood collection tubes. One tube is required for test or profiles unless otherwise indicated. Example: Lipid Profile #2 requires 2 red stopper tubes (Red x 2). Coagulation Profile requires 1 lavender and 1 blue (lav/blue) stopper tubes.

R = routine collection (5:30 A.M.-7:30 A.M.). Requests must be in laboratory by 0130 hours.

T = today requests to be performed on the next scheduled run today.

DT = draw specimen today, perform the test on next scheduled run (usually the next day).

S = stat requests, collect specimen and perform test as soon as possible. Results phoned or printed out on patient unit.

(1) (2) (3) (4) = relative cost of laboratory test or test profile when ordered in the mode identified. Example: A serum potassium (1) ordered as a single test is 1/2 as expensive as electrolytes (2). It is no more expensive, however, to order the electrolyte profile which includes 4 tests than it is to order 2 of the electrolyte tests. Profiles will not be split to accommodate stat work.

Figure 8–10. Panels of tests that can be used to tailor different kinds of profiles, general or specific. (From Cole GW: Biochemical test profiles and laboratory system design. Hum Pathol 11:432, 1980.)

CHEMISTRY					HEMATOLOGY					
THYROID	(RED)	(3)	R	DT	BLOOD CELL(CBC)	(LAV.)	(1)	R	T	S
T$_3$ UPTAKE		(2)	R	DT	PCV		(1)	R	T	S
T$_4$ TOTAL		(2)	R	DT	HEMOGLOBIN		(1)	R	T	S
					RED CELL COUNT		(1)	R	T	S
TRIIODOTHYRONINE	(RED)	(3)	R	DT	INDICIES		(1)	R	T	S
IRON	(RED)	(1.5)	R	DT	WHITE CELL COUNT		(1)	R	T	S
IRON		(1)	R	DT	CBC #2	(LAV.)	(2)	R	T	S
IRON BINDING CAP					BLOOD CELL PROFILE		(1)	R	T	S
PHARMACEUTICALS	(RED)				DIFFERENTIAL WBC		(1)	R	T	S
PHENOBARBITAL		(2)	R	DT	CBC #3	(LAV.)	(2)	R	T	S
DIGOXIN		(2)	R	DT	BLOOD CELL PROFILE		(1)	R	T	S
DILANTIN		(2)	R	DT	PLATELET COUNT		(1)	R	T	S
PROCAINAMIDE		(2)	R	DT	CBC #4	(LAV.)	(3)	R	T	S
QUINIDINE		(2)	R	DT	BLOOD CELL PROFILE		(1)	R	T	S
SALICYLATE		(1)	R	DT	DIFFERENTIAL WBC		(1)	R	T	S
					PLATELET COUNT		(1)	R	T	S
IMMUNOLOGY					RETICULOCYTES	(LAV.)	(1)	R	T	
					SEDIMENTATION RATE	(BLUE)	(1)	R	T	
NEWBORN SCREEN	(RED)	(3)			HAPTOGLOBIN ELECTRO.		(2)	R	DT	
CORD BLOOD (SEND TO LAB)		(2)	R	DT		(RED)				
OR 1.5ML. VENOUS BLOOD		(3)			HAPTOGLOBIN AND					
OR 24 CAPILLARY TUBES		(3)			METHEMALBUMIN					
FUNGUS SCREEN	(RED)	(1)	R	DT	HEMOGLOBINOPATHY(LAV. X2)		(3)	R	DT	
HISTOPLASMOSIS					HEMOGLOBIN					
COCCIDIOMYCOSIS					ELECTROPHORESIS		(2)	R	DT	
BLASTOMYCOSIS					A$_2$ HEMOGLOBIN		(1)	R	DT	
IMMUNOELECTROPHORESIS		(2)	R	DT	FETAL HEMOGLOBIN		(1)	R	DT	
	(RED)				SICKLE CELL PREP		(1)	R	T	S
IMMUNOGLOBULINS	(RED)	(2)	R	DT	COAGULATION(LAV./BLUE)		(3)	R	T	S
IGG		(1)	R	DT	PROTHROMBIN TIME		(1)	R	T	S
IGA		(1)	R	DT		(BLUE)				
IGM		(1)	R	DT	PARTIAL THROMB TIME		(1)	R	T	S
RA LATEX(QUANT.)	(RED)	(1)	R	DT		(BLUE)				
ANA	(RED)	(2)	R	DT	PLATELET COUNT		(1)	R	T	S
LE PREP*	(RED)	(1)	R	T		(LAV.)				
URIC ACID (URICASE)	(RED)	(1)	R	DT	FIBRINOGEN		(1)	R	T	S
HB$_s$Ag	(RED)	(2)	R	DT		(BLUE)				
HB$_s$Ag ANTIBODY	(RED)	(2)	R	DT	CLOT LYSIS	(SPECIAL)	(2)	R	T	S
MONO SPOT TEST	(RED)	(1)	R	DT	FIBRIN SPLIT PROD.		(1)	R	T	S
FTA ABSORBED	(RED)	(1.5)	R	DT		(SPECIAL)				
					CLOTTING TIME	(SPECIAL)	(1)	R	T	S

*SPECIMEN AND/OR REQUEST MUST BE IN LAB BEFORE 2:00 P.M.
COLLECT IN A PLAIN RED STOPPER TUBE (V.#3200U) NOT CORVAC

Figure 8–11. Panels of tests that can be used to tailor different kinds of profiles, general or specific. (From Cole GW: Biochemical test profiles and laboratory system design. Hum Pathol 11:433, 1980.)

```
                              LUFKIN MEDICAL LABS
              450 MEDICAL ARTS BUILDING, MINNEAPOLIS 55402,   PHONE 612/335-2136




M                                             06-17  RUN NO. 152
AGE  60 MALE
NORMAL RANGES ASSUME PATIENT IS WALKING

TEST RESULTS

   CALCIUM      7.7       PHOSPHORUS    4.2      GLUCOSE     109.0
   BUN         37.0       URIC ACID     5.6      CHOLESTROL  177.0
   TOTAL PROT   5.4       LDH         149.0      SGOT         27.0
   ALBUMIN      2.8       BILIRUBIN      .4      ALK PTASE    86.0


ABNORMAL TEST            VALUE           NORMAL RANGE
   CALCIUM      LO         7.7           8.6 -  10.2
   PHOSPHORUS   HI         4.2           2.2 -   4.1
   BUN          HI        37.0           7.0 -  25.0
   TOTAL PROT   LO         5.4           6.1 -   7.7
   ALBUMIN      LO         2.8           3.3 -   5.1



      POSSIBLE DIAGNOSTIC PROBLEMS

   RENAL INSUFFICIENCY
      LO:  CALCIUM      TOTAL PROT  ALBUMIN
      HI:  PHOSPHORUS  BUN

   PRERENAL AZOTEMIA (CHF, SHOCK, ETC.)
      LO:  CALCIUM      TOTAL PROT  ALBUMIN
      HI:  PHOSPHORUS  BUN

   PANCREATITIS
      LO:  CALCIUM      TOTAL PROT  ALBUMIN
      HI:  BUN

   MALABSORPTION OR MALNUTRITION
      LO:  CALCIUM      TOTAL PROT  ALBUMIN

   REGIONAL ENTERITIS
      LO:  CALCIUM      TOTAL PROT  ALBUMIN

   NEPHROTIC SYNDROME
      LO:  TOTAL PROT  ALBUMIN
      HI:  BUN

   ULCERATIVE COLITIS, INTESTINAL OBSTRUCTION, ETC
      LO:  CALCIUM      TOTAL PROT  ALBUMIN

   LEUKEMIA OR OTHER MYELOPROLIFERATIVE DISORDERS
      LO:  CALCIUM      TOTAL PROT  ALBUMIN
```

Figure 8–12. Computer-assisted interpretive report. (From Reece RL, Hobbie RK: Computer evaluation of chemistry values: A reporting and diagnostic aid. Am J Clin Pathol. 57:666, 1972.)

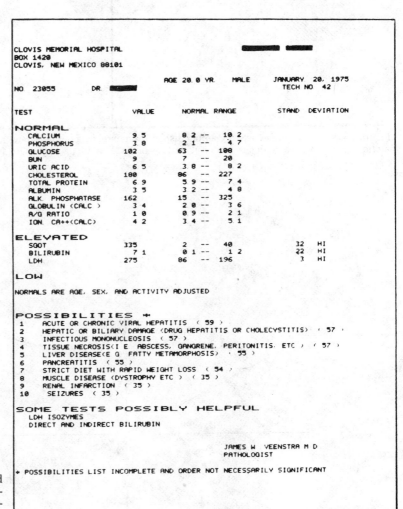

Figure 8–13. Computer-assisted interpretive report. (From Veenstra JW: Routine automated interpretation of chemistry profiles. Laboratory Medicine 6:51, 1975.)

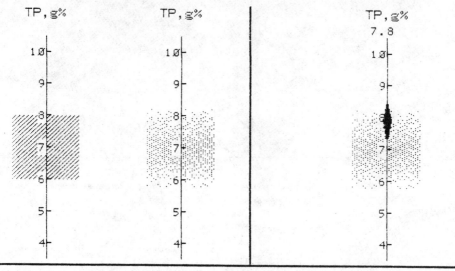

Figure 8–14. Computer-assisted graphic display of reference population with superimposed display of an analytic value and its confidence limits. (Courtesy of B. T. Williams, M.D., Regional Health Resources Center, Urbana, Ill.)

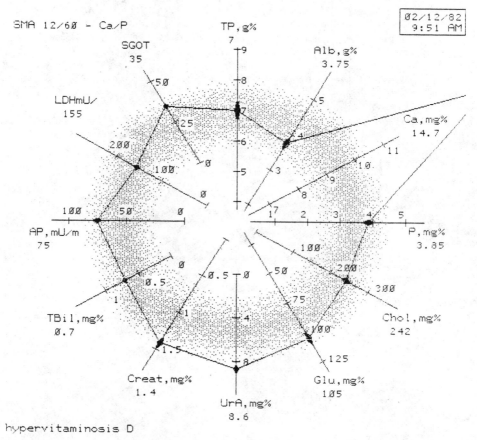

Figure 8–15. Computer-assisted radial plot of 12-channel chemistry test results. (Courtesy of B. T. Williams, M.D., Regional Health Resources Center, Urbana, Ill.)

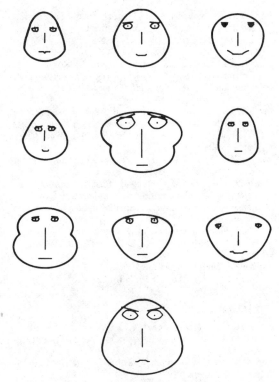

Figure 8–16. Computer-assisted graphic display of biochemical test results showing faces, which depict results of various individuals. (From Robertson EA, Van Steirteghem AC, Byrkit JE, Young DA: Biochemical individuality and the recognition of personal profiles with a computer. Clin Chem 26:32, 1980.)

files based on a pathologist's review (23 per cent in the survey of Speicher and Smith, 1980). Others have devised computer-assisted interpretive reports (Figs. 8–12 and 8–13. Good reviews of computer-assisted interpretive reporting are available by Hobbie and Reece (1981) and Elevitch (1982).

The SMA 6/60 and 12/60 (Technicon Instruments Corporation, Tarrytown, NY) biochemical profiles use graphic displays of test results as a method of interpretive reporting (Figs. 8–6 through 8–8). In this regard, a vector plot of chemistry test results appears promising (Figs. 8–14 and 8–15). Robertson and associates (1980) designed a system for displaying biochemical test results that produces graphic displays in the form of computer-drawn faces (Table 8–12 and Fig. 8–16).

Table 8–12. FACIAL FEATURES CONTROLLED BY TEST RESULTS*

Radius to corner of face
Angle of radius to horizontal
Vertical size of face
Eccentricity of upper face
Eccentricity of lower face
Length of nose
Vertical position of mouth
Curvature of mouth
Width of mouth
Vertical location of eyes
Separation of eyes
Slant of eyes
Eccentricity of eyes
Size of eyes
Position of pupils
Vertical position of eyebrows
Slant of eyebrows
Size of eyebrows

The purpose of this table is simply to tell the reader which facial features were varied. An "esthetically reasonable" range was chosen for an individual feature, the results of the corresponding test were scaled with a linear transform ($y = a + bx$) so that the transformed test results fell within the "esthetically reasonable" range.

*From Robertson EA, Van Steirteghem AC, Byrkit JE, et al: Biochemical individuality and the recognition of personal profiles with a computer. Clin Chem 26:32, 1980.

REFERENCES

Value of Screening

Altshuler CH: The problem: Assuring appropriate transfer and utilization of laboratory information. In Werner M: Consultation in Laboratory Medicine by Pathologists. Chicago, American Society of Clinical Pathologists, 1980, pp 49–55.

Altshuler CH, Bareta J, Cafaro AF, et al: The PALI and SLIC systems. CRC Crit Rev Clin Lab Sci 3:379–402, 1972.

Babb RR: An evaluation of the executive health examination. West J Med 133:260–263, 1980.

Burke MD: Clinical problem solving and laboratory investigation: Contribution to laboratory medicine. In Stefanini M, Benson ES (eds): Progress in Clinical Pathology, Volume VIII. New York, Grune & Stratton, Inc, 1981, pp 1–24.

Collen MF: Cost effectiveness of multiphasic health testing. In Young DS, Nipper H, Uddin D, et al (eds): Clinician and Chemist: The Relationship of the Laboratory to the Physician. Washington, DC, American Association for Clinical Chemistry, Inc, 1979, pp 121–130.

Durbridge TC, Edwards RG: The validity of screening. In Benson ES, Rubin M (eds): Logic and Economics of Clinical Laboratory Use. New York, Elsevier, North Holland, Inc., 1978, pp 197–202.

Durbridge TC, Edwards F, Edwards RG, et al: Evaluation of benefits of screening tests done immediately on admission to hospital. Clin Chem 22:968–971, 1976.

Galen RS: Multiphasic screening and biochemical profiles: State of the art, 1975. In Stefanini M, Isenberg HD (eds): Progress in Clinical Pathology. Vol VI. New York, Grune & Stratton, Inc., 1975, pp 83–110.

Pribor HC: Biochemical profiling. Laboratory Management, January 1980, pp 27–30.

Pribor HC: Profiling: Another look. Laboratory Management, February 1981, pp 23–25.

Sackett D, Holland WW: Controversy in the detection of disease. Lancet 2:357–359, 1975.

Werner M, Altshuler CH: Utility of multiphasic biochemical screening and systematic laboratory investigations. Clin Chem 25:509–511, 1979.

Werner M, Altshuler CH: Cost effectiveness of multiphasic screening: Old controversies and a new rationale. Hum Pathol 12:111–117, 1981.

Wheeler LA, Brecher G, Sheiner LB: Clinical laboratory use in the evaluation of anemia. JAMA 238:2709–2714, 1977.

Inflammation

Daniels JC, Larson DL, Abston S, et al: Serum protein profiles in thermal burns: II. Protease inhibitors, complement factors, and C-reactive protein. J Trauma 14:153–162, 1974.

Deodhar SD, Valenzuela R: C-reactive protein: New findings and specific applications. Laboratory Management, June 1981, pp 47–53.

Evans MI, Hajj SN, DeVoe LD, et al: C-reactive protein as a predictor of infectious morbidity with premature rupture of membranes. Am J Obstet Gynecol 138:648–652, 1980.

Fischer CL, Gill CW: Acute-phase proteins. In Ritzmann SE, Daniels JC (eds): Serum Protein Abnormalities. Diagnostic and Clinical Aspects. Boston, Little, Brown & Company, 1975, pp 331–350.

Friedman RB, Anderson RE, Entine SM, et al: Effects of disease on clinical laboratory tests. Clin Chem 26:1D–476D, 1980.

Gambino SR (ed): A CRP supplement. Lab Report for Physicians 4(1):1–5, 1982.

Gambino SR, DiRe JJ, Monteleone M, et al: The Westergren sedimentation rate, using K₃EDTA. Am J Clin Pathol 43:173–180, 1965.

Gewurz H, Mold C, Siegel J, et al: C-reactive protein and the acute phase response. In Stollerman GH (ed): Advances in Internal Medicine. Chicago, Year Book Publishers, Inc, 1982, pp 345–372.

Gill WG, Bush S, Burleigh WM, et al: An evaluation of a C-reactive protein assay using a rate immu-nonephelometric procedure. Am J Clin Pathol 75:50–55, 1981.

Jodal U, Hanson LA: Sequential determination of C-reactive protein in acute childhood pyelonephritis. Acta Pediatr Scand 65:319–324, 1976.

McCarthy PL, Frank AL, Ablow RC, et al: Value of C-reactive protein in the differentiation of bacterial and viral pneumonia. J Pediatr 92:454–456, 1978.

Pepys MB, Druguet M, Klass HJ, et al: Ciba Foundation Symposium 46. Immunology of the Gut. New York, Elsevier, Excerpta Medica, North-Holland, 1977, pp 283–304.

Robbins SL, Cotran RS: Inflammation. In Robbins SL, Cotran RS (eds): Pathologic Basis of Disease, ed 2. Philadelphia, WB Saunders Company, 1979, pp 55–90.

Smith SJ, Bos G, Esseveld MR, et al: Acute phase proteins from the liver and enzymes from myocardial infarction: A quantitative relationship. Clin Chim Acta 81:75–85, 1977.

Swaim WR: The Westergren vs. the zeta sedimentation ratio test. JAMA 245:1161–1162, 1981.

Walsh L, Davies P, McConkey B: Relationship between erythrocyte sedimentation rate and serum C-reactive protein in rheumatoid arthritis. Ann Rheum Dis 38:362–363, 1979.

Whicher JT: The role of the acute phase proteins. Diagnostic Medicine, May/June 1981, pp 52–69.

Whicher JT, Bell AM, Southall PJ: Inflammation: Measurements in clinical management. Diagnostic Medicine, July/August 1981, pp 62–80.

Pregnancy

Bates HM: Ectopic pregnancy: RIA for the beta-hCG subunit. Laboratory Management, February 1981, pp 27–28.

Bish DJ: Routine pregnancy testing is a must! Lab, 79. June 1979, pp 8–10.

Horwitz CA: Pregnancy tests 1980: Advantages and limitations. Laboratory Medicine 11:620–623, 1980.

Keller PJ: Human chorionic gonadotropin. Contrib Gynecol Obstet 2:92–113, 1976.

Milwidsky A, Adoni, A. Miodovnik M, et al: Human chorionic gonadotrophin (beta-subunit) in the early diagnosis of ectopic pregnancy. Obstet Gynecol 51:725–726, 1978.

Park RC: Pregnancy testing: An update. Newsletter, Armed Forces District, The American College of Obstetricians and Gynecologists, Vol III, No 3, 1980.

Pelosi MA, Apuzzio J, Harrigan JT: What to expect from the new generation of pregnancy tests. Cont Ob/Gyn 17:233–246, 1981.

Schwartz RO, DiPietro DL: Beta-hCG as a diagnostic aid for suspected ectopic pregnancy. Obstet Gynecol 56:197–203, 1980.

Multiphasic Screening by Chemistry Tests

Altshuler CH, Bareta J, Cafaro AF, et al: The PALI and SLIC systems. CRC Crit Rev Clin Lab Sci 3:379–402, 1972.

Beeler MF: Interpretations in Clinical Chemistry. Chicago, American Society of Clinical Pathologists, 1979.

Beeler MF, Catrou PG: Interpretation of the biochemical profile. ASCP Check Sample, Clinical Chemistry No. CC-120. Chicago, American Society of Clinical Pathologists, 1979.

Cole GW: Biochemical test profiles and laboratory system design. Hum Pathol 11:424–434, 1980.

Elevitch FR: Computer-assisted clinical laboratory

interpretive reports. Laboratory Medicine 13:45–47, 1982.

Grams RR, Lezotte D: Unlimited volumes of laboratory data. J Med Syst 2:343–345, 1978.

Grams RR, Lezotte D, Gudat JC: Establishing a multivariate clinical laboratory data base. J Med Syst 2:355–362, 1978.

Henry JB, Howanitz PJ: Organ panels and the relationship of the laboratory to the physician. In Jones RJ, Palulonis RM (eds): Chicago, American Medical Association, 1980, p 29.

Hobbie RK, Reece RL: Interpretive reporting by computer. Hum Pathol 12:127–134, 1981.

Lufkin N, Chadbourn W, Popowich J, et al: A portfolio of patterns. Lufkin Medical Laboratories Letter, May 1969, pp 19–22.

Preston JA, Troxel DB: Biochemical Profiling in Diagnostic Medicine. Tarrytown, NY, Technicon Instruments Corporation, 1971.

Reece RL, Hobbie RK: Computer evaluation of chemistry values: A reporting and diagnostic aid. Am J Clin Pathol 57:664–675, 1972.

Robertson EA, Van Steirteghem AC, Byrkit JE, et al: Biochemical individuality and the recognition of personal profiles with a computer. Clin Chem 26:30–36, 1980.

Speicher CE, Smith JW: Interpretive reporting in clinical pathology. JAMA 243:1556–1560, 1980.

Veenstra JW: Routine automated interpretation of chemistry profiles. Laboratory Medicine 6:50–52, 1975.

Ward PCJ: Chemical profiles of disease. Hum Pathol 4:47–65, 1973.

Wolf PL: Interpretation of Biochemical Multitest Profiles: An analysis of 100 important conditions. New York, Masson Publishing USA, Inc, 1977.

CHAPTER 9

THE UNEXPECTED TEST RESULT

HOW DO UNEXPECTED TEST
  RESULTS OCCUR?
EXAMPLES OF ABNORMAL TEST
  RESULTS
  Unexplained Elevation of Serum
    ALP Levels
  Unexplained Elevation of Serum
    Calcium Levels

HOW DO UNEXPECTED TEST
RESULTS OCCUR?

This chapter is concerned with the subproblem of finding the explanation for an unexpected test result rather than solving a clinical subproblem in the context of a particular set of signs and symptoms. These unexpected test results, which may be within or outside the reference intervals, can arise in the course of multiphasic screening or in the course of working up a particular clinical subproblem. Our examples of the unexplained elevation of serum alkaline phosphatase (ALP) and of serum calcium will illustrate how to work up unexpected findings for other analytes in a timely, decisive, and cost-effective manner.

The unexpected test result can arise in two ways:

1. Minor "abnormalities" are a common occurrence during screening. The chances for an abnormality increase in direct proportion to the number of tests performed (Table 9–1). Frequently, these test results are statistical outliers in patients who are free of disease. Sometimes, however, a test result lying outside the reference interval can serve as a clue to an unexpected or occult disease process. The follow-up of statistical outliers in patients who are free of disease has been criticized as a waste of money and is used as an argument against screening.

2. Unexpected test results also occur during the course of a clinical workup when laboratory results are not consistent with the diagnoses under consideration.

Table 9–1. PERCENTAGE OF PERSONS EXPECTED TO BE NORMAL FOR A NUMBER OF TESTS, EACH USING $\bar{x} \pm 2s$ NORMAL RANGE*

Number of Different Tests	Persons Expected to Be Normal for All Tests Undertaken (%)
1	95.45
2	91.11
3	86.96
4	83.00
5	79.23
6	75.62
7	72.18
8	68.90
9	65.76
10	62.77
11	59.91
12	57.19

*From Barnett RN: Clinical Laboratory Statistics. Boston, Little, Brown & Co, 1979, p 171.

For these two situations, it is useful to have an approach for solving the problem of an unexpected test result. Is the patient free of disease, or is the elevation a clue to occult disease? An advantage of the programmed accelerated laboratory investigation (PALI) of Altshuler and co-workers (1972) is that it provides automatic follow-up of unexpected abnormal test results.

Before the advent of screening by laboratory tests, the problem of the unexplained abnormal test result was less common. Physicians made diagnoses and initiated treatment on the basis of a history and physical examination supplemented by appropriate laboratory studies. The history and physical examination generated hypotheses, and laboratory tests were sometimes used to confirm or exclude these hypotheses. The introduction of screening reversed this sequence of data gathering. When part of a routine hospital admission battery, multiple laboratory tests may now be performed even in the absence of a physician's request. Physicians may also order a large number of studies to discover occult abnormalities or preclinical disease without specific hypotheses in mind (Morrow, 1975).

If screening results in an unexplained abnormal test result in the absence of signs or symptoms, the physician must either ignore the finding or consider diagnostic or therapeutic measures. Morrow (1975) labeled the patient's state of health in which no signs and symptoms are present except for an unexplained abnormal test result as "iatrogenesis imperfecta." Rang (1972) described the Ulysses syndrome, which consists of a previously healthy person's emerging from a routine periodic health examination with a false-positive test result. Like Ulysses, the patient must pass through a long journey of investigative procedures before returning to the previous state of health.

A study by Schneiderman and colleagues (1972) concluded that some physicians tend to pay little attention to the abnormal results of screening tests; rarely did abnormal results lead to positive diagnoses. Other studies showed the same tendency (Altshuler, 1980; Wheeler et al., 1977). (See Chapter 8 on the value of screening.)

An unexplained abnormal test result sometimes ignored by physicians is an elevated serum ALP in the absence of other findings. An investigative workup often leads to no diagnosis whatsoever—and sometimes at great expense. In our experience, a group of physicians have routinely followed up unexplained elevations of serum ALP by ordering determinations of serum ALP isoenzymes, liver scintiscans, and bone survey radiologic studies.

We propose a general approach to determine whether unexplained abnormalities are indicative of disease:

1. Repeat the measurement.
   a. Prepare the patient properly.
   b. Obtain a proper sample.
   c. Ensure appropriate specimen handling.
   d. Practice good laboratory methodology.
2. Use the correct reference interval.
3. Consider possible drug-metabolite interferences.
4. Consider differential diagnoses.
5. Proceed with follow-up studies if appropriate.

This approach is illustrated by the following examples of unexplained elevations of serum ALP and serum calcium. Information in Part 3 will describe the approach to unexpected results of other common tests.

EXAMPLES OF ABNORMAL TEST RESULTS

UNEXPLAINED ELEVATION OF SERUM ALP LEVELS

Definition and Significance

Elevated ALP frequently occurs in the course of multiphasic screening or in the laboratory workup of a particular disease. Although it is sometimes found in patients free of disease, an elevated serum ALP can have pathologic meaning and serve as a clue to serious disease of the heart, lungs, gastrointestinal tract, kidneys, liver, spleen, and bones as well as to neoplastic disease. A decrease in serum ALP can also have pathologic significance.

Pathophysiology

Elevated serum ALP levels can occur in various conditions:

1. During the reparative phase of an acute myocardial infarct lasting from 4 to 10 days after the onset of infarction. The elevation is

presumed to arise from the vascular endothelium of the repair tissue. Congestive heart failure can elevate the serum level of liver ALP. (See the discussion of acute myocardial infarction in Chapter 10.) The reparative phase of an acute pulmonary infarct can be associated with an elevation of serum ALP that lasts 1 to 2 weeks after the onset of infarction. The ALP is believed to originate in the vascular endothelium of the reparative tissue. (See the discussion of pulmonary embolism in Chapter 11.)

2. Presence of lesions of the stomach and small intestine. If the small intestinal lesion produces malabsorption, serum bone ALP can be elevated secondary to vitamin D deficiency. (See the discussion of malabsorption in Chapter 13.)

3. In acute infarction of the kidneys or spleen, secondary to repair.

4. In hepatic disease, especially of an obstructive nature. (See the discussion of liver function tests, cholestasis, and hyperbilirubinemia in Chapter 15.)

5. In osseous disease when there is increased activity of osteoblasts.

6. In pregnancy, as a result of placental ALP. (See the discussion of pregnancy in Chapter 8.)

7. Rarely, the production of ectopic ALP by a neoplasm (Regan or Nagao isoenzyme). Neoplastic ALP tends to resemble placental ALP.

Clinical Contexts

Diagnosis.   When there is an unexpected elevation of serum ALP, we should search for signs and symptoms of disease in organs that can be associated with a high serum ALP—namely, heart, lungs, liver, spleen, kidneys, gastrointestinal tract, bones, placenta—as well as neoplasms. We should also consider drugs that can elevate serum ALP levels.

Management.   An elevated serum ALP level can be used to follow the course of a disease and its response to therapy, for example, following the response of a prostatic carcinoma with osteoblastic metastases treated with chemotherapy. (See the discussion of prostatic carcinoma in Chapter 12.)

Screening.   Elevated serum ALP can be discovered in the course of multiphasic screening. (See Chapter 8.)

Strategy

Test Sequence.   The strategy for an unexplained elevation of serum ALP is as follows:

1. Repeat the serum ALP measurement, using the best method available.
2. Use the correct reference interval.
3. Obtain a serum gamma-glutamyl transpeptidase (GGT) level.
4. Consider possible drug-metabolite interferences.
5. Consider differential diagnoses.
6. If history and physical examination suggest disease, and other laboratory studies are outside the reference intervals, proceed with the following measures:
   a. Order a determination of serum ALP isoenzymes.
   b. Perform bone survey radiologic studies.
   c. Do a liver scintiscan.

Patient Preparation.   Ideally, the patient should be fasting in order to obviate an elevated level after meals. This tendency is accentuated in patients of blood groups O and B who are secretors. Serum ALP is slightly higher in the standing versus recumbent position.

Specimen Collection and Handling.   Avoid hemolysis; a small amount of ALP is present in erythrocytes. If possible, perform the analysis within 24 hours because serum ALP can increase with storage. Use only serum or heparinized plasma.

Methodology.   Consult the laboratory for methodology, reference intervals, and potential sources of interference. Use a good method for ALP such as that of Bowers and McComb (1976) with *para*-nitrophenylphosphate as the substrate.

Interpretation

Diagnosis.   There is a sequence of questions to answer in the diagnostic interpretation of an unexplained elevation of serum ALP (Fig. 9–1):

1. Is the elevation caused by errors in patient preparation, specimen collection and handling, or laboratory procedure or by the use of an inappropriate reference interval?
2. If 1. is not the case, can elevation be due to drug-metabolite interference?
3. If 1. and 2. are not the case, what diseases

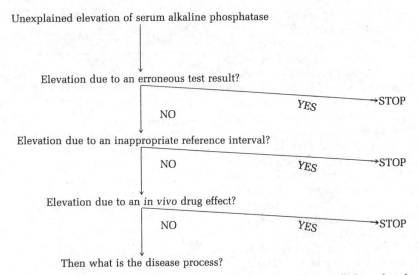

Figure 9–1. Diagnostic reasoning for an unexplained elevation of serum alkaline phosphatase

or disorders can cause an elevated serum ALP level?

4. What additional procedures can help identify the pathologic cause of an elevated serum ALP level?

In the following discussion, a strategy for answering each of these questions is described.

1. Is the elevation caused by errors in patient preparation, specimen collection and handling, or laboratory procedure or by the use of an inappropriate reference interval?

McComb and colleagues (1979) wrote a comprehensive text on ALP; see Chapter 9 in their book for a discussion on the clinical use of serum ALP measurements. An article on the significance of elevated and decreased serum ALP levels is available by Wolf (1978).

Unexplained elevations of serum ALP levels can be due to errors in obtaining the specimen or in performing the measurement. Therefore, the serum ALP measurement should be repeated to verify that the test result is not due to improper procedures. Standards and controls for the ALP test run should be acceptable. Next, it is important to use reference intervals that are appropriate for the particular method used to measure serum ALP and to be aware of differences that are due to age and sex. Growing children and pregnant women have elevated levels of serum ALP. Munan and associates (1979) determined reference intervals for serum ALP by SMA 12/60 analysis (Technicon Instruments Corpora-

tion, Tarrytown, NY) with results in U/liter at 37°C. The 97.5 percentiles, or upper reference limits, for males and females by age group are given in Table 9–2.

It is preferable to compare an individual's resulting serum ALP level with that level obtained in a previous state of health. Statland and colleagues (1976) cited a CV of 3.5 per cent for intraindividual variation for serum ALP compared with a 24.8 per cent for interindividual variation.

There is a small but definite increase in serum ALP following meals, particularly those high in fat. This rise is caused by entry of intestinal ALP into the circulation and is ac-

Table 9–2. UPPER REFERENCE LIMITS FOR SERUM ALKALINE PHOSPHATASE*

| Age Group (Yr) | Upper Reference Limit (U/liter) | |
	Males	Females
10–14	325	339
15–19	182	176
20–24	102	98
25–34	109	100
35–44	122	112
45–54	139	121
55–64	159	132
65–74	161	172
75+	227	199

*Adapted from Munan L, Kelly A, Petitclerc C: Population survey enzyme patterns: Age–sex dependencies. In McComb RB, Bowers GN Jr, Posen S (eds): Alkaline Phosphatase, New York, Plenum Press, 1979, p 528.

centuated in subjects having blood groups B and O who are secretors (Wolf, 1978). Therefore, when repeating a serum ALP measurement to verify accuracy, it is worthwhile to draw a specimen after the patient has fasted. If the patient stands for longer than 30 minutes slightly higher serum ALP levels will result than if the patient reclines (Statland et al., 1974).

Only serum or heparinized plasma, preferably free of hemolysis, should be used for ALP measurements. The cells should be separated within 1 to 2 hours of collection. Minimal hemolysis is probably acceptable, since the concentration of ALP in erythrocytes is only about six times that of serum using the phenylphosphate method. Oxalate, citrate, fluoride, and EDTA inhibit the enzyme (Henry et al., 1974). Fresh human serum ALP can increase spuriously following storage (1 per cent during a working day and 5 per cent during 4 days) with or without refrigeration (Massion and Frankenfeld, 1972). Therefore, the repeat serum ALP measurement should be performed promptly.

2. Can the elevated serum ALP level be due to drug-metabolite interference?

A large number of drugs can increase serum ALP levels secondary to cholestatic or hepatocellular disease (McComb et al., 1979; Schiff, 1975; Young, 1975). Examples include chlorpromazine, methyltestosterone, and estrogenic and progestational agents. Serum albumin extracted from human placental tissue contains a large amount of ALP and intravenous administration of this product will elevate the level.

Part 3 presents a list of drugs that can elevate serum ALP. This compilation illustrates the extensive information on drug interferences available in the work of Young and associates (1975).

3. What diseases or disorders can elevate the serum ALP level?

A number of diseases can elevate serum ALP (Table 9–3); (see Friedman et al., 1980; McComb et al., 1979; and Wolf, 1978). It is important to remember that most patients with multiple myeloma have normal serum ALP levels.

Wolf (1978) found that in hepatic disease the level of serum ALP can give a clue to the kind of disorder present (a decision level), with the highest levels (a 20- to 25-fold increase) occurring in primary biliary cirrhosis or carcinoma, metastatic or primary. (See Chapter 15.)

Table 9–3. DISEASES AND DISORDERS THAT CAN ELEVATE SERUM ALKALINE PHOSPHATASE (ALP)*

Cardiovascular
Cardiac failure (hepatic ALP from congestion)
Organization of myocardial infarct (ALP from angioblastic proliferation)

Respiratory
Organization of pulmonary infarct (ALP from angioblastic proliferation)

Urinary
Chronic renal failure (bone ALP)
Nephrotic syndrome (?)
Organization of renal infarct (ALP from angioblastic proliferation)

Gastrointestinal
Erosive or ulcerative lesion of small intestine, stomach, or colon (intestinal ALP)
Malabsorption (bone ALP from vitamin D deficiency)

Pancreatic
Acute pancreatitis (hepatic ALP)
Carcinoma of head of pancreas (hepatic ALP)
Chronic pancreatitis (hepatic or bone ALP from vitamin D deficiency)
Cystic fibrosis (hepatic or bone ALP due to vitamin D deficiency)

Hepatobiliary
Any kind of liver disease, especially with cholestasis (hepatic ALP)

Hematologic
Leukemia (?)
Myelofibrosis (?)

Endocrine
Acromegaly (bone ALP)
Adrenal cortical hyperfunction (bone ALP)
Diabetes mellitus with ketoacidosis (?)
Hyperparathyroidism (bone ALP)
Hyperthyroidism (bone ALP)
Hypothyroidism (bone ALP)

Infections
Many infections, especially with bone or liver disease (bone or liver ALP)

Musculoskeletal
Osteoblastic bone lesions (bone ALP)
Osteomalacia (bone ALP)
Rhabdomyolysis (bone ALP ?)
Rickets (bone ALP)

Neoplasia
Neoplastic production (Regan or Nagao isoenzyme) (ectopic ALP)
Tumors involving bone or liver (bone or liver ALP)

Miscellaneous
Familial hyperphosphatasemia (liver ALP ?)
Unexplained elevation (?)

*Proposed pathologic mechanism for the elevations follows in parentheses.

4. What additional procedures can help to identify the pathologic cause of an elevated serum ALP level?

Determining the levels of serum ALP isoenzymes, serum GGT, and urinary hydroxyproline is helpful. Determinations of serum GGT offer greater diagnostic sensitivity and specificity for liver disease than those for serum leucine aminopeptidase and 5'-nucleotidase (Gambino, 1979). Serum GGT is invariably elevated in liver disease but rarely in bone disease. Urinary excretion of hydroxyproline is often elevated in bone disease. The requirement of a timed urine collection limits the utility and convenience of urinary hydroxyproline measurements.

Modestly elevated levels of serum ALP not due to specimen errors, test performance errors, or drugs when correct reference intervals have been used should be considered for further follow-up studies. A serum GGT test is inexpensive and should be done. However, unless the serum ALP is markedly elevated, it is our opinion that expensive further studies should not be routinely done in the absence of positive clues to the presence of disease obtained from the clinical history, physical examination, or other laboratory evaluations.

Management. The use of the elevated serum ALP strategy in management can be illustrated by this example. A woman returns for evaluation 1 year after having had a total hysterectomy for an early carcinoma of the uterine cervix. During the evaluation, a multichannel chemistry profile reveals an isolated elevation of serum ALP. Other laboratory studies, as well as the clinical history and physical examination, are within normal limits. The physician is faced with the dilemma of either ignoring the elevated serum ALP level, with the accompanying risk of missing occult metastatic disease, or admitting her to the hospital and performing follow-up studies (using serum ALP isoenzymes, a liver scintiscan, and bone survey radiographic tests).

Our personal experience with this dilemma stimulated us to develop a strategy to help decide whether or not the elevated serum ALP is indicative of disease. The merit of this strategy is that it enables the physician either to determine quickly that the elevated serum ALP is not a reflection of disease or to proceed with follow-up studies with confidence that they are necessary. This strategy can serve as a model to resolve other unexplained laboratory test results (Speicher, 1981).

Test Requests and Reports

Test Requests. The execution of this strategy can be offered by the laboratory as a clinical problem-solving service. A repeat ALP and serum GGT measurement can be performed.

Interpretive Reports. A consultative interpretive report can be sent to the requesting physician. This report would help to determine whether or not the elevated ALP level is indicative of disease. Figure 9–2 shows the report used for serum ALP isoenzymes.

UNEXPLAINED ELEVATION OF SERUM CALCIUM LEVELS

Definition and Significance

An elevated serum calcium level is another example of an unexplained abnormal test result that occasionally occurs during screening. Heath and colleagues (1980) cite the Mayo Clinic experience during the period that followed introduction of a 12-channel chemistry profile in mid-1974. After the beginning of automated blood testing, about half of 51 patients found to have hypercalcemia had symptoms related to hyperparathyroidism, whereas prior to automated testing, 80 per cent of patients with hypercalcemia had problems related to hypersecretion of the parathyroid glands. Thus, 26 asymptomatic patients showed unexplained elevations of serum calcium, whereas in the prior 9 ½ years, only seven asymptomatic patients had shown unexplained elevations of serum calcium.

If the situation at the Mayo Clinic is extrapolated nationwide, 35,000 to 86,000 new cases of patients with unexplained elevations of serum calcium would be discovered annually in the United States. Depending upon whether these patients undergo operations for hyperparathyroidism (the median cost of surgery in 1977 was $1,700) or are followed up (the cost of an annual checkup in 1977 was $315), unexplained elevations of serum calcium would boost national medical costs by $60 million to $146 million annually (Bishop, 1980). The prevalence of hypercalcemia varies from 0.1 to 2.9 per cent, depending on the population, number of serum calcium measurements per person, laboratory methods, and definition of the reference interval for serum calcium concentration (Christensson et al., 1976).

Whether or not to perform parathyroidec-

Form 9245
468213

OHIO STATE UNIVERSITY HOSPITALS
CLINICAL CHEMISTRY LABORATORY

ALKALINE PHOSPHATASE
ISOENZYMES
REPORT FORM

Date Requested:_____

TOTAL ALKALINE PHOSPHATASE ACTIVITY: _____U/liter

NORMAL:	FEMALES:	30-72	U/liter
	MALES:	30-94	U/liter
	CHILDREN:	100-240	U/liter (with increases to 300 U/liter during growth spurts in males)

ISOENZYMES:

BONE_____

LIVER I _____

LIVER II _____

BILIARY _____

INTESTINAL _____

PLACENTAL _____

OTHER_____

SIGNATURE _____ DATE

INTERPRETATION

1. NORMAL:
   Most individuals normally have only bone and liver I isoenzymes in their serum.

2. BONE:
   An increase of bone isozyme is indicative of increased osteoblastic activity. Small increases may be observed on resumption of ambulation following prolonged bed rest.

3. LIVER I:
   Liver I isozyme is normally secreted by liver into the circulation, and increased serum levels are due to enhanced biosynthesis and/or secretion, or to hepatic congestion and decreased clearance of the enzyme. Liver I enzyme also occurs in vascular endothelium, and serum levels may be increased slightly due to vasculitis.

4. LIVER II:
   Liver II isozyme is an intracellular enzyme that is not normally secreted. Its presence in serum is believed to be indicative of parenchymal cell damage.

5. BILIARY:
   Biliary phosphatase is formed in the biliary tree and is normally secreted in bile. Its presence in serum may be indicative of cholestasis.

6. INTESTINAL:
   Some patients with intestinal disease have intestinal phosphatase in their serum, but many such patients do not, and the significance of increased serum levels of this isoenzyme is not fully known. Some individuals of blood type O or B normally have a small amount of intestinal phosphatase, particularly after meals.

7. PLACENTAL:
   Placental phosphatase occurs in serum during the first trimester of pregnancy, and increases throughout pregnancy. Liver I isozyme may also increase moderately during pregnancy.

8. UNIDENTIFIED:
   A variety of "unidentified" isozymes may occur, and are frequently found to be of neoplastic origin. Some of these isoenzymes are heat stable and may be useful in monitoring a patient's progress.

9. DRUG EFFECTS:
   Hepatotoxic drugs may cause increased total alkaline phosphatase due to increased liver I and biliary isozymes. A listing of drugs that affect alkaline phosphatase is given in: "Effect of Drugs on Clinical Laboratory Tests." Clin. Chem. 21:1D-432D (1975).

   Some albumin preparations (Plasmonate) contain a heat stable phosphatase in sufficient amount to increase serum levels.

Figure 9–2. Intrepretive report for alkaline phosphatase isoenzymes. (Courtesy of Ohio State University Hospitals.)

tomy in every case of mild, asymptomatic hypercalcemia is debatable. Heath and colleagues (1980) found that asymptomatic hypercalcemic patients discovered by screening tend to have high blood pressure, perhaps secondary to nephropathy. (See the discussion of hypertension in Chapter 10.) Some authorities believe that until further clinical studies are completed, it is best to recommend parathyroidectomy to all patients with asymptomatic hypercalcemia because the procedure is curative and because renal damage can occur in some patients who are not treated. Fifteen to 18 per cent of patients will need surgery within 5 years because of organic progression or anxiety and as a result of the burden of intensive medical follow-up (Coe and Favus, 1980; Hodgson, 1981). Bilezikian (1982) reviewed non-surgical alternatives to the therapy of mild, chronic hypercalcemia resulting from primary hyperparathyroidism. Reviews are available on hypercalcemic disorders (Lee, 1978) and hyperparathyroidism (Potts, 1980).

Pathophysiology

Total serum calcium, as measured in the clinical laboratory, represents the sum of three fractions: One is bound to protein, a second forms diffusible calcium complexes (e.g., calcium citrate), and a third consists of ionized calcium. For clinical purposes, approximately 50 per cent of the total serum calcium concentration can be taken as an approximation of the ionized calcium fraction. The overwhelming majority of disorders of calcium homeostasis are related to disturbances in the concentration of serum ionized calcium. The day-to-day fluctuations in total serum calcium concentration are almost totally accounted for by changes in the fraction bound to protein (mostly albumin). Serum ionized calcium is maintained within a very narrow range. In practice, a change in serum albumin concentration of 1 gm/100 ml can be expected to result in a change of total serum calcium concentration of approximately 0.8 mg/100 ml in the same direction below or above the middle of the reference interval (Lancet editorial, 1979; Lee et al., 1978). Alkalosis decreases the concentration of serum ionized calcium, and acidosis increases it.

The pathophysiologic mechanisms governing serum levels of ionized calcium are related to complex interrelated variables that include the

Table 9–4. CAUSES OF HYPERCALCEMIA*

Neoplasms
 Skeletal metastases
 Increased production of parathyroid hormone (PTH)
  or PTH-like factors
  Coexistent hyperparathyroidism
  Ectopic PTH secretion
   (pseudohyperparathyroidism)
 Non-PTH hypercalcemic factors
  Osteolytic phytosterols
  Prostaglandins
  Osteoclast activating factors
  Vasoactive intestinal peptides (VIP)
 Neoplasm-related complications
  Dehydration
  Acute immobilization
  Therapeutic agents: estrogens, androgens,
   progestins, tamoxifen
  Adrenal insufficiency secondary to tumor
   metastases
  Hyperproteinemia

Hyperparathyroidism
 Primary hyperparathyroidism
  Idiopathic
  Familial
  Association with:
   Extraparathyroid neoplasia
   Thyrotoxicosis
   Multiple endocrine abnormalities
 Hypercalcemic secondary hyperparathyroidism
  Renal failure:
   Acute
   Chronic
  Post-renal transplant
  Osteomalacia associated with malabsorption
  Post-resection of bone or soft tissue tumors
   associated with vitamin D-resistant
   osteomalacia and rickets

Non-parathyroid endocrinopathies
 Hyperthyroidism
 Hypothyroidism
 Hypoadrenocorticism
 Pheochromocytoma
 Acromegaly

Possible increased sensitivity to vitamin D
 Granulomatous disease: sarcoidosis, tuberculosis,
  histoplasmosis, coccidioidomycosis
 Idiopathic infantile hypercalcemia

Miscellaneous
 Physiologic hypercalcemia
 Immobilization
 Other hypercalcemic conditions in children
 Acute renal failure, usually associated with
  rhabdomyolysis
 Chronic renal failure
 Phosphorus depletion in uremic patients
 Hypophosphatasia
 Generalized periostitis

---

*Adapted from Lee DBN, Zawada ET, Kleeman CR: The pathophysiology and clinical aspects of hypercalcemic disorders. West J Med 129:286, 1978.

rate of excretion of parathyroid hormone, the rate of movement of calcium in and out of bone, the rate of absorption of calcium from the gastrointestinal tract, and the rate of excretion of calcium in the urine. Table 9–4 classifies the causes of hypercalcemia.

Clinical Contexts

Diagnosis. When presented with an unexplained elevation of serum calcium, the physician should search for signs and symptoms of disease that may be associated with a high serum calcium level only (Fig. 9–3). Hypertension or mild nephropathy may be the only finding (Heath et al., 1980). If the serum calcium level is greater than 15 mg/100 ml, especially in the presence of symptoms, and if the electrocardiogram exhibits a short QT interval, immediate therapy directed at lowering the serum calcium level is necessary (Barnett, 1980).

Management. Serum calcium may be used to follow the course of hypercalcemic and hypocalcemic disorders and their response to therapy, e.g., as in following the response of serum calcium after surgical removal of a parathyroid adenoma. A serum calcium level should be interpreted with knowledge of the serum albumin level.

Screening. An elevated serum calcium level is discovered during the course of screening, with a prevalence of 0.1 to 2.9 per cent (Christensson et al., 1976).

Strategy

Test Sequence. The strategy for an unexplained elevation of serum calcium is as follows:

1. Perform at least three measurements of serum calcium by the original method and by a second method. Use the reference method if possible.

2. Use the correct reference interval.

3. Obtain serum measurements of the following: albumin and globulins by protein electrophoresis, ALP, creatinine, electrolytes, magnesium, phosphorus, and urea nitrogen.

4. Consider drug-metabolite interferences.

5. Consider the differential diagnosis. Barnett (1980) suggests that further studies include

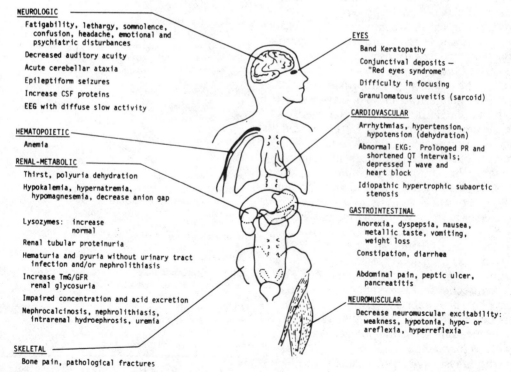

Figure 9–3. Clinical features associated with hypercalcemia. (From Lee DBN, Zawada ET, Kleeman CR: The pathophysiology and clinical aspects of hypercalcemic disorders. West J Med 129:302, 1978.)

a careful history and physical examination, complete blood count, ESR, thyroid function tests, x-ray study of the chest, intravenous pyelogram, and skeletal survey x-ray studies.

6. Measure urine calcium and creatinine on random urine samples and calculate the renal calcium-creatinine clearance ratio as follows: renal calcium clearance-creatinine clearance = UCa × SCr/SCa × UCr where Ca is calcium, Cr is creatinine, U is urine, and S is serum.

7. Reserve measurement of serum parathyroid hormone for cases of hypercalcemia that remain unexplained after a thorough workup (Wong and Freier, 1982).

Patient Preparation. No special procedures are required. Posture affects serum protein concentrations, and ambulatory patients can have slightly higher serum calcium levels than recumbent patients (Statland and Winkel, 1981). (See Part 3 for chemistry and hematology tests.)

Specimen Collection and Handling. Perform calcium measurements promptly. Use serum or heparinized plasma, and avoid other anticoagulants. Do not use cork stoppers, for they can contain calcium and cause spurious elevations as much as 9.9 mg/100 ml higher than the true serum value (Schwartz, 1973). Do not apply a tourniquet or allow muscular exercise of the limb chosen for venipuncture, since venous occlusion or muscular exercise can artifactually cause an elevation (Radcliff et al., 1962). Try to prevent hemolysis and lipemia. Carefully draw an early-morning blood specimen after the patient has fasted. (See Part 3.)

Methodology. Consult the laboratory for methodology, accuracy and precision, reference intervals, and potential sources of interference. The reference method for serum calcium measurement is atomic absorption. However, the automated methods for measuring serum calcium that are in widespread use are accurate and reproducible. Precision of both atomic absorption and automated methods is approximately ±3 per cent. Measure serum parathyroid hormone by a radioimmunoassay specific for the carboxy-terminal end of the molecule. (See Part 3.)

Interpretation

Diagnosis. There is a sequence of questions to answer in the diagnostic workup and interpretation of an unexplained elevation of the serum calcium level:

1. Is the elevation caused by errors in patient preparation, specimen collection and handling, or laboratory procedure or by the use of an inappropriate reference interval?

2. If 1. is not the case, can the elevation be due to drug-metabolite interference?

3. If 1. and 2. are not the case, what diseases or disorders can cause an elevated serum calcium level?

4. What additional procedures can help identify the pathologic cause of an elevated serum calcium level?

See Wong and Freier (1982) for an algorithm for use of laboratory tests in the differential diagnosis of the cause of hypercalcemia.

In the following discussion, a strategy for answering each of these questions is described:

1. Is the elevation caused by errors in patient preparation, specimen collection and handling, or laboratory procedure, or by the use of an inappropriate reference interval?

A widely quoted reference interval for total serum calcium is 8.5 to 10.5 mg/100 ml. Patients with calcium levels above 11.0 mg/100 ml are arbitrarily regarded as in need of operation (*Lancet* editorial, 1980). Erroneous measurements can result from clerical and methodologic mistakes as well as from poor patient preparation and poor specimen collection and handling. An elevated serum calcium level should be measured repeatedly, by atomic absorption if possible, to exclude technical or clerical errors.

Serum calcium is the only common chemical analyte for which the precision of existing laboratory methodologies does not meet medical decision needs. A practical way to improve precision is by repeated analyses. For example, repeating a serum calcium measurement on the same sample four times will halve the standard deviation of the method as follows (Copeland, 1980). (See Chapter 6.)

$$\text{average SD} = \frac{\text{individual SD}}{\sqrt{\text{number of measurements}}}$$

Obtain a serum specimen after the patient has fasted. Avoid using a tourniquet; the patient's fist should not be clenched. Perform measurements without delay. A simultaneous measurement of serum albumin should be done, and the reference interval for serum calcium should be adjusted up or down according to the ratio of 0.8 mg/100 ml of serum calcium for every 1 gm/100 ml of serum albumin below or above the middle of the reference interval (Lee, 1978; *Lancet* editorial, 1979). Measurement of serum albumin and globulins by protein electrophoresis will identify patients with gammopathies who should be investigated for multiple myeloma (monoclonal gammopathy) or sarcoidosis (increased gamma globulins).

Ideally, an individual's serum calcium level should be compared with baseline serum calcium levels obtained in a previous state of health. If this is not possible, obtain an appropriate reference interval derived from a similar reference population using the same well-controlled analytic procedure with similar methods of specimen collection and handling. Remember that when the patient is in the recumbent position, serum calcium levels will be slightly lower. Serum levels of phosphorus, ALP, urea nitrogen, creatinine, electrolytes, and magnesium outside their reference intervals favor a pathologic cause for an elevated serum calcium level.

2. Can the elevated serum calcium level be due to drug-metabolite interference?

Certain pharmacologic agents can cause hypercalcemia, such as vitamin D and its metabolites, vitamin A, milk and alkali, thiazide diuretics, calcium, and lithium (Lee et al., 1978). Conditions in which serum calcium is elevated include hyperlipemia and hyperproteinemia. See Part 3 for a list of drugs and other prelaboratory variables that can elevate the serum calcium level as based on the work of Young and associates (1975).

3. What diseases or disorders can elevate the serum calcium level?

Neoplastic disease metastatic to bone is the most common cause of hypercalcemia encountered in hospital practice (Lafferty, 1966; Lee et al., 1978). The malignancies most frequently complicated by hypercalcemia are cancers of the breast, lung, and kidney (Wong and Freier, 1982). Artifactual hypercalcemia (asymptomatic) can occasionally occur in multiple myeloma (Annesley et al., 1982).

In general, severe hypercalcemia (greater than 14 mg/100 ml) suggests non-parathyroid causes and usually malignant conditions. Hypercalcemia due to hyperparathyroidism is usually milder. If hypercalcemia is documented for more than 1 year, especially with a history of renal stones or peptic ulcers, primary hyperparathyroidism is likely and malignancy is unlikely (Wong and Freier, 1982). Part 3 describes diseases that can cause hypercalcemia based on the work of Friedman and colleagues (1980) and others.

4. What additional procedures can help identify the pathologic cause of an elevated serum calcium level?

The ratio of chloride to phosphorus should be calculated to aid in distinguishing primary hyperparathyroidism from other causes of hypercalcemia. Palmer and associates (1974) studied serum chloride and phosphate concentrations in 52 hypercalcemic patients. The chloride values were high (mean 107 mEq/liter) in 25 hyperparathyroid patients; chloride was low (mean 98 mEq/liter) and phosphate higher (mean 4.5 mg/100 ml) in the 27 patients with hypercalcemia from other causes. The chloride-phosphate ratio ranged from 31.8 to 80 in patients with hyperparathyroidism, 96 per cent of the values being higher than 33; and from 17.7 to 32.3 in subjects with hypercalcemia from other causes, 92 per cent of values being lower than 30.

In another series of patients with possible ectopic parathyroid hormone–producing tumors, 80 per cent had chloride-phosphate ratios in the range of primary hyperparathyroidism (Lafferty, 1966). A chloride-phosphate ratio of less than 33 (especially less than 29) is a signal that the hypercalcemia is not the result of uncomplicated primary hyperparathyroidism (Wong and Freier, 1982). Briccetti and Bleich (1975) suggest that if the serum chloride is greater than 104 mEq/liter in hypercalcemic patients, it is probable that the hypercalcemia is caused by hyperparathyroidism. A serum chloride less than 100 mEq/liter is inconsistent with primary hyperparathyroidism (Wong and Freier, 1982).

If the elevated serum calcium level is accompanied by an elevated serum ALP level, diseases such as hyperparathyroidism, hyperthyroidism, osteoblastic bone lesions, or malignancy may be a factor. A serum ALP greater than twice the upper reference limit is unlikely to indicate uncomplicated primary hyperparathyroidism (Wong and Freier, 1982).

Elevations of serum urea nitrogen (SUN) and creatinine can provide a clue to the nephropathy of mild hyperparathyroidism (Heath, et al., 1980).

Serum potassium levels were low in 33 of 103 patients (32 per cent) with hypercalcemia. A higher prevalence (52.3 per cent) of hypokalemia was found in patients with hypercalcemia associated with malignant disease than in those with primary hyperparathyroidism (16.9 per cent). In addition, the degree and frequency of hypokalemia were greater at higher levels of serum calcium (Aldinger and Samaan, 1977).

Lee and associates (1978) tabulated differential diagnostic indices for hypercalcemia resulting from excess parathyroid hormone compared with other causes (Table 9–5).

Urine calcium levels more than 400 mg per day in subjects on a normal diet are consistent with hyperparathyroidism. Familial hypocalciuric hypercalcemia is a rare disease that can mimic hyperparathyroidism. Patients with this disease do not respond to parathyroidectomy and can be distinguished by their low renal calcium creatinine clearance ratio of less than 0.01 (Marx et al., 1980).

Most laboratory evaluations of hypercalcemia hinge on whether or not the elevated serum calcium level is due to excessive parathyroid hormone production. Figure 9–4 shows how measurement of parathyroid hormone can discriminate among normal patients, those with tumor hypercalcemia, hypoparathyroidism, pseudohypoparathyroidism, chronic renal

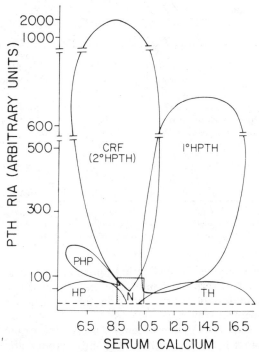

Figure 9–4. Schematic illustrating results seen when simultaneous measurements of immunoreactive parathyroid hormone *(PTH RIA)* and serum calcium are made in normal subjects *(N)* and in patients with tumor hypercalcemia *(TH)*, hypoparathyroidism *(HP)*, pseudohypothyroidism *(PHP)*, chronic renal failure with secondary hyperparathyroidism [CRF(2° HPTH)], and primary hyperparathyroidism 1° HPTH). Enclosed areas indicate the range of values typical for each class of subject measured. Note overlap of regions and interrupted scales. (From Potts JT Jr: Disorders of parathyroid glands. In Isselbacher KJ, Adams RD, Braunwald E, et al (eds): Harrison's Principles of Internal Medicine, ed. 9. Copyright © 1980, McGraw-Hill, Inc, New York, p 1836. Used by permission of McGraw-Hill Book Company.)

failure with secondary hyperparathyroidism, and those with primary hyperparathyroidism (Kao, 1982). Table 9–6 presents laboratory test results for diagnosing primary hyperparathyroidism in hospital patients with hypercalcemia.

Management. Repeated measurements of serum calcium and albumin can be used to assess the course of hypercalcemia or its response to therapy (parathyroidectomy).

Table 9–5. LABORATORY DIFFERENTIAL DIAGNOSTIC INDICES BETWEEN PTH–DEPENDENT AND NON-PTH–DEPENDENT CAUSES OF HYPERCALCEMIA*

Indices	PTH–Dependent	Non-PTH–Dependent
Serum calcium	<14 mg/dl	>14 mg/dl
Azotemia	Usually absent	Usually present
Serum phosphorus	↓	N— ↑
Serum bicarbonate	N— ↓	N— ↑
Serum chloride (mEq/liter) / Serum phosphorus (mg/dl)	>32	<32
Tubular reabsorption of calcium	↑	↓
Tubular reabsorption of phosphate	↓	↑
Urinary cAMP	↑	↓
Steroid suppression test	Serum calcium no change	Serum calcium ↓

Key:
↑ = Increase; ↓ = decrease; cAMP = cyclic adenosine monophosphate; N = normal; PTH = parathyroid hormone.

*From Lee DBN, Zawada ET, Kleeman CR: The pathophysiology and clinical aspects of hypercalcemic disorders. West J Med 129:302, 1978.

Test Requests and Reports

Test Requests. Properly designed request forms can help to ensure appropriate labora-

Table 9–6. SENSITIVITY, SPECIFICITY, AND PREDICTIVE VALUE OF LABORATORY TEST RESULTS IN DIAGNOSIS OF PRIMARY HYPERPARATHYROIDISM IN HOSPITALIZED HYPERCALCEMIC PATIENTS*

Laboratory Test Results	Sensitivity in No. (%) of Patients	Specificity in No. (%) of Patients	Predictive Value, %	
			Positive	*Negative*
Chloride ≥ 100 mmol/liter	40/41 (97.6)	21/41 (51.2)	17.7	99.5
Chloride-phosphorus ratio ≥ 33	39/41 (95.1)	22/41 (53.3)	18.1	99.0
Chloride-phosphorus ratio ≥ 29	41/41 (100)	16/41 (39.0)	15.0	100.0
Alkaline phosphatase < 370 units/liter	37/37 (100)	21/41 (52.5)	18.8	100.0
Parathyroid hormone > 90 µL Eq/ml	18/18 (100)	11/15 (73.3)	28.7	100.0
Parathyroid hormone > 180 µL Eq/ml	10/18 (55.6)	15/15 (100)	100.0	95.4

*From Wong ET, Freier EF: The differential diagnosis of hypercalcemia: An algorithm for more effective use of laboratory tests. *JAMA* 247:79, 1982. Copyright 1982, American Medical Association.
†Prevalence of primary hyperparathyroidism was 9.7 per cent of all hospitalized hypercalcemic patients.

tory studies for evaluating unexplained elevations of serum calcium. The execution of systematic laboratory testing in this regard is a problem-solving service.

Figure 9–5 shows Henry's use of the organ panel for the parathyroid glands. Henry and Howanitz (1980) gave the rationale for this panel as follows:

A prospective study of 1,630 asymptomatic adult patients in a Mayo Clinic series showed 1.4% of the patients with hypercalcemia diagnosed as having hyperparathyroidism. Serum calcium is the best diagnostic test for primary hyperparathyroidism. Serum phosphorus is included to distinguish primary hyperparathyroidism from other forms of hypercalcemia and an alkaline phosphatase is used as an indicator of bone involvement. It is recommended that this panel be used on three successive occasions to evaluate patients for primary hyperparathyroidism. If the diagnosis of primary hyperparathyroidism is still not forthcoming, we then recommend the measurement of parathyroid hormone (PTH) by a radioimmunoassay (RIA) specific for the carboxyl-terminal end of the molecule. It has been demonstrated that RIAs which are specific for the carboxyl-terminal region of the PTH molecule are far superior to those which are directed to the amino-terminal region of PTH for the separation of normal patients from those with primary hyperparathyroidism.

Interpretive Reports. An interpretive report of test results from the execution of the strategy can be sent to the requesting physician. This report should address whether or not the elevated serum calcium level is pathologic and whether or not it is parathyroid hormone–dependent.

Only 1 per cent of laboratory directors in our survey use interpretive reports for hyperparathyroidism; however, 23 per cent use them for screening, which includes the problem of hypercalcemia (Speicher and Smith, 1980). This is a promising area for interpretive reporting, owing to the availability of a good data base for using discriminant functions in differential diagnosis (Watson et al., 1980). When PTH is measured, a two-dimensional graphic report, similar to that shown in Figure 9–4, is useful (Arnaud et al., 1971; Kao, 1982).

Wong and Freier (1982) reported that in

PARATHYROID				
Calcium Total mEq/L	4.5–5.4			
Alkaline Phosphatase IU/L	Adult 4–13 Child 13–20			
Inorganic Phosphorus mg/dl	Adult 2.0–5.2 Child 4.0–7.0			

Figure 9–5. Organ panel for parathyroid glands. (From Henry JB, Murphy J: Effective utilization of clinical laboratories. In Henry JB (ed): Clinical Diagnosis and Management by Laboratory Methods, ed. 16. Philadelphia, WB Saunders Company, 1979, p 2042.)

using a linear discriminant function derived from four laboratory tests (serum calcium, chloride, ALP, and parathyroid hormone), 29 of 30 patients (96.7 per cent) were classified correctly into hyperparathyroid and non-parathyroid groups. The hydrocortisone suppression test and discriminant analysis each achieved a diagnostic accuracy of about 93 per cent in 48 patients with either non-parathyroid malignant disease or hyperparathyroidism without osteitis fibrosis. When both tests pointed to the same diagnosis, they were wrong in less than 1 per cent of cases (Watson et al., 1980). A computer program that evaluates patients with hypercalcemia has been devised (Briccetti and Bleich, 1975).

REFERENCES

How Unexpected Test Results Occur

Altshuler CH: The problem: Assuring appropriate transfer and utilization of laboratory information. In Werner, M: Clinical Consultation in Laboratory Medicine by Pathologists. Chicago, American Society of Clinical Pathologists, 1980, pp 49–55.

Altshuler CH, Bareta J, Cafaro AF, et al: The PALI and SLIC systems. CRC Crit Rev Clin Lab Sci 3:379–402, 1972.

Morrow G: Iatrogenesis imperfecta—A new pediatric problem. Pediatrics 55:453–455, 1975.

Rang M: The Ulysses syndrome. Can Med Assoc J 106:122–123, 1972.

Schneiderman LJ, DeSalvo L, Baylor S, et al: The "abnormal" screening laboratory results: Its effect on physician and patient. Arch Intern Med 129:88–90, 1972.

Wheeler LA, Brecher G, Sheiner LB: Clinical laboratory use in the evaluation of anemia. JAMA 238:2709–2714, 1977.

Unexplained Elevation of Serum Alkaline Phosphatase

Bowers GN Jr, McComb RB: Determination of alkaline phosphatase using a continuous monitoring procedure. In Tietz NW (ed): Fundamentals of Clinical Chemistry, ed 2. Philadelphia, WB Saunders Company, 1976, pp 606–609.

Friedman RB, Anderson RE, Entine SM, et al: Effects of diseases on clinical laboratory tests. Clin Chem 26:35D-38D, 1980.

Gambino R: Gamma glutamic transpeptidase—An underused test. Lab Report for Physicians, November 1979, pp 2–4.

Henry RJ, Cannon DC, Winkelman JW (eds): Clinical Chemistry: Principles and Techniques. Hagerstown, Md, Harper & Row, 1974, p 927.

Massion CG, Frankenfeld, JK: Alkaline phosphatase: Lability in fresh and frozen human serum, and in lyophilized control material. Clin Chem 18:366–373, 1972.

McComb RB, Bowers GN, Posen S: Alkaline Phosphatase. New York, Plenum Press, 1979, pp 525–786.

Munan L, Kelly A, Petitclerc C: Population serum enzyme patterns: Age-sex dependencies. In McComb RB, Bowers GN, Posen S (eds): Alkaline Phosphatase, New York, Plenum Press, 1979, p 528.

Schiff L: Diseases of the Liver, ed 4. Philadelphia, JB Lippincott Company, 1975, pp 604–710.

Speicher CE: Unexplained elevation of serum alkaline phosphatase. Clinical Chemistry No CC 81-2 (CC-128). Chicago, American Society of Clinical Pathologists, 1981.

Statland BE, Bokelund H, Winkel P: Factors contributing to intra-individual variation of serum constituents: 4. Effects of posture and tourniquet application on variation of serum constituents in healthy subjects. Clin Chem 20:1513–1519, 1974.

Statland BE, Winkel P, Killingsworth LM: Factors contributing to intra-individual variation of serum constituents: 6. Physiologic day-to-day concentrations of ten specific proteins in sera of healthy subjects. Clin Chem 22:1635–1638, 1976.

Wolf PL: Clinical significance of an increased or decreased serum alkaline phosphatase level. Arch Pathol Lab Med 102:497–501, 1978.

Young DS, Pestaner LC, Gibberman V: Effects of drugs on clinical laboratory tests. Clin Chem 21:246D–248D, 1975.

Unexplained Elevation of Serum Calcium

Aldinger KA, Samaan NA: Hypokalemia with hypercalcemia. Prevalence and significance in treatment. Ann Intern Med 87:571–573, 1977.

Annesley TM, Burritt MF, Kyle RA: Artifactual hypercalcemia in multiple myeloma. Mayo Clin Proc 57:572–575, 1982.

Arnaud CD, Tsao HS, Littledike T: Radioimmunoassay of human parathyroid hormone in serum. J Clin Invest 50:21–34, 1971.

Barnett R: Parathyroid hormone and calcium abnormalities, editorial. West J Med 132:525–526, 1980.

Bilezikian JP: The medical management of primary hyperparathyroidism. Ann Int Med 96:198–202, 1982.

Bishop JE: Soaring medical costs and the Mayo "epidemic," editorial. Wall Street Journal, February 26, 1980, p 18.

Briccetti AB, Bleich HL: A computer program that evaluates patients with hypercalcemia. J Clin Endocrinol Metab 41:365–372, 1975.

Christensson T, Hellström K, Wengle B, et al: Prevalence of hypercalcemia in a health screening in Stockholm. Acta Med Scand 200:131–137, 1976.

Coe FL, Favus MJ: Does mild, asymptomatic hyperparathyroidism require surgery?, editorial. N Engl J Med 302:224–225, 1980.

Copeland BE, Hoyt LH: Clinical chemistry. In Jones RJ, Palulonis RM (eds): Laboratory Tests in Medical Practice. Chicago, American Medical Association, 1980, pp 77–94.

Diagnosis and treatment of primary hyperparathyroidism, editorial. Lancet 1:1339–1340, 1980.

Friedman RB, Anderson RE, Entine SM, et al: Effects of diseases on clinical laboratory tests. 26:61D-62D, 1980.

Heath H, Hodgson SF, Kennedy MA: Primary hyperparathyroidism: Incidence, morbidity, and potential economic impact in a community. N Engl J Med 302:189–193, 1980.

Henry JB, Howanitz PJ: Organ panels and the relationship of the laboratory to the physician. In Jones RJ, Palulonis RM (eds): Laboratory Tests in Medical Practice. Chicago, American Medical Association, 1980, pp 29.

Hodgson SF, Heath H: Asymptomatic primary hyperparathyroidism: Treat or follow?, editorial. Mayo Clin Proc 56:521–522, 1981.

Kao PC: Parathyroid hormone assay. Mayo Clin Proc 57:596–597, 1982.

Lafferty FW: Pseudohyperparathyroidism. Medicine 45:247–260, 1966.

Lee DBN, Zawada ET, Kleeman CR: The pathophysiology and clinical aspects of hypercalcemic disorders. West J Med 129:278–320, 1978.

Marx SV, Stock JL, Attie MF, et al: Familial hypocalciuric hypercalcemia: Recognition among patients referred after unsuccessful parathyroid exploration. Ann Intern Med 92:351–356, 1980.

Palmer FJ, Nelson JC, Bacchus H: The chloride-phosphate ratio in hypercalcemia. Ann Intern Med 80:200–204, 1974.

Potts JT Jr: Disorders of parathyroid glands. In Isselbacher KJ, Adams RD, Braunwald E, et al: Harrison's Principles of Internal Medicine, ed. 9. New York, McGraw-Hill Book Company, 1980, pp 1832–1843.

Radcliff FJ, Baume PE, Jones WO: Effect of venous stasis and muscular exercise on total serum calcium concentration. Lancet 2:1249–1251, 1962.

Schwartz MK: Interferences in diagnostic biochemical procedures. Adv Clin Chem 16:1–45, 1973.

Serum calcium, editorial. Lancet 1:858–859, 1979.

Speicher CE, Smith JW: Interpretive reporting in clinical pathology. JAMA 243:1556–1560, 1980.

Statland BE, Winkel P: Response of clinical chemistry quantity values to selected physical, dietary, and smoking activities. In Stefanini M, Benson ES (eds): Progress in Clinical Pathology. Volume VIII. New York, Grune & Stratton, Inc, 1981, pp 25–44.

Watson L, Moxham J, Fraser P: Hydrocortisone suppression test and discriminant analysis in differential diagnosis of hypercalcemia. Lancet 1:1320–1325, 1980.

Wong ET, Freier EF: The differential diagnosis of hypercalcemia: An algorithm for more effective use of laboratory tests. JAMA 247:75–80, 1982.

Young DS, Pestaner LC, Gibberman V: Effects of drugs on clinical laboratory tests. Clin Chem 21:273D, 1975.

CHAPTER 10

CARDIOVASCULAR SUBPROBLEMS

CORONARY HEART DISEASE

The term *coronary heart disease* implies damage to heart muscle caused by obstruction of the coronary arterial blood supply. The obstruction can be gradual or sudden, partial or complete. Gradual, partial obstructions cause angina pectoris. Sudden, complete obstructions cause myocardial infarction. Intermediate obstructions cause clinical episodes intermediate between angina pectoris and myocardial infarction.

There are a number of mechanisms by which obstruction of the coronary arterial blood supply occurs:

1. Atherosclerosis with or without thrombi—by far the most common situation. (Risk factors for ischemic heart disease are discussed later in this chapter.)

2. Coronary arterial spasm, syphilitic aortitis, dissecting aneurysm of the aorta.

3. Embolism. The emboli can arise from a number of possible sources, such as thrombi, atheromatous plaques, bacterial vegetations, and tumors (Robbins and Cotran, 1979).

ACUTE MYOCARDIAL INFARCTION

Definition and Significance

Acute myocardial infarction is necrosis of cardiac muscle secondary to a sudden interruption of the arterial blood supply to the heart. It is the most dramatic and significant complication of atherosclerosis. Together with stroke, it is the primary cause of morbidity and mortality in adults. It is important not only to diagnose acute myocardial infarction accurately when it is present but also to exclude it when it is absent. The psychologic and economic penalties of diagnosing acute myocardial infarction when it is not present are great.

Pathophysiology

Oliva (1981) reviewed the pathophysiology of acute myocardial infarction and postulated a dynamic interaction among damaged intima, platelet aggregates, and arterial spasm as a prelude to coronary arterial thrombosis. Regardless of the mechanism for arterial obstruction, the development and resolution of an acute myocardial infarction may be described in three stages.

155

1. Development of necrosis (4 to 10 days).
2. Plateau of maximal necrosis.
3. Resolution or healing of the necrotic tissue (approximately 6 weeks) (Robbins and Cotran, 1979).

The necrotic muscle releases its contents into the bloodstream, and serum concentrations of SGOT, CPK, LDH, and myoglobin rise as a result. Myoglobin is also increased in the urine. Theoretically, larger infarctions should produce greater elevations of these analytes. However, in practice, these proportional elevations do not always occur. After infarction, serum and urinary myoglobin concentrations increase earlier than those of serum CPK (Rosano et al., 1977; Saranchak and Bernstein, 1974). Serum CPK increases in 3 to 6 hours; SGOT, in 3 to 8 hours; and serum LDH, slightly later.

Although serum myoglobin, CPK, SGOT, and LDH have good diagnostic sensitivity for the presence of acute myocardial infarction, they lack diagnostic specificity because they are found in many other tissues. CPK is highest in skeletal muscle, but appreciable amounts are found in cardiac muscle, brain, thyroid, and lung tissue, with only trace amounts in other tissues. Very little CPK can be detected in liver and erythrocytes. SGOT is highest in the heart, liver, skeletal muscle, and kidney, with smaller amounts in the pancreas, spleen, and lung. A minimal concentration of SGOT—about ten times the serum activity—is present in erythrocytes. LDH is common to virtually all human tissues.

CPK is a dimer with a molecular weight of approximately 86,000 daltons consisting of two subunits of either the B or M type. There are three dimers or isoenzymes of CPK in human tissues: CPK-MM, CPK-MB, and CPK-BB. CPK catalyzes the following reversible reaction:

$$\text{ATP} + \text{creatine} \underset{}{\overset{\text{CPK}}{\rightleftharpoons}} \text{ADP} + \begin{matrix}\text{creatine}\\\text{phosphate}\end{matrix}$$

LDH is a tetramer with a molecular weight of approximately 135,000 daltons consisting of two subunits of either the H or M type. There are five tetramers or isoenzymes of LDH: LDH-1 (HHHH), LDH-2 (HHHM), LDH-3 (HHMM), LDH-4 (HMMM), and LDH-5 (MMMM). LDH catalyzes the following reversible reaction:

$$\text{L-lactate} + \text{NAD}^+ \underset{}{\overset{\text{LDH}}{\rightleftharpoons}}$$
$$\text{pyruvate} + \text{NADH} + \text{H}^+$$

Other changes occur in the blood of patients with acute myocardial infarction such as leukocytosis, increased erythrocyte sedimentation rate, and elevated C-reactive protein. These changes are sensitive but very non-specific and do little to separate acute myocardial infarction from other inflammatory disorders. (See the discussion of inflammation in Chapter 8.)

Clinical Contexts

Diagnosis. Clinical laboratory studies are often used to confirm an impression of acute myocardial infarction. Frequently, the clinical picture is clear, such as when the patient presents with sudden, crushing anterior chest pain radiating to the left shoulder, arm, or jaw and the electrocardiogram shows new QRS changes accompanied by evolutionary ST segment and T-wave changes. Sometimes, however, the location, severity, and duration of the pain are atypical. Or there may be no pain, and the patient can present with acute pulmonary edema, shock, or cardiac arrest. The electrocardiogram can be equivocal or obscured by left or right bundle-branch block, left or right ventricular hypertrophy, or previous infarction. The electrocardiogram has a sensitivity of 63 to 82 per cent and a specificity of 100 per cent for acute myocardial infarction (Lott and Stang, 1980). The experience of the clinician and the clarity of the clinical picture and electrocardiogram determine to what extent laboratory studies are necessary to confirm or exclude the presence of acute myocardial infarction (Wagner, 1980; Willerson, 1982).

The clinical impression may indicate other conditions if acute myocardial infarction is first ruled out. Other diagnoses include angina pectoris, pericarditis, pulmonary embolism, dissecting aneurysm of the aorta, esophagitis with esophageal spasm, acute pancreatitis, and acute biliary tract disease.

Another clinical subproblem is the exclusion of acute myocardial infarction in a patient who has recently undergone heart surgery.

Management. A higher mortality and greater morbidity are associated with larger infarctions; thus, as a prognostic guide, knowledge of the size of the infarction is important. Knowing the amount of myocardium damaged

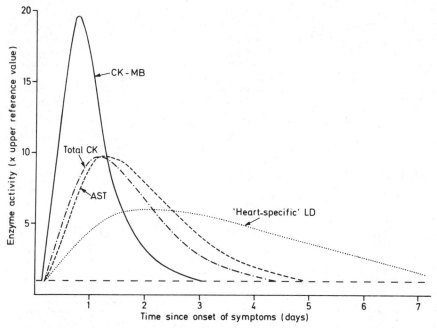

Figure 10–1. Changes in serum enzyme activity after myocardial infarction. (From Hearse DJ, Lewis, J. (eds): Enzymes in Cardiology: Diagnosis and Research. New York, John Wiley & Sons, Inc, 1979, p 223. Reprinted by permission.) (AST = SGOT; "heart-specific" LD = LDH-1 > LDH-2; CK = CPK.)

is necessary to gauge therapy appropriately (Rude, 1981).

Screening. Screening for acute myocardial infarction in the absence of clinical signs and symptoms is not indicated.

Strategy

Test Sequence. The most effective test sequence for confirming or excluding a diagnosis of acute myocardial infarction is the parallel and serial measurement of CPK and LDH enzymes and isoenzymes in blood samples drawn at the time of admission and every 12 hours for the first 48 hours (Galen, 1975, 1978; Roe, 1977a). Measurements at 12-hour intervals are frequent enough to detect transient elevations of isoenzymes, and a duration of 48 hours is long enough to detect LDH isoenzyme elevations (Irvin et al., 1980; Lott and Stang, 1980). (See Figure 10–1 and Table 10–1.) Other sequences have been suggested (e.g., three samples with the first on admission and the second and third at 6 to 13 hours and 24 to 37 hours, respectively). This permits a drawing schedule with collection of samples at 7 A.M., 12 noon, 5 P.M., and 10 P.M. (Helena Laboratories, 1977). Sampling at intervals of 6 to 12 hours will usually lead to detection of

even small subendocardial infarcts (Roberts and Sobel, 1978). Lupovitch and Kaplan (1980) have measured CPK and LDH isoenzymes at the time of hospital admission and at 8-hour intervals for the ensuing 48-hour period.

Any new clinical episode that raises the possibility of reinfarction or extension of existing infarction requires initiating a new series of CPK and LDH isoenzyme studies. These should be drawn at the time of the clinical episode and every 12 hours for the next 48 hours.

Stat CPK and LDH isoenzyme measurements are not usually required because a single stat determination of these isoenzymes can miss the characteristic CPK-MB band and LDH 1-2 changes (Fig. 10–1). These findings can be observed only through serial studies. Therefore, whether or not to admit a patient with a possible acute myocardial infarction must be a conservative decision based on clinical findings; however, if aggressive therapy—such as surgical reperfusion—is contemplated, stat CPK and LDH measurements may be required (Rude et al., 1981).

Because serial CPK and LDH isoenzyme studies are expensive and time consuming, many laboratories elect not to measure isoen-

Table 10–1. RELATIVE PREDICTIVE VALUES OF VARIOUS STRATEGIES FOR THE DIAGNOSIS OF ACUTE MYOCARDIAL INFARCTION

Strategy	Predictive Value	Comment
Serial measurement of CPK and LDH serum isoenzymes	Very good (essentially 100% in coronary unit)	Combines the magnitude of elevations and temporal sequence of alterations with the organ specificity of isoenzymes
Serial measurement of total CPK, SGOT, LDH serum enzymes	Good	Magnitude of elevations and temporal sequence of alterations increases predictive value over a single measurement
Single measurement of CPK and LDH serum isoenzymes	Moderately good	In spite of better organ specificity, there is still non-specificity secondary to elevations by a variety of diseases and disorders
Single measurement of total CPK, SGOT, and LDH serum enzymes	Moderate	Non-specificity secondary to elevations by numerous diseases, drugs, and miscellaneous factors
Leukocyte count, ESR, and C-reactive proteins	Poor	Does not discriminate between myocardial infarction and other inflammations

zymes unless total CPK and total LDH are elevated. Although this policy is reasonable as a way of keeping the number of isoenzyme studies under control, it should be understood that small infarcts occasionally occur that affect the isoenzyme patterns but that do not elevate the total enzyme values (Guzy, 1977). Therefore, if clinical indications are strong, isoenzymes should be measured whether or not total CPK and total LDH are elevated. To avoid missing small infarctions, Baillie (1977) recommends isoenzyme studies on patients whose results are in the top 33 per cent of the normal range of total CPK. Of 419 patients admitted to a coronary-care unit for acute myocardial infarction, 69 (16 per cent) had elevated serum CPK-MB in the absence of an elevated total serum CPK (Dillon et al., 1982).

Some investigators have advocated obtaining serum or urine myoglobin concentrations by RIA as an additional useful measurement in diagnosing acute myocardial infarction (Saranchak and Bernstein, 1974). Measurement of myoglobin appears to be high in diagnostic sensitivity but lacking in diagnostic specificity (Rosano et al., 1977). Although the magnitude of elevations and temporal sequence of serial myoglobin elevations in concert with the clinical findings may confer good predictive value for acute myocardial infarction, we believe that myoglobin studies may be of more potential value in excluding such a diagnosis than in

confirming it. An RIA for serum CPK-MB of high diagnostic sensitivity appears promising for excluding acute myocardial infarction (Dillon et al., 1982).

If the appropriate series of CPK and LDH studies have been performed and only LDH 1-2 changes are present with absence of CPK-MB, a definite diagnosis cannot be confirmed. In an effort to rule out other causes of LDH 1-2 changes (e.g., hemolytic anemia), some investigators have suggested measuring serum haptoglobin. Serum haptoglobin tends to be normal in acute myocardial infarction and decreased in hemolytic anemia. It is interesting that in vitro hemolysis will not produce the LDH 1-2 "flip" (Lott and Stang, 1980). Whether or not the ratio of LDH-1 to LDH-2 increases enough to produce an actual flip appears to be related to sampling times, methodology, and other variables (Bruns et al., 1981).

Using a rapid, highly sensitive nephelometric immunoprecipitin technique, Marchand and associates (1980) performed serum haptoglobin assays in 100 patients after hospital admission in whom the prevalence of hemolysis was 24 per cent. Using a serum haptoglobin limit of 25 mg/100 ml or less as indicative of hemolysis, the sensitivity (83 per cent) and specificity (96 per cent) are high providing a predictive value for hemolytic disease of 87 per cent.

Patient Preparation. Intramuscular injections should be avoided because they can elevate serum CPK.

Specimen Collection and Handling. Care is necessary to preserve the integrity of CPK and LDH isoenzymes. For maximal stability, CPK isoenzymes stored at any temperature require the presence of a suitable sulfhydryl compound. Dilution of CPK can result in increased activity (Guzy, 1977). A slight degree of hemolysis will not affect CPK determinations. CPK-MM is the most stable dimer and CPK-BB the most unstable. The serum sample should be promptly refrigerated at 4°C and should be run within 24 hours. With refrigeration at 4°C, CPK-MB is relatively stable (Lott and Stang, 1980).

Serum specimens for LDH can be stored at room temperature at 25°C for 48 hours with little loss of activity (6 per cent or less). LDH isoenzymes keep best at room temperature and should be measured within 24 hours (Lott and Stang, 1980). Hemolyzed sera should not be used, since erythrocytes contain 150 times more LDH than serum. Thus, it is best to separate serum from red blood cells as soon as possible.

In summary, CPK and LDH isoenzymes can be determined on the same sample, provided that a non-hemolyzed serum is promptly separated from the red blood cells. The separated serum should be split into two portions: The one for CPK isoenzymes should be quickly refrigerated at 4°C, and the other for LDH isoenzymes should be held at room temperature. CPK and LDH isoenzyme analyses should be run as soon as possible, optimally within 24 hours. With this protocol, we have not found it necessary to use preservatives.

Methodology. Consult the laboratory concerning the methods used for measuring serum CPK and LDH enzymes, reference intervals, accuracy and precision, and potential sources of interference.

CPK isoenzymes can be measured by electrophoresis, ion-exchange chromatography, immunologic inhibition, selective activation, and RIA (Galen, 1978). RIA is the most sensitive method, being able to detect as few as 0.01 units (Dillon et al., 1982). In our experience, electrophoresis has been technically satisfactory, giving good separation and clinically reliable results. Enzymatically inactive serum CPK-B protein (CPK-Bi) is reported to be not only a sensitive test for myocardial infarction but also a predictor of

risk of subsequent infarction for patients suffering with chest pain syndrome (Galen, 1981).

LDH isoenzymes can be measured by electrophoresis, heat inactivation, substrate inhibition, chromatography, and immunochemistry. We have chosen electrophoresis because it gives good separation and provides the greatest diagnostic information.

Interpretation

Diagnosis. When a series of CPK and LDH isoenzymes studies is performed, as in the sequence outlined in the section on strategy, the combination of a CPK-MB isoenzyme band, followed by an LDH-1 equal to or greater than LDH-2 (the so-called "flipped" LDH), is highly predictive (essentially 100 per cent in a coronary care unit) of acute myocardial infarction (Table 10–2). In healthy persons, LDH-2 is greater than LDH-1.

If a quantitative method for serum CPK-MB is used (e.g., immunoassay), look for a rise and fall in the absolute amount of serum CPK-MB as well as an increase in its percentage of the total serum CPK (Gambino, 1980, 1981). The upper reference limit for serum CPK-MB in a healthy population is 2 to 4 U/liter, and the upper reference limit for its percentage of the total is 5 per cent (Dillon, 1982).

The term flipped LDH was coined to highlight the LDH-1 > LDH-2 changes (Galen, 1975). With some methods, a clear-cut flip may be absent following a small myocardial infarction (Bruns, 1981; Gambino, 1981). CPK-MB and LDH flip do not have to be visible in the same sample. The flipped LDH never precedes the appearance of CPK-MB. Neither the presence of CPK-MB alone nor the LDH flip alone is diagnostic of acute myocardial infarction, for each can be caused by other diseases or disorders. On the other hand, no disorder is known that produces the combination of CPK-MB and LDH flip in the temporal sequence that is seen in acute myocardial infarction.

It is interesting that even though CPK-MB per se does not have 100 per cent diagnostic specificity to confirm a diagnosis of acute myocardial infarction, it does have the diagnostic sensitivity to exclude this diagnosis with a high degree of certainty if it is absent (Table 10–2). This makes it a slightly better test for excluding than confirming a diagnosis of acute myocardial infarction.

Other possible causes of an elevated serum

Table 10–2. SENSITIVITY AND SPECIFICITY OF CPK-MB AND INCREASED RATIO OF LDH-1 TO LDH-2 IN POPULATIONS WITH A HIGH PREVALENCE OF ACUTE MYOCARDIAL INFARCTION*

Prevalence	CPK		CPK-MB		LDH		Increased LDH-1/LDH-2	
	Sensitivity %	Specificity %	Sensitivity %	Specificity %	Sensitivity %	Specificity %	Sensitivity %	Specificity %
27/61(44%)	100	—	97	—†	—	—	91	—†
91/328(28%)	98	85	100	99†	—	—	90	95†
51/212(24%)	100	85	94	100†	—	—	—	—
46/96(48%)	—	—	100	93†	—	—	78	99†
47/100(47%)	94	72	100	92‡	—	—	—	—
80/151(53%)	100	65	96	100†	—	—	—	—
87/201(43%)	93	76	98	97‡	91	80	86	90
192/401(48%)	97	78	100	98†	97	81	—	—
34/143(24%)	94	57	70	95§	—	—	—	—
44/98(45%)	—	—	100	86†	—	—	70	94†
101/228(44%)	—	—	—	100§	—	—	100	91†
173/370(47%)	100	86	99	98†	—	—	—	—
28/71(39%)	100	88	96	93§	—	—	61	98†
29/67(43%)	100	60	100	100‖	100	39	—	—
1449/2525(57%)	98	75	98	97†	—	—	75	97
(Average of above studies)			85	95‡ 96§				

*Adapted from Lott JA, Stang JM: Serum enzymes and isoenzymes in the diagnosis and differential diagnosis of myocardial ischemia and necrosis. Clin Chem 26(9):1244, 1980.
†Electrophoresis.
‡Chromatography.
§Immunoinhibition.
‖Electrophoresis followed by elution and fluorescence.

CPK-MB are given in Table 10–3. Additional potential causes of an elevated serum LDH-1 to LDH-2 ratio that can produce an actual flip are hemolysis and renal infarction (Gambino, 1980).

When performing serial CPK and LDH isoenzyme studies to confirm or exclude acute myocardial infarction, we should be alert to the possibility of other coexisting diseases or disorders that can affect concentrations. The presence of LDH-5, for instance, is said to be indicative of right-sided heart failure with hepatic congestion. An elevated SGPT has a similar meaning. Gambino (1979) suggested that the elevated SGPT is related to poor perfusion of the liver and not to an increase in hepatic venous pressure. For example, elevated SGPT was not found in patients with pulmonary emboli in the absence of low cardiac output, nor has elevated SGPT correlated with the presence at autopsy of chronic passive congestion of the liver.

Cohen and Kaplan (1978) reported four patients with striking transaminase elevations whose initial diagnosis was hepatitis but who were later shown to have central hepatic necrosis associated with left ventricular failure. Signs of right-sided heart failure were absent.

The candidate for general surgery can be evaluated for acute myocardial infarction in the same manner as a medical patient. However, the predictive value of the strategy may be lower in surgical patients because of a lower prevalence of acute myocardial infarction. Patients who have undergone cardiac surgery represent a greater challenge to the physician's ability to distinguish acute myocardial infarction from isoenzyme elevations secondary to cardiac manipulation (Roe, 1977*a*). This is because serum isoenzyme elevations do not provide a basis for distinguishing infarcted cardiac muscle from muscle injured at surgery.

Chronic heart disease, electric cardioversion for heart rhythm disturbances, coronary catheterization, pulmonary embolism, and exercise usually do not produce increases of CPK-MB. Because CPK-MB is present in skeletal muscle in low levels of activity, substantial injury to skeletal muscle can elevate the serum CPK-MB level (Lott and Stang, 1980).

See Figure 10–2 for an overview of the interpretation of the results of serum enzyme and isoenzyme studies for acute myocardial infarction. Table 10–4 summarizes the results of common chemistry and hematology tests.

Table 10–3. POSSIBLE CAUSES FOR ELEVATION OF SERUM CPK-MB OTHER THAN ACUTE MYOCARDIAL INFARCTION*

Cardiovascular System
  Angina pectoris
  Atrial fibrillation
  Cardiac catheterization
  Cardiac trauma
  Cardiopulmonary resuscitation
  Cardioversion
  Congestive heart failure
  Coronary insufficiency
  Tachyarrhythmias
Respiratory System
  Pulmonary embolism
Endocrine System
  Hypothyroidism
Musculoskeletal System
  Dermatomyositis
  Multiple trauma
  Muscular dystrophy
  Myoglobinuria
  Polymyositis
  Rhabdomyolysis
  Viral myositis
Miscellaneous Causes
  Carbon monoxide poisoning
  Malignant hyperthermia
  Marathon running
  Peripartum period
  Reye's syndrome

*Compiled from Dillon MC, Calbreath DF, Dixon AM, et al.: Diagnostic problems in acute myocardial infarction: CK-MB in the absence of abnormally elevated total creatine kinase levels. Arch Intern Med 142:33–38, 1982; Guzy PM: Creatine phosphokinase—MB (CPK-MB) and the diagnosis of myocardial infarction. West J Med 127:455–460, 1977; Siegel AJ, Silverman LM, Holman L: Elevated creatine kinase MB isoenzyme levels in marathon runners. JAMA 246:2049–2051, 1981.

Management. Serum CPK elevations greater than eight times the upper reference limit or serum SGOT elevations greater than five times the upper reference limit are associated with large infarcts. Mortality is reportedly increased twofold to threefold within a year after infarction (Basta and Coyle, 1980). Lower values do not guarantee a more favorable prognosis. Methods for estimating the size of infarctions by CPK and CPK-MB measurements appear promising (Roberts, 1979; Roberts and Sobel, 1978; Roe, 1977*b*; Rude et al., 1981).

The presence of mitochondrial creatine kinase (a CPK isoenzyme bound to mitochondria, which by electrophoresis migrates cathodic to CPK-MM) is a poor prognostic sign. It

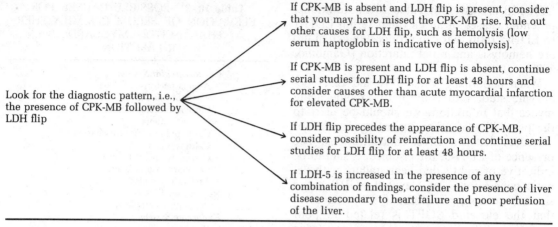

Look for the diagnostic pattern, i.e., the presence of CPK-MB followed by LDH flip

If CPK-MB is absent and LDH flip is present, consider that you may have missed the CPK-MB rise. Rule out other causes for LDH flip, such as hemolysis (low serum haptoglobin is indicative of hemolysis).

If CPK-MB is present and LDH flip is absent, continue serial studies for LDH flip for at least 48 hours and consider causes other than acute myocardial infarction for elevated CPK-MB.

If LDH flip precedes the appearance of CPK-MB, consider possibility of reinfarction and continue serial studies for LDH flip for at least 48 hours.

If LDH-5 is increased in the presence of any combination of findings, consider the presence of liver disease secondary to heart failure and poor perfusion of the liver.

Figure 10–2. Interpretation of studies for the subproblem of acute myocardial infarction. (LDH flip = LDH-1 ≥ LDH-2.)

Table 10–4. COMMON LABORATORY TEST RESULTS IN ACUTE MYOCARDIAL INFARCTION*

Laboratory Test	Value	Pathophysiologic Factors
Chemistry (Serum)		
Bilirubin, total	—	
Calcium, total	—	
Carbon dioxide	—	
Chloride	—	
Cholesterol	↑	May be a predisposing risk factor; can increase related to the stress of the acute illness
Creatine phosphokinase	↑	Related to the infarcted cardiac muscle—CPK-MB
Creatinine	↑	In approximately 50 per cent of patients
Glucose	↑	May be a predisposing risk factor; can increase according to the stress of the acute illness
Lactic dehydrogenase	↑	Related to the infarcted cardiac muscle—LDH-1 and LDH-2; LDH-5 rises with heart failure and poor liver perfusion
Phosphatase, alkaline	↑	Associated with repair of infarcted myocardium
Phosphorus, inorganic	—	
Potassium	—	
Proteins, total	—	
Proteins, albumin	↓	In approximately 20 per cent of patients at the time of initial hospitalization
Sodium	↓	Frequently found; seems to correlate with degree of myocardial involvement
Transaminase, aspartate amino	↑	Related to the infarcted cardiac muscle
Urea nitrogen	↑	In approximately one third of patients at the time of initial hospitalization. Majority show an elevation during hospitalization
Uric acid	↑	May be a predisposing minor risk factor; if very elevated can indicate poor prognosis as a result of tissue hypoxia
Hematology (Blood)		
Hemoglobin	—	
Hematocrit	↑	Small increase related to an early blood volume decrease
	↓	The small early increase may be followed by a small decrease
Leukocyte count, total	↑	Related to the inflammatory response secondary to the infarct
Platelet count	—	

Key:
— = No change; ↑ = can be increased; ↓ = can be decreased.

*Based on information from Friedman, RB, Anderson RE, Entine SM, et al: Effects of diseases on clinical laboratory tests. Clin Chem 26:1D–476D, 1980; Wolf PL: Interpretation of Biochemical Multitest Profiles: An Analysis of 100 Important Conditions. New York, Masson Publishing USA, Inc, 1977; Woolliscroft JO, Colfer H, Fox IH: Hyperuricemia in acute illness: A poor prognostic sign. Am J Med 72:58–62, 1982.

CARDIAC INJURY I				
Creatine Phosphokinase (CPK)/IU/L	Male 55–170 Female 30–135			
Lactic Dehydrogenase IU/L	71–207			
CARDIAC INJURY II				
Lactic Dehydrogenase Isoenzymes	See Special Report			
Creatine Phosphokinase Isoenzymes	See Special Report			

Figure 10–3. Organ panels for cardiac injury. (From Henry JB, Murphy J: Effective utilization of clinical laboratories. In Henry JB (ed): Clinical Diagnosis and Management by Laboratory Methods, ed. 16. Philadelphia, WB Saunders Company, 1979, p 2044).

was found in eight patients in shock, six of whom died within 12 days (Bark, 1980).

Woolliscroft and associates (1982) suggest that marked hyperuricemia, as an indicator of severe tissue hypoxia at the height of an illness, may predict a fatal outcome. Six of 16 patients with acute cardiovascular disease died (three of the six had acute myocardial infarction). These six had a mean serum urate level of 11.1 mg/100 ml (range, 6.6 to 15.5 mg/100 ml) and reached a peak mean value of 20.7 mg/100 ml (range, 13.6 to 33.0 mg/100 ml).

Preliminary data indicate that CPK-Bi can predict the risk of subsequent infarction for patients suffering from chest pain syndrome (Galen, 1981). Schroeder and associates (1980) reported that patients admitted to their coronary-care unit with acute ischemic chest pain without a myocardial infarction had a 6- to 24-month prognosis similar to that of patients who had actual infarction.

Test Requests and Reports

Test Requests. The execution of the test sequence for confirming or excluding a diagnosis of acute myocardial infarction can be offered by the laboratory as a clinical problem-solving service. Henry devised two organ panels for cardiac injury (Fig. 10–3). Henry and Howanitz (1980) gave the rationale for these panels as follows:

Cardiac Injury Panel No. 1. CK is elevated in 95% of patients with acute myocardial infarction. Almost 100% of the patients with myocardial infarction have elevated LDH. Serum CK rises within six hours after the onset of chest pain, with serum LDH rising by 48 hours. If one or both of these enzymes is elevated, the isoenzymes are determined. This panel has been especially useful in an emergency room setting.

Cardiac Injury Panel No. 2. The MB isoenzyme CK is almost specific for heart muscle and coupled with the isoenzyme pattern of LDH, in which fast-moving isoenzyme 1 is greater than isoenzyme 2, we have a powerful tool in the diagnosis of acute myocardial infarction.

Interpretive Reports. The results of the strategy can be collated and returned to the attending physician in the form of an interpretive report (Fig. 10–4). Of the pathologists we surveyed (Speicher and Smith, 1980), 31 per cent were practicing interpretive reporting for cardiac injury.

Galen and Gambino (1978) modified the computer program of Reece and Hobbie (1972; 1974) to include the diagnosis of acute myocardial infarction. This program was run on the Columbia University Computer Center IBM 360/91–360/75 coupled system. They wrote another computer-assisted isoenzyme interpretation program capable of deciding whether or not given isoenzyme results are diagnostic of acute myocardial infarction. The program was written in an advanced version of BASIC and is interactive.

Lupovitch and Kaplan (1980) developed interpretive reports that address not only the diagnosis of the infarct but also an estimate of its size in gram-equivalents of myocardium. The system is based on a programmable calculator and is programmed in BASIC.

ATHEROSCLEROSIS

Atherosclerosis, a condition in which material is deposited within the intima of the large arteries of the body, is a specific variety of arteriosclerosis. The basic lesion—the atheroma—consists of a raised focal fibrofatty plaque within the intima, having a core of lipid

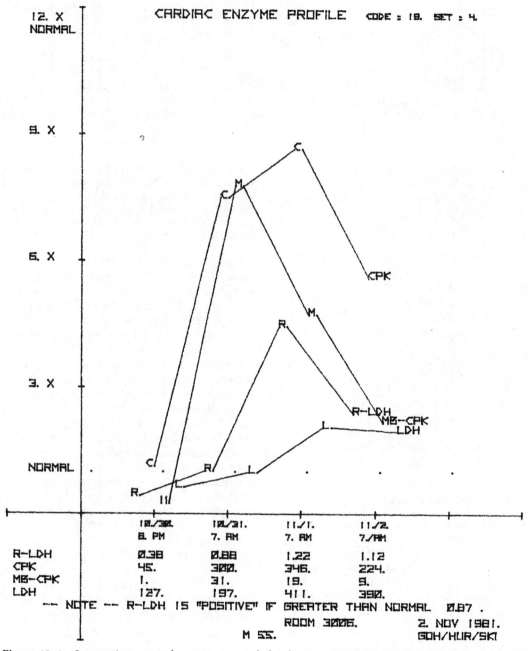

Figure 10–4. Interpretive report for acute myocardial infarction. (R-LDH = LDH-1 is increased >LDH-2.) (Courtesy of J. T. Gohmann, M.D., Portsmouth, Ohio.)

(mainly cholesterol, usually complexed to proteins and cholesterol esters) and a covering fibrous cap. These atheromata, or plaques, project into the lumen of an artery and compromise the blood flow. The decrease in the blood flow can vary in degree from minimal through severe. Sometimes the obstruction to blood flow is complete. When complete obstruction occurs, there is often a thrombus superimposed on an atherosclerotic plaque (Robbins and Cotran, 1979).

The significance of atherosclerosis is related to the importance of the organs affected by decreased or obstructed blood flow. In the brain, atherosclerosis causes strokes; in the heart, ischemic heart disease; and in the legs, intermittent claudication.

RISK OF ISCHEMIC HEART DISEASE

Definition and Significance

Because ischemic heart disease is a life-threatening complication of atherosclerosis, we chose to express the risk of developing atherosclerosis and its complications in terms of the clinical subproblem, risk of ischemic heart disease. It should be understood that the risk factors for the atherosclerotic complications of stroke and intermittent claudication of the legs are essentially the same as for ischemic heart disease. It thus follows that by identifying and decreasing the risk factors for ischemic heart disease, we should also be simultaneously identifying and decreasing those for stroke and intermittent claudication, though perhaps not to the same degree.

The purpose of assessing the risk of ischemic heart disease is to determine the extent of risk and to decrease the unfavorable risk factors. The hypothesis that favorable manipulation of adverse risk factors decreases the propensity to develop ischemic heart disease has not been proved conclusively; however, early studies support this belief.

Risk factors for ischemic heart disease can be categorized as major and minor, as shown in Table 10–5. The effects of age, sex, serum cholesterol, serum high-density lipoprotein (HDL) cholesterol, systolic blood pressure, cigarette smoking, glucose tolerance, and left ventricular hypertrophy on risk can be quantified according to data developed in the Framingham study (Dawber, 1975). These risk

Table 10–5. RISK FACTORS CONTRIBUTING TO ISCHEMIC HEART DISEASE

Major Factors	Minor Factors
High cholesterol	Physical inactivity
Low HDL cholesterol	Obesity
Hypertension	Stress
Cigarette smoking	Hyperuricemia
Glucose intolerance	Elevated triglyceride
Left ventricular hypertrophy	

factors have been distributed in tabular form by the American Heart Association (Coronary Risk Handbook, 1973).

Prevention of acute pancreatitis is another reason to treat hyperlipemia. Severe elevation of serum triglyceride levels can provoke acute pancreatitis, and reduction of serum triglyceride (below 1000 mg/100 ml) can prevent further attacks (Cameron et al., 1974). (See the discussion of acute pancreatitis in Chapter 14.)

Pathophysiology

The pathogenesis of atherosclerosis is not fully understood. Historically, there are two major hypotheses (Kottke and Subbiah, 1978). One theory stresses the importance of thrombosis in the development of atherosclerosis; the other emphasizes the accumulation of lipids in the intima of the large arteries. The true pathogenesis probably involves a complex interaction of both of these mechanisms. Even though the pathogenesis is unclear, a pragmatic approach to the care of millions of patients at risk for this disease demands diagnosis and treatment based on the best available evidence.

With respect to the lipid accumulation theory, clinical studies have demonstrated a striking correlation between elevated serum cholesterol and an increased incidence of ischemic heart disease (Kannel, 1979). In addition, serum HDL cholesterol has been shown to be inversely correlated with the incidence of ischemic heart disease (Castelli et al., 1977; Gordon et al., 1977). Evidence for a positive relationship between elevated serum triglycerides, i.e., serum very-low-density lipoproteins (VLDL), and an increased incidence of ischemic heart disease is weak and not as conclusive as for cholesterol (Hulley et al., 1980). Yet certain authorities have been convinced that it exists (Levy, 1973). The relationship between serum cholesterol, HDL cholesterol, and ischemic heart disease has been quantified (Castelli et al., 1977; Kannel et al., 1971).

Clinical Contexts

Diagnosis. Assessment of risk of ischemic heart disease does not constitute a diagnosis and therefore is not performed to confirm or exclude a diagnosis. However, this subproblem often arises when a patient is hospitalized with a variety of diseases, including acute myocardial infarction. It is inappropriate to assess risk factors in a hospitalized patient who is being stressed by an acute disease process. It is unrealistic to expect serum cholesterol, serum HDL cholesterol, and systolic blood pressure to be basal during a period of stress.

Management. Assessment of risk factors is performed as a prognostic and therapeutic guide to determine whether they can be favorably modified in order to lower the chance of ischemic heart disease. Once an increased risk is documented, assessment of risk factors is repeated as necessary to determine how the risk changes as these factors are modified. A 6-week period is appropriate to determine the effectiveness of a new dietary or drug regimen before serum lipids are remeasured (Margolis, 1978).

Screening. It is appropriate to assess risk factors for ischemic heart disease as a targeted screening procedure. Ideally, screening antedates clinical disease, but it can also be useful in a stable period after signs or symptoms of ischemic heart disease appear. The age at which screening should first be performed is debatable. Fatty deposits, termed *fatty streaks,* are present in the aorta of all infants over the age of 1 year and begin to appear in the coronary arteries at age 10. Glueck and colleagues (1971) advocated measurement of cholesterol in the cord blood of newborn infants. Familial hypercholesterolemia can be identified in the first year of life (Margolis, 1978).

We believe that all young adults are suitable candidates for screening. When there is a positive family history of ischemic heart disease or hyperlipemia, screening should be performed in childhood. When serum triglyceride levels are normal in childhood, serum lipids should be evaluated at a later age, since serum triglyceride levels are not usually elevated before the age of 20 years (Margolis, 1978).

Strategy

Test Sequence. The best test sequence for assessment of risk factors is to measure total serum cholesterol and serum HDL cholesterol and to interpret the results in concert with information about other risk factors (age, sex, systolic blood pressure, cigarette smoking, left ventricular hypertrophy, and glucose intolerance) (Table 10–5). If serum cholesterol and/or HDL cholesterol are outside the reference intervals, they should be remeasured together with a serum triglyceride test on a specimen taken after fasting. If the values are still outside the reference intervals, the subproblem of the etiology of hyperlipidemia should be addressed (Fig. 10–5).

Patient Preparation. Serum cholesterol and serum HDL cholesterol should not be measured in outpatients or inpatients who are being stressed by acute disease. This is especially true if the results are being used to quantify risk as defined in the Framingham study. In order for the Framingham data to be useful, the patient should be from a similar population sample under basal or usual conditions. Basal conditions, according to Rifkind (1974), include the following:

1. Conventional Western diet.
2. Steady weight.
3. No acute illness.
4. No lipid-lowering or lipid-influencing drugs.

Although feeding has little effect on serum cholesterol and HDL cholesterol levels, it has a marked effect on the serum triglyceride level. Therefore, if serum triglycerides are measured, the serum should be drawn after a 12- to 16-hour fast of water only. Serum lipid concentration can drop approximately 10 per cent in patients who assume a recumbent position after standing (Tan et al., 1973).

Because serum cholesterol, HDL cholesterol, and triglycerides are all subject to physiologic and analytic variation, it is worthwhile to measure them at least two and preferably three times before making management decisions. These measurements should be taken at intervals at least a week apart. This series of measurements not only documents hyperlipemia but also serves as a baseline against which therapy can be evaluated (Margolis, 1978).

Specimen Collection and Handling. We recommend using serum or plasma for lipid studies. If plasma is used, it should be anticoagulated with either EDTA or heparin. EDTA is preferred. Hemolysis should be avoided.

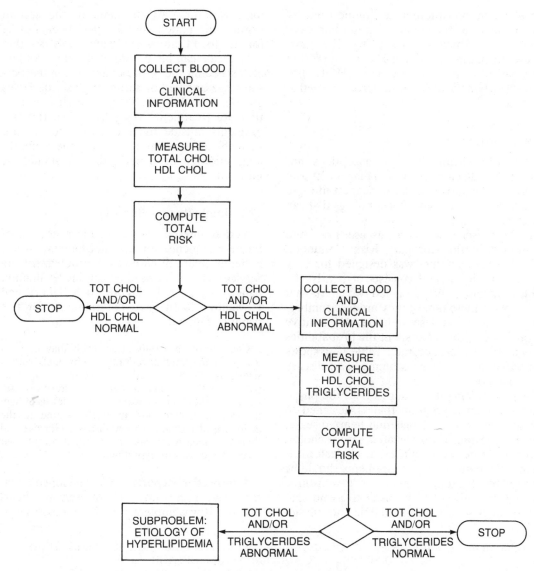

Figure 10–5. Strategy for assessing risk of ischemic heart disease.

Highly lipemic, turbid, non-fasting specimens for cholesterol and HDL cholesterol measurements should be stored overnight at 4°C, and the clear serum or plasma used for analysis. If samples are not analyzed immediately, they can be stored at 4°C for up to 1 to 2 weeks. Samples should not be frozen, since the freeze-thaw cycle destroys lipoprotein structure and decreases lipoprotein resolution on agarose gel.

Methodology. Consult the laboratory concerning its methods for measuring serum cholesterol, HDL cholesterol, and triglycerides and for reference intervals, accuracy and precision, and potential sources of interference.

Serum cholesterol can be measured by colorimetric, chromatographic, enzymatic, and automated direct methods. Colorimetry (i.e., the Abell-Kendall procedure or the Schoenheimer-Sperry method), chromatography, and enzyme studies can all give good results. Automated direct methods can overestimate serum cholesterol by 30 to 40 mg/100 ml (Tamir et al., 1979).

Serum triglycerides can be measured by colorimetry and enzyme studies. The wide variety of methods still in use to measure serum and plasma triglyceride levels suggests that no one technique is completely satisfactory (Tamir et al., 1979). Serum HDL cholesterol can be measured by precipitation techniques and by enzymatic measurement after lipoprotein electrophoresis (Jenny et al., 1978). We have measured plasma cholesterol and triglyceride enzymatically and have estimated HDL cholesterol enzymatically after lipoprotein electrophoresis.

Interpretation

Risk of ischemic heart disease does not constitute a diagnosis. It is a management tool to assess prognosis in order to suggest lifestyle modifications (diet, smoking) or drugs that can reduce risk.

Risk of ischemic heart disease has been quantified in the Coronary Risk Handbook (1973). This pamphlet was designed for easy use by physicians and consists of nearly 100 tables. Brittain (1982) designed two charts that can replace these tables; they are less cumbersome to use and also indicate the relative importance of the factors, but the probabilities may be slightly less accurate. Table 10–6 shows the variation of risk for ischemic heart disease in a man 40 years of age.

After assessing the patient's risk, the physician can plan a program that is designed to reduce the chance of ischemic heart disease. We believe that if an elevated serum cholesterol or depressed serum HDL cholesterol is found, the pathologic measurements should be verified by repeating them at least two or three times (Margolis, 1978) in order to avoid spurious values secondary to analytic and physiologic variation. At the time of the second testing, the patient should have been fasting for 12 to 14 hours on water only so that triglyceride can be measured. Cholesterol levels exceeding the 95th percentile for the person's age and sex or serum triglyceride levels greater than 300 mg/100 ml are clear indications for treatment (Margolis, 1978). If measurements outside the reference intervals are verified, the strategy for solving the subproblem, etiology of hyperlipidemia, should be initiated.

Test Requests and Reports

Test Requests. We offer the execution of the test sequence for the subproblem, risk of ischemic heart disease, as a problem-solving service. Henry devised a cardiac evaluation panel, as shown in Figure 10–6. Henry and Howanitz (1980) gave the rationale for this panel as follows:

Cholesterol and triglyceride levels may be used to screen for lipid disorders in individuals with a strong family history of atherosclerosis or those patients with evidence of coronary artery disease. Recent studies have indicated that the levels of high density lipoproteins are inversely related to the incidence of coronary artery disease. Glucose and thyroxine measurements are included to rule out secondary causes of hyperlipidemia.

Interpretive Reports. We developed an interpretive report for risk of ischemic heart disease. It was implemented by our associates,

Table 10–6. COMPARISON OF QUANTIFIABLE RISK FACTORS FOR ISCHEMIC HEART DISEASE IN A MAN 40 YEARS OF AGE

Years from now	Risk for Ischemic Heart Disease per 1000 Patients (All Columns)							
2 years	2	3	7	12	7	8	11	169
4 years	3	7	15	35	17	19	28	368
6 years	7	16	32	75	37	38	51	528
8 years	10	22	40	89	47	51	65	604
Least-risk factors	*	—	—	—	—	—	—	—
Systolic hypertension	—	175 mm Hg	—	—	—	—	—	+
Glucose intolerance	—	—	+	—	—	—	—	+
Hypercholesterolemia	—	—	—	350 mg/100 ml	—	—	—	+
Low HDL cholesterol	—	—	—	—	35 mg/100 ml	—	—	+
Cigarette smoking	—	—	—	—	—	+	—	+
Left ventricular hypertrophy	—	—	—	—	—	—	+	+

*This is the column of least risk: Systolic blood pressure is less than 105 mm Hg, serum cholesterol less than 185 mg/100 ml, and the serum HDL cholesterol is 45 mg/100 ml. Glucose intolerance, cigarette smoking, and left ventricular hypertrophy are not present.

CARDIAC EVALUATION				
Cholesterol mg/dl	Age 20–30 130–230			
Triglyceride mg/dl	10–160			
T$_4$-RIA µg/dl	5.5–12.3			
Glucose mg/dl	65–115			
Uric Acid mg/dl	Male 2.1–7.8 Female 2.0–6.4			
HDL Cholesterol mg/dl	40–75			

Figure 10–6. Cardiac evaluation panel. (Adapted from Henry JB, Murphy J: Effective utilization of clinical laboratories. In Henry JB (ed): Clinical Diagnosis and Management by Laboratory Methods, ed. 16. Philadelphia, WB Saunders Company, 1979, p 2044.)

Newman and McNair (1979) (Fig. 10–7). The program is written in extended BASIC on a small microcomputer using the Framingham data for age, sex, serum cholesterol, serum HDL cholesterol, systolic blood pressure, cigarette smoking, left ventricular hypertrophy, and glucose intolerance.

Bruce and associates (1981) demonstrated the feasibility of computer reporting and interpretation of symptom-limited exercise testing data. They presented measurements of cardiovascular impairment and gave estimates of probabilities of subsequent primary and secondary coronary heart disease based on prior Seattle Heart Watch experience. Risk factors (e.g., smoking, cholesterol, hypertension) are included in the data base, and a graphic display of the functional impairment and risk is provided by computer printout.

ETIOLOGY OF HYPERLIPIDEMIA

Definition and Significance

If the serum cholesterol and/or triglyceride levels are elevated, the cause can sometimes be determined. This inquiry constitutes the subproblem, etiology of hyperlipidemia. It is often difficult to decide which levels are pathologic. As with levels of blood pressure, increasing levels of serum cholesterol are related in a linear fashion to increasing risk of atherosclerosis and its complications. Reference intervals for serum cholesterol (the intervals found from surveys of given populations) are usually significantly higher than ideal intervals (values at which risk of atherosclerosis is min-

imal) (Elliott, 1979; Wright, 1976). Once it has been determined that the serum cholesterol or triglyceride level is elevated, it is useful to determine whether the patient has a primary (genetic) hyperlipidemia or a hyperlipidemia secondary to another disease such as diabetes mellitus or hypothyroidism. It is only by accurately determining the etiology of hyperlipidemia that an effective management program can be designed. Lipoprotein phenotyping may be helpful in accomplishing this determination.

Pathophysiology

Lipids (cholesterol, phospholipids, and triglycerides) are carried in the serum in combination with protein. Without protein, lipids are not soluble in aqueous solutions. These combinations of lipids and protein are referred to as *lipoproteins*. All of the lipoproteins contain cholesterol, phospholipids, and triglycerides. However, the proportions are different (Fig. 10–8).

Chylomicrons are composed of about 95 per cent neutral fat or triglyceride, but they do carry some cholesterol, protein, and phospholipids. Chylomicrons are elevated after meals; normal individuals require 12 to 16 hours to clear chylomicrons from serum completely. It is not clear whether chylomicrons contribute to atherosclerosis.

Very-low-density lipoproteins (VLDLs) are rich in triglycerides, with a triglyceride-to-cholesterol ratio of approximately 5:1. They have more cholesterol and fewer triglycerides than do chylomicrons, and they also carry phospho-

FORM 3352-REV. 2-68
(461001)

THE OHIO STATE UNIVERSITY HOSPITALS
GENERAL CONSULTATION REQUEST

Outpatient: John J.
OSUH#:123456789
Age: 55

TO _____LIPIDS LAB_____ DATE ___JULY 11, 1979___
(PHYSICIAN AND/OR SERVICE)

☒ OUTPATIENT ☐ INPATIENT

PROVISIONAL DIAGNOSIS:

REASON FOR REFERRAL: EVALUATION OF RISK FOR CORONARY HEART DISEASE

PATIENT NAME: OUTPATIENT, JOHN J. ____
OSUH ID#: 123456789
SEX: XX MALE, ____ FEMALE
AGE: 55 YEARS
SYSTOLIC B.P.: 150 MM HG, ____ NA (138 MM HG WILL BE ASSUMED)
DOES PATIENT SMOKE CIGARETTES: XX YES, ___ NO, ___ NA (NO WILL BE ASSUMED)
IS LEFT VENTRICULAR HYPERTROPHY BY ECG
    PRESENT: ___ YES, XX NO, ___ NA (NO WILL BE ASSUMED)
IS GLUCOSE INTOLERANCE PRESENT: ___ YES, XX NO, ___ NA (NO WILL BE ASSUMED)
IS THIS A FASTING SPECIMEN: ___ YES, XX NO.

_____(USE REVERSE SIDE IF NECESSARY)_____ M.D.

REPORT AND OPINION OF CONSULTANT

DATE ___JULY 12, 1979___

SERUM TOTAL CHOLESTEROL: 340 MG/DL
HDL CHOLESTEROL: 39 MG/DL
TRIGLYCERIDES: FASTING SPECIMEN REQUIRED

RISK FACTOR OF CORONARY HEART DISEASE
IN 2 YEARS = 84 PER THOUSAND
IN 4 YEARS = 179 PER THOUSAND
IN 6 YEARS = 250 PER THOUSAND
IN 8 YEARS = 313 PER THOUSAND

IF SERUM TOTAL CHOLESTEROL DROPS TO 253 MG/DL
    THEN RISK IN 2 YEARS = 52 PER THOUSAND
IF HDL CHOLESTEROL RISES TO 50 MG/DL
    THEN RISK IN 2 YEARS = 56 PER THOUSAND
IF SYSTOLIC B.P. DROPS TO 138 MM HG
    THEN RISK IN 2 YEARS = 74 PER THOUSAND
IF THE PATIENT STOPS SMOKING
    THEN RISK IN 2 YEARS = 50 PER THOUSAND
IF ALL FOUR OF THE ABOVE ARE CHANGED AS DESCRIBED
    THEN RISK IN 2 YEARS = 18 PER THOUSAND

FOR ALL PATIENTS WITH TOTAL CHOLESTEROL OVER 300 MG/DL AND/OR HDL CHOLESTEROL UNDER 40,
IT IS RECOMMENDED THAT A 12 TO 14 HOUR FASTING SPECIMEN BE SUBMITTED FOR REPEAT ANALYSIS
AND POSSIBLE LIPOPROTEIN PHENOTYPING.

_____(USE REVERSE SIDE IF NECESSARY)_____ M.D.

FORM – #24004

1-4 \ \ \ \ \ \ \ \ \ \ \ \ \ \ \ \ \ \ \ CONSULTS

Figure 10–7. Interpretive report for risk of ischemic heart disease. (Courtesy Ohio State University Hospitals.)

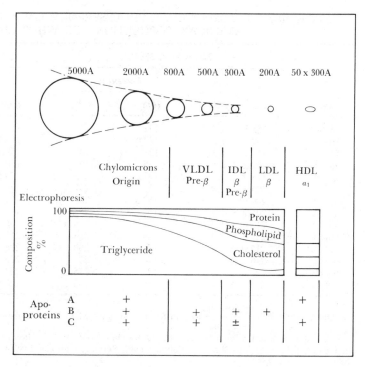

Figure 10–8. Classification of plasma lipoproteins by physical and chemical properties. (From Bierman EL: Hyperproteinemia. Kalamazoo, Mich., The Upjohn Company, 1976, p 4.)

lipids and protein. Increased serum VLDLs probably contribute to an increased risk of atherosclerosis (Levy, 1973).

Low-density lipoproteins (LDLs) contain the major portion of serum cholesterol as well as protein, phospholipid, and a little triglyceride. Increased levels of serum LDLs are generally considered to contribute significantly to atherosclerosis (Fredrickson, 1978).

High-density lipoproteins (HDLs) contain mainly protein as well as some cholesterol, phospholipid, and a little triglyceride. The cholesterol, even though small in amount, may be significant. There is evidence that a normal or high level of serum HDL may be important in lowering risk of atherosclerosis either by preventing other types of cholesterol from being deposited in the walls of arteries or by actually removing cholesterol from arterial walls (Castelli et al., 1977; Gordon et al., 1977). Fredrickson and associates (1978) give an excellent overall review of hyperlipoproteinemia.

Clinical Contexts

Diagnosis. The etiology of hyperlipidemia should be investigated whenever the serum total cholesterol or triglyceride level is elevated after a 12- to 16-hour fast in a properly prepared patient. Elevation of serum triglycerides without elevated serum cholesterol in a nonfasting specimen is not a reason for investigating the etiology of hyperlipidemia because the elevated serum triglyceride may be secondary to a meal.

Deciding whether or not the serum total cholesterol and triglycerides are elevated is complicated by a lack of good reference intervals for these analytes. Tables 10–7 and 10–8 give age- and sex-adjusted reference intervals for serum and plasma total cholesterol and triglyceride levels. We believe it is reasonable to investigate the etiology of hyperlipidemia whenever the serum total cholesterol or triglyceride level is elevated above the 90th percentile. Even reduction of levels that are within the reference intervals can be helpful in lowering risk. The physician should search for evidence of a disorder or drug that can cause the hyperlipidemia (Table 10–9). Serum HDL cholesterol, as a risk factor, should be evaluated when it is low. Our reference interval for men is 25 to 65 mg/100 ml; for females, 32 to 79 mg/100 ml.

Management. After classifying the hyperlipidemia according to Frederickson (1978) (Table 10–10), decide whether it is primary or

Table 10–7. PLASMA TOTAL CHOLESTEROL (mg/dl)* IN 11 FREE-LIVING NORTH AMERICAN POPULATIONS OF WHITE PARTICIPANTS†

Age	Males (n = 3580)			Females (n = 3413)		
	Mean ± SEM	Percentiles		Mean ± SEM	Percentiles	
		10th	90th		10th	90th
5–9	155.3 ± 1.8	131	183	164.0 ± 1.8	135	189
10–14	160.9 ± 1.5	132	191	160.1 ± 1.5	131	191
15–19	153.1 ± 1.4	123	183	159.5 ± 1.6	126	198
20–24	162.2 ± 2.5	126	197	170.3 ± 2.5	132	220
25–29	178.7 ± 2.1	137	223	179.5 ± 1.7	142	217
30–34	193.1 ± 1.8	152	237	179.2 ± 1.7	141	215
35–39	200.6 ± 1.9	157	248	189.6 ± 2.1	149	233
40–44	205.2 ± 1.9	161	251	197.5 ± 1.9	156	241
45–49	213.4 ± 1.9	171	258	206.2 ± 2.0	162	256
50–54	213.2 ± 1.9	168	263	217.3 ± 2.4	171	267
55–59	215.0 ± 2.2	172	260	228.7 ± 2.4	182	278
60–64	216.6 ± 3.3	170	262	232.3 ± 3.7	186	282
65–69	221.0 ± 3.8	174	275	234.1 ± 4.0	179	282
70+	210.3 ± 3.4	160	253	224.5 ± 2.8	181	268

*Multiply by $0.026 \frac{mmol \cdot dl}{liter \cdot mg}$ to transform to SI units; SEM = Standard error of the mean.

†The Lipid Research Clinics Population Studies Data Book: Vol. I. The Prevalence Study. From The U.S. Department of Health, Education and Welfare: Public Health Service, National Institutes of Health, Pub. No. NIH-791527, July 1979, p. 52.

Table 10–8. PLASMA TOTAL TRIGLYCERIDES (mg/dl)* IN 11 FREE-LIVING NORTH AMERICAN POPULATIONS OF WHITE PARTICIPANTS†

Age	Males (n = 3580)			Females (n = 3413)		
	Mean ± SEM	Percentiles		Mean ± SEM	Percentiles	
		10th	90th		10th	90th
5–9	51.9 ± 1.7	34	70	63.8 ± 2.5	37	103
10–14	63.4 ± 1.6	37	94	72.0 ± 1.7	44	104
15–19	78.2 ± 2.4	43	125	72.8 ± 1.9	40	112
20–24	89.3 ± 3.7	50	146	87.3 ± 2.9	42	135
25–29	104.2 ± 4.2	51	171	87.4 ± 2.8	45	137
30–34	122.1 ± 3.7	57	214	86.0 ± 2.8	45	140
35–39	140.8 ± 5.5	58	250	98.3 ± 3.2	47	170
40–44	152.4 ± 6.9	69	252	98.1 ± 2.6	51	161
45–49	143.4 ± 5.9	65	218	112.5 ± 3.4	55	180
50–54	153.4 ± 5.5	75	244	116.0 ± 3.4	58	190
55–59	134.3 ± 4.2	70	210	133.1 ± 4.8	65	229
60–64	130.6 ± 8.7	65	193	132.1 ± 9.1	66	210
65–69	138.6 ± 11.1	61	227	136.5 ± 6.8	64	221
70+	132.8 ± 7.2	71	202	128.3 ± 6.5	68	189

*Multiply by $0.026 \frac{mmol \cdot dl}{liter \cdot mg}$ to transform to SI units; SEM = Standard error of the mean.

†The Lipid Research Clinics Population Studies Data Book: Vol. I. The Prevalence Study. From the U.S. Department of Health, Education, and Welfare: Public Health Service, National Institutes of Health. Pub. No. NIH-791527, July 1979, p. 58.

Table 10–9. SECONDARY HYPERLIPOPROTEINEMIAS*

		Morphology				
Cause†	*I* *Chylos‡*	*V* *Chylos‡* *Pre-β§*	*IV* *Pre-β§*	*III‖* *Broad-β*	*II-A¶* β	*II-B* β + *Pre-β§*
Diabetes						
Severe	+	+				
Moderate		±	±	±		±
Mild		±	±	±		
Renal disease						
Nephrotic syndrome		±	±		±	±
Uremia		±	±			
Alcohol		±	±			
Corticosteroid Treatment						
High dose	±	±				
Low dose			±		±	±
Estrogen or oral contraceptive treatment		±	±			
Hypothyroidism		+	+	+	+	+
Dysglobulinemia	+	+				

*Modified from Bierman EL: Hyperlipoproteinemia. Kalamazoo, Mich., The Upjohn Company, 1976, p 9.
†See text for additional causes
‡Chylomicrons
§Pre-β = Pre-beta lipoproteins.
‖Broad-β = Broad-beta lipoproteins.
¶β = beta lipoproteins.

secondary. If it is secondary, treat the underlying disease; if primary, devise a management plan for lowering the serum lipids and screen family members for hyperlipidemia.

During the therapy of patients with hyperlipidemia and hyperlipoproteinemia, serum and plasma total cholesterol, serum HDL cholesterol, and serum or plasma triglycerides should be measured (after a fast of 12 to 16 hours) at the time of each office visit. If triglycerides have not been elevated, it is possible to use a specimen from a fed or fasting patient. Values for serum total cholesterol and serum HDL cholesterol can be used together with information from the history and physical examination to assess risk of ischemic heart

Table 10–10. CLASSIFICATION OF HYPERLIPOPROTEINEMIA*

		Morphology				
Pathophysiology	*I* *Chylos†*	*V* *Chylos†* *Pre-β‡*	*IV* *Pre-β‡*	*III* *Broad-β§*	*II-A* β‖	*II-B* β‖ + *Pre-β‡*
↓ Removal						
LPL¶ deficiency	+	+				
LPL¶ depletion		+	+			+
Remnant accumulation				+		
? ↓ LDL# removal					+	+
Production ↑		+	+		+	+

*Modified from Bierman EL: Hyperlipoproteinemia. Kalamazoo, Mich., The Upjohn Company, 1976, p 8.
†Chylomicrons.
‡Broad-β = broad-beta lipoproteins
‖β = beta lipoproteins
¶LPL = lipoprotein-lipase
#LDL = low-density lipoproteins

disease. Values for serum total cholesterol, HDL cholesterol, and triglycerides can be used to assess the effectiveness of the therapeutic regimen.

Screening. The etiology of hyperlipidemia as a clinical subproblem is addressed only if hyperlipidemia is documented to be present by measuring serum and plasma total cholesterol and triglycerides after a 12- to 16-hour fast.

Strategy

Test Sequence. After measuring fasting total cholesterol and triglyceride (by a 12- to 16-hour fast, water only) and determining that cholesterol and/or triglyceride are above the 90th percentile, the physician can initiate phenotyping. Fredrickson's phenotypes (1978) can sometimes provide a clue to the etiology of the hyperlipoproteinemia.

Patient Preparation. Rifkind (1974) considers adequate patient preparation to be:

1. A conventional Western diet.
2. Steady weight.
3. No acute illness (defer sampling at least 6 weeks after myocardial infarction).
4. No lipid-lowering or lipid-influencing drugs.
5. Fasting for 12 to 16 hours on water only.

These conditions make it impossible to study the etiology of hyperlipidemia in hospitalized patients, and we recommend outpatient evaluation. If the fasting serum total cholesterol and triglyceride levels are elevated while the patient is hospitalized, wait until after recovery to begin further investigations.

Specimen Collection and Handling. The requirements are the same as for the clinical subproblem of risk of ischemic heart disease. See the discussion earlier in this chapter.

Methodology. Lipoprotein phenotyping can be done by three techniques, all of which require quantitative measurement of total serum or plasma cholesterol and trigylcerides:

1. Use of a nomogram together with a physical examination of serum that has been standing overnight at 4°C in a refrigerator (Fredrickson, 1972). This is called the "refrigerator test."
2. Lipoprotein electrophoresis.
3. Ultracentrifugation.

Some investigators recommend the abandonment of lipoprotein electrophoresis and even lipoprotein phenotyping for the management of hyperlipidemia. Certainly, lipoprotein electrophoresis is not required in the workup of every patient with hyperlipoproteinemia (Fredrickson, 1972, 1978; Immarino, 1974; Steinberg, 1973). We perform the refrigerator test in conjunction with lipoprotein electrophoresis on agarose gel and reserve ultracentrifugation for cases that cannot be phenotyped by these methods.

Interpretation

If a secondary hyperlipoproteinemia is diagnosed, remove the offending drug (e.g., estrogen, oral contraceptives, glucocorticoids, alcohol) or treat the underlying disease (e.g., hypothyroidism, diabetes mellitus, chronic renal failure, nephrotic syndrome, multiple myeloma, obstructive liver disease, acute porphyria, glycogen storage disease) (Margolis, 1978) (see Part 3 for effects of drugs and diseases on serum cholesterol). If a primary hyperlipoproteinemia is diagnosed, institute appropriate therapy.

In either primary or secondary hyperlipoproteinemia, the patient should be followed by measuring serum or plasma cholesterol, HDL cholesterol, and triglyceride levels as described in the subproblem, risk of ischemic heart disease. A 6-week period is generally sufficient to determine the effectiveness of either a dietary or drug regimen (Margolis, 1978); it is thus unnecessary to measure serum lipids very frequently (i.e., every week).

Test Requests and Reports

Test Requests. The laboratory can assist the attending physician in solving the clinical subproblem, etiology of hyperlipidemia, by executing the test sequence for etiology of hyperlipidemia as well as strategies for secondary causes of hyperlipidemia. (See the discussions of cholestasis in Chapter 15 and of diabetes mellitus in Chapter 16 for strategies to diagnose these causes of secondary hyperlipidemia.)

Interpretive Reports. Test results can be collated and returned to the attending physician in the form of an interpretive report.

HYPERTENSION

Hypertension is an elevation of systolic or diastolic blood pressure above the upper reference limits. According to Feinstein (1973) (see Chapter 2), it can be classified as a functional disorder of the cardiovascular system. Because up to 25 per cent of the United States population may be affected—blacks almost twice as often as whites (Chobanian, 1980)—and because it kills people by contributing to heart failure, renal failure, and stroke, it presents physicians with an important diagnostic and management challenge. The following discussion focuses on the clinical subproblems that arise in the hypertensive patient.

As with serum cholesterol levels, there is no sharp demarcation between blood pressure (BP) levels that are or are not associated with increased morbidity and mortality. Risk increases in a linear fashion with increasing levels of systolic or diastolic BP (Lew, 1973). Even modest BP elevations above the upper reference limits are associated with risk (Kannel, 1976). The World Health Organization (WHO, 1959) defines hypertension as follows:

Normal blood pressure: 139 mm Hg or less systolic, 89 mm Hg or less diastolic.

High blood pressure: 160 mm Hg or greater systolic, 95 mm Hg or greater diastolic.

For practical purposes, adult BP of less than 140/90 is not associated with hypertensive risk; between 140/90 and 160/95 is considered borderline elevated; and more than or equal to 160/95 is hypertensive (Chobanian, 1980). In children these limits are lower (Blumenthal, 1977; Kilcoyne, 1975). Kaplan(1982) believes the WHO criteria may be set too high and that they should vary with age and sex.

Pickering and associates (1982) monitored BP every 15 minutes using a non-invasive ambulatory BP recorder during 24 hours in 25 subjects with normal BP, 25 with borderline hypertension, and 25 with established essential hypertension. The 24-hour recording in all three groups showed the highest BP figures at work and the lowest during sleep. Pressures recorded in the physician's office gave good predictions of the average 24-hour pressure in normal and established hypertensive subjects but not in the borderline group; in such patients, 24-hour monitoring may be of particular value in establishing the need for treatment.

The Veterans Administration Cooperative Study Group on Antihypertensive Agents clearly determined that treatment of patients having mean diastolic BP values averaging between 115 and 129 mm Hg is beneficial (1967). This same group demonstrated beneficial effects in the treatment of patients whose mean diastolic pressure averaged between 90 and 114 mm Hg (1970). The results were confirmed by the 5-year findings of the hypertension detection and follow-up program (1979).

Moser (1977) provides a good source for guidance concerning the detection and management of the hypertensive patient. The benefits of treating every hypertensive patient—especially those with borderline hypertension—when balanced against the drug side effects, are not agreed upon by all (Alderman, 1977). Stratification of risk according to average 24-hour BP measurements is needed, though it may be many years before this information becomes available (Pickering et al., 1982).

EVALUATION OF THE HYPERTENSIVE PATIENT

Definition and Significance

Every patient with hypertension, whether benign or malignant, primary or secondary, should have a laboratory evaluation. This evaluation is performed for these reasons (Burke, 1980; Simpson, 1978):

1. To provide baseline data for use in subsequent drug therapy.
2. To search for other risk factors.
3. To look for target organ damage.
4. To find a specific cause.

The evaluation of patients who are young or who have severe hypertension should be vigorously pursued. We shall refer to these key studies as the clinical subproblem, evaluation of the hypertensive patient.

Pathophysiology

Hypertension of unknown etiology is referred to as *primary* or *essential*. Most diagnosed cases of hypertension are placed in this category.

Secondary hypertension has a variety of etiologies. These are addressed later in this chapter.

Many factors, genetic as well as environmental, are important in the etiology and pathophysiology of primary hypertension. Cardiac output, systemic vascular resistance, blood volume, sympathetic and central nervous system activity, and the renin-angiotensin-aldosterone system are all contributing factors. There are several sources for a discussion of this complex topic (Burke, 1980; Kaplan, 1982).

Patients with primary hypertension can be divided into three groups, based on the clinical course of their disease:

1. *Labile hypertension* occurs when the patient has elevated BP levels at some times but not at others. The significance of this type of hypertension in terms of morbidity and mortality is under debate.

2. *Benign hypertension* usually begins insidiously in the fourth decade, and the patient often remains free of symptoms for 10 to 15 years. Atherosclerosis is the main complication, with approximately 50 per cent dying of congestive heart failure, 20 per cent of cerebrovascular accident, and 30 per cent of other causes such as acute myocardial infarction.

3. *Malignant hypertension* presents with a rapidly rising or sustained elevated diastolic pressure, usually over 130 mm Hg. Vascular changes lead to progressive disease of the brain, eyes, and kidneys. Renal failure and hypertensive encephalopathy are the life-threatening complications, and untreated patients usually die in less than a year.

Clinical Contexts

Diagnosis. Evaluation of the hypertensive patient is not performed to confirm a clinical impression or to exclude a diagnosis, since the initial diagnosis of hypertension has already been made. Rather, effort should be directed at detection of the etiology and effective management. A thorough history, physical examination, and laboratory evaluation should be performed.

Drug and dietary causes of hypertension should be specifically ruled out, including:

1. Oral contraceptives and estrogens.
2. Steroids.
3. Thyroid hormones.
4. Monamine oxidase (MAO) inhibitors with tyramine.
5. Sympathomimetics (e.g., amphetamines, cold remedies).
6. Licorice excess.

Though some laboratory studies are directed at the detection of end-organ damage (e.g., serum creatinine and urea nitrogen to detect renal damage), others offer diagnostic clues concerning the etiology of secondary hypertension (e.g., fasting blood sugar to detect pheochromocytoma and Cushing's syndrome). The presence of end-organ damage supports the diagnosis of hypertension in those patients with borderline BP values.

Management. Assessment of end-organ damage, particularly a deterioration in renal function, is an important objective of the strategy. This information affects prognosis and therapy. Evaluation of the hypertensive patient can be used to monitor the effect of antihypertensive drugs on the serum potassium as well as idiosyncratic drug reactions reflected in the complete blood count. Baseline renal tests are useful in monitoring deterioration of kidney function.

Screening. Evaluation of the hypertensive patient is an example of targeted screening. It should be performed for each hypertensive patient regardless of clinical signs and symptoms.

Strategy

Test Sequence. Table 10–11 lists the tests we recommend for the evaluation of the hypertensive patient. Chobanian (1980) suggests a urine culture on at least one occasion as well as laboratory assays to detect pheochromocytoma. Henry and Howanitz (1980) suggest a determination of creatinine clearance in the

Table 10–11. RECOMMENDED TESTS FOR LABORATORY EVALUATION OF THE HYPERTENSIVE PATIENT*

Complete blood count
Fasting serum sugar
Serum urea nitrogen
Serum creatinine
Serum potassium
Serum calcium
Serum uric acid
Urinalysis
Electrocardiogram
Assessment of other risk factors (see text)
Exclusion of causes of hypertension (see text)

*Moser (1977) recommends only the following basic laboratory tests: hemoglobin or hematocrit; urinalysis; serum potassium, creatinine or urea nitrogen; and electrocardiogram. However, with the advent of multichannel chemistry and hematology instrumentation, it has often been less expensive to obtain biochemical and hematology profiles, which include all of our tests and more, than to obtain tests individually. (Moser M: Report of the Joint National Committee on Detection, Evaluation, and Treatment of High Blood Pressure: A cooperative study. JAMA 237:255–261, 1977.)

hypertension panel for a more sensitive indicator of renal deterioration than that given by serum creatinine.

A complete blood count is performed to exclude anemia, which can further stress the heart. It is also useful to know the leukocyte count as a baseline for monitoring drug therapy. An elevated fasting blood glucose is helpful to detect diabetes mellitus (another important risk factor for ischemic heart disease) and can be a clue to the presence of Cushing's syndrome and pheochromocytoma. Serum urea nitrogen (SUN) and creatinine studies are complementary and can detect end-organ damage in the kidney or serve as a clue to primary renal disease, such as pyelonephritis or glomerulonephritis. A depressed serum potassium level can serve as a clue to adrenocortical disorders as well as a baseline for monitoring drug therapy. Knowing the serum calcium level can aid in detecting reversible hypertension secondary to hypercalcemia (Blum et al., 1977; Waeber et al., 1982).

If the laboratory offers a biochemical profile that includes all the suggested serum chemistry tests, it may be less expensive to order the profile rather than to order each chemistry test individually. Elevation of serum uric acid is considered a minor risk factor and is present in approximately 25 per cent of untreated hypertensive populations (*Lancet* editorial, 1981). A urinalysis and electrocardiogram are useful to detect existing kidney or heart disease and to serve as baseline studies. Other risk factors for atherosclerosis should be assessed, as discussed earlier in this chapter, and secondary causes of hypertension should be excluded. (See the discussion of etiology of hypertension later in this chapter.)

There is no consensus concerning the kinds or frequency of tests that should be performed to monitor hypertensive patients. Intervals for testing vary from 3 months to 1 year, and the kinds of tests recommended depend on the therapy used, e.g., serum potassium to monitor the effects of thiazides and liver function tests to monitor the effects of methyldopa.

Patient Preparation. If a serum glucose is obtained, an overnight fast (water only for 10 to 16 hours) is preferred for detection of diabetes mellitus. (See the discussion in Chapter 16 and Part 3 for chemistry and hematology tests.)

Specimen Collection and Handling. The specimen for urinalysis should be collected in a suitable, clean container. All studies should be accomplished expeditiously (see Part 3).

Methodology. Consult the laboratory about methodologies, reference intervals, accuracy and precision, and potential sources of interference. The urinalysis should be performed on a fresh specimen, which should be inspected for appearance, specific gravity, pH, protein, glucose, ketones, blood, bilirubin, and sediment. There should be a quality control program for the urinalysis (see Part 3).

Interpretation

Diagnosis. Performance of the hypertension evaluation panel on every hypertensive patient is designed to detect diabetes mellitus, renal disease, and general abnormalities of the hematopoietic system.

The reference interval for a fasting glucose is 60 to 115 mg/100 ml. Morning fasting values above 140 mg/100 ml are regarded as diabetic. Values above 115 mg/100 ml and certainly above 140 mg/100 ml can be a clue to the presence of pheochromocytoma, Cushing's syndrome, and acromegaly (National Diabetes Data Group, 1979). (See Chapter 16.) Testing for SUN, creatinine, and potassium has been described.

Information concerning the existence or development of end-organ (renal) damage can be determined from the SUN, creatinine, potassium, and complete blood count. Because SUN varies with prerenal disorders (dehydration, shock, diminished blood volume, and congestive heart failure) and postrenal disorders (urinary tract obstruction) as well as renal disease, it is not as specific as serum creatinine in diagnosing renal disease. Cole (1979) says that while a SUN level above 27 mg/100 ml is consistent with prerenal, renal, or postrenal disease, a value above 44 mg/100 ml is suggestive of renal disease. A serum creatinine level above 1.3 mg/100 ml for males and 1.0 mg/100 ml for females is indicative of renal disease (values are method-dependent). However, there is much overlap between creatinine levels in healthy patients and patients with renal damage. Serum potassium is elevated in severe renal failure. In patients with borderline elevations of serum creatinine, creatinine clearance is a more sensitive and specific indicator of renal damage. Hypokalemia can be a clue to aldosteronism.

Urinalysis can detect and help diagnose

HYPERTENSION				
Creatinine mg/dl	0.6–1.2			
Creatinine Clearance ml/min	80–120			
Urinary Free Cortisol mcg/24 hr	20–90			
Metanephrines µg/mg creatinine	Less than 1.82			
Chloride mEq/L	98–109			
CO$_2$ Content mM/L	24–30			
Sodium mEq/L	135–145			
Potassium mEq/L	4.0–4.8			
Glucose mg/dl	65–115			

Figure 10–9. Organ panel for hypertension. (From Henry JB, Murphy, J: Effective utilization of clinical laboratories. In Henry JB (ed): Clinical Diagnosis and Management by Laboratory Methods, ed. 16. Philadelphia, WB Saunders Company, 1979, p 2044.)

renal disease by finding urinary protein, erythrocytes, and leukocytes, as well as by identifying various kinds of casts in the urinary sediment.

Management. Some of the tests in the hypertension evaluation panel are useful for monitoring the adverse effects of antihypertensive therapy. For instance, the complete blood count can detect drug reaction by anemia, leukopenia, or thrombocytopenia, whereas low serum potassium may result from thiazide diuretics. The SUN and creatinine levels serve to monitor end-organ damage in the kidneys.

Test Requests and Reports

Test Requests. The execution of the test sequence for the evaluation of the hypertensive patient can be offered as a problem-solving service. Figure 10–9 gives Henry's panel of tests for hypertension. Henry and Howanitz (1980) gave the rationale for this panel as follows:

The best single determination for the diagnosis of pheochromocytoma is the urinary metanephrine. It is important to have a sensitive and specific test for this entity which is a surgically correctable form of hypertension. Gitlow in his experience with more than 16,000 patients improved the diagnostic reliability of this determination. Urinary free cortisol has achieved excellent sensitivity for the evaluation of hypercortisolism, while today fasting blood glucose is the most reliable indicator of diabetes mellitus. A creatinine clearance and serum electrolytes are included for the evaluation of renal function, which may be altered secondarily or primarily by hypertension. The study of Woods revealed that renin profiling as a way of identifying volume and vasodilator constrictive components of hypertension leaves much to be desired; current evidence suggests that drug treatment is best administered in an empiric fashion, diuretics first, an adrenergic blocking agent second, and vasodilator therapy third. For this reason, we do not advocate renin measurements.

Interpretive Reports. A report of the test results can be sent to the attending physician. This report could address evidence of end-organ damage and clues to secondary causes of the hypertension. DeGoulet and co-workers (1980) devised a computer-assisted hypertension management system called ARTEMIS. At a total annual cost of $11 per patient, this system helped to achieve a high rate of compliance at one year (81.3 per cent) by providing patients with updated editions of their personal summary reports as well as by sending periodical letters of recall to them and to their physicians.

ETIOLOGY OF SECONDARY HYPERTENSION

Definition and Significance

Most hypertensive patients have primary or essential hypertension. The remainder have secondary hypertension. Some causes of secondary hypertension are curable, but others are not. It is important to search for curable causes. Although the total cost of searching for every curable cause in every patient is prohibitive, young patients (under 35 years), those with abrupt onset of hypertension, and those with a negative family history for essential hypertension should receive a more thorough diagnostic evaluation. In addition to the tests in our evaluation strategy, these patients can be studied by a chest roentgenogram, rapid-sequence intravenous pyelogram (IVP), and laboratory tests for hyper- and hypothyroidism, pheochromocytoma, renovascular hypertension, and so on. Table 10–12 lists the causes of hypertension. Table 10–13 shows the prevalence of various forms of hypertension in the general population and in specialized referral clinics.

The laboratory plays a major role in the diagnosis of secondary causes of hypertension, as shown in Table 10–12. However, in this book, we address only Cushing's syndrome and pheochromocytoma (see Chapter 16).

Clinical Contexts

Since excessive cost prohibits laboratory evaluations for all potentially curable causes

Table 10–12. CLASSIFICATION OF HYPERTENSION BY ETIOLOGY*

A. Essential hypertension
B. Renal
  1. Parenchymal
    Acute glomerulonephritis
    Chronic nephritis, glomerulonephritis,
      pyelonephritis, heredity, irradiation, lupus
      erythematosus
    Polycystic kidney disease
    Hydronephrosis
    Renin-producing tumor
    Diabetic nephropathy (Kimmelstiel-Wilson)
  2. Renovascular
    Fibromuscular arterial stenosis
    Atherosclerotic arterial stenosis
    Renal infarctions
    Polyarteritis
  3. Trauma
    Perirenal hematoma
    Renal arterial thrombosis
    Renal arterial dissection
C. Endocrine
  1. Thyroid
    Hyperthyroidism
    Hypothyroidism
  2. Adrenal
    Pheochromocytoma
    Primary aldosteronism
      Adenoma
      Hyperplasia
      Glucocorticoid suppressible
      hyperaldosteronism
    Congenital adrenal hyperplasia
      11-β Hydroxylation deficiency
      17-α Hydroxylation deficiency
    Cushing's disease
  3. Parathyroid hyperparathyroidism

D. Neurogenic
    Respiratory acidosis (carbon dioxide retention)
    Brain tumor
    Encephalitis
    Bulbar poliomyelitis
    Familial dysautonomia
    Acute porphyria
    Quadriplegia ("micturitional crisis")
    Extra-adrenal chromaffin tumors
      Paragangliomas
      Von Recklinghausen's disease
E. Mechanical interference with flow
    AV fistulas (Paget's disease, patent ductus arteriosus)
    Aortic insufficiency
    Coarctation of the aorta
    Atherosclerotic systolic hypertension
F. Exogenous
  1. Poisoning
    Lead
    Thalium
  2. Medication
    Sympathetic amines
    MAO inhibitor combined with ephedrine or tyramine (including tyramine-rich foods, cheese, red wine)
    Birth control pills
    Prednisone—high doses
  3. Food
    Licorice ingestion
  4. Iatrogenic
    Volume overload in marginal renal insufficiency
G. Toxemia of pregnancy
H. Miscellaneous
    Polycythemia
      Rubra vera
      "Stress," Gaisbock's syndrome
    Burns
    Carcinoid syndrome

*From Julius S, Classification of hypertension, In Genest J, Koiu E, Kuchel O (eds): Hypertension: Physiopathy and Treatment. Copyright © 1977 by McGraw-Hill, Inc. Used by permission of McGraw-Hill Book Company, New York, p. 10.

Table 10–13. PREVALENCE OF VARIOUS FORMS OF HYPERTENSION IN THE GENERAL POPULATION AND IN SPECIALIZED REFERRAL CLINICS*†

Diagnosis	General Population, %	Specialty Clinic, %
Essential hypertension	92–94	65–85
Renal hypertension		
Parenchymal	2–3	4–5
Renovascular	1–2	4–16
Endocrine hypertension		
Primary aldosteronism	0.3	0.5–12
Cushing's syndrome	<0.1	0.2
Pheochromocytoma	<0.1	0.2
Oral contraceptive–induced	2–4	1–2
Miscellaneous	0.2	1

*Estimates based on a number of reports in the literature.

†From Williams GH, Jagger PI, Braunwald E: In Harrison's Principles of Internal Medicine. Copyright © 1980 by McGraw-Hill, Inc. Used by permission of McGraw Hill Book Company, New York, p 1168.

of hypertension in each patient, it is useful for physicians to know the clinical and laboratory features of all the curable causes. When any of these features are present in a hypertensive patient, the physician should proceed with the appropriate laboratory evaluation. This approach will detect most curable causes of hypertension with less cost than evaluating all patients with hypertension (Burke, 1980).

There are many strategies for finding the cause of secondary hypertension. Figure 16–4 gives a number of options for approaching the diagnosis of pheochromocytoma.

Pathophysiology

See Chapter 16 for a discussion of Cushing's syndrome and pheochromocytoma. Burke (1980) and Kaplan (1982) reviewed the pathophysiology of hypertension.

Strategy

Burke (1980) included test strategies for initial evaluation of all hypertensive patients as well as for the following causes of secondary hypertension: pheochromocytoma, renovascular hypertension, and primary aldosteronism. Maronde (1975) described an approach to the diagnostic workup of the hypertensive patient. See Chapter 16.

Interpretation

See Chapter 16, Burke (1980), and Kaplan (1982).

Test Requests and Reports

See Chapter 16.

REFERENCES

Coronary Heart Disease

Baillie EE: CK Isoenzymes. ASCP Technical Improvement Service, Number 30, Chicago, Illinois, American Society of Clinical Pathologists, 1977.

Bark CJ: Mitochondrial creatine kinase. A poor prognostic sign. JAMA 243:2058–2060, 1980.

Basta LL, Coyle JF: Ischemic heart disease. In Conn HF, Conn RB (eds): Current Diagnosis, ed 6. Philadelphia, WB Saunders Company, 1980, pp 345–354.

Bruns DE, Emerson JC, Intemann S, et al: Lactate dehydrogenase isoenzyme-1: Changes during the first day after acute myocardial infarction. Clin Chem 27:1821–1823, 1981.

Cohen JA, Kaplan MM: Left-sided heart failure presenting as hepatitis. Gastroenterology 74:583–587, 1978.

Dillon MC, Calbreath DF, Dixon AM, et al: Diagnostic problems in acute myocardial infarction: CK-MB in the absence of abnormally elevated total creatine kinase levels. Arch Intern Med 142:33–38, 1982.

Galen RS: The enzyme diagnosis of myocardial infarction. Hum Pathol 6:141–155, 1975.

Galen RS: Isoenzymes, part three. Which method to choose. Diagnostic Medicine, August 1978, pp 42–63.

Galen RS: CK Isoenzymes—What next? Diagnostic Medicine, July/August 1981, pp 9–12.

Galen RS, Gambino SR: Cardiac profile: A practical guide for the use of CPK and LDH isoenzymes. Beaumont, Tex, Helena Laboratories, 1978.

Gambino R (ed): An unexpected elevation of SGPT. Lab Report for Physicians 1:5, 1979.

Gambino R (ed): LDH isoenzymes. Lab Report for Physicians 2:7–8, 1980.

Gambino R (ed): LDH. Lab Report for Physicians 3:96, 1981.

Guzy PM: Creatine phosphokinase—MB (CPK-MB) and the diagnosis of myocardial infarction. West J Med 127:455–460, 1977.

Helena Laboratories: Methodology: CPK-LDH isoenzyme testing, the definitive cardiac profile. Beaumont, Tex, June 1977.

Henry JB, Howanitz PJ: Organ panels and the relationship of the laboratory to the physician. In Jones RJ, Palulonis RM (eds): Laboratory Tests in Medical Practice. Chicago, American Medical Association, 1980, p 32.

Irvin RG, Cobb FR, Roe CR: Acute myocardial infarction and MB creatine phosphokinase: Relationship between onset of symptoms of infarction and appearance and disappearance of enzyme. Arch Intern Med 140:329–334, 1980.

Lott JA, Stang JM: Serum enzymes and isoenzymes in the diagnosis and differential diagnosis of myocardial ischemia and necrosis. Clin Chem 26:1241–1250, 1980.

Lupovitch A, Kaplan AG: Interpretive reporting of laboratory data: Biochemical profile of an acute myocardial infarct. Am J Clin Pathol 73:767–773, 1980.

Marchand A, Galen RS, Van Lente F: The predictive value of serum haptoglobin in hemolytic disease. JAMA 243:1909–1911, 1980.

Oliva PB: Pathophysiology of acute myocardial infarction, 1981. Ann Intern Med 94:236–250, 1981.

Reece RL: Using a computer to interpret multiphasic screening results. Geriatrics 29:51–59, 1974.

Reece RL, Hobbie RK: Computer evaluation of chemistry values: A reporting and diagnostic aid. Am J Clin Pathol 57:664–675, 1972.

Robbins SL, Cotran RS: Ischemic heart disease. In Robbins SL, Cotran RS (eds): Pathologic Basis of Disease, ed 2. Philadelphia, WB Saunders Company, 1979, pp 648–662.

Roberts R: Can we clinically measure infarction size? JAMA 242:183–185, 1979.

Roberts R, Sobel BE: Creatine kinase isoenzymes in the assessment of heart disease. Am Heart J 95:521–528, 1978.

Roe CR: Diagnosis of myocardial infarction by serum isoenzyme analysis. Ann Clin Lab Sci 7:201–208, 1977a.

Roe CR: Validity of estimating myocardial infarct size from serial measurements of enzyme activity in serum. Clin Chem 23:1807–1812, 1977b.

Rosano TG, Sanders LA, Johnson ES, et al: Myoglobin concentrations and muscle-enzyme activities in serum after myocardial infarction and cardiac arrhythmia. Clin Chem 23:868–870, 1977.

Rude RE, Muller JE, Braunwald E: Efforts to limit the size of myocardial infarcts. Ann Intern Med 95:736–761, 1981.

Saranchak HJ, Bernstein SH: A new diagnostic test for acute myocardial infarction. JAMA 228:1251–1255, 1974.

Schroeder JS, Lamb IH, Hu M: Do patients in whom myocardial infarction has been ruled out have a better prognosis after hospitalization than those surviving infarction? N Engl J Med 303:1–5, 1980.

Speicher CE, Smith JW: Interpretive reporting in clinical pathology. JAMA 243:1556–1560, 1980.

Wagner GS: Optimal use of serum enzyme levels in the diagnosis of acute myocardial infarction. Arch Intern Med 140:317–319, 1980.

Willerson JT: Acute myocardial infarction. In Wyngaarden JB, Smith LH (eds). Cecil Textbook of Medicine, ed 16. Philadelphia, WB Saunders Company, 1982, pp 247–256.

Woolliscroft JO, Colfer H, Fox IH: Hyperuricemia in acute illness: A poor prognostic sign. Am J Med 72:58–62, 1982.

Atherosclerosis

Brittain E: Probability of coronary heart disease developing. West J Med 136:86–89, 1982.

Bruce RA, Hossack KF, Belanger L, et al: A computer terminal program to evaluate cardiovascular functional limits and estimate coronary event risks. West J Med 135:342–350, 1981.

Cameron JL, Capuzzi DM, Zuidema GD, et al: Acute pancreatitis with hyperlipemia: Evidence for a persistent defect in lipid metabolism. Am J Med 56:482–487, 1974.

Castelli WP, Doyle JT, Gordon T, et al: HDL cholesterol and other lipids in coronary heart disease: the cooperative lipoprotein phenotyping study. Circulation 55:767–772, 1977.

Coronary Risk Handbook—Estimating Risk of Coronary Heart Disease in Practice. New York, American Heart Association, 1973.

Dawber, TR: Risk factors for atherosclerotic disease. Technical Bulletin, Upjohn Company, 1975.

Elliott J: An "ideal" serum cholesterol level? JAMA 241:1979–2000, 1979.

Frederickson DS: A physician's guide to hyperlipidemia. Modern Concepts of Cardiovascular Disease 41:31–36, 1972.

Fredrickson DS, Goldstein JL, Brown MS: The familial hyperlipoproteinemias. In Stanbury JB, Wyngaarden JB, Fredrickson DS (eds): The Metabolic Basis of Inherited Disease, ed 4. New York, McGraw-Hill Book Company, Inc, 1978, pp 604–655.

Glueck CJ, Heckman F, Schoenfeld M, et al: Neonatal familial type II hyperlipoproteinemia: Cord blood cholesterol in 1800 births. Metabolism 20:597–608, 1971.

Gordon T, Castelli WP, Hjortland MC, et al: High density lipoprotein as a protective factor against coronary heart disease: The Framingham study. Am J Med 62:707–714, 1977.

Henry JB, Howanitz PJ: Organ panels and the relationship of the laboratory to the physician. In Jones RJ, Palulonis RM (eds): Laboratory Tests in Medical Practice. Chicago, American Medical Association, 1980, p 32.

Hulley SB, Rosenman RH, Bawol RD, et al: Epidemiology as a guide to clinical decisions: The association between triglyceride and coronary heart disease. N Engl J Med 302:1383–1389, 1980.

Immarino RM: Whither lipoprotein electrophoresis. Hum Pathol 5:626–628, 1974.

Jenny RW, Newman HAI, Saat YA: A new method for the quantitation of alpha-lipoprotein cholesterol. Clin Chem 24:1025, 1978.

Kannel WB, Castelli WP, Gordon T: Cholesterol in the prediction of atherosclerotic disease. New perspectives based on the Framingham study. Ann Intern Med 90:85–91, 1979.

Kannel WB, Garcia MJ, McNamara PM, et al: Serum lipid precursors of coronary heart disease. Hum Pathol 2:129–151, 1971.

Kottke BA, Subbiah, MTR: Pathogenesis of atherosclerosis. Concepts based on animal models. Mayo Clin Proc 53:35–48, 1978.

Levy RL: Triglycerides as a risk factor in coronary artery disease. JAMA 224:1770, 1973.

Margolis S: Treatment of hyperlipemia. JAMA 239:2696–2698, 1978.

Newman HAI, McNair MW: HDL cholesterol and total risk for coronary heart disease. OSU Dept of Path Clin Lab Update. Vol 1, No 3, Sept 1979.

Rifkind BM: As quoted in: Lipid prognosticators of atherosclerotic disease. Laboratory Management, February 1974, pp 17–21.

Robbins SL, Cotran RS: Atherosclerosis. In Robbins SL, Cotran RS (eds): Pathologic Basis of Disease, ed 2. Philadelphia, WB Saunders Company, 1979, pp 598–611.

Steinberg D: Maintenance of eulipemic state in patient with type 4 hyperlipoproteinemia, letter. JAMA 226:573–574, 1973.

Tamir I, Rifkind BM, Levy RI: Measurement of lipids and evaluation of lipid disorders. In Henry JB: Clinical Diagnosis and Management by Laboratory Methods, ed 16. Philadelphia, WB Saunders Company, 1979, pp 189–227.

Tan MH, Wilmshurst EG, Gleason RE, et al: Effect of posture on serum lipids. N Engl J Med 289:416–419, 1973.

Wright IS: Correct levels of serum cholesterol: Average vs normal vs optimal. JAMA 236:261–262, 1976.

Hypertension

Alderman MH: High blood pressure: Do we really know whom to treat and how? N Engl J Med 296:753–755, 1977.

Blum M, Kirsten M, Worth MH: Reversible hypertension: Caused by the hypercalcemia of hyperparathyroidism, vitamin D toxicity, and calcium infusion. JAMA 237:262–263, 1977.

Blumenthal S, Epps RP, Heavenrich, R, et al: Report of the task force on blood pressure control in children. Pediatrics 59(suppl): 797–820, 1977.

Burke MD: Hypertension: Diagnostic test strategies. CRC Crit Rev Clin Lab Sci 13:279–320, 1980.

Chobanian AV: Hypertension. In Conn HF, Conn RB (eds): Current Diagnosis, ed 6. Philadelphia, WB Saunders Company, 1980, pp 354–360.

Cole GW: The clinical usefulness of multiple result ranges for a laboratory test, as exemplified by serum urea nitrogen. In Young DS, Uddin D, Nipper H, et al (eds): Clinician and Chemist: The Relationship of the Laboratory to the Physician. Washington, American Association for Clinical Chemistry, 1979, pp 265–272.

DeGoulet P, Menard J, Berger C, et al: Hypertension management: The computer as a participant. Am J Med 68:559–567, 1980.

Feinstein AR: An Analysis of diagnostic reasoning: 1. The domains and disorders of clinical macrobiology. Yale J Biol Med 46:212–232, 1973.

Henry JB, Howanitz PJ: Organ panels and the relationship of the laboratory to the physician. In Jones RJ, Palulonis RM (eds): Laboratory Tests in Medical Practice. Chicago, American Medical Association, 1980, p 32.

Hypertension and uric acid, editorial. Lancet 1:365–366, 1981.

Hypertension Detection and Follow-up Program Cooperative Group: Five-year Findings of the Hypertension Detection and Follow-up Program: 1. Reduction in mortality of persons with high blood pressure, including mild hypertension: JAMA 242:2562–2571, 1979.

Kannel WB: Some lessons in cardiovascular epidemiology from Framingham. Am J Cardiol 37:269–282, 1976.

Kaplan NM: Clinical Hypertension, ed 3. Baltimore, Williams and Wilkins, 1982.

Kilcoyne MM: Adolescent hypertension, editorial. Am J Med 58:735–739, 1975.

Lew EA: High blood pressure, other risk factors and longevity. Am J Med 55:281–294, 1973.

Maronde RF: The hypertensive patient, an algorithm for diagnostic work-up. JAMA 233:997–1000, 1975.

Moser M: Report of the Joint National Committee on Detection, Evaluation, and Treatment of High Blood Pressure: A cooperative study. JAMA 237:255–261, 1977.

National Diabetes Data Group: Classification and diagnosis of diabetes mellitus and other categories of glucose intolerance. Diabetes 28:1039–1057, 1979.

Pickering TG, Harshfield GA, Kleinert HD, et al: Blood pressure during normal daily activities, sleep, and exercise. Comparison of values in normal and hypertensive subjects. JAMA 247:992–996, 1982.

Simpson F: Hypertension. Br Med J 2:882–883, 1978.

Veterans Administration Cooperative Study Group on Antihypertensive Agents: Effects of treatment on morbidity in hypertension: Results in patients with diastolic blood pressures averaging 115 through 129 mm Hg. JAMA 202:1028–1034, 1967.

Veterans Administration Cooperative Study Group on Antihypertensive Agents: Effects of treatment on morbidity in hypertension: II. Results in patients with diastolic blood pressure averaging 90 through 114 mm Hg. JAMA 213:1143–1152, 1970.

Waeber B, Brunner HR, Burckhardt P, et al: Hypertension in a patient with hypercalcemia. Arch Intern Med 142:143–145, 1982.

World Health Organization. Hypertension and coronary heart disease: Classification and criteria for epidemiological studies. WHO Technical Report Series No. 168, Geneva, 1959.

CHAPTER 11

RESPIRATORY SUBPROBLEMS

PULMONARY AIRWAY DISEASE
  Chronic Obstructive Lung Disease
PULMONARY VASCULAR
  DISEASE
  Acute Pulmonary Embolism
PLEURAL DISEASE
  Etiology of Pleural Effusion

PULMONARY AIRWAY DISEASE

CHRONIC OBSTRUCTIVE PULMONARY DISEASE

Definition and Significance

The term *chronic obstructive pulmonary disease* (COPD) refers to a group of disorders characterized by a combination of bronchial obstruction and emphysema. The bronchial obstruction may be due to chronic bronchitis, bronchial asthma, or bronchiectasis. The spectrum of presentations includes some patients who have bronchial obstruction predominantly, others showing emphysema primarily, and others with a combination of these (Miller, 1981). COPD should be distinguished from upper-airway (larynx, trachea) obstruction caused by foreign bodies, tumors, secretions, or inflammation (Spivak and Barnes, 1978).

The etiology of COPD is closely related to inhalation of tobacco smoke and environmental pollutants. Occasional patients are at much higher risk of developing COPD as a result of inborn metabolic errors such as alpha$_1$-antitrypsin deficiency and cystic fibrosis. (See the discussions of these two conditions in Chapter 17.) Homozygous alpha$_1$-antitrypsin deficiency occurs in one in 4000 persons; heterozygous alpha$_1$-antitrypsin deficiency occurs in 2 to 8 per cent of the population (Morse, 1978). The prevalence of cystic fibrosis at birth is one patient for every 1600 to 2000 live-born infants (Scully et al., 1981). Additional host factors include increased serum IgE and "atopy," as well as an individual's inherent reactivity to stimuli that tend to produce bronchoconstriction (Burrows, 1981; Fanta and Ingram, 1981).

COPD is a major cause of disability in older subjects, ranking behind heart disease and schizophrenia in the United States, according to social security statistics. The mortality rate in the United States is increasing and probably approaches that from lung cancer (Burrows, 1982).

Pathophysiology

Chronic bronchitis is characterized by persistent, excess production of respiratory tract mucus. Emphysema is characterized by destruction of alveolar walls, leading to a reduced number of enlarged air spaces. This results in an increased residual volume of air in the lungs after maximal expiration and in interference with diffusing capacity with associated abnormalities of arterial PO_2 and PCO_2 (Robbins and Cotran, 1979; Snider, 1981).

The most characteristic pathophysiologic feature of COPD is increased airway resistance. This can be quantified by two pulmonary function tests known as the FEV_1 and the FVC. After a full inspiration, the FEV_1 is the volume of air that can be forcibly exhaled in 1 second; the FVC is the total volume that can be forcibly exhaled. The FEV_1-FVC ratio in a healthy population is about 0.8 or greater (Burrows, 1982).

A timed spirogram enables the volume exhaled from the lungs over some interval of time to be measured. If the flow is plotted against the volume exhaled, a maximum expiratory-flow volume (MEFV) curve can be obtained. This curve can be used to measure instantaneous flow at a given point in exhalation; e.g., Vmax 75 per cent is the flow achieved after exhaling 75 per cent of the FVC. The Vmax 75 per cent is considered a more sensitive indicator of airway dysfunction than the FEV_1, which measures flow earlier in expiration and is more dependent on effort. However, because the Vmax 75 per cent shows wider variability than the FEV_1 and requires greater patient cooperation, the FEV_1 is the more important clinical test for assessing the severity of an airway obstructive disorder (Burrows, 1981).

Clinical Contexts

Diagnosis. Patients with COPD present most commonly between 55 and 65 years of age. It is much more common in males than females, the ratio being 9:1, but this may reflect only differences in smoking habits (Burrows, 1982). Young patients in their 20s and 30s rarely have accumulated enough years of smoking exposure to have COPD. If these patients have presenting symptoms of severe dyspnea, other diagnoses should be considered, such as bronchiectasis, asthma, alpha₁-antitrypsin deficiency, and cystic fibrosis. (See Chapter 17 for discussions of the latter two conditions.) COPD is often inaccurately over-diagnosed and is used as a catch-all category for patients with cough or dyspnea or both (Neff, 1980).

The most frequent feature of COPD is dyspnea. Other symptoms include cough, expectoration, wheezing, recurrent respiratory infections, and even weakness or weight loss.

Physical findings include obstructed bronchi, overinflation of lungs, low diaphragm, and an increased area of cardiac dullness. Labored breathing, cyanosis, and slight dependent edema can be present. Pulmonary hypertension and cor pulmonale can occur. When emphysematous elements of COPD predominate, patients have been called type A; when obstructive elements predominate, patients have been called type B. Type A patients often hyperventilate and maintain reasonably normal PO_2, earning the name "pink puffers." Type B patients commonly have cyanosis and congestive heart failure, earning the name "blue bloaters" (Burrows, 1982).

Management. Laboratory studies, such as the FEV_1, FVC, and arterial blood gas measurements, can be useful for evaluating response to therapy and prognosis.

Classic childhood asthma tends to remit during adolescence, making testing less useful for prognosis. Only 25 per cent of childhood asthmatics continue to have symptoms as adults. A minority of patients whose asthma begins after age 35 appear to show subsequent complete remission. In the average patient with chronic obstructive bronchitis, there is a loss of FEV_1 in the range of 50 to 75 ml per year, two to three times the average rate of decline for non-smokers. Continued smoking accelerates the deterioration (Burrows, 1981). The best guide to prognosis appears to be the amount of predicted FEV_1 obtained following administration of a bronchodilator (Traver et al., 1979).

Strategy

Test Sequence. Measurements of forced expiratory volume exhaled in the FEV_1 and of FVC, together with determinations of arterial blood gases and a complete blood count, are essential. These can be supplemented with a chest radiograph, a lung scan, and an electrocardiogram.

Patient Preparation. No special procedures are required for measuring FEV_1 and FVC or arterial blood gases. (See Part 3 for chemistry and hematology tests.)

Specimen Collection and Handling. Collect a heparinized arterial blood sample for blood gases anaerobically, place it in ice water, and obtain the measurements promptly (in less than 30 minutes). If a plastic syringe is used, it should be gastight and should not permit

Table 11–1. OPERATING CHARACTERISTICS OF CONVENTIONAL SPIROMETRIC TESTS IN SMOKERS*

Test	Cutoff Point†	Young, Minimally Symptomatic or <20 Pack-Year Smokers		Middle-Aged, Moderately Symptomatic or >20 Pack-Year Smokers	
		Sensitivity	Specificity	Sensitivity	Specificity
FEV_1‡	<80	4–13	95%	11–43	90
FEV_1/forced vital capacity	<80	9–12	90%	21–47	90
Maximum midexpiratory flow rate	<80	20	80%	20–38	80

*From Griner PF, Mayewski RJ, Mushlin AI, et al: Selection and interpretation of diagnostic tests and procedures. Principles and applications. Ann Int Med 94:578, 1981.
†Per cent of predicted normals based on regression analysis of height, sex, and age.
‡FEV_1 = Forced expiratory volume in 1 second.

diffusion and exchange of gases (Tietz, 1976). (See Part 3.)

Methodology. Consult the laboratory for its methodologies, reference intervals, accuracy and precision, and sources of interference. (See Part 3.)

Interpretation

Diagnosis. Griner and associates (1981) calculated the sensitivity and specificity of conventional spirometric tests in smokers (Table 11–1). For the young smoker in whom the diagnosis of COPD is suspected, a history of dyspnea on exertion, chronic cough, sputum production, or wheezing is about as sensitive as currently available spirometric pulmonary function tests. Griner's group pointed out that

the FEV_1 can be made more sensitive by changing the cutoff point to less than 90 per cent of the value for a healthy population instead of less than 80 per cent. The "trade-off," of course, is a significant decrease in specificity.

When COPD is moderate to severe, however, the conventional spirometric test results are more likely to show a pathologic condition. Therefore, when a smoker presents with severe respiratory symptoms, conventional spirometric tests can be of value in confirming or excluding the presence of COPD (Table 11–1 and Fig. 11–1). Table 11–2 gives the results of some common laboratory tests in COPD.

Management. Table 11–3 shows the relationship between the patient's initial postbronchodilator per cent-predicted FEV_1 and approximate mortality.

Figure 11–1. Predictive values for the results of forced expiratory flow volume in severely symptomatic smoking patients. Examples assume a prior estimate of chronic obstructive lung disease to be at least 50 per cent in this population. Patients correctly classified as having chronic obstructive lung disease = 50/55 = 91 per cent positive predictive value. Patients correctly classified as not having chronic obstructive lung disease = 45/45 = 100 per cent = negative predictive value. Total patients correctly classified 95/100 = 95 per cent. (From Griner PF, Mayewski RJ, Mushlin AI, et al: Greenland P: Selection and interpretation of diagnostic tests and procedures; Principles and applications. Ann Intern Med 94:579, 1981.)

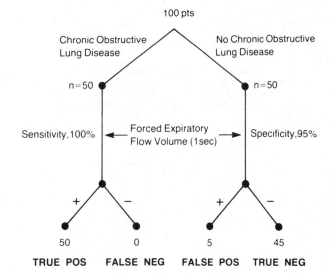

Table 11–2. COMMON LABORATORY TEST RESULTS IN CHRONIC OBSTRUCTIVE PULMONARY DISEASE*

Laboratory Test	Value	Pathophysiologic Factors
Chemistry (Serum)		
Bilirubin, total	—	
Calcium, total	—	
Carbon dioxide	↑	Increases in P_{CO_2} and in bicarbonate caused by compensated respiratory acidosis
Chloride	↓	Reciprocal decrease in chloride follows the increase in bicarbonate
Cholesterol	↓	Decrease in decompensated patients correlates with degree of hypoxemia
Creatine phosphokinase	—	
Creatinine	—	
Glucose	—	
Lactic dehydrogenase	—	
Phosphatase, alkaline	—	
Phosphorus, inorganic	—	
Potassium	↑	Related to the presence of acidosis
	↓	Suggests a coexisting primary metabolic alkalosis
Proteins, total	—	
Proteins, albumin	—	
Sodium	—	
Transaminase, aspartate amino	—	
Urea nitrogen	—	
Uric acid	—	
Hematology (Blood)		
Hemoglobin	↑	Polycythemia secondary to hypoxemia
	↓	High prevalence of peptic ulcer with bleeding
Hematocrit	↑	Polycythemia secondary to hypoxemia
	↓	High prevalence of peptic ulcer with bleeding
Leukocyte count, total	↑	Related to the presence of inflammation
Platelet count	—	

Key:
— = No change; ↑ = can be increased; ↓ = can be decreased.

*Based on information from Friedman RB, Anderson RE, Entine, SM, et al: Effects of diseases on clinical laboratory tests. Clin Chem 26:1D–476D, 1980; Wolf PL: Interpretation of Biochemical Multitest Profiles: An Analysis of 100 Important Conditions. New York, Masson Publishing Company, Inc, 1977.

Table 11–3. APPROXIMATE MORTALITY RATES IN RELATIONSHIP TO INITIAL POSTBRONCHODILATOR PER CENT PREDICTED FEV_1 (%pbFEV$_1$)*

Initial %pbFEV$_1$	Approximate Mortality (%)			
	2 years	5 years	10 years	15 years
Subjects under 65 years of age				
<20	55	90	90	>95
20 to 29	35	70	90	>95
30 to 39	15	55	80	93
40 to 49	10	10	60	70
50 to 59	5	5	45	65
60 +	<1	5	15	35
Subjects aged 65 years or older				
<40	40	70	>95	—
40 +	15	30	15	—

*From Burrows B: An overview of obstructive lung diseases. Med Clin North Am 65:468, 1981.

Test Requests and Reports

Test Requests. The execution of the test sequence for COPD may be offered to the ordering physician as a problem-solving service. Henry's pulmonary panel is an example of a problem-solving test profile that addresses the general issue of any kind of pulmonary disease rather than COPD specifically (Fig. 11–2). Henry and Howanitz (1980) gave the rationale for this panel as follows:

Functional disturbances of ventilation are reflected primarily by elevation of PCO_2 while defects in respiration reveal hypoxemia (depression of PO_2 and O_2 saturation). Chronic obstructive airways disease is often associated with ventilation and diffusion defects (elevated PCO_2 and decreased PO_2). A CBC is included to determine the severity of secondary polycythemia, which may be present.

PULMONARY				
Blood pH units	Art. 7.38–7.44 Ven. 7.36–7.41			
Blood PCO$_2$ mmHg	Art. 35–40 Ven. 40–45			
Blood PO$_2$ mmHg	Art. 95–100			
Oxygen Saturation Percent	Art. 94–100 Ven. 60–85			
CO$_2$ Content mM/L	24–30			
Sodium mEq/L	135–145			
Potassium mEq/L	4.0–4.8			
Chloride mmol/L	98–109			
Urea Nitrogen (BUN) mg/dl	8–18			
Glucose mg/dl	65–115			
CBC	See Hematology Report Form			

Figure 11–2. Pulmonary panel. (From Henry JB, Murphy J: Effective utilization of clinical laboratories. In Henry JB (ed): Clinical Diagnosis and Management by Laboratory Methods, ed. 16. Philadelphia, WB Saunders Company, 1979, p 2043.)

```
OHIO STATE U HOSPITALS                            PRINTED  1:36 PM        10/15/82
PULMONARY FUNCTIONS REPORT      ASSN # 1234       TEST   CONDUCTED        10/15/82
PT. NAME                        PHONE             REFER BY
ADDRESS                                                           PB          755
MRN                             ADM. # ____       ROOM # ____     SMOKE HX     18
AGE        35 YRS               SEX    M          RACE   C        HCT          42
BSA        1.94 M2              HEIGHT  72 IN      WEIGHT  160 LB  PT COOP:  GOOD
DIAGNOSIS: D.I.P.                                 DATE PREVIOUS TEST      09/11/82
```

		PRE/DILATOR		POST/DILATOR	
MECHANICS OF BREATHING (BTPS)	PRED	ACTUAL	%PRED	ACTUAL	%PRED
FORCED VITAL CAPACITY (FVC) L	5.41	4.80	89		
1.0 SEC FORCED EXP. VOL. (FEV1.0) L	4.36	3.23	74*		
FEV 1.0 % FVC		67*			
FEV 3.0 % FVC	⟩=95%	88			
FORCED MID EXP. FLOW (FEF25-75) LPS	5.26	2.20	42*		
PEAK FLOW (PF) LPS	9.99	9.5	95		
MAX VOLUNTARY VENT. (MVV) LPM					
LUNG VOLUMES (BTPS)					
SLOW VITAL CAPACITY (SVC) L	5.41	4.80	89		
EXPIRATORY RESERVE VOL (ERV) L	2.16	1.59	74*		
FUNC. RES. CAP. (FRC) L (N2 W.O.)	4.25	4.03	95		
RESIDUAL VOLUME (RV) L	2.08	2.44	117		
TOTAL LUNG CAP. (TLC) L	7.52	7.24	96		
RV/TLC RATIO, %	27.72	34	123*		
DIFFUSING CAPACITY					
DLCO SINGLE BREATH ML/MIN/MM HG	37.70	21.7	58*		
VA	7.52	6.97	93		
DLCO/VA	⟩=3.9	3.11			

```
DIST. INSP. GAS
  % N2 INCR 750-1250 ML            ⟨=2%
  CLOSING VOL. (CV)/VC, %

ART BLOOD GAS ANALYSIS               PRED       ROOM AIR         100% - O2
  PH                              7.35-7.45
  PO2, MM HG
  PCO2, MM HG                       35-41
  ACTUAL BICARB., MEQ/L             24-28
  ALV.-ART. O2 DIFFERENCE
  PHYSIO. SHUNT, (QS/AT), %          ⟨8%
```

INTERPRETATIONS: (PRELIMINARY)   * = OUTSIDE NORMAL RANGE

    THE PATTERN IS ONE OF A MINIMAL OBSTRUCTIVE VENTILATORY DEFECT
    THERE IS A MODERATE DECREASE IN THE DIFFUSING CAPACITY
    THE DLCO° IS REDUCED OUT OF PROPORTION TO THE MEASURED TLC[+]

COMMENTS:


```
TECHNOLOGIST _____    M.D. _____
  °DLCO = Diffusion Capacity for Carbon Monoxide
  +TLC  = Total Lung Capacity
```

Figure 11–3. Computer-assisted interpretive report for pulmonary function tests. (Courtesy of Ohio State University Hospitals.)

Interpretive Reports. The results of the tests can be collated and returned to the attending physician in the form of an interpretive report. For the panel illustrated in Figure 11–2, the results can be entered directly on the request form. Figure 11–3 shows a computer-assisted interpretive report for pulmonary function tests.

PULMONARY VASCULAR DISEASE

ACUTE PULMONARY EMBOLISM

Definition and Significance

Pulmonary embolism is the occlusion of one or more vessels of the pulmonary arterial tree by a previously detached thrombus or some foreign material from a source extrinsic to the lung. A single embolus is the exception rather than the rule.

Pulmonary embolism can cause pulmonary infarction, which is necrosis of lung parenchyma resulting from interference with its blood supply. However, only a minority of clinically significant pulmonary emboli result in pulmonary infarction (less than 10 per cent) (Soloff and Rodman, 1967a). Infarction is usually seen in patients who have pre-existing pulmonary or cardiac disease, i.e., compromised airways or systemic blood flow (Moser, 1980).

Most pulmonary emboli originate from thrombi, especially those originating in the deep veins of the lower extremities. Occasionally, non-thrombotic materials are the source of emboli, such as amniotic fluid, fat, bone marrow, tumor, air, or particulate matter from an intravenous injection.

Acute pulmonary embolism is an important problem. It occurs often and is frequently a cause of death. Figure 11–4 gives the incidence and outcome of pulmonary embolism in the United States. Routine autopsies have detected recent or old thromboemboli in the lungs of some 30 per cent of patients who died in hospitals; emboli can be demonstrated in over 60 per cent of autopsy cases by special techniques (Freiman et al., 1965). Just as remarkable as this high prevalence is the fact that 70 to 90 per cent of the recent emboli discovered at autopsy are not diagnosed antemortem (Moser, 1980).

Pathophysiology

A pulmonary embolus can be single or multiple and can vary in size from one that blocks the bifurcation of the pulmonary artery (saddle embolus) to those that block fine branches of the pulmonary artery. If enough of the pulmonary arterial bed is blocked, mechanical obstruction follows, with dilation of the pulmonary artery, cor pulmonale, and liver congestion. With massive embolism (greater than 50 per cent occlusion), 90 per cent of patients die within an hour or two.

In 30 to 40 per cent of patients with pulmonary embolism there is associated pleural effusion (Rosenow, 1981). (See the discussion of the etiology of pleural effusion later in this chapter.)

Emboli that reach smaller arteries go more frequently to lower than upper lobes and more often to the right than the left lung. Although the continuing circulation through the bronchial arteries is often sufficient to prevent infarction, if the lung is congested, infected, or hypoventilated, infarction is more likely to occur.

Figure 11–4. Incidence of pulmonary embolism per year in the United States. (From Dalen, J. E., Alpert, JS: Natural history of pulmonary embolism. Prog Cardiovasc Dis 17:261, 1975. By permission of Grune & Stratton.)

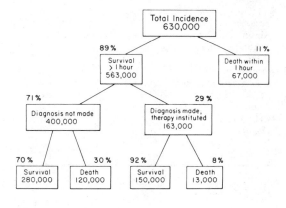

Table 11–4. SIGNS AND SYMPTOMS OF 327 PATIENTS WITH PULMONARY EMBOLISM*

	Total Series N = 327	Massive Emboli N = 197	vs	Submassive Emboli N = 130
Symptoms				
Chest pain	83†	79		89§
Pleuritic	74	67		82¶
Non-pleuritic	14	16		13
Dyspnea	84	85		82
Apprehension	59	65¶		50
Cough	53	53		52
Hemoptysis	30	23		40¶
Sweats	27	29		23
Syncope	13	20‖		4
Signs				
Respirations > 16/min	92	95		87
Rales	58.	57		60
↑ S_2P‡	53	58§		45
Pulse > 100/min	44	48		38
Temperature > 37.8°C	43	43		42
Phlebitis	32	36		26
Gallop	34	39¶		25
Diaphoresis	36	42¶		27
Edema	24	23		25
Murmur	28	28		27
Cyanosis	19	25‖		9
Associated Conditions				
Current venous disease	45	47		42
Immobilization	58	60		55
Congestive heart failure and chronic lung disease	38	36		40
Malignant neoplasm	6	8		5

*Adapted from Bell WR: Pulmonary embolism: Progress and problems. Am J Med 72:182, 1982.

†All figures are percentages.

‡ ↑ S_2P = Increased intensity of the pulmonic component of the second heart sound.

§Statistically significant (p <0.05).

¶Statistically significant (p <0.01).

‖Statistically significant (p <0.001).

Based on chi-square test with continuity correction.

Infarctions cause necrosis of the pulmonary parenchyma (see the discussion of inflammation in Chapter 8), involve the pleura, and take a number of days to resolve. Pleural effusions associated with infarctions tend to be bloody. About two-thirds of the patients show resolution of the infarct in 6 weeks, and approximately 20 per cent in 5 weeks (Soloff and Rodman, 1967a; Spivak and Barnes, 1978).

Clinical Contexts

Diagnosis. Patients with massive pulmonary embolism exhibit sudden dyspnea, tachypnea, cyanosis, substernal oppressive pain, right-sided cardiac dilatation and failure, tachycardia, restlessness, anxiety, syncope, convulsions, and hypotension. Patients with submassive pulmonary embolism (less than 50 per cent occlusion) show dyspnea, worsening of an underlying cardiac or pulmonary disease, and possibly all the features of massive embolism (Table 11–4).

The features of pulmonary infarction are as follows: no pain to pleuritic pain, hemoptysis, cough, dyspnea, fever, tachycardia, pleural friction rub, areas of dullness or flatness on percussion, and diminished breath sounds (Bell et al., 1977; Soloff and Rodman, 1967b).

Table 11–5 presents predisposing factors for pulmonary embolism. When these factors are present, the index of suspicion for pulmonary embolism should be high. According to Rosenow and colleagues (1981), five techniques

Table 11–5. PREDISPOSING FACTORS IN 167 PATIENTS WITH PULMONARY EMBOLIZATION*

Condition	% Total Patients	Condition	% Total Patients
Thrombophlebitis	39.5	Angina	5.4
Venous varicosity and insufficiency	15.0	Congestive heart failure	17.4
Peripheral arterial disease	4.8	Arrhythmia	16.2
Recent immobilization from fracture (casting)	15.0	Rheumatic heart disease	1.2
		Other heart disease	9.0
Bed rest	32.4	Primary pulmonary disease	7.8
Recent surgery	31.2	Dehydration	3.6
Recent termination of pregnancy	1.2	Diabetes mellitus	8.4
Pelvic disease	6.0	Malignancy	7.2
Obesity	30.0	Hemoglobinopathy	1.2
Cerebrovascular disease	6.6	Polycythemia	0.0
Hypertension	10.2	No predisposing etiology	6.0
Nephrotic syndrome	0.6		
Myocardial infarction	12.0		

*Adapted from Bell WR, Simon TL, DeMets DL: The clinical features of submassive and massive pulmonary emboli. Am J Med 62:357, 1977.

are valuable in the diagnosis of venous thrombosis:

1. Venous Doppler examination.
2. Plethysmography.
3. Fibrinogen leg scanning.
4. Radionuclide venography.
5. Venography.

Management. Baseline laboratory studies can be helpful in following the course of pulmonary embolism and infarction.

Screening. It is not appropriate to screen for pulmonary embolism and infarction in the absence of clinical features of disease or predisposing factors.

Strategy

Test Sequence. Perform the following procedures:

1. Obtain serial and parallel measurements of the following:
   a. Arterial blood gases.
   b. Complete blood count.
   c. Serum bilirubin, LDH, and transaminases.
   d. ESR. Consider C-reactive protein (CRP). (See the discussion of inflammation in Chapter 8.)
2. Obtain a perfusion lung scan (rarely false negative, commonly false positive). A simultaneous ventilation-perfusion lung scan will considerably increase the specificity of the perfusion lung scan by detection of ventilation to perfusion mismatching (a ventilation-perfusion mismatch).
3. Consider pulmonary angiography with awareness of some morbidity (4 per cent) and mortality (less than 0.2 per cent) (some false-negative results, essentially no false-positive results) in the following situations (Rosenow et al., 1981):
   a. When probability of the diagnosis of pulmonary embolism is intermediate or low using the ventilation-perfusion lung scan and when the clinical picture is suspicious for pulmonary embolism.
   b. When there is suspected pulmonary embolism in the presence of parenchymal lung disease and congestive failure, which compromise the utility of the ventilation-perfusion lung scan.
   c. When there is probable pulmonary embolism and high risk for the use of anticoagulants or when caval ligation is being considered.
   d. When there is a past history of unconfirmed "recurrent pulmonary emboli."
   e. In the case of probable massive pulmonary embolism, when the use of expensive and potentially hazardous fibrinolytic therapy or pulmonary embolectomy is being considered.
4. If there is a requirement to distinguish pulmonary embolism from acute myocardial infarction, see the discussion of acute myocardial infarction (Chapter 10).

Patient Preparation. No special preparation is required for arterial blood gases, ESR, CRP, electrocardiogram, chest roentgenograms, lung scan, or angiography. However, angiography should be done within 24 to 72 hours after onset of the suspected pulmonary embolism; otherwise, resolution of the clots will make interpretation of the angiogram difficult (Rosenow et al., 1981). (See Part 3 for chemistry and hematology tests.)

Specimen Collection and Handling. Collect a sample for blood gases anaerobically, place it in ice water, and obtain the measurements promptly (in less than 30 minutes). If a plastic syringe is used, it should be gastight and should not permit diffusion and exchange of gases (Tietz, 1976). Collect the ESR sample in citrate. A clot tube will suffice for CRP. (See Part 3.)

Methodology. Consult the laboratory for its methodologies, reference intervals, accuracy and precision, and potential sources of interference. (See Part 3.)

Interpretation

Diagnosis. Table 11–4 shows sensitivity of symptoms, signs, and associated conditions in patients with pulmonary embolism. As noted in this table, the three most sensitive parameters for pulmonary embolism are chest pain (83 per cent), dyspnea (84 per cent), and tachypnea (92 per cent). The most sensitive laboratory studies are a pathologic electrocardiogram (85 per cent) and an arterial PO_2 of less than 90 mm Hg (95 per cent) (Rosnow et al., 1981).

Perfusion lung scanning rarely gives false-negative results but can give false-positive findings in chronic obstructive pulmonary disease, asthma, pneumonia, lung cysts, bronchiectasis, and atelectasis. A ventilation-perfusion mismatch on a simultaneous ventilation-perfusion lung scan is considered diagnostic for pulmonary embolism. False negatives occur with angiography when the emboli are in smaller than second-order arteries, but there are few false positives (Spivak and Barnes, 1978).

McNeil (1980) showed how simultaneous ventilation-perfusion lung scans can be coupled with the clinical likelihood of pulmonary embolism to obtain probabilistic estimates of pulmonary embolism in particular patients. An excellent review of the use of the radionuclide ventilation-perfusion lung scan in the diagnosis and management of pulmonary embolism is available by Rosenow and colleagues (1981). This review also discusses the advantages of various methods of diagnosing deep venous thrombosis, i.e., physical examination, contrast venography, isotope venography, ^{125}I fibrinogen uptake, plethysmography, and Doppler ultrasound blood flow detection.

An analysis was made of how a diagnosis was arrived at in 60 consecutive patients with suspected pulmonary embolism (Herlev Hospital Study Group, 1979). The results suggest that radiologists were biased by the clinical information when interpreting the lung scans and that physicians in turn believed implicitly in the lung scan report when they made the final diagnosis. The agreement between the first and second readings of the lung scans was unsatisfactory, and the radiologic findings did not correlate with the clinical and lung scan assessments.

Wacker and associates (1961) first suggested that the triad of an elevated serum LDH, an elevated serum bilirubin, and an SGOT that was not elevated might be diagnostic for pulmonary infarction. However, this triad was present in only 12 per cent of patients with pulmonary emboli proved by angiography (Szucs et al., 1971). The triad of an elevated serum LDH, elevated serum bilirubin, and a low arterial P_{O_2} may have a sensitivity of 50 per cent and a specificity of nearly 100 per cent. Four patients with large pulmonary emboli confirmed at autopsy had low arterial P_{O_2} (42 to 71 mm Hg) while breathing room air. Their total serum LDH was moderately elevated (334 to 562 U/liter), and their serum total bilirubin was mildly elevated (1.8 to 3.9 mg/100 ml) and had a large unconjugated component (half or more of the total) (Gambino, 1981). Further evaluation of the effectiveness of the triad of elevated serum LDH, elevated serum bilirubin, and low arterial P_{O_2} is necessary.

A leukocytosis or elevation of the ESR is consistent with pulmonary infarction, as a reflection of inflammation in and around the infarction. An elevation in CRP would have the same significance (Moser, 1980). However, an elevated ESR or CRP is not specific for infarction. (See the discussion of inflammation in Chapter 8.)

The electrocardiogram shows pathologic changes at one time or another in up to 85 per cent of patients with acute pulmonary embolism. However, these changes are notoriously transient and very non-specific. The chest roentgenogram has a sensitivity of 70 to 85 per cent and is slightly more specific than the electrocardiogram. (Rosenow et al., 1981).

Konttinen and associates (1974) evaluated serum enzyme determinations in 33 patients with pulmonary embolism. The level of SGOT was elevated in one third, and LDH was elevated in two thirds of the patients. Serum LDH isoenzymes were substantially LDH-1 and LDH-5, indicating extrapulmonary sources of enzyme, such as erythrocytes and liver. The elevation of LDH-1 is presumably due to hemolysis of red blood cells trapped in the infarcted area of the lung, whereas the elevation of LDH-5 is almost certainly due to centrilobular hepatic damage secondary to heart failure and depressed cardiac output. This elevated LDH-5 is usually accompanied by elevated serum SGOT and SGPT. Serum CPK was elevated in 5 of 22 patients studied, and its elevation was totally due to CPK-MM. The increased CPK activity occasionally described in the serum of patients with pulmonary infarction is unlikely to have arisen from lung tissue, which contains little CPK. The rises are more likely to be due to intramuscular injections or associated disease (Smith, 1979).

Light and Bell (1974) studied serum LDH and fibrinogen-fibrin degradation products in pulmonary embolism in 35 patients. Levels of serum LDH tended to be maximal during the 48 hours following embolization. The serum fibrinogen-fibrin degradation products were elevated or borderline in 20 per cent of the patients. Single measurements of serum LDH, and fibrinogen-fibrin degradation products, performed when the diagnosis is suspected, are not reliable tests for pulmonary emboli.

Circulating DNA has been studied as a possible test for the diagnosis of pulmonary embolism (sensitivity 83 per cent) (Sipes et al., 1978). However, a study by Lippman and colleagues (1982) demonstrated that plasma DNA was not helpful in the differential diag-

Table 11–6. COMMON LABORATORY TEST RESULTS IN PULMONARY EMBOLISM AND INFARCTION*

Laboratory Test	Value	Pathophysiologic Factors
Chemistry (Serum)		
Bilirubin, total	↑	Unconjugated type originating from degraded erythrocytes
Calcium, total	—	
Carbon dioxide	—	
Chloride	—	
Cholesterol	—	
Creatine phosphokinase	↑	Unlikely to have arisen from lung tissue, but CPK-BB is present in lung tissue
Creatinine	—	
Glucose	↑	Elevated in 45 per cent of patients at time of hospitalization; possibly related to stress
Lactic dehydrogenase	↑	From degraded erythrocytes, LDH-1 or LDH-2; or from the liver if there is heart failure, LDH-4, or LDH-5
Phosphatase, alkaline	↑	Originates from damaged vascular endothelium and proliferating vascular endothelial cells during healing
Phosphorus, inorganic	—	
Potassium	—	
Proteins, total	—	
Proteins, albumin	—	
Sodium	—	
Transaminase, aspartate amino	↑	Prevalence of elevation 0 to 30 per cent. Originates from degraded erythrocytes and from the liver if there is heart failure
Urea nitrogen	—	
Uric acid	↑	Related to necrosis of lung tissue and increase in cell turnover from this lesion
Hematology (Blood)		
Hemoglobin	—	
Hematocrit	—	
Leukocyte count, total	↑	Usually normal in pulmonary embolism and elevated with pulmonary infarction
Platelet count	↑	May be increased as a predisposing cause for thrombosis

Key:
— = No change; ↑ = can be increased; ↓ = can be decreased.
*Based on information from Friedman RB, Anderson RE, Entine SM, et al: Effects of diseases on clinical laboratory tests. Clin Chem 26:1D–476D, 1980; Wolf PL: Interpretation of Biochemical Multitest Profiles: An Analysis of 100 Important Conditions. New York, Masson Publishing Company, Inc, 1977.

nosis of pulmonary embolism; that is, there was no significant difference in plasma DNA between patients with pulmonary embolism and hospitalized sick patients in the control group.

Table 11–6 gives the results of common laboratory tests in pulmonary embolism and infarction.

Management. Baseline studies can be helpful in following the course of pulmonary embolism and infarction.

Test Requests and Reports

Test Requests. The execution of the test sequence for acute pulmonary embolism can be offered to the ordering physician as a problem-solving service. Henry's pulmonary panel can be used to order the arterial blood gases, a complete blood count, and some additional serum chemistries (Fig. 11–2). (See the discussion of chronic obstructive pulmonary disease earlier in this chapter.)

Interpretive Report. The results of the tests can be collated and returned to the attending physician in the form of an interpretive report.

PLEURAL DISEASE

ETIOLOGY OF PLEURAL EFFUSION

Definition and Significance

Pleural effusion consists of excess fluid in either the right or left pleural cavity. Clinically, the term includes any fluid within the pleural cavity. However, it is normal to have a small amount of pleural fluid present in each pleural cavity. This fluid is located between the visceral and parietal pleurae and serves to lubricate these surfaces as they move over one another.

Detection of a pleural effusion depends on the sensitivity of the method used. The diagnostic sensitivities of various methods of detection are as follows:

1. Clinical history: Detects very large effusions (respiratory distress, pleuritic pain).

2. Physical examination: Detects only large effusions (diminished chest movement, decreased to absent breath sounds, dullness to percussion, mediastinal shift).

3. Routine posteroanterior chest roentgenogram: Detects 300 ml effusion.

Table 11–7. CAUSES OF PLEURAL EFFUSIONS*

Transudates
  Congestive heart failure
  Cirrhosis with ascites
  Nephrotic syndrome
  Hypoalbuminemia
  Peritoneal dialysis
  Atelectasis, acute
  Superior vena cava obstruction
  Subclavian catheter misplacement
  Early mediastinal malignancy

Exudates
  Parapneumonic effusion (bacterial pneumonia)
  Pulmonary infarction
  Malignancy (direct pleural involvement, late
    mediastinal involvement)
  Viral disease
  Connective tissue disease (lupus, rheumatoid, mixed)
  Tuberculosis
  Fungal disease
  Parasitic disease (*Entamoeba histolytica, Paragonimus westermani*)
  Gastrointestinal disease (pancreatitis, esophageal
    rupture, subphrenic abscess)
  Drug reaction (nitrofurantoin, methysergide)
  Asbestosis
  Meigs' syndrome
  Postmyocardial infarction and postcardiac surgical
    operation
  Trapped lung
  Lymphatic abnormality
  Uremic pleurisy
  Atelectasis, chronic
  Chylothorax
  Sarcoidosis

*From Sahn SA: The differential diagnosis of pleural effusions. West J Med 137:103, 1982.

4. Ultrasonic chest examination: Detects 3 to 5 ml of loculated pleural fluid (Gryminski et al., 1976).

Detection of a minimal amount of fluid in the pleural cavity of a patient may not be pathologically significant, since up to 15 ml can be identified in the pleural cavity of about 10 per cent of a healthy population (Black, 1972). However, once a pleural effusion is documented in the context of clinical features of disease, the burden of proof is on the attending physician to determine the etiology of the effusion.

Defining the etiology of a pleural effusion usually involves aspiration of the fluid (thoracentesis), which can then be used for diagnostic purposes. If the effusion is large, aspiration of the fluid will achieve a therapeutic benefit because it will relieve respiratory distress.

In the subproblem of etiology of pleural effusion, we discuss how laboratory studies can be optimally used to arrive at a specific diagnosis. At the Mayo Clinic, Leuallen and Carr (1955) studied 436 patients with pleural effusion. They found that neoplasms caused the effusions in about half the cases. The other half were divided among congestive heart failure, infections, and miscellaneous or indeterminate causes.

Ryan and co-workers (1981) followed 51 patients with pleural effusion of indeterminate cause at thoracotomy. Thirty-one (60.8 per cent) had no recurrence of the effusion over a 1½- to 15-year follow-up. In 18 patients (35.3 per cent), the cause of the effusion became apparent after 12 days to 6 years: 13 patients had a malignancy, three had collagen-vascular disease, and one patient each had the yellow-nail syndrome and mitral stenosis. Two patients died shortly after thoracotomy, with death not clearly related to the pleural effusion.

Table 11–7 gives the causes of pleural effusions. Pleural effusions (*Lancet* editorial, 1982) can occur in viral pneumonia—20 per cent of patients (Fine et al., 1970)—and in asbestosis—21 per cent of patients (Gaensler and Kaplan, 1971). Knowledge of the physiology of pleural fluid formation and analysis of the cellular content and chemistry of these effusions, in conjunction with the history, physical examination, and ancillary laboratory data, should enable a clinician to reach a presumptive or definitive diagnosis in about 90 per cent of patients with pleural effusions (Sahn, 1982).

Pathophysiology

Normally, pleural fluid is produced by the parietal pleura and absorbed by the visceral pleura. Five mechanisms have been linked etiologically to the pathologic accumulation of pleural fluid (Sahn, 1981):

1. Increased hydrostatic pressure, as in congestive heart failure.
2. Increased capillary permeability, as in pneumonia or any type of pleurisy.
3. Decreased oncotic pressure, as in hypoalbuminemia.
4. Increased intrapleural negative pressure, as in atelectasis.
5. Impaired lymphatic drainage of the pleural space, such as in mediastinal carcinomatosis.

Transudative peritoneal fluid can cross the diaphragm to the pleural space. This fluid can move into the pleural space through defects in the diaphragm or through diaphragmatic lymphatics. The protein concentration of pleural fluid transudates can be greater than expected in the presence of impaired lymphatic drainage, vascular stasis, or capillary damage. Pleural fluid exudates are caused by diseases that either increase pleural capillary permeability or interfere with the lymphatic drainage of the pleural space (Black, 1972).

Clinical Contexts

Diagnosis. The evaluation of a patient with pleural effusion generally includes a complete clinical examination, appropriate blood tests and roentgenograms, and studies of the pleural fluid. The evaluation may include a needle biopsy of the pleura and open thoracotomy (Black, 1981).The history and physical examination will often reveal the cause of a pleural effusion, e.g., congestive heart failure. Whenever a diagnostic dilemma associated with a pleural effusion exists, thoracentesis should be performed. This not only provides fluid for examination but also relieves associated respiratory distress if the effusion is large. Thoracentesis is a benign procedure, only rarely resulting in pneumothorax and hemothorax.

In a series of 436 cases of pleural effusions, 50.9 per cent were in the right pleural space, 45.2 per cent were in the left pleural space, and 3.9 per cent were bilateral (Leuallen and Carr, 1955).

Management. Clinical laboratory studies of a pleural effusion can serve as baseline studies to follow progress of disease or response to therapy.

Screening. Pleural fluid examination is obviously not a screening procedure.

Strategy

Test Sequence. Once pleural fluid is obtained, perform at least the following studies:

1. Quantity of fluid.
2. Gross description of fluid.
   a. Clear.
   b. Turbid.
   c. Milky.
   d. Hemorrhagic.
   e. Purulent.
   f. Putrid or foul-smelling.
3. Pleural fluid protein and LDH levels.
4. Serum protein and LDH concentrations if serum is available.

If the pleural fluid is transudative in nature, no further laboratory studies on the pleural fluid are useful. If the pleural fluid is exudative in nature or if the clinical findings suggest an inflammatory or neoplastic process, perform the following studies:

1. Cytology.
2. Cultures: bacterial, acid-fast, and fungal.

Some authors (Storey et al., 1976) suggest that routine cultures be omitted.

Consider performing the following measurements on the pleural fluid if clinically indicated:

1. Cell counts: Erythrocyte, leukocyte, and leukocyte differential.
2. Serum and pleural fluid glucose.
3. Amylase.
4. pH.
5. Chromosome analysis.
6. Lipid studies: Triglycerides and lipoprotein electrophoresis.
7. Rheumatoid factor.
8. Mesothelial cell count.

If laboratory studies in concert with the clinical history, physical examination, and radiographic studies do not yield the cause of a pleural exudate, it may be necessary to perform a pleural biopsy or even a thoracotomy to achieve a definitive diagnosis.

Patient Preparation. For the most accurate interpretation of the pleural fluid glucose level, thoracentesis should be carried out while a patient is in a fasting state; a serum glucose determination should be obtained at the same time (Sahn, 1982). (See Part 3 for chemistry and hematology tests.)

Specimen Collection and Handling. Collect pleural fluid for appropriate tests and one tube of venous blood as follows:

1. Pleural fluid for chemistry tests: 10 ml, heparinized. Glucose can decrease if the fluid is not frozen or preserved with fluoride.

2. Venous blood for chemistry tests: One clot tube. Glucose can decrease if the serum is not frozen or preserved with fluoride.

3. Pleural fluid for cytology: 25 to 50 ml, heparinized.

4. Pleural fluid for bacterial cultures: 10 ml, heparinized.

5. Pleural fluid for acid-fast and fungal cultures: 10 ml, heparinized (a larger quantity, i.e., 50 ml, increases the sensitivity for culturing acid-fast bacilli).

6. Pleural fluid for hematology tests: 1 EDTA tube.

7. Pleural fluid for pH: Several ml collected anaerobically, iced, and quickly sent to the laboratory.

8. Pleural fluid for miscellaneous tests: 10 ml, heparinized.

These samples should be delivered to the laboratory immediately. (See Part 3.)

Methodology. Consult the laboratory for its methodologies, reference intervals, accuracy and precision, and potential sources of interference. (See Part 3.)

Interpretation

Diagnosis. It is important to divide pleural effusions into two principal types, transudates and exudates. Table 11–8 gives criteria for making this distinction. Based on experience, we believe that these are effective criteria for distinguishing transudates from exudates.

The presence of a bloody fluid (greater than 10,000 erythrocytes/mm³) or a leukocyte count greater than 1000/mm³ does not reliably distinguish a pleural transudate from a pleural exudate (Light, Erozan, et al., 1973). On the basis of a study of 50 samples of pleural fluid collected from consecutive patients in a thoracic clinic, Dines and associates (1975) concluded that counts of pleural fluid erythrocytes, leukocytes, and differential leukocytes have no specificity and no usefulness in the differential diagnosis of the origin of the effusion.

If a pleural effusion is a transudate, the pleural surfaces are not diseased and the ac-

Table 11–8. CRITERIA DISTINGUISHING PLEURAL FLUID TRANSUDATES FROM EXUDATES

Test	Transudate	Exudate
Specific gravity*	<1.016	>1.016
Protein*	<3.0 gm/100 ml	>3.0 gm/100 ml
Pleural fluid LDH†	<200 IU/liter‡	>200 IU/liter‡
Pleural fluid-to-serum protein ratio†	<0.5	>0.5
Pleural fluid-to-serum LDH ratio†	<0.6	>0.6

*These criteria misclassify 8 per cent of transudates and 11 per cent of exudates.

†These criteria misclassify fewer transudates and exudates than pleural fluid specific gravity and protein. When any one of these criteria indicate an exudate, conclude that the fluid is an exudate. When all three of these criteria are in agreement, misclassifications will be as few as 1 to 2 per cent, according to Light and colleagues (1972).

‡Where upper reference limit for serum is 300 IU/liter.

cumulation of excess fluid is due either to decreased oncotic pressure or to increased hydrostatic pressure. Table 11–9 gives the prevalence of various kinds of transudates and exudates in a series of 150 patients with pleural effusion. Once an effusion has been classified as a transudate, no further laboratory studies on the pleural fluid are useful. If a pleural

Table 11–9. CAUSES OF 150 PLEURAL EFFUSIONS*

Effusions		Number
Transudates		47
Congestive heart failure	39	
Other transudates	8	
Cirrhosis	5	
Nephrosis	3	
Exudates		103
Malignancy	43	
Effusions associated with pneumonia	26	
Tuberculosis	14	
Other exudates	20	
Pancreatitis	6	
Pulmonary infarction	5	
Postmyocardial infarction (Dressler's) syndrome	3	
Systemic lupus erythematosus	1	
Rheumatoid pleuritis	1	
Pleural actinomycosis	1	
Trauma	2	
Infectious hepatitis	1	

*Adapted from Light RW, MacGregor MI, Luchsinger PC, et al: Pleural effusions: The diagnostic separation of transudates and exudates. Ann Int Med 77:508, 1972.

effusion is an exudate, additional laboratory studies on the pleural fluid are required to ascertain the nature of the pleural disease. A parapneumonic effusion is any pleural effusion associated with a bacterial pneumonia or lung abscess. Table 11–10 indicates the pleural fluid findings in a variety of common diseases.

Pleural fluid exudates can have the following characteristics:

1. **Observation:** The fluid can be turbid, milky, hemorrhagic, or purulent. Turbid fluid due to a large number of leukocytes can be distinguished from turbid fluid due to increased lipids by centrifugation. If the turbidity clears, the turbidity is due to leukocytes. With chylothorax, chylomicrons produce a whitish layer on top of the centrifuged fluid (Sahn, 1982). Fluid accompanying a mesothelioma can be viscous and hemorrhagic. Anaerobic bacterial infections of the pleurae can produce fluid having a foul odor.

2. **Cytology and pleural biopsy:** Most patients with malignant pleural disease will have malignant cells demonstrable by cytologic evaluation. Cytologic study has a higher diagnostic yield than pleural biopsy in malignant disease of the pleurae but a lower diagnostic yield than pleural biopsy in tuberculous disease of the pleurae. Conversely, pleural biopsy has a lower yield than cytologic study in malignant pleural disease but a higher yield in tuberculous pleurisy (Frist, 1979). Vladutiu and associates (1981) suggested that cytologic examination combined with orosomucoid and carcinoembryonic antigen (CEA) quantitation in pleural fluid has considerable value for the diagnosis of malignant pleural effusions (74 per cent sensitivity for orosomucoid assay alone; 36 per cent sensitivity and 95 per cent specificity for CEA assay alone; 86 per cent sensitivity for CEA and orosomucoid assays together; 46 per cent sensitivity for cytology alone). The most common primary tumors metastasizing to the pleurae are those of the lung, breast, stomach, and ovary (Sahn, 1982).

3. **Hematology:**
   a. **Erythrocyte count:** A pink-tinged pleural fluid can be caused by a small number of erythrocytes (greater than 10,000/mm³). Small numbers of erythrocytes can be found in all types of effusions (transudates and exudates).

Bloody pleural fluid, with erythrocyte counts greater than 100,000/mm³, has a high predictive value for malignant pleural disease, pulmonary infarction, or trauma (Light, Erozan, et al., 1973). Pleural effusions associated with pulmonary embolism are usually bloody when there is infarction and less commonly when there is no infarction (Rosenow et al., 1981). Effusions due to pneumonia are not usually bloody. Bloody fluid from a traumatic tap is typically non-uniform in distribution in sequential samples of the pleural effusion and frequently clears with aspiration. In addition, a traumatic thoracentesis fluid can clot within several minutes, whereas pleural fluid present for several hours to days will become defibrinated and will not form a good clot (Sahn, 1981).

   b. **Leukocyte count:** More than 80 per cent of pleural transudates, but less than 20 per cent of exudates, have leukocyte counts of less than 1000/mm³. Pneumonia is present in 50 per cent of patients who have an effusion with leukocyte counts greater than 10,000/mm³. The remaining 50 per cent of patients with effusions that have leukocyte counts greater than 10,000/mm³ have diseases such as pulmonary infarction, pancreatitis, postmyocardial infarction syndrome, and systemic lupus erythematosus.

   c. **Leukocyte differential count:** Differential leukocyte counts in tuberculous effusions usually have more than 50 per cent small lymphocytes. A count greater than 50 per cent is also the most common pattern for malignant effusions. A count greater than 50 per cent lymphocytes is a very uncommon pattern for non-tuberculous, non-malignant fluids. A predominance of polymorphonuclear leukocytes is usually associated with pneumonia, pancreatitis, and pulmonary infarction and can be seen in effusions caused by tumor or collagen vascular disease. A predominance of polymorphonuclear leukocytes can occasionally be found in malignant effusions. Tuberculous effusions characteristically have fewer than 1 per cent mesothelial cells, whereas most non-tuberculous effusions have

Table 11–10. PLEURAL FLUID CHARACTERISTICS IN COMMON DISEASES*

Diagnosis	Appearance	Total Leukocytes (per µl)	Predominant Leukocytes	RBC (per µl)	Protein	Glucose	LDH	Amylase	pH	Comment
Transudates										
Congestive heart failure	Clear, straw-colored	<1000	M	0–1000	PF/S<0.5	PF = S	PF/S< 0.6 <200 IU/L	≤S	>7.40	Usually presence of biventricular failure
Cirrhosis	Clear, straw-colored	<500	M	<1000	PF/S<0.5	PF = S	PF/S<0.6 <200 IU/L	≤S	>7.40	Incidence 5% of cirrhotic patients with ascites
Exudates										
Parapneumonic (uncomplicated)	Turbid	5000–25,000	P	<5000	PF/S>0.5	PF = S	PF/S>0.6	≤S	>7.30	Resolves with antibiotics only
Empyema	Turbid to purulent	25,000–100,000	P	<5000	PF/S>0.5	0–60 mg/dl PF/S<0.5	PF/S>0.6 some >1000 IU/L	≤S	<7.30	Requires tube drainage
Pulmonary infarction	Straw-colored to bloody	5000–15,000	P	1000–100,000	PF/S>0.5	PF = S	PF/S>0.6	≤S	>7.30	Small effusion with basal alveolar infiltrate and elevated diaphragm
Tuberculosis	Straw-colored to serosanguineous	5000–10,000	M	<10,000	PF/S>0.5	PF = S or <60 mg/dl	PF/S>0.6	≤S	<or>7.30	Positive PPD, AFB stain and culture of pleural tissue often diagnostic
Rheumatoid disease	Turbid, green to yellow	1000–20,000	M or P	<1000	PF/S>0.5	<30 mg/dl	Often > 1000 IU/L	≤S	<7.30	Men, rheumatoid nodules, low pleural fluid complement
Carcinoma	Turbid to bloody	<10,000	M	1000 to several 100,000	PF/S>0.5	PF = S or <60 mg/dl	PF/S>0.6	≤S	<or>7.30	Cytology and pleural biopsy enable diagnosis in 80%
Pancreatitis	Turbid	5000–20,000	P	1000–10,000	PF/S>0.5	PF = S	PF/S>0.6	PF/S>2	>7.30	Occurs in 6% of cases of pancreatitis: left sided in 70%

Key:
RBC = red blood cells; LDH = lactate dehydrogenase; M = mononuclear; PF = pleural fluid; S = serum; P = polymorphonuclear; PPD = tuberculin skin test with purified protein derivative; AFB = acid-fast bacilli.

*Reproduced with permission from Sahn SA: Pulmonary disease. In Reller LB, et al (eds): Clinical Internal Medicine. Boston, Little, Brown & Company, 1979, pp 106–107.

greater than 5 per cent mesothelial cells (Light, Erozan, et al., 1973). Pleural fluid eosinophilia is not specific for any particular disease (Metzger et al., 1974).

4. **Chemistry tests:** As noted in Table 11–8, determinations of pleural fluid protein and LDH levels are of considerable help in distinguishing a transudate from an exudate, particularly when considered together with serum protein and LDH levels. Pleural fluid glucose concentration is over 60 mg/ 100 ml in the majority of tuberculous and malignant fluids. A pleural fluid glucose level below 60 mg/100 ml or 40 mg/100 ml less than the serum glucose level suggests bacterial disease or rheumatoid pleuritis but can also be seen with tuberculous or neoplastic disease. Pleural fluid glucose concentration is usually above 60 mg/100 ml in effusions resulting from lupus erythematosus. Pleural fluid amylase is above the serum upper reference limit for healthy persons in pancreatitis, pancreatic tumor, and occasionally pneumonia. (See the discussion of acute pancreatitis in Chapter 14.) It is below the serum upper reference limit in transudates, tuberculous effusions, and other exudates (Light and Ball, 1973). Besides pancreatitis pleural fluid amylase can be elevated secondary to esophageal rupture with escape of salivary amylase (Sherr et al., 1972). It can also be elevated with pancreatic pseudocyst and, rarely, with primary or metastatic carcinoma of the lung (Sahn, 1982).

5. **Microbiologic cultures:** Cultures for anaerobic organisms, fungi, and acid-fast bacilli require special handling. Because acid-fast bacilli are frequently sparse in number, the likelihood of a positive result can be increased by culturing larger volumes of fluid.

6. **Other helpful facts:**
   a. A pH less than 7.20 is often present in empyema and parapneumonic effusions that require drainage with a chest tube (Light, Girard, et al., 1980; Light, MacGregor, et al., 1973; Potts, 1976). Parapneumonic effusion with a pH over 7.30 usually resolves with antibiotic therapy alone. A pleural fluid pH less than 7.30 suggests that the fluid is an exudate and that the differential diagnosis is narrowed to empyema, malignancy, rheumatoid pleurisy, lupus pleuritis, tuberculosis, and esophageal rupture (Sahn, 1982).

   b. Chromosome analysis can be useful in the diagnosis of malignant pleural effusions (Dewald et al., 1976).
   c. Hepatitis B surface antigen is present in the pleural effusions accompanying hepatitis B (Merrill et al., 1977).
   d. Besides rheumatoid pleuritis, rheumatoid factor can be elevated above a titer of 1:160 in bacterial pneumonia, carcinoma, and tuberculosis (Levine et al., 1968).
   e. Triglycerides in pleural fluid, two to eight times the serum level, are consistent with chylothorax. Lipoprotein electrophoresis of a chylous effusion will show markedly elevated chylomicrons (Roy and Carr, 1967), and the fluid will stain positive with Sudan III. The most common cause of chylous effusion is malignancy, usually lymphoma. Other causes are surgical procedures and trauma. Chyliform (chylouslike) effusions are long-standing effusions seen in tuberculosis pleurisy, trapped lung, or rheumatoid pleurisy and are characterized by high levels of cholesterol (resulting from cellular degeneration), low levels of triglyceride, absence of chylomicrons, and negative staining with Sudan III (Sahn, 1982).
   f. Hyaluronate measurements in pleural fluid can be helpful in the diagnosis of pleural mesothelioma.
   g. Complement in pleural fluid is lower in lupus erythematosus and rheumatoid arthritis compared with malignant disease (Hunder et al., 1972).

Test Requests and Reports

Test Requests. A test sequence for the etiology of pleural effusion can be offered by the laboratory, which is directed at discriminating between transudates and exudates. If the effusion is identified as a transudate and the clinical findings are consistent, the laboratory studies may stop. If the effusion is identified as an exudate, the test sequence is directed at the etiology of the exudate. Of course, the test sequence is always carried out in the context of the patient's clinical picture.

Interpretive Report. The results of the tests can be collated and returned to the attending physician in the form of an interpretive report.

REFERENCES

Chronic Obstructive Pulmonary Disease

Burrows B: Chronic airways disease. In Wyngaarden JB, Smith LH, (eds): Cecil Textbook of Medicine, ed 16. Philadelphia, WB Saunders Company, 1982, pp. 363–371.

Burrows B: An overview of obstructive lung diseases. Med Clin North Am 65:455–471, 1981.

Fanta CH, Ingram RH: Airway responsiveness and chronic airway obstruction. Med Clin North Am 65:473–487, 1981.

Griner PF, Mayewski RJ, Mushlin AI, et al: Selection and interpretation of diagnostic tests and procedures. Principles and applications. Ann Intern Med 94:453–600, 1981.

Henry JB, Howanitz PJ: Organ panels and the relationship of the laboratory to the physician. In Jones RJ, Palulonis RM (eds.) Laboratory Tests in Medical Practice. Chicago, American Medical Association, 1980, p 31.

Miller WF: Chronic obstructive pulmonary disease. Hospital Practice, February 1981, pp 89–106.

Morse JO: Alpha-1-antitrypsin deficiency. N Engl J Med 299:1045–1048, 1099–1105, 1978.

Neff TA: The diagnosis and management of chronic obstructive lung disease. Cleveland Clinic Quarterly 47:17–24, 1980.

Robbins SL, Cotran RS: Chronic obstructive pulmonary disease. In Robbins SL, Cotran RS (eds): Pathologic Basis of Disease, ed 2. Philadelphia, WB Saunders Company, 1979, pp 827–836.

Scully RE, Galdabini JJ, McNeely BU (eds): Case records of the Massachusetts General Hospital. Case 14-1981. N Engl J Med 304:831–836, 1981.

Snider GL: Pathogenesis of emphysema and chronic bronchitis. Med Clin North Am 65:647–665, 1981.

Spivak JL, Barnes HV: Mechanical upper airway obstruction. In Spivak JL, Barnes HD: Manual of Clinical Problems in Internal Medicine, ed 2. Boston, Little, Brown & Company, 1978, pp 445–446.

Tietz NW: Electrolytes. In Tietz NW (ed): Fundamentals of Clinical Chemistry, ed 2. Philadelphia, WB Saunders Company, 1976, pp 873–899.

Traver GA, Cline MG, Burrows B: Predictors of mortality in COPD: A 15-year follow-up study. Am Rev Respir Dis 119:895–902, 1979.

Pulmonary Embolism

Bell WR, Simon TL, DeMets DL: The clinical features of submassive and massive pulmonary emboli. Am J Med 62:355–360, 1977.

Freiman DG, Suyemoto J, Weesler S: Frequency of pulmonary thromboembolism in man. N Engl J Med 272:1278–1280, 1965.

Gambino R (ed): Lab rounds: Low PaO_2, high LDH, and elevated bilirubin. Lab Report for Physicians 3:77–78, 1981.

Herlev Hospital Study Group: Diagnostic decision—Process in suspected pulmonary embolism. Lancet 1:1336–1338, 1979.

Konttinen A, Somer H, Auvinen S: Serum enzymes and isozymes. Extrapulmonary sources in acute pulmonary embolism. Arch Intern Med 133:243–246, 1974.

Light RW, Bell WR: LDH and fibrinogen-fibrin degradation products in pulmonary embolism. Arch Intern Med 133:372–375, 1974.

Lippman ML, Morgan L, Fein A, et al: Plasma and serum concentration of DNA in pulmonary thromboembolism. Ann Rev Respir Dis 125:416–419, 1982.

McNeil BJ: Ventilation-perfusion studies and the diagnosis of pulmonary embolism: Concise communication. J Nucl Med 21:319–323, 1980.

Moser KM: Diagnosis and management of pulmonary embolism. Hospital Practice, October 1980, pp 57–68.

Rosenow EC III, Osmundson PJ, Brown ML: Pulmonary embolism. Mayo Clin Proc 56:161–178, 1981.

Sipes JN, Suratt PM, Teates CD, et al: A prospective study of plasma DNA in the diagnosis of pulmonary embolism. Am Rev Respir Dis 118:475–478, 1978.

Smith AF: Enzymes and routine diagnosis. In Hearse DJ, deLeirus J (eds): Enzymes in Cardiology. New York, John Wiley & Sons, 1979, pp 199–246.

Soloff LA, Rodman T: Acute pulmonary embolism: I. Review. Am Heart J 74:710–724, 1967a.

Soloff LA, Rodman T: Acute pulmonary embolism: II. Clinical. Am Heart J 74:829–847, 1967b.

Spivak JL, Barnes HV: Pulmonary embolism. In Spivak JL, Barnes HV: Manual of Clinical Problems in Internal Medicine. Boston, Little, Brown & Company, 1978, pp 15–19.

Szucs MM, Brooks HL, Grossman W, et al: Diagnostic sensitivity of laboratory findings in acute pulmonary embolism. Ann Intern Med 74:161–166, 1971.

Tietz NW: Electrolytes. In Tietz NW (ed): Fundamentals of Clinical Chemistry, ed 2. Philadelphia, WB Saunders Company, 1976, pp 873–899.

Wacker WE, Rosenthal M, Snodgrass PJ, et al: A triad for the diagnosis of pulmonary embolism and infarction. JAMA 178:8–13, 1961.

Etiology of Pleural Effusion

Black LF: The pleural space and pleural fluid. Mayo Clin Proc 47:493–506, 1972.

Black LF: Pleural effusions, editorial. Mayo Clin Proc 56:201–202, 1981.

Dewald GD, Dines DE, Weiland LH, et al: Usefulness of chromosome examinations in the diagnosis of malignant pleural effusions. N Engl J Med 295:1494–1500, 1976.

Dines DE, Pierre RV, Franzen SJ: The value of cells in the pleural fluid in the differential diagnosis. Mayo Clin Proc 50:571–572, 1975.

Fine NL, Smith LR, Sheedy PF: Frequency of pleural effusions in mycoplasma and viral pneumonias. N Engl J Med 283:790–793, 1970.

Frist B, Kahan AV, Koss LG: Comparison of the diagnostic value of biopsies of the pleura and cytologic evaluation of pleural fluids. Am J Clin Pathol 72:48–51, 1979.

Gaensler EA, Kaplan AI: Asbestos pleural effusion. Ann Intern Med 74:178–191, 1971.

Gryminski J, Krakowka P, Lypacewicz G: The diagnosis of pleural effusion by ultrasonic and radiologic techniques. Chest 70:33–37, 1976.

Hunder GG, McDuffie FC, Hepper NGG: Pleural fluid complement in systemic lupus erythematosus and rheumatoid arthritis. Ann Intern Med 76:357–363, 1972.

Leuallen EC, Carr DT: Pleural effusion. A statistical study of 436 patients. N Engl J Med 252:79–83, 1955.

Levine H, Szanto M, Grieble HG, et al: Rheumatoid factor in nonrheumatoid pleural effusions. Ann Intern Med 69:487–492, 1968.

Light RW, Ball WC: Glucose and amylase in pleural effusions. JAMA 225:257–260, 1973.

Light RW, Erozan YS, Ball WC: Cells in pleural fluid. Their value in differential diagnosis. Arch Intern Med 132:854–860, 1973.

Light RW, Girard WM, Jenkinson SG, et al: Parapneumonic effusions. Am J Med 69:507–512, 1980.

Light RW, MacGregor MI, Ball WC, et al: Diagnostic significance of pleural fluid pH and PCO_2. Chest 64:591–596, 1973.

Light RW, MacGregor MI, Luchsinger PC, et al: Pleural effusions: The diagnostic separation of transudates and exudates. Ann Intern Med 77:507–513, 1972.

Merrill WD, Farris JR, Rounds O: Hepatitis antigen in pleural effusion, letter. Ann Intern Med 87:120, 1977.

Metzger AL, Coyne M, Stephen L, et al: In vivo LE cell formation in peritonitis due to systemic lupus erythematosus. J Rheum 1:130–133, 1974.

Mysterious pleural effusions, editorial: Lancet 1:1226, 1982.

Potts DE, Levin DC, Sahn SA: Pleural fluid pH in parapneumonic effusions. Chest 70:328–331, 1976.

Rosenow EC III, Osmundson PJ, Brown ML: Pulmonary embolism. Mayo Clin Proc 56:161–178, 1981.

Roy PH, Carr DT, Payne WS: The problem of chylothorax. Mayo Clin Proc 42:457–467, 1967.

Ryan CJ, Rodgers RF, Unni KK, et al: The outcome of patients with pleural effusion of indeterminate cause at thoracotomy. Mayo Clin Proc 56:145–149, 1981.

Sahn SA: Pleural manifestations of pulmonary disease. Hospital Practice, March 1981, pp 73–89.

Sahn SA: The differential diagnosis of pleural effusions. West J Med 137:99–108, 1982.

Sherr HP, Light RW, Merson MH, et al: Origin of pleural fluid amylase in esophageal rupture. Ann Intern Med 76:985–986, 1972.

Storey DD, Dines DE, Coles DT: Pleural effusion: A diagnostic dilemma. JAMA 236:2183–2186, 1976.

Vladutiu AO, Brason FW, Adler RH: Differential diagnosis of pleural effusions. Clinical usefulness of cell marker quantitation. Chest 79:297–301, 1981.

CHAPTER 12

GENITOURINARY SUBPROBLEMS

KIDNEY DISEASE
  Acute Renal Failure
PROSTATIC DISEASE
  Prostatic Carcinoma

KIDNEY DISEASE

ACUTE RENAL FAILURE

Definition and Significance

Acute renal failure is characterized by an abrupt accumulation of nitrogenous wastes *(azotemia)*. The failure is due to intrinsic kidney disease that is not readily reversed despite correction of hemodynamic or obstructive factors (Schrier, 1981). Patients may be classified as *oliguric* (urine output less than 400 ml/day) or *non-oliguric* (urine output greater than 800 ml/day). The azotemia is manifested by accumulation of urea nitrogen, creatinine, and uric acid, and there is retention of phosphate and sulfate ions. Depending on diet, sodium and magnesium ions can also accumulate. Metabolic acidosis with elevation of the serum potassium level can occur. There is frequently a bleeding tendency and a normochromic, normocytic anemia with a depression of the serum calcium level. If the renal failure becomes chronic, osteodystrophy and peripheral neuropathy can occur (Maffly, 1980).

If the renal failure occurs suddenly, over a period of days to weeks, it is *acute*. If it occurs slowly, over a period of months to years, it is *chronic*. Division of renal failure into acute and chronic varieties is helpful in arriving at the cause, for the differential diagnoses of acute and chronic renal failure differ.

Acute azotemia may be prerenal, renal, or postrenal. Prerenal failure is characterized by azotemia secondary to inadequate perfusion of the kidneys and is reversible within 24 hours if the systemic cause of the renal hypoperfusion is corrected. Postrenal failure is characterized by azotemia resulting from mechanical obstruction distal to the kidneys; in this case, renal function may be restored or improved if the obstruction is removed.

Acute renal failure is a diagnosis of exclusion. First, postrenal and prerenal causes of azotemia must be excluded; then the exact etiology of acute renal failure must be determined. The causes of acute renal failure are given in Table 12–1.

Pathophysiology

Acute azotemia may result from several causes:

1. *Prerenal:* A fall in blood pressure or obstruction of the renal arteries and veins.

202

Table 12–1. SPECIFIC DISORDERS THAT CAUSE ACUTE RENAL FAILURE*

Ischemic Disorders
Major trauma
Massive hemorrhage
Compartmental syndrome
Septic shock
Transfusion reactions
Myoglobinuria
Postpartum hemorrhage
Cardiac, aortic, and biliary surgery
Pancreatitis, gastroenteritis

Nephrotoxicities, Including Hypersensitivity Reactions to
Heavy metals: mercury, arsenic, lead, bismuth, uranium, cadmium
Organic solvents: carbon tetrachloride, ethylene glycol
X-ray contrast media (particularly in diabetic patients)
Pesticides
Fungicides
Antibiotics: aminoglycosides, penicillins, tetracyclines, amphotericin
Other agents: phenytoin, phenylbutazone, uric acid, calcium

Diseases of Glomeruli and Small Blood Vessels
Acute poststreptococcal glomerulonephritis
Systemic lupus erythematosus
Polyarteritis nodosa
Schönlein-Henoch purpura
Subacute bacterial endocarditis
Serum sickness
Goodpasture's syndrome
Malignant hypertension
Hemolytic-uremic syndrome
Drug-related vasculitis
Abruptio placentae, abortion with or without gram-negative sepsis, postpartum renal failure
Rapidly progressive glomerulonephritis of unknown etiology

Major Blood Vessel Diseases
Renal artery thrombosis, embolism, or stenosis
Bilateral renal vein thrombosis

*From Schrier RW: Acute renal failure: Pathogenesis, diagnosis, and management. Hospital Practice, March 1981, p 101.

2. *Renal:* Acute tubular necrosis and other parenchymal diseases, such as bilateral renal cortical necrosis, glomerulitis, papillary necrosis, end-stage chronic renal disease, and miscellaneous causes, e.g., hypercalcemia, hyperuricemia, multiple myeloma, and homograft rejection.

3. *Postrenal:* Urinary tract obstruction, e.g., benign prostatic hypertrophy.

The pathophysiologic mechanisms for acute azotemia secondary to intrinsic renal disease have not been fully elucidated. There appears to be a complex interaction of several factors that include the following (Fig. 12–1):

1. Decreased blood flow to the renal cortex with a secondary decrease in the glomerular filtration rate (GFR).

2. Acute tubular necrosis.

3. Obstruction of the tubules by cellular debris and protein pigments, e.g, hemoglobin or myoglobin.

Acute renal failure is a special form of acute azotemia resulting from intrinsic renal disease that is potentially reversible in an interval ranging from several days to several weeks. A detailed discussion of acute renal failure, including its pathophysiology, is available by Finn (1979) and Levinsky (1977).

Clinical Contexts

Diagnosis. The clinical picture of acute renal failure is characterized by the signs and symptoms of the primary disorder (Table 12–1). Oliguria is usually present. Acute renal failure is accompanied by an abrupt reduction of renal function and a rising serum urea nitrogen (SUN) level and creatinine (azotemia). Depending on the time the patient is first seen and the kind of therapy administered, there can be varying degrees of acid-base, electrolyte, and fluid balance complications: metabolic acidosis; elevated levels of serum potassium, phosphate, and sulfate; and a depressed level of serum calcium.

Acute renal failure usually follows the inciting cause by several hours to 2 days. Oliguria may be absent. Anderson and colleagues (1977) suggested that non-oliguric acute renal failure occurs considerably more often than is generally appreciated; yet, in most instances scant amounts of urine are passed. Complete absence of urinary output—*anuria*—suggests bilateral renal artery occlusion, obstructive uropathy, acute cortical necrosis, or rapidly progressive glomerulonephritis (Maffly, 1980).

Acute renal failure is usually marked by an *oliguric phase* lasting a few hours to 3 or more weeks (sometimes over 2 months); a *diuretic phase* lasting a few days to a week or longer, and a *recovery phase* characterized by a progressive rise in glomerular filtration rate and restoration of acid-base, electrolyte, and fluid balances to normal.

The clinical picture of organ system involvement plus azotemia is called *uremia*. The features of uremia include the following:

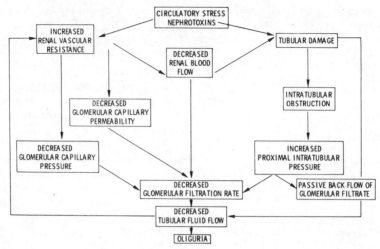

Figure 12–1. Schema of interrelated events that may follow acute circulatory or toxic renal damage. Alterations in glomerular capillary pressure, permeability, and blood flow lead directly to a reduction in filtration and urine formation, obstruction of the tubules retards the flow of filtrate and promotes leakage back across damaged epithelium. The factors, derived from various experimental models, are not mutually exclusive nor are all necessarily present; moreover, they probably vary in importance between different models and from time to time in the same model. (From Finn, WF: Acute renal failure. In Earley LE, Gottschalk CW (eds): Strauss and Welt's Diseases of the Kidney, ed 3, Boston, Little, Brown & Company, 1979, p 178.)

1. *Gastrointestinal:* Anorexia, nausea, and thirst (if water is withheld).

2. *Central nervous system:* Asterixis, convulsions, and coma.

3. *Cardiovascular:* Cardiac output, blood pressure, and electrocardiographic changes.

The diagnostic workup of acute renal failure is concerned with distinguishing renal causes of acute azotemia from prerenal and postrenal causes. Early recognition and treatment of prenenal azotemia can prevent its progression to acute renal failure. If a renal cause is present, its specific etiology should be determined. In addition, the patient should be studied for the presence of an underlying chronic renal disease.

Management. Acute renal failure can be managed by careful monitoring of water balance, electrolytes, minerals, and calories. Appropriate drugs and dialysis are used as necessary. Laboratory measurements provide data necessary for effective management. Non-oliguric acute renal failure (urine volume > 800 ml/day) is a more benign disease than oliguric renal failure; i.e., more than 50% of patients can be managed without hemodialysis (Schrier, 1982).

Screening. In the absence of clinical features (e.g., shock, crush injury, incompatible blood transfusion, or oliguria), there is no need to screen for acute renal failure.

Strategy

Test Sequence. Azotemia can be documented by measuring SUN and creatinine. The following studies are useful to confirm and characterize the severity of the azotemia and to determine its etiology:

1. Sodium, potassium, chloride, carbon dioxide, calcium, magnesium, phosphorus (PO_4), and uric acid.

2. Complete blood count.

3. Urine volume, sediment, osmolality, sodium, urea nitrogen, creatinine.

After an obstructive basis for acute azotemia has been excluded by clinical testing, acute renal failure may be distinguished from prerenal causes of acute azotemia by the following (Miller, 1978; Schrier, 1979).

1. Urine osmolality.

2. Urine sodium.

3. Ratio of urine urea nitrogen to serum urea nitrogen.

4. Ratio of urine creatinine to serum creatinine.

5. Renal failure index (urinary sodium concentration ÷ U/P creatinine concentration).

6. Fractional excretion of filtered sodium (U/P sodium concentration ÷ U/P creatinine concentration × 100).

The logic of this strategy has been discussed

by Harrington and Cohen (1975). They have indicated the therapeutic importance of vigorously excluding both prerenal and postrenal disorders, for which specific therapy is often curative, before one assumes the presence of intrinsic renal disease, for which immediate, specific treatment is only rarely available.

Patient Preparation. No special preparation is required for serum and urine osmolality tests and routine urinalysis. (See Part 3 for chemistry and hematology tests.)

Specimen Collection and Handling. The urine should be collected in a clean container and promptly analyzed. (See Part 3.)

Methodology. Consult the laboratory concerning its specific methodologies, accuracy and precision, reference intervals, and potential sources of interference. (See Part 3.)

Interpretation

Diagnosis. If the laboratory tests establish the presence of acute azotemia (a sudden elevation of serum creatinine above 2 mg/100 ml and urea nitrogen above 25 mg/100 ml), the next step is to exclude a postrenal cause and prerenal cause. A postrenal cause can be excluded by ruling out an obstructive uropathy; a prerenal cause can be excluded by clinical information, radiographic studies, and the use of urinary indices as given in Table 12–2.

A postrenal cause for acute azotemia may be excluded by working up the patient for an enlarged prostate, palpable bladder, large residual urine volume, hydronephrotic kidneys, ureteral obstruction, history of renal calculi, and so forth. Usually, no urine sediment abnormalities are found in postrenal azotemia (Schrier, 1981). Patients with urinary tract obstruction have urinary indices that are indistinguishable from those of patients with acute renal failure (Schrier, 1982). If an obstruction is found and if it is relieved, a brisk diuresis ensues which can be as high as 6 to 8 liters per hour. Salt and water losses can be significant and, if not compensated for, can result in shock. Hypokalemia can occur (Spivak and Barnes, 1978).

A prerenal cause for acute azotemia (i.e., volume depletion, congestive heart failure, or severe liver disease) may be excluded by the clinical context and by measuring serum and urine analytes and computing indices (Del Greco and Krumlovksy, 1981; Finn, 1979; Miller et al., 1978); see Table 12–2.

Table 12–2. INDICES FOR DISTINGUISHING PRERENAL FROM OLIGURIC ACUTE RENAL FAILURE*

Index†	Units/Formula	Prerenal	Renal
Uosm	mosm/kg H_2O	>500	<350
Urine sodium	mEq/l	<20	>40
Urine/plasma urea nitrogen	—	>8	<3
Urine/plasma creatinine	—	>40	<20
Renal failure index	$U_{Na}/U/P_{CR}$	<1	>1
Fractional excretion of filtered sodium	$\dfrac{U/P_{Na}}{U/P_{CR}} \times 100$	<1	>1

*Adapted from Miller TR, Anderson RJ, Linas SL, et al: Urinary diagnostic indices in acute renal failure: A prospective study. Ann Intern Med 89:49, 1978.

†If the urine osmolality, urine sodium, U/P urea nitrogen and U/P creatinine do not clearly indicate prerenal azotemia or acute renal failure, then rely on the renal failure index and the fractional exception of filtered sodium (these last two indices function less well in nonoliguric renal failure, 6 per cent and 10 per cent false negatives respectively).

A rising serum creatinine level above 2.5 mg/100 ml strongly suggests established renal failure as opposed to prerenal azotemia. The SUN:creatinine ratio is usually 10 to 15:1 in renal parenchymal disease but is greater than 20:1 in prerenal azotemia and urinary tract obstruction (Contiguglia et al., 1979). Usually, no urine sediment abnormalities are found in prerenal azotemia (Schrier, 1981). Najarian (1980) believed that acute tubular necrosis may be distinguished from prerenal azotemia by the "sniff test." He found that urine from patients with acute tubular necrosis had very little odor, whereas urine from patients with prerenal azotemia had a disagreeable odor resulting from concentrated urinary chemicals.

Errors in using urinary indices are possible if we rely completely on laboratory test results. These values must always be interpreted in the context of the history and physical examination (Bricker, 1979), as the following paragraphs describe.

Acute renal failure secondary to volume depletion (prerenal failure) can progress to acute tubular necrosis; if the urine was examined prior to the advent of acute tubular necrosis, it will have been low in sodium and have a high ratio of urine creatinine to serum creatinine.

In acute tubular necrosis, there may be a

profound stimulus to sodium retention. For example, a patient with burns may have oliguria, a glomerular filtration rate below 1 ml per minute, and a creatinine U/P ratio of less than 10, but virtually no sodium in the urine. A low urinary sodium level has also been seen in acute tubular necrosis after major cardiac surgery and mercury poisoning.

With regard to urinary indices, patients with acute glomerulonephritis appear similar to prerenal patients and must be distinguished by the clinical history and urinalysis. The indices are of no value in distinguishing obstructive uropathy from renal causes (Miller, 1978).

If prerenal and postrenal causes for acute renal azotemia are excluded, the patient should be studied to determine the specific etiology of the renal disease. A careful workup

should be directed at the detection of causes listed in Table 12–1. Clues may be obtained from test results, e.g., acute renal failure secondary to hypercalcemia or hyperuricemia or to rhabdomyolysis with hypokalemia, hypophosphatemia and elevated CPK.

The presence of underlying chronic renal disease is suggested by kidneys that are small as shown by x-ray films or by ultrasound. Hypertension, proteinuria, nocturia, anemia, hypocalcemia, hyperphosphatemia, and acidosis, which are more pronounced than that observed in the usual acute renal failure patient, suggest chronic renal disease. Generally, the SUN must increase above 40 mg/100 ml and serum creatinine above 4 mg/100 ml before the anion gap is increased (Emmett and Narins, 1977). In addition, the urine in chronic

Table 12–3. COMMON LABORATORY TEST RESULTS IN ACUTE RENAL FAILURE*

Laboratory Test	Value	Pathophysiologic Factors
Chemistry (Serum)		
Bilirubin, total	—	
Calcium, total	↑	Can be a cause of acute renal failure
	↓	Electrolyte change related to decreased renal function
Carbon dioxide	↓	Related to metabolic acidosis
Chloride	↑	Cause?
Cholesterol	—	
Creatine phosphokinase	↑	When acute renal failure is due to rhabdomyolysis
Creatinine	↑	Related to decreased renal clearance
Glucose	↑	Common finding
Lactic dehydrogenase	↑	In 75 per cent of patients at initial hospitalization
Phosphatase, alkaline	—	
Phosphorus, inorganic	↑	Related to decreased renal clearance
	↓	Can be a cause of rhabdomyolysis with acute renal failure
Potassium	↑	Related to decreased excretion during oliguric phase.
	↓	Can occur early in renal failure related to diarrhea, vomiting, or urinary loss; can occur in relation to large urinary excretion in diuretic stage; can be a cause of rhabdomyolysis with acute renal failure
Proteins, total	—	
Proteins, albumin	—	
Sodium	↓	Often decreased in second week
Transaminase, aspartate amino	↑	In 65 per cent of patients at initial hospitalization
Urea nitrogen	↑	Related to decreased renal clearance
Uric acid	↑	Related to decreased renal clearance; can be a cause of acute renal failure
Hematology (Blood)		
Hemoglobin	↓	Related to renal failure
Hematocrit	↓	Related to renal failure
Leukocyte count, total	↑	In 65 per cent of patients at initial hospitalization; not necessarily related to infection
Platelet count	↓	Related to peripheral destruction, e.g., disseminated intravascular coagulation

Key:
— = No change; ↑ = can be increased; ↓ = can be decreased.

*Based on information from Friedman RB, Anderson RE, Entine SM, et al: Effects of diseases on clinical laboratory tests. Clin Chem 26:1D–476D, 1980; Del Greco F, Krumlovsky FA: Role of the laboratory in management of acute and chronic renal failure. Ann Clin Lab Sci 11:283–291, 1981.

renal failure will sometimes contain only an occasional discrete cast, whereas many granular casts are commonly seen in the urine from patients with acute renal failure (Maffly, 1980).

In acute cortical necrosis, selective renal arteriography can demonstrate a characteristic arterial pattern and irregular cortical perfusion defects.

If necessary for diagnosis, a percutaneous biopsy should be performed. Although the renal morphology of a patient with acute renal failure can be essentially normal, renal biopsy can be of value if it reveals the presence of some specific lesion, e.g., acute cortical necrosis or proliferative glomerulonephritis.

If the urine sediment contains eosinophils, acute interstitial nephritis should be suspected. Red blood cell casts suggest glomerulonephritis or vasculitis (Schrier, 1981). A positive urine dipstick test for occult blood is compatible with the presence of either hemoglobin or myoglobin, which can be associated with transfusion reactions or muscle injury, respectively. The serum is often pink or red in the presence of hemoglobinuria and straw-colored in the presence of myoglobinuria. This is because free hemoglobin is bound to haptoglobin and becomes elevated in the serum, whereas free myoglobin is immediately cleared by the kidneys (Bradley et al., 1979). See Table 12–3 for the results of common laboratory tests in acute renal failure.

Management. Laboratory measurements of SUN, creatinine, uric acid, electrolytes, and other analytes are of critical importance for following the course of acute renal failure and guiding effective therapy.

Test Requests and Reports

Test Requests. The laboratory can offer the appropriate tests and computation of indices listed in Table 12–2 as a problem-solving service directed toward the differentiation of prerenal and renal causes of acute renal failure. Henry's renal panel is another example of a group of laboratory tests designed to diagnose and manage renal disease (Fig. 12–2). Henry and Howanitz (1980) gave the rationale for this renal panel as follows:

BUN is useful in following patients with end stage renal disease undergoing dialysis since it reflects effectiveness of dialysis better than serum creatinine. However, serum creatinine is a better single screening test for renal function since it is virtually unaffected by protein ingestion, or metabolism and dehydration. Serum creatinine combined with the urine creatinine can be used to calculate the creatinine clearance—the most practical method for determining glomerular filtration rate. Serum albumin and total protein are included as an indication of severity of any proteinuria, while urine culture and urinalysis are used to detect an infection which may further compromise renal function.

Serum osmolality is very useful in following hypo- and hypernatremic states, which are usually associated with hypo- and hyperosmolality, respectively, as well as disturbances of water balance. In severe diabetes mellitus a serum osmolality is helpful in forewarning the physician against hyperosmolality, which may lead to intracellular dehydration, convulsions, and death. Urine osmolality is the most accurate method for assessing urine concentration since renal and pituitary disturbances in function reflect changes in osmolality (number of solute particles), rather than specific gravity (mass of solute particles). Both serum and urine osmolality measurements generate the U/P ratio (normal 4/1) which, with the urine volume, permit calculation of free water clearance. Knowledge of free water clearance aids in the management of postoperative patients, patients with cardiac failure, cirrhosis, Addison's disease, and polyuric syndromes, and those in other situations, such as dialysis.

Interpretive Reports. The test results and calculated indices can differentiate prerenal and renal causes of acute azotemia and may be returned to the attending physician in the form of an interpretive report. A clear advantage is that the data are collated and all mathematical calculations are already accomplished. In the case of Henry's renal panel (Fig. 12–2), an interpretive comment concerning the renal panel test results can also be made. Computer-aided management of acute renal failure using decision analysis has been described (Gorry et al., 1973).

PROSTATIC DISEASE

PROSTATIC CARCINOMA

Definition and Significance

Prostatic carcinoma is an adenocarcinoma of the glandular epithelium of the prostate and the third leading cause of cancer deaths among men in the United States. It primarily affects men over the age of 50, and the etiology is unknown. Each year there are 42,000 new cases of prostatic carcinoma in the United

RENAL				
Urea Nitrogen (BUN) mg/dl	8–18			
Creatinine mg/dl	0.6–1.2			
Creatinine Clearance ml/min	80–120			
Total Osmolality Serum mOsm/kg	285–295			
Osmolality Urine mOsm/kg	300–1000			
Osmolal Clearance ml/min				
Free Water Clearance ml/min				
Sodium mEq/L	135–145			
Potassium mEq/L	4.0–4.8			
Chloride mEq/L	98–109			
CO_2 Content mM/L	24–30			
Inorganic Phosphorus mg/dl	Adult 2.0–5.2 Child 4.0–7.0			
Calcium mEq/L	4.5–5.4			
Glucose mg/dl	65–115			
Uric Acid mg/dl	Female 2.0–6.4 Male 2.1–7.8			
Albumin gm/dl	Age 15–35 3.44–5.64 Age 35–55 3.22–5.10			
Total Proteins gm/dl	6.7–8.3			
Urinalysis	See Microscopy Report Sheet			
Urine Culture & Colony Count	See Bacteriology Report Sheet			

Figure 12–2.   Renal panel. (From Henry JB, Murphy J: Effective utilization of clinical laboratories. In Henry JB (ed): Clinical Diagnosis and Management by Laboratory Methods, ed 16. Philadelphia, WB Saunders Company, 1979, p 2044.)

States with 17,000 deaths per year. Roughly 30 per cent, or 12,000, of the new cases are potentially curable when first discovered (Klein, 1979).

The extent of prostatic carcinoma can be classified according to the schema listed in Table 12–4 (Murphy et al., 1978).

Pathophysiology

Prostatic carcinoma frequently arises in the posterior lobe of the prostate, but it can arise in any site where there is active glandular epithelium. The natural history of the disease is invasion through the prostatic capsule into the surrounding pelvic tissue. Following this, the tumor often metastasizes to bone, particularly the pelvis, spine, femora, and ribs. Some tumors spread widely to viscera, particularly the lungs, liver, and adrenal glands. The bony metastases can be osteolytic, but osteoblastic lesions are more common and in males point strongly to prostatic carcinoma (Robbins and Cotran, 1979).

Prostatic carcinoma, like normal prostatic glandular epithelium, secretes acid phosphatase. Since the malignant glandular epithelium of prostatic carcinoma has no ducts to drain secretions, it is believed that accumulations of acid phosphatase diffuse into adjacent interstitial compartments and thereby enter the blood stream (Murphy et al., 1978). Elevation of serum acid phosphatase is used as a diagnostic test for prostatic carcinoma.

Prostatic carcinoma confined to the prostate gland frequently does not cause an elevation of serum acid phosphatase. Conversely, because acid phosphatase comprises a number of isoenzymes present in erythrocytes, platelets, leukocytes, reticuloendothelial cells, liver, spleen, and kidney, as well as prostate, there are a number of extraprostatic diseases that

Table 12–4. STAGING OF PROSTATIC CARCINOMA*

Stage	Description
A (I)	Occult, incidental
B (II)	Confined within the prostate gland
C (III)	Periprostatic (outside the prostatic capsule)
D (IV)	Metastatic

*From Murphy GP, Karr, J, Chu TM: Prostatic acid phosphatase: Where are we? Ca—A Cancer Journal for Clinicians 28:261, 1978.

can cause an elevated serum acid phosphatase. In fact, even some benign diseases and disorders of the prostate, such as infarction, can cause an elevation. Digital rectal examination of the prostate does not elevate the serum acid phosphatase (Daar, 1981; Johnson, 1979; Phatak, 1982) as had been reported previously (Hock, 1949; Kendall, 1961).

Osteoblastic bone lesions secondary to metastatic prostatic carcinoma are associated with an elevation of serum alkaline phosphatase (ALP). Presumably, the source of the increased ALP is the osteoblasts themselves.

Besides measurement of serum acid phosphatase and ALP, other procedures useful in the diagnosis and staging of prostatic carcinoma include radionuclide bone scanning, skeletal radiography, lymphangiography, pelvic lymphadenectomy, and biopsies for tissue diagnosis. Direct measurement of bone marrow acid phosphatase has been evaluated as a method of documenting metastases to bone. A good review of carcinoma of the prostate is available by Catalona and Scott (1978) and Klein (1979).

Clinical Contexts

Diagnosis. Clinical features of prostatic carcinoma include symptoms of bladder outlet obstruction, a hard prostate on digital rectal examination, back pain, pathologic fractures secondary to metastases, and symptoms and signs of renal insufficiency secondary to urinary tract obstruction (Krupp, 1978). (See the discussion of acute renal failure earlier in this chapter.)

Sometimes the clinical picture is consistent with diseases other than prostatic carcinoma, such as benign prostatic hypertrophy, or bone lesions not due to metastatic prostatic carcinoma. In these situations, prostatic carcinoma must be excluded.

Management. After the diagnosis of prostatic carcinoma is confirmed, appropriate therapy should be instituted. The effects of castration and chemotherapy on prostatic carcinoma may be monitored by following serial determinations of serum acid phosphatase and ALP.

Screening. Prostatic carcinoma can exist in the absence of the clinical features just mentioned. Because prostatic carcinoma is such a common disease in men over the age of 50 years, it frequently can be present in an occult form. It would be useful to have a screening test for prostatic carcinoma that would have the diagnostic sensitivity to detect occult disease. When screening is done for the presence of prostatic carcinoma, the method having the greatest diagnostic sensitivity should ordinarily be used. False-positive results can be a significant problem, since they can be eliminated only by further studies.

Strategy

Diurnal (Doe, 1965) and circadian (Batsakis, 1967) variations in serum acid phosphatase have been reported to occur, but these findings have not been corroborated (Johnson, 1979). Nevertheless, we believe that serial measurement of acid phosphatase on several successive days is appropriate.

Measurement of serum ALP is useful because elevations can provide indirect evidence of the presence of prostatic carcinoma metastic to the liver and/or bone. Parallel and serial measurements of serum acid and alkaline phosphatase provide an objective method of evaluating the response of prostatic carcinoma to surgical or medical therapy.

Measurement of bone marrow acid phosphatase as a means of documenting bone metastases is of limited value (Rosenberg and Grabstald, 1980).

Test Sequence. To determine which screening test is most accurate in detecting prostatic cancer, Guinan and colleagues (1980) evaluated ten diagnostic procedures in 300 elderly men with symptoms of urinary tract obstruction and a high prevalence of prostatic cancer (Table 12–5). Their data demonstrate that a skillful digital rectal examination is still the most effective test for detection of prostatic carcinoma.

In light of these findings, we believe the best strategy to detect prostatic cancer should include a careful digital rectal examination followed by measurement of serum acid phosphatase. Measurement of serum ALP should be done with the realization that a positive test result depends on the presence of prostatic carcinoma that is already metastic to bone and/or liver. A serum immunoassay usually has greater sensitivity than a colorimetric method. It is also more specific for the prostatic isoenzyme.

A SUN and creatinine determination can be useful for detecting postrenal obstruction, and a serum calcium and phosphorus measurement can aid in detecting metastases to bone.

Patient Preparation. Although not essential (Daar, 1981; Johnson, 1979; Phatak, 1982), it is still preferable, if possible, to draw the blood sample for acid phosphatase before examining the prostate. (See Chapter 9 and Part 3 for additional discussion of serum ALP and other chemistry tests.)

Specimen Collection and Handling. Pros-

Table 12–5. RESULTS OF SCREENING TESTS FOR PROSTATE CANCER*

Test	No. of Patients	Sensitivity	Specificity	Predictive Value Positive Test	Predictive Value Negative Test	Efficiency‖
Rectal examination	300	0.69	0.89	67	91	85
Acid phosphatase—enzyme	300	0.56	0.94	72	88	84
Acid phosphatase—RIA†	100	0.20	0.85	29	78	70
Acid phosphatase—CIEP‡	100	0.20	0.95	56	80	78
Urine cytology before massage	202	0.17	0.98	67	80	79
Prostatic-secretion cytology after massage	211	0.29	0.98	78	82	81
Urine cytology after massage	209	0.22	0.98	71	81	80
Aspiration cytology	200	0.55	0.91	65	88	83
Lactic dehydrogenase V/I ratio§	132	0.47	0.82	44	83	73
Leukocyte-adherence inhibition	113	0.50	0.79	43	83	72

*From Guinan P, Bush I, Ray V, et al: The accuracy of the rectal examination in the diagnosis of prostate carcinoma. N Engl J Med 303:501, 1980. Reprinted by permission.

†RIA = Radioimmunoassay.

‡CIEP = Counterimmunoelectrophoresis.

§V/I ratio = LDH-5 isoenzyme ≥ LDH-I isoenzyme in prostatic fluid

‖Efficiency = $\dfrac{\text{true positives} + \text{true negatives}}{\text{total tested}} \times 100$

tatic acid phosphatase is rapidly destroyed at room temperature. Serum should be quickly separated from erythrocytes and assayed immediately. Hemolysis should be avoided. If the assay is delayed, the serum should be frozen. The addition of disodium citrate monohydrate at a level of 10 mg/ml of serum or three drops of 6 molar acetic acid per 5 ml of serum will lower the pH and stabilize the enzyme. At this lower pH, serum acid phosphatase will be preserved for several hours at room temperature and up to a week if refrigerated. Fluoride and oxalate ions, as well as heparin, inhibit enzyme activity and should be avoided (Katchmar and Moss, 1976).

Immunoassay has the advantage of measuring inactive as well as active prostatic acid phosphatase (Foti et al., 1977). This assay is not affected by hemolysis.(See Chapter 9 and Part 3.)

Methodology. The colorimetric enzymatic method of choice uses thymolphthalein monophosphate as the substrate (Roy et al., 1971). This substrate has greater analytic specificity for prostatic acid phosphatase than other substrates. We use this substrate. (See Chapter 9 and Part 3.)

Newer methods employing RIA, counterimmunoelectrophoresis (CIEP), and fluorescent immunoassay promise greater diagnostic sensitivity. This increased sensitivity may be accompanied by a decrease in diagnostic specificity. Griffiths (1980) compared the diagnostic sensitivity of three methods, one by RIA, and the other two by enzymatic assay. His finding that the RIA is more sensitive than the enzyme assay conflicts with the work of Guinan and associates (1980). Another study (Flüchter et al., 1982) supports Griffiths' findings, and it is likely that immunoassays are more sensitive.

Consult the laboratory about its methodologies, accuracy and precision, reference intervals, and potential sources of interference.

Interpretation

Diagnosis. The use of serum acid phosphatase for diagnosing prostatic carcinoma should be made with knowledge of the diagnostic sensitivity and diagnostic specificity of the particular method being employed (Table 12–5). The predictive value of a positive or negative test for elevated serum acid phosphatase depends not only on the diagnostic sensitivity and specificity of the method used but also on the prevalence of prostatic carcinoma in the population being studied. The prevalence of prostatic cancer in men studied by Guinan and associates, urologists (1980), was 23 per cent. Because their patients were referred, the prevalence of prostatic cancer in the general population may be expected to be lower. This lower prevalence would, of course, result in a decreased predictive value and efficiency of digital rectal examination and serum acid phosphatase measurement as screening tests for prostatic cancer.

Serum ALP is elevated in 90 per cent of patients with bone metastases (Wallach, 1978). Levels of ALP can be elevated in patients without bone metastases. Marked elevations occur with bone metastases.

Carcinoembryonic antigen (CEA) can be elevated in almost 35 per cent of all patients with proven prostatic cancer (Rosenberg and Grabstald, 1980). Other laboratory test results that can be elevated or depressed in prostatic carcinoma are given in Table 12–6.

Management. Serum acid and alkaline phosphatase measurements are good management tests for following response to therapy. Increased serum acid phosphatase shows a pronounced fall in activity within 3 to 4 days after castration or within 2 weeks after estrogen therapy has begun. It can fall to a normal level or remain slightly elevated. Failure to fall corresponds to failure of clinical response that occurs in 10 per cent of patients. A good response to castration or estrogen therapy results in a rise in ALP that peaks at approximately 3 months and then declines. Recurrence of bone metastases causes a new rise in ALP (Wallach, 1978).

Test Requests and Reports

Test Requests. The execution of laboratory tests germane to the diagnosis and management of prostatic carcinoma may be offered by the laboratory as a problem-solving service. Henry's prostatic organ panel is an example of such an approach (Fig. 12–3). He and Howanitz (1980) gave the rationale for the panel as follows:

Elevated serum acid phosphatase is a hallmark of prostatic carcinoma which has spread beyond the capsule. The effect of nonprostatic acid phosphatase is minimal by employing specific substrates now available. To increase the sensitivity of serum acid

Table 12–6. COMMON LABORATORY TEST RESULTS IN PROSTATIC CARCINOMA*

Laboratory Test	Value	Pathophysiologic Factors
Chemistry (Serum)		
Bilirubin, total	—	
Calcium, total	↑	Mild. In 10 per cent of patients with metastases to bone
Carbon dioxide	—	
Chloride	—	
Cholesterol	↑	Cause?
	↓	Cause?
Creatine phosphokinase	—	
Creatinine	↑	Related to postrenal azotemia in advanced disease
Glucose	↑	In approximtely 35 per cent of patients at initial hospitalization
Lactic dehydrogenase	↑	In approximately 25 per cent of patients at initial hospitalization; may be related to tumor mass in advanced carcinoma; isoenzyme is LDH-5
Phosphatase, alkaline	↑	In 90 per cent of patients with bone metastases; liver metastases can also cause elevation
Phosphorus, inorganic	↓	In approximately 35 per cent of patients at initial hospitalization
Potassium	—	
Proteins, total	—	
Proteins, albumin	↓	In approximtely 35 per cent of patients at initial hospitalization
Sodium	—	
Transaminase, aspartate amino	↑	In approximately 25 per cent of patients at initial hospitalization
Urea nitrogen	↑	Related to postrenal azotemia in advanced disease
Uric acid	↑	In approximately 40 per cent of patients at initial hospitalization
Hematology (Blood)		
Hemoglobin	↓	In approximately 40 per cent of patients at initial hospitalization
Hematocrit	↓	In approximately 40 per cent of patients at initial hospitalization
Leukocyte count, total	—	
Platelet count	—	

Key:
— = No change; ↑ = can be increased; ↓ = can be decreased.
*Based on information from Friedman RB, Anderson RE, Entine SM, et al: Effects of diseases on clinical laboratory tests. Clin Chem 26:1D–476D, 1980; Wallach J: Interpretation of Diagnostic Tests, ed 3 Boston, Little, Brown & Company, 1978.

PROSTATIC				
Acid Phosphatase IU/L	0–0.8			
Creatinine mg/dl	0.6–1.2			
Calcium mEq/L	4.5–5.4			
Alkaline Phosphatase IU/L	Adult 4–13			
Phosphorus mg/dl	Adult 2.0–5.2			

Figure 12–3. Prostatic organ panel. (From Henry JB, Murphy J: Effective utilization of clinical laboratories. In Henry JB (ed): Clinical Diagnosis and Management by Laboratory Methods, ed 16. Philadelphia, WB Saunders Company, 1979, p 2042.)

phosphatase in detecting prostatic cancer, we also perform an RIA. A rise in serum acid phosphatase level has been noted, however, in some cases following rectal examination. Calcium and alkaline phosphatase values are useful in evaluating the possibility of metastatic spread to bone. This screen also includes renal function determinations since there is a high incidence of renal disease associated with prostatism.

Interpretive Reports. A well-designed interpretive report can help to convey the complete information content of the test results for the prostatic carcinoma test sequence.

REFERENCES

Acute Renal Failure

Anderson RJ, Linas SL, Berns AS, et al: Nonoliguric acute renal failure. N Engl J Med 296:1134–1138, 1977.

Bradley M, Schumann GB, Ward PCJ: Examination of urine. In Henry JB (ed): Clinical Diagnosis and Management by Laboratory Methods, ed 16. Philadelphia, WB Saunders Company, 1979, pp 559–634.

Bricker NS: Acute renal failure. In Beeson PB, McDermott W, Wyngaarden JB (eds): Cecil Textbook of Medicine, ed 15. Philadelphia, WB Saunders Company, 1979, pp 1367–1375.

Contiguglia SR, Mishell JL, Klein MH: Renal and urinary tract disorders. In Friedman HH (ed): Problem-Oriented Medical Diagnosis, ed 2. Boston, Little Brown & Company, 1979, pp 214–227.

Del Greco F, Krumlovsky FA: Role of the laboratory in management of acute and chronic renal failure. Ann Clin Lab Sci 11:283–291, 1981.

Emmett M, Narins RG: Clinical use of the anion gap. Medicine 56:38–54, 1977.

Finn WF: Acute renal failure. In Earley LE, Gottschalk CW (eds): Strauss and Welt's Diseases of the Kidney,

ed 3. Boston, Little Brown & Company, 1979, pp 167–210.

Gorry GA, Kassirer JP, Essig A, et al: Decision analysis as the basis for computer-aided management of acute renal failure. Am J Med 55:473–484, 1973.

Harrington JT, Cohen JJ: Acute oliguria. N Engl J Med 292:89–91, 1975.

Henry JB, Howanitz PJ: Organ panels and the relationship of the laboratory to the physician. In Jones RJ, Palulonis RM (eds): Laboratory Tests in Medical Practice. Chicago, American Medical Association, 1980, p 33–34.

Levinsky NG: Pathophysiology of acute renal failure. N Engl J Med 296:1453–1458, 1977.

Maffly RH: Renal failure and tubular dysfunction. In Rubenstein E, Federman DD: Scientific American Medicine. New York, Scientific American, Inc, 1980, pp 10 II–1 to 10 II–43.

Miller TR, Anderson RJ, Linas SL, et al: Urinary diagnostic indices in acute renal failure: A prospective study. Ann Intern Med 99:47–50, 1978.

Najarian, JS: The diagnostic importance of the odor of urine, letter. N Engl J Med 303:1128, 1980.

Schrier RW: Acute renal failure. Kidney International 15:205–216, 1979.

Schrier RW: Acute renal failure: Pathogenesis, diagnosis, and management. Hospital Practice, March 1981, pp 93–112.

Schrier RW: Acute renal failure. JAMA 247:2518–2525, 1982.

Spivak JL, Barnes HV: Manual of Clinical Problems in Internal Medicine. Boston, Little, Brown & Company, 1978.

Prostatic Carcinoma

Batsakis JG, Briere RD: Interpretive Enzymology. Springfield, Ill, Charles C Thomas, 1967.

Catalona WJ, Scott WW: Carcinoma of the prostate: A review. J Urol 119:1–8, 1978.

Daar AS, Merrill CR, Moola SM, et al: Rectal examination and acid phosphatase: evidence for persistence of a myth. Brit Med J 282:1378–1379, 1981.

Doe RP, Seal US; Acid phosphatase in urology. Surg Clin N Amer 45:1455–1466, 1965.

Flüchter SH, Bichler KH, Hartzmann R, et al: Clinical

value of different methods for determination of acid phosphatase in prostatic cancer. Urol Int 37:79–86, 1982.

Foti AG, Cooper JF, Herschman H, et al: Detection of prostatic cancer by solid-phase radioimmunoassay of serum prostatic acid phosphatase. N Engl J Med 297:1357–1361, 1977.

Griffiths JC: Prostate-specific acid phosphatase: Re-evaluation of radioimmunoassay in diagnosing prostatic disease. Clin Chem 26:433–436, 1980.

Guinan P, Bush I, Ray V, et al: The accuracy of the rectal examination in the diagnosis of prostate carcinoma. N Engl J Med 303:499–503, 1980.

Henry JB, Howanitz PJ: Organ panels and the relationship of the laboratory to the physician. In Jones RJ, Palulonis RM (eds): Laboratory Tests in Medical Practice. Chicago, American Medical Association, 1980, p 30.

Hock E, Tessier RN: Elevation of serum acid phosphatase following prostatic massage. J Urol 62:488–491, 1949.

Johnson CD, Costa D, Castro JE: Acid phosphatase after examination of the prostate. Br J Urol 51:218–223, 1979.

Kachmar JF, Moss DW; Acid phosphatase in serum. In Tietz NW (ed): Fundamentals of Clinical Chemistry. Philadelphia, WB Saunders Company, 1976, pp 613–618.

Kendall AR: Acid phosphatase elevation following prostatic examination in the earlier diagnosis of prostatic carcinoma. J Urol 86:442–449, 1961.

Klein LA: Prostatic carcinoma. N Engl J Med 300:824–833, 1979.

Krupp MA: Carcinoma of the prostate. In Krupp MA, Chatton MJ (eds): Current Medical Diagnosis and Treatment. Los Altos, Cal, Lange Medical Publications, 1978, pp 562–563.

Murphy GP, Karr J, Chu TM: Prostatic acid phosphatase: Where are we? CA: A Cancer Journal for Clinicians 28:258–264, 1978.

Phatak PS, James N: Acid phosphatase after examination of the prostate. Ann Clin Biochem 19:195–196, 1982.

Robbins SL, Cotran RS: Carcinoma of prostate. In Robbins SL, Cotran RS (eds): Pathologic Basis of Disease. Philadelphia, WB Saunders Company, 1979, pp 1235–1240.

Rosenberg G, Grabstald H: Prostatic cancer. In Conn HF, Conn RB (eds): Current Diagnosis 6. Philadelphia, WB Saunders Company, 1980, pp 831–836.

Roy AV, Brower ME, Hayden JE: Sodium thymolphthalein monophosphate: A new acid phosphatase substrate with greater specificity for the prostatic enzyme in serum. Clin Chem 17:1093–1102, 1971.

Wallach JW: Interpretation of Diagnostic Tests ed 3. Boston, Little, Brown & Company, 1978, p 452.

CHAPTER 13

GASTROINTESTINAL SUBPROBLEMS

GASTRIC AND DUODENAL DISEASE

GASTRIC ANALYSIS AND ACID-PEPTIC DISEASE OF STOMACH AND DUODENUM

Definition and Significance

Acid-peptic disease of the stomach and duodenum consists of disorders of the gastrointestinal tract in which gastric analysis provides useful diagnostic and management information. These disorders include (Beeler, 1978):

1. Peptic ulcer.
2. Gastric carcinoma.
3. Pernicious anemia.
4. The Zollinger-Ellison syndrome.

Gastric analysis also provides determination of the completeness of surgical vagotomy.

Additional reasons for laboratory study of gastric contents include cytologic examination for carcinoma, diagnosis of pulmonary tuberculosis, and identification of the toxic agent in a patient with an overdose of drugs or poisons. These latter three reasons are not discussed in this chapter.

Peptic ulcer is said to affect as many as 10 per cent of the population at one time or another. This condition causes significant morbidity as a result of pain and discomfort, which can seriously affect a patient's enjoyment of life and perhaps even the ability to work. Complications such as obstruction, perforation, and hemorrhage can result in severe disease and even death. The incidence of peptic ulcer may be decreasing (Grossman et al., 1981).

Gastric carcinoma is one of the most common lethal malignancies. In the United States, it causes about 15,000 deaths each year. Less than 10 per cent of patients survive 5 years.

Any chance of survival depends on early diagnosis.

Pernicious anemia is a disease caused by vitamin B_{12} deficiency secondary to a lack of intrinsic factor associated with gastric atrophy. Its manifestations include macrocytic anemia and demyelination of nerves, typically involving the posterior and lateral columns of the spinal cord. Untreated pernicious anemia causes serious disability and even death. The prevalence of pernicious anemia at age 40 is 0.02 per cent and between the age of 50 and 60, 0.5 per cent.

The Zollinger-Ellison syndrome is characterized by ulceration of the upper gastrointestinal tract, marked increase of gastric acid secretion, and non-beta islet-cell tumors of the pancreas that secrete gastrin. Occasionally, the site of excess gastrin secretion can be extrapancreatic, such as the stomach or duodenum. It is estimated that excess gastrin secretion may account for 0.1 to 1 per cent of peptic ulcers. The Zollinger-Ellison syndrome is a debilitating disease. Moreover, the majority of pancreatic gastrinomas are malignant.

Pathophysiology

Stimuli to gastric secretion occur in three phases (Cannon, 1979):
1. *Cephalic or neurogenic phase*: Mediated through the vagus nerves.
2. *Gastric phase*: Mediated by gastrin secreted by the gastric antrum.
3. *Intestinal phase*: Mediated by humoral substances secreted by the duodenum.
Beeler (1978) has provided the following information regarding pathophysiology and the completeness of surgical vagotomy.

Peptic ulcers are sharply "punched-out" chronic ulcerations usually located in the stomach and duodenum. They are causally related to injury of the mucosa secondary to gastric secretions containing hydrochloric acid and proteolytic enzymes. Peptic ulcer disease is a heterogeneous group of diseases with multiple genetic and environmental causes (Grossman et al., 1981). Patients with gastric ulcers can secrete normal or reduced acid and volume of gastric juice. Patients with duodenal ulcers are generally hypersecretors of acid and volume. Anacidity after stimulation rarely occurs with a benign peptic ulcer.

Measuring gastric secretion for the purpose of diagnosing *gastric carcinoma* is considered less helpful than it has been in the past. Most patients with gastric cancer secrete some acid, and only 20 per cent of patients with gastric carcinoma have stimulant-fast anacidity.

Inadequate gastric secretion of intrinsic factor is found in *pernicious anemia* and is associated with gastric atrophy with stimulant-fast anacidity. Anacidity is present in 15 per cent of people between 40 and 60 years of age and in 25 per cent of those between 60 and 70.

Patients with the *Zollinger-Ellison syndrome* usually have very high secretions of acid and volume of gastric juice associated with high levels of serum gastrin. (See the discussion of the Zollinger-Ellison syndrome later in this chapter.)

Since hypoglycemic stimulation of gastric acid secretion is mediated through intact vagus nerves, the completeness of *surgical vagotomy* may be evaluated by measuring the stimulant effect of parenteral insulin on gastric acid secretion.

Clinical Contexts

Diagnosis. Peptic ulcer disease has the following clinical features: sharply localized epigastric pain, nausea, excessive salivation, and relief of pain by food or antacids. Anorexia and spontaneous vomiting are more commonly associated with gastric ulcer (Walsh, 1979).

Many diseases can produce epigastric pain. The list includes other diseases of the stomach, liver, gallbladder, and pancreas as well as diseases of intrathoracic structures such as pleuritis or myocardial infarction.

Gastric carcinoma often has no distinctive clinical features, especially in early cases.

The presentation of pernicious anemia can relate more to the symptoms and signs of anemia and demyelination of the posterior and lateral tracts of the spinal cord than to gastrointestinal findings.

The Zollinger-Ellison syndrome is an uncommon variant of peptic ulcer disease (discussed later in this chapter).

Management. The only management indication for gastric analysis in acid-peptic disease of the stomach and duodenum is to determine the completeness of surgical vagotomy.

Screening. Since 80 per cent of individuals with gastric carcinoma have some free acid, stimulant-fast anacidity is not a reliable screening test for gastric cancer (Beeler, 1978). However, except for the few patients with juvenile pernicious anemia who have free acid but lack intrinsic factor, the absence of stimulant-fast anacidity will effectively exclude the diagnosis of pernicious anemia.

Strategy

Test Sequence. Gastric analysis is time consuming for the physician who performs the intubation and supervises the procedure. In addition, it is an unpleasant experience for the patient. Therefore, gastric analysis should be performed only for clear-cut indications that involve acid-peptic disease of the stomach and duodenum (Beeler, 1978; Cannon, 1979):

1. To document anacidity for the diagnosis of pernicious anemia or gastric carcinoma.

2. To measure acid output when peptic ulcer is suspected.

3. To document the hypersecretory state of the Zollinger-Ellison syndrome.

4. To determine the completeness of surgical vagotomy by the insulin test.

Other reasons for study of gastric contents, e.g., cytologic examination, diagnosis of tuberculosis, and identification of drugs and poisons, are excluded from this discussion.

Patient Preparation. The patient must be properly prepared for gastric analysis (Cannon, 1979); (Malagelada et al., 1982). Minimum requirements include an overnight fast of 12 hours and withdrawal of medications that influence gastric secretion, such as antacids, anticholinergic drugs, reserpine, alcohol, adrenergic blocking agents, and adrenocorticosteroids. The patient must also be free of the sight or odor of food and must not be subjected to stimuli that produce strong emotional reactions.

After intubation, the residual volume of gastric secretion is collected. Gastric secretion is collected for 2 hours. The first hour represents basal gastric secretion. The second hour represents stimulated gastric secretion and is collected after the administration of histamine, pentagastrin, or betazole (Histalog).

The insulin-hypoglycemia test is performed by collecting gastric secretion for 2 hours before and after administering insulin. Hypoglycemia (serum glucose less than 50 mg/100 ml) must be documented.

Specimen Collection and Handling. Specimens should be collected in chemically clean tubes and analyzed immediately.

Methodology. Consult the laboratory for its methodology. A good discussion of methodology is available by Cannon (1979) and Malagelada et al. (1982). The volume in milliliters, titratable acidity in mEq/liter, and pH are measured on the residual gastric secretion, the basal gastric secretion, and the stimulated gastric secretion. Maximal acid output refers to the acid output in mEq/hour that occurs in the second poststimulant hour. Older terms, such as "free acid," "combined acid," and "total acid" as well as "maximal histamine response," "peak acid output," "achlorhydria," and "hypochlorhydria," are confusing and best avoided.

Anacidity is defined as the failure of the pH to fall below 6.0 rather than 3.5. With this definition, virtually all adult patients with pernicious anemia will demonstrate anacidity. (Cannon, 1979; Wallach, 1978).

Interpretation

Diagnosis. Table 13–1 lists decision levels for gastric analysis results in health and disease. As shown, data concerning acid output are not sufficient to make a firm diagnosis. The following correlations are generally accepted:

1. High acid output is compatible with duo-

Table 13–1. DECISION LEVELS FOR GASTRIC ANALYSIS RESULTS*

1 hour basal acid	
< 2 mEq	Normal, gastric ulcer, or carcinoma
2–5 mEq	Normal, gastric or duodenal ulcer
> 5 mEq	Duodenal ulcer
> 20 mEq	Zollinger-Ellison syndrome

1 hour after stimulation (histamine or betazole hydrochloride)	
0 mEq	Anacidity, gastritis, gastric carcinoma
1–20 mEq	Normal, gastric ulcer, or carcinoma
20–35 mEq	Duodenal ulcer
35–60 mEq	Duodenal ulcer, high normal, Zollinger-Ellison syndrome
> 60 mEq	Zollinger-Ellison syndrome

Ratio of basal acid to poststimulation outputs	
20%	Normal, gastric ulcer, or carcinoma
20–40%	Gastric or duodenal ulcer
40–60%	Duodenal ulcer, Zollinger-Ellison syndrome
> 60%	Zollinger-Ellison syndrome

*Adapted from Wallach J: Interpretation of Diagnostic Tests: A Handbook Synopsis of Laboratory Medicine, 3rd ed. Boston, Little, Brown & Company, 1978, p 143.

denal and prepyloric ulcer or Zollinger-Ellison syndrome.

2. Stimulant-fast anacidity is compatible with pernicious anemia and gastric carcinoma.

3. High ratio of basal acid output to maximum acid output (>40 per cent or basal acid secretion >10 mEq/hr) is compatible with the Zollinger-Ellison syndrome.

See Table 13–2 for common laboratory test results in acid-peptic disease of the stomach and duodenum.

Management. The patient may be considered to be completely vagotomized if the acid output after insulin administration is less than the acid output before insulin. The insulin test is valid only if the serum glucose falls below 50 mg/100 ml at some point in the test, which

will usually be 30 minutes after insulin administration. Furthermore, the test is valid only if the stomach has been shown capable of secreting hydrochloric acid. Incomplete vagotomy is suggested if:

1. The acid output in the 2-hour postinsulin period exceeds that of the 2-hour basal period by more than 0.5 mEq.

2. The acid output is greater than 2 mEq in either basal hour (Cannon, 1979).

Test Requests and Reports

Test Requests. The performance of gastric analysis can be offered by the laboratory as a problem-solving service. The upper portion of the form in Figure 13–1 shows a request for

Table 13–2. COMMON LABORATORY TEST RESULTS IN PEPTIC ULCER, SITE UNSPECIFIED*

Laboratory Test	Value	Pathophysiologic Factors
Chemistry (Serum)		
Bilirubin, total	—	
Calcium, total	↑	Can increase secondary to excessive intake of milk and alkali. Peptic ulcer common in hyperparathyroidism; can also increase with vomiting and dehydration
Carbon dioxide	↑	Reciprocal increase of bicarbonate in response to low chloride
Chloride	↓	Related to vomiting of acid-rich gastric contents; occurs especially with pyloric obstruction
Cholesterol	—	
Creatine phosphokinase	—	
Creatinine	—	
Glucose	↓	A high frequency of spontaneous hypoglycemia
Lactic dehydrogenase	—	
Phosphatase, alkaline	↑	Caused by entry of alkaline phosphatase of the intestinal type into the bloodstream
Phosphorus, inorganic	—	
Potassium	↓	Related to amount of vomiting
Proteins, total	↑	Related to vomiting and dehydation
Proteins, albumin	↑	Related to vomiting and dehydration
Sodium	↓	Related to amount of vomiting
Transaminase, aspartate amino	—	
Urea nitrogen	↑	Related to hemorrhage into the gastrointestinal tract with absorption of protein converted to urea nitrogen by intestinal bacteria
Uric acid	—	
Hematology (Blood)		
Hemoglobin	↓	Related to blood loss
Hematocrit	↓	Related to blood loss
Leukocyte count, total	↑	Increased with shift to left related to perforation, massive hemorrhage, and toxic or infectious complications; erythrocyte sedimentation rate and acute-phase reactants can also increase
Platlet count	—	

Key:
— = No change; ↑ = can be increased; ↓ = can be decreased.
*Based on information from Friedman RB, Anderson RE, Entine SM, et al: Effects of disease on clinical laboratory tests. Clin Chem 26:1D–476D, 1980; Wolf PL: Interpretation of Biochemical Multitest Profiles: An Analysis of 100 Important Conditions. New York, Masson Publishing, Inc. 1977.

BRISTOL HOSPITAL LABORATORY

BH 340 7/77

Date   Location   Doctor

Pt. Identification   Clinical Impression:

X-Ray:

Active Bleeding? _____
Obstruction? _____
Medications? _____

Prior Surgery? _____

Repeat Gastric Analysis? _____

Baseline Values

Time	Volume	Blood	Bile	pH	Titratable Acidity	Acid Output
Fasting Residual	ml				mEq/L	mEq
15min					mEq/L	mEq
30min					mEq/L	mEq
45min					mEq/L	mEq
60min					mEq/L	mEq

Add 15, 30, 45 & 60 min. = Basal Acid Output = _____ mEq/hr.

Post Histologue Stimulation   1.5 mg sub-cut per Kg

Time	Volume	Blood	Bile	pH	Titratable Acidity	Acid Output
30min					mEq/L	mEq
60 min					mEq/L	mEq
90 min					mEq/L	mEq
120min					mEq/L	mEq

Maximal Output

Add Output for greatest hour interval _____ mmEq/L

Achlorhydria — Anacidity
pH > 6 No change
with stimulation.

Zollinger — Ellison Syndrome
High basal acid output
Ratio of basal to maximal
output over 60%.

INTERPRETATION

CONDITION	SEX	NUMBER OF PATIENTS	ACID OUTPUT (mEq. hour) Basal	Maximal
Controls	Male	35	4.2	22.6
	Female	26	1.8	15.2
Medical students	Male	145	5.3	26.7
	Female	16	3.3	21.4
Duodenal ulcer	Male	256	7.1	35.2
	Female	64	4.2	25.7
Gastric ulcer	Male	117	2.9	19.6
	Female	43	1.6	13.1
Gastric carcinoma	Male	74	1.5	6.7
	Female	32	0.7	3.0
Jejunal ulcer	Male	10	7.9	25.1
	Female	4	5.5	16.4

Tech _____ and _____ Date

GASTRIC ANALYSIS

Figure 13–1. Request and report form for gastric analysis. (Courtesy of L. S. Kish, M.D., Bristol, Connecticut.)

gastric analysis where the attending physician can enter a clinical impression and other important information.

Interpretive Reports. Figure 13–1 shows this same form serving as an interpretive report. The form contains not only test results but also reference intervals and decision levels. There is a place for an interpretive comment.

ZOLLINGER-ELLISON SYNDROME

Definition and Significance

The Zollinger-Ellison (1955) syndrome consists of peptic ulceration that is intractable to medical treatment, gastric hypersecretion, and diarrhea caused by gastrin-secreting pancreatic non-beta islet-cell lesions. The ulcers usually occur in the stomach and duodenum, and only 25 per cent occur in atypical locations for peptic ulcers not belonging to the Zollinger-Ellison syndrome, such as the jejunum. Approximately 60 per cent of the islet-cell lesions are malignant and 40 per cent are benign. Among the benign lesions, 30 per cent are adenomas and 10 per cent are hyperplasias. Occasionally, the gastrin-secreting lesion is located in an extrapancreatic site such as the duodenum.

The lesions of the Zollinger-Ellison syndrome can be part of a hereditary multiple-endocrine neoplasia (MEN) syndrome with tumors of the parathyroid glands, pituitary, and adrenal gland as well as of the pancreas (Table 13–3). See Chapter 9 for a discussion of hypercalcemia and hyperparathyroidism and Chapter 16 for disorders of the adrenal gland.

Pathophysiology

Secretion of gastrin by the gastric antrum is stimulated by the vagus nerves during the cephalic phase of gastric secretion, by increased gastric pH, by antral distention, and by the presence of food and its digested products in the stomach. Emptying of the stomach and decreased gastric pH inhibit secretion of gastrin. There is still some doubt whether the delta cell of the pancreatic islets is clearly the source of gastrin and the origin of gastrinoma (Robbins and Cotran, 1979).

Clinical Contexts

Diagnosis. The clinical features of the Zollinger-Ellison syndrome are peptic ulceration refractory to medical treatment, recurrence of ulcer after an ulcer operation, gastric hypersecretion, and diarrhea. The syndrome occurs in all age groups but is diagnosed most often between the third and fifth decades. The number of patients with peptic ulcer who have the Zollinger-Ellison syndrome is unknown but is probably less than 1 per cent (Walsh, 1979). (See the discussion of gastric analysis earlier in this chapter.)

Management. Once diagnosed, the condition is usually treated by total gastrectomy. Laboratory studies may be used to document the recurrence of neoplastic tissue by demonstrating a rise in the serum gastrin level. Cimetidine can provide control in most patients with gastrinoma and its therapeutic role is under debate (Clain, 1982).

Screening. Laboratory studies are not used to screen for the Zollinger-Ellison syndrome in the absence of clinical features suggestive of the disease. When these features are present, a serum gastrin level of 100 pg/ml or more would separate nearly all patients with the syndrome from most nongastrinoma subjects (Ippoliti, 1977).

Strategy

Test Sequence. Serum gastrin should be measured when the clinical features of the syndrome are present and in any of the following situations (Wallach, 1978):

1. Basal acid secretion >10 mEq/hr in patients with intact stomachs.

2. Ratio of basal to poststimulation gastric acid output >40 per cent in patients with intact stomachs.

3. All patients with recurrent ulceration after surgery for duodenal ulcer.

4. All patients with duodenal ulcer for whom elective gastric surgery is planned.

Table 13–3. MULTIPLE ENDOCRINE NEOPLASIA (MEN) SYNDROMES*

Lesions	MEN I	MEN IIa	MEN IIb
Pituitary	+ + + +	0	0
Medullary carcinoma of thyroid	+	+ + + +	+ + + +
Parathyroid	+ + + +	+ +	+
Adrenal cortex	+ + + +	+	+
Pheochromocytoma	0	+ + + +	+ + + +
Pancreas	+ + + +	0	0
Peptic ulcer	+ + + +	0	0
Mucocutaneous neuromas	0	0	+ + + +

*From Robbins SL, Cotran RS: Pathologic Basis of Disease. Philadelphia, WB Saunders Company 1979, p 1112.

When basal serum gastrin levels are elevated, a secretin stimulation test should be performed. A calcium stimulation test may also be used. Secretin appears to have these advantages over calcium (Deveney et al., 1977):

1. Secretin has no demonstrated harmful side effects; calcium is potentially dangerous to the cardiovascular system.

2. The secretin test can be done in 15 to 30 minutes; 3 to 4 hours are required with calcium.

3. The separation of those with and those without gastrinoma is more clear-cut with secretin than with calcium.

4. Fewer false negatives are likely with secretin.

Measurement of gastric acid secretion did not add any diagnostic advantage to the estimation of fasting serum gastrin alone (Malagelada et al., 1982a).

Patient Preparation. The secretin stimulation test is performed by giving secretin, 2 U/kg body weight, as an intravenous bolus injection. Blood for serum gastrin levels is drawn before injection and at 2, 5, 10, 15, 30, and 60 minutes afterward. The best source of natural secretin has been the Gastrointestinal Hormone Resources, Karolinska Institute, Stockholm, Sweden (Deveney et al., 1977; Malagelada et al., 1982b).

Specimen Collection and Handling. Blood samples for gastrin levels are collected in tubes containing no preservatives (heparin will interfere). Plasma is unsuitable for analysis. Serum specimens must be frozen immediately to prevent destruction of gastrin by proteolytic enzymes.

Methodology. Serum gastrin is measured by radioimmunoassay (RIA) (McGuigan and Trudeau, 1968). Consult the laboratory for its methodology, accuracy and precision, reference intervals, decision levels, and potential sources of interference.

Interpretation

Diagnosis. A basal serum gastrin concentration greater than 500 pg/ml in a patient who secretes excess gastric acid and is not in renal failure is highly suggestive for gastrinoma. Basal serum gastrin levels above 100 pg/ml but below 500 pg/ml are compatible with gastrinoma. About 40 per cent of patients with the Zollinger-Ellison syndrome will have a fasting serum gastrin concentration of 100 to 500

Table 13–4. NON-TUMOROUS CAUSES OF HYPERGASTRINEMIA*

Pernicious anemia
Chronic gastritis (atrophic)
Massive small intestinal resection (short bowel syndrome)
Syndrome of retained gastric antrum (hyperchlorhydria)
Antral G-cell hyperplasia (hyperchlorhydria)
Renal failure

*From Gottlieb AJ, Zamkoff KW, Jastremski MS, et al (eds): The Whole Internist Catalog. A Compendium of Clues to Diagnosis and Management. Philadelphia, WB Saunders Company, 1980, p 277.

pg/ml, whereas about 10 per cent of peptic ulcer patients without evidence of gastrinoma have a fasting gastrin concentration in that range (Ippoliti, 1977). These decision levels can differ for various RIAs performed in different laboratories (Malagelada et al., 1982a). Other causes of hypergastrinemia are given in Table 13–4. A basal serum gastrin level greater than 1000 pg/ml in the presence of gastric acid secretion does not require a secretin test for confirmation of gastrinoma, for other causes of hypergastrinemia do not produce these levels (Clain, 1982).

An increase in serum gastrin of greater than 110 pg/ml over the basal level after secretin stimulation and of 395 pg/ml after calcium stimulation is diagnostic of gastrinoma. Although patients with pernicious anemia can have high basal serum gastrin levels and elevated gastrin levels after stimulation with calcium, their secretin stimulation tests are always negative (Table 13–5). Using these criteria, there were no false-positive tests with either calcium or secretin among 65 patients. False-negative results may occasionally be seen with either secretin or calcium stimulation, but less often with secretin. False-negative results with secretin occur with a frequency of about 5 per cent (Deveney et al., 1977). False-positive responses to secretin have not been reported (Ippoliti, 1977).

McGuigan and Wolfe (1980) used an increase of 200 pg/ml as their decision level in the secretin stimulation test. Malagelada and associates (1982b) reported that the peak gastrin level after secretin (500 pg/ml), in contrast to an absolute increase over the basal serum gastrin level, proved to be the best indicator of a positive response (100 per cent sensitive and 100 per cent specific in their series). Early cases are more likely to give false-negative results, and on follow-up, false-negative results

Table 13–5. FASTING AND STIMULATED SERUM GASTRIN LEVELS IN VARIOUS STATES*

State	Fasting Gastrin Level	Gastrin Level Following Challenge		
		Calcium	*Secretin*	*Test Meal*
Normal	Normal	Normal	Normal	Elevated
Zollinger-Ellison syndrome	Markedly elevated	Elevated	Elevated	Normal or elevated
Duodenal ulcer	Normal	Normal	Normal	Markedly elevated
Pernicious anemia	Elevated	Elevated	Normal	Elevated

*From Broussard LA, Frings CS: Interpretation of serum gastrin levels (clinical forum). Laboratory Management 21:21, 1979.

can convert to positive results. Reference intervals and decision levels for the secretin and calcium stimulation tests can vary for different laboratories. The results of common laboratory tests in the Zollinger-Ellison syndrome are given in Table 13–6.

Management. If a gastrinoma is totally re-

sected by surgery, basal serum gastrin levels should drop to baseline values. The patient may then be followed with serum gastrin measurements. If the serum gastrin concentration rises above baseline, it is indicative of recurrent tumor.

Stabile and associates (1980) reported that

Table 13–6. COMMON LABORATORY TEST RESULTS IN THE ZOLLINGER-ELLISON SYNDROME*

Laboratory Test	Value†	Pathophysiologic Factors
Chemistry (Serum)		
Bilirubin, total	—	
Calcium, total	↑	Multiple endocrine neoplasia (MEN) with hyperparathyroidism
	↓	Related to deficiency of vitamin D with calcium malabsorption
Carbon dioxide	—	
Chloride	—	
Cholesterol	—	
Creatine phosphokinase	—	
Creatinine	—	
Glucose	↑	MEN with pheochromocytoma
Lactic dehydrogenase	—	
Phosphatase, alkaline	↑	An indication of vitamin D deficiency with calcium malabsorption
Phosphorus, inorganic	↓	An indication of vitamin D deficiency with calcium malabsorption
Potassium	↓	Related to severe diarrhea
Proteins, total	—	
Proteins, albumin	↓	Related to malabsorption
Sodium	—	
Transaminase, aspartate amino	—	
Urea nitrogen	—	
Uric acid	—	
Hematology (Blood)		
Hemoglobin	—	
Hematocrit	—	
Leukocyte count, total	—	
Platelet count	—	

Key:
— = No change; ↑ = can be increased; ↓ = can be decreased.
*Based on information from Friedman RB, Anderson RE, Entine SM, et al: Effects of disease on clinical laboratory tests. Clin Chem 26:1D–476D, 1980; Carbone JV, Brandborg LL, Silverman S Jr.: Zollinger-Ellison syndrome. In Krupp MA, Chatton MJ (eds): Current Medical Diagnosis 1978. Los Altos, Cal, Lange Medical Publications, 1978, pp 358–359.
†These test results can occur in addition to the ones noted for peptic ulcer (see Table 13–2).

basal serum gastrin levels greater than 1500 pg/ml were found only in patients with metastases to lymph nodes or liver, whereas levels greater than 8000 pg/ml indicated massive liver replacement by tumor. Basal serum levels of alpha-subunit human chorionic gonadotropin (alpha-hCG) were elevated (>7 ng/ml) in four of 20 patients with metastatic gastrinoma and low in all 16 patients with benign disease. The results suggest that serum gastrin and alpha-hCG levels may be useful in assessing the biologic behavior of gastrinomas and in planning appropriate surgical and non-surgical treatment. hCG and its subunits have been shown to be sensitive and specific markers for islet-cell carcinoma (Kahn et al., 1977).

Test Requests and Reports

Test Requests. The laboratory can offer a problem-solving service for the diagnosis of the Zollinger-Ellison syndrome. This may be ordered and executed when the physician believes it is indicated.

Interpretive Reports. The results of the tests may be returned to the ordering physician in the form of an interpretive report. Figure 13–2 is an example of a graphic report for secretin and calcium stimulation tests in a patient with the Zollinger-Ellison syndrome.

INTESTINAL DISEASE

MALABSORPTION

Definition and Significance

Malabsorption is a term used to indicate defective absorption of nutrients by the small intestine. These nutrients include fats, proteins, carbohydrates, vitamins, and minerals, individually or in combination. The defective absorption may be due to intestinal, biliary, or pancreatic disease. In biliary or pancreatic disease, the intestine may be normal and the disorder is more appropriately called *maldigestion*. When the defective absorption is due to intestinal disease, the disorder is sometimes referred to as *malassimilation* (Beeler, 1978).

If malabsorption is present, another subproblem, etiology of malabsorption must be solved, except for distinguishing among intestinal, biliary and pancreatic causes, etiology of malabsorption will not be addressed in detail in the following discussion.

Pathophysiology

Impaired digestion and absorption of fats, proteins, carbohydrates, vitamins, minerals, and water are caused by a wide variety of

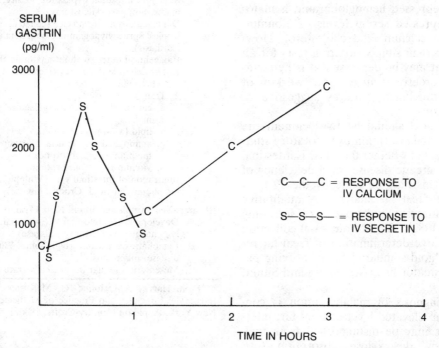

Figure 13–2. Secretin and calcium stimulation tests in a patient with the Zollinger-Ellison syndrome.

pathophysiologic derangements, which are categorized in Table 13–7.

Clinical Contexts

Diagnosis. The clinical features of malabsorption and maldigestion include weight loss, anorexia, abdominal distention, borborygmus, muscle wasting, and abnormal yellow to gray, greasy, soft stools that may be increased in number. These stools are difficult to flush (Gray, 1982). In addition, edema, ascites, skeletal disorders, peripheral and circumoral paresthesias, tetany, and, rarely, convulsions may be observed (Glickman, 1982).

Intestinal deficiencies of lactase or sucrase lead to distention, slight nausea, and frothy diarrhea 30 minutes to 2 hours after ingesting the offending carbohydrate.

Management. The degree of severity of each deficiency as well as response to therapy can be followed by laboratory studies.

Screening. Screening for malabsorption by laboratory studies in the absence of clinical features is not indicated.

Strategy

Test Sequence. A large number of laboratory test results can be outside the reference intervals in the malabsorption syndrome, for example, depressed hemoglobin and hematocrit and depressed serum levels of albumin, vitamin B_{12}, calcium, and cholesterol. However, rather than simply ordering tests for all analytes that may be depressed, it is better to pursue an orderly strategy for a workup of patients with clinical features suggestive of malabsorption.

The first goal should be to document the presence of malabsorption by laboratory studies, regardless of whether the cause is intestinal disease, pancreatic disease, or a deficiency of bile salts. This may be done by the 72-hour quantitative fecal fat analysis. A qualitative fecal fat analalysis may be used as a screening test (Gray, 1982). The 72-hour stool collection for quantitative determination of fecal fat remains the "gold standard" for identifying patients with steatorrhea (Rosenberg and Sitnin, 1981).

If the diagnosis of malabsorption is confirmed by an elevated level of fecal fat, intestinal causes may be distinguished from maldigestion by the xylose absorption test.

Table 13–7. PATHOPHYSIOLOGIC CLASSIFICATION OF MALABSORPTION*

I. Failure of Digestion (Intraluminal Phase)
  A. Decreased pancreatic enzymes
    1. Pancreatic insufficiency (pancreatitis, cystic fibrosis, protein deficiency, and pancreatic cancer)
    2. Inactivation of pancreatic enzymes by gastric hypersecretion (Zollinger-Ellison syndrome and ileal resection)
    3. Failure to convert proenzyme to active form (enterokinase and trypsinogen deficiencies)
  B. Impaired bile acid micelle formation
    1. Impaired bile acid synthesis (severe hepatocellular disease)
    2. Interrupted enterohepatic circulation (ileal resection, bile duct obstruction, or biliary cirrhosis)
    3. Bile acid deconjugation (bacterial overgrowth)
      a. stasis due to motor abnormality (scleroderma, intestinal pseudo-obstruction, diabetic visceral neuropathy)
      b. stasis due to anatomic abnormalities (multiple diverticula, strictures, and blind loops including long afferent loop of a gastrojejunostomy)
      c. small bowel contamination (gastrocolic and jejunocolic fistula)
  C. Inadequate mixing of food, bile, and pancreatic enzymes (gastrojejunostomy)

II. Failure of Absorption (Mucosal Phase)
  A. Inadequate absorptive surface (intestinal resection, intestinal bypass for obesity, inadvertent gastro-ileostomy)
  B. Damaged absorbing surface (celiac disease, tropical sprue, hypogammaglobulinemia, giardiasis)
  C. Biochemical defect without anatomic alteration
    1. Disaccharide deficiency (lactase and sucrase deficiency)
    2. Transport deficiency
      a. carbohydrate (glucose-galactose malabsorption)
      b. lipid (a-β-lipoproteinemia)
      c. amino acids (cystinuria, Hartnup's disease, methionine malabsorption)
      d. vitamin B_{12} malabsorption
  D. Infiltration of intestinal wall (Whipple's disease, lymphoma, amyloid, Crohn's disease)

III. Impaired Lymph and Blood Flow (Transit Phase)
  A. Developmental abnormality (intestinal lymphangiectasia, Milroy's disease)
  B. Lymphatic obstruction (lymphoma, Whipple's disease, tuberculosis)
  C. Mesenteric vascular insufficiency (rare if ever)

*From Harvey AM, Johns RJ, McKusick VA, et al (eds): The Principles and Practice of Medicine, 20th ed. New York, Appleton-Century-Crofts, 1980, p 681.

Physiologic absorption of xylose excludes intestinal disease and suggests maldigestion. Defective absorption of xylose suggests intestinal disease or a combination of intestinal disease and maldigestion.

Studies to determine the specific etiology of intestinal disease include roentgenograms and biopsy of the small intestine. Studies to determine the specific etiology of maldigestion include the secretin test for the pancreas (see Chapter 14) and liver function tests and the bile salt breath test for bile salt deficiency syndromes (see Chapter 15).

The sequence of decisions and requests for these tests is given in Figure 13–3. Several popular absorptive tests (serum carotene, vitamin A absorption, and ^{131}I-triglyceride) may be done. However, they are not very sensitive or specific.

Patient Preparation. The procedures are as follows (Gray, 1982; Spivak and Barnes, 1978):

1. *Quantitative fecal fat analysis*: The patient should ingest 60 to 100 gm of fat per day and collect stool for 72 hours. The following conditions are important:
   a. Give the patient a 60- to 100-gm fat diet for 3 to 5 days prior to and during the 72-hour collection period.
   b. Bowel movements should occur daily.
   c. Stool collection should be complete.
   d. Ingestion of castor, mineral, and nut oils should be eliminated and suppositories should not be used.
   Microscopic examination of a homogenized stool specimen using Sudan 3 as the fat stain or determination of fecal dry weight per 24 hours can be successful as screening tests for increased fecal fat excretion (Gambino, 1981).
2. *Xylose absorption test*: The patient ingests 25 gm of xylose and collects urine for the next 5 hours. It is important that the patient ingest approximately 500 ml of water during the first 3 hours of the collection period to ensure adequate urinary filtration of the xylose.
3. *Small intestine roentgenogram*: No special preparation is needed.
4. *Small intestine biopsy*: No special preparation is needed.
5. *Secretin test*: See the discussion of chronic pancreatitis in Chapter 14.
6. *Bile salt breath test*: No special preparation is needed.

Specimen Collection and Handling. Specimens for fecal fat may be collected in individual glass or plastic containers or in one large tarred container (clean paint cans work well). Wax-coated containers should not be used. During the collection period, the fecal specimens should be refrigerated. Contamination of feces with urine should be avoided. Any obvious foreign matter should be removed before proceeding with the analysis.

If serum carotene and vitamin A are measured, a fasting blood sample should be used. The serum should be protected from hemolysis and light and analyzed immediately or promptly frozen at −10°C, at which temperature vitamin A is stable for at least 2 weeks.

Methodology. Both gravimetric and titrimetric methods provide reliable measurements of quantitative fecal fat. Sudan 3 is satisfactory for staining neutral fat for the qualitative fecal fat test. Simko (1981) described acceptable screening tests for increased fecal excretion using either staining with Sudan 3 or dry weight of stool. The key to successful use of the Sudan 3 staining method is to convert the soaps in the stool to free fatty acids using heat and acetic acid. Soaps do not take up the Sudan dye, whereas free fatty acids do.

Consult the laboratory for its methodologies, accuracy and precision, reference intervals, and potential sources of interference.

Interpretation

Diagnosis. Malabsorption is present if the patient excretes over 6 gm of fat per day. Brooks (1972) reported that the presence of greater than three globules of neutral fat per microscopic high-power field or presence of fat globules greater than 75 microns in diameter is compatible with the malabsorption syndrome. Table 13–8 gives Simko's (1981) data for interpreting fecal fat studies. Reference intervals for serum carotenes are 40 to 200 μg/100 ml; for serum vitamin A, 15 to 60 μg/100 ml. Low serum levels for these two analytes are compatible with the malabsorption syndrome. If malabsorption is present, it may be due to either a disease of the intestine itself or secondary to biliary or pancreatic disease. Remember that fecal fat excretion is normal in disaccharidase (lactase and sucrase) deficiency.

If the xylose absorption test shows low serum or urine levels (less than 25 mg/100 ml

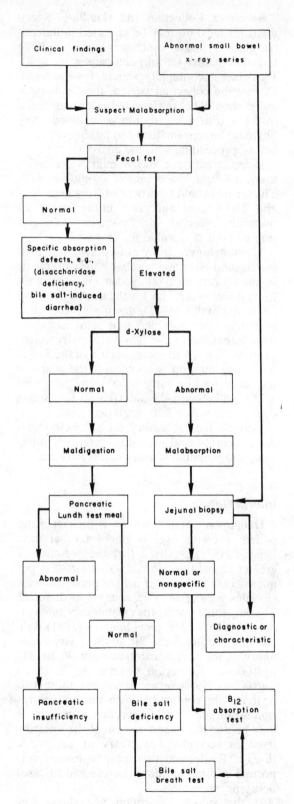

Figure 13–3. Sequence for evaluating malabsorption. (Adapted from Harvey AM, Johns RJ, McKusick, VA, et al (eds): The Principles and Practice of Medicine, 20th ed, 1980, p. 683. Courtesy of Appleton-Century-Crofts, Publishing Division of Prentice-Hall, Inc, Englewood Cliffs, NJ).

Table 13–8. FECAL FAT DATA IN PATIENTS WHO EXCRETE MORE OR LESS THAN 6 GRAMS IN 24 HOURS*

Test	Normal Excreters (< 6 gm/24 hr)	Abnormal Excreters (> 6 gm/24 hr)	p
Fecal fat (gm/24 hr)	1.9 ± 0.4 S.E.	17.4 ± 2.6 S.E.	< 0.001
Number of fat droplets (per hpf†)	2.5 ± 0.8	26.6 ± 4.0	< 0.001
Wet weight of stool (gm/24 hr)	186.0 ± 34.0	297.0 ± 44.0	< 0.01
Dry weight of stool (gm/24 hr)	20.5 ± 4.6	45.2 ± 4.2	< 0.001

*From Gambino R (ed): Fecal fat: Lab Report for Physicians. 3:58 1981; Simko, V: Fecal fat microscopy; Am J Gastroenterol 75:206, 1981.
†Per high-power field.

elevation of the serum level 1 to 2 hours after ingestion of 25 gm of xylose or less than 6 gm of xylose in the urine within 5 hours after ingestion of 25 gm of xylose), intestinal disease alone or in combination with maldigestion is present. If the xylose absorption test shows greater than 25 mg/100 ml elevation of the serum level or greater than 6 gm of xylose in the urine within five hours, the intestine is normal and maldigestion is present. False-positive xylose absorption tests occasionally occur in the following situations (Gray, 1982):

1. Decreased renal function in patients over 60 years of age or patient of any age with renal disease.

2. Patients with increased extracellular fluid, particularly with ascites or massive edema.

In patients with decreased renal function, only serum levels should be used in the interpretation of xylose absorption.

Table 13–9 lists some diseases of the small intestine that can cause malabsorption (Perera et al., 1975).

If xylose absorption is normal, consider chronic pancreatitis with exocrine deficiency (see the discussion of chronic pancreatitis in Chapter 14) or bile salt deficiency syndromes (see the discussion of cholestasis in Chapter 15). Bile salt deficiency syndromes, which include bacterial overgrowth related to jejunal diverticula or stasis associated with regional enteritis, diabetic enteropathy, or scleroderma (Rosenberg et al., 1967), may be diagnosed by the bile salt breath test. In this test, a small dose of conjugated glycocholic acid ^{14}C is ingested. If there is bacterial overgrowth in the small intestine, radioactive glycine, radioactive

CO_2 or both will be liberated, transported through the intestinal wall, and excreted by the lungs as $^{14}CO_2$. ($^{14}CO_2$ excretion to ten times the upper reference limit for a healthy population) (Glickman, 1982).

Table 13–10 summarizes the results of common laboratory tests in malabsorption.

Management. The severity of steatorrhea and response to therapy can be gauged by repeated measurements of fecal fat.

Test Requests and Reports

Test Requests. The execution of the test sequence for malabsorption may be offered by the laboratory as a problem-solving service.

Table 13–9. CAUSES OF MALABSORPTION CLASSIFIED BY SMALL INTESTINAL BIOPSY

Celiac sprue and uncommon causes of malabsorption showing the same pathologic changes as celiac sprue
  Celiac sprue
  Unclassified sprue (refractory sprue)
  Tropical sprue syndrome
  Infectious gastroenteritis
  Stasis syndrome
  Kwashiorkor
Malabsorption with diagnostic pathologic changes
  Whipple's disease
  Abetalipoproteinemia (acanthocytosis)
  Collagenous sprue
  Primary intestinal lymphoma with malabsorption
  Eosinophilic gastroenteritis
  Giardiasis
  Coccidiosis
  Stronglyoidiasis
  Primary or secondary lymphangiectasia
  Immunodeficiency

Table 13–10. RESULTS OF COMMON LABORATORY TESTS IN MALABSORPTION, CAUSE UNSPECIFIED*

Laboratory Test	Value	Pathophysiologic Factors
Chemistry (Serum)		
Bilirubin, total	↓	Related to decreased protein and albumin
Calcium, total	↓	May be related to a decreased albumin or vitamin D deficiency with decreased calcium absorption
Carbon dioxide	↑ ↓	Chronic diarrhea can result in either metabolic acidosis or metabolic alkalosis
Chloride	↑ ↓	Reciprocal changes to bicarbonate can occur
Cholesterol	↓	Related to lipid malabsorption
Creatine phosphokinase	—	
Creatinine	—	
Glucose	—	
Lactic dehydrogenase	↑	Related to decreased vitamin B_{12} absorption with megaloblastic anemia and intramedullary death of megaloblasts
Phosphatase, alkaline	↑	An indication of vitamin D deficiency with decreased absorption of calcium and osteomalacia
Phosphorus, inorganic	↓	Related to decreased absorption
Potassium	↓	Diarrhea?
Proteins, total	↓	Related to protein malabsorption
Proteins, albumin	↓	A feature of the marked hypoproteinemia that can occur
Sodium	↓	Diarrhea?
Transaminase, aspartate amino	↑	Same cause as lactic dehydrogenase but elevation is smaller
Urea nitrogen	—	
Uric acid	↓	Related to decreased protein and albumin
Hematology (Blood)		
Hemoglobin	↓	Related to multiple deficiencies
Hematocrit	↓	Related to multiple deficiencies
Leukocyte count, total	—	
Platelet count	—	

Key:
— = No change; ↑ = can be increased; ↓ = can be decreased.

*Information from Friedman RB, Anderson RE, Entine SM, et al: Effects of disease on clinical laboratory tests. Clin Chem 26:1D–476D, 1980; Wolf PL: Interpretation of Biochemical Multitest Profiles: An Analysis of 100 Important Conditions. New York, Masson Publishing, Inc. 1977.

MALABSORPTION				
Fecal Fat gm, day	2–5			
Xylose Tolerance Urine gm/5 hr	5.3–7.7			
Calcium Total mEq/L	4.5–5.4			
Carotene µg/dl	50–360			
Albumin gm/dl	Age 15–35 3.44–5.64 Age 35–55 3.22–5.10			
Total Proteins gm/dl	6.78–8.3			
Folic Acid ng/ml	5–21			
Electrophoresis	See Chemistry Report Form			

Figure 13–4. Malabsorption panel. (From Henry JB, Murphy J: Effective utilization of clinical laboratories. In Henry JB (ed): Clinical Diagnosis and Management by Laboratory Methods, ed. 16. Philadelphia, WB Saunders Company, 1979, p 2043.)

The test request form can offer this strategy as an alternative to the protocol of individual tests.

Figure 13–4 presents a malabsorption panel that has been devised by Henry. He and Howanitz (1980) gave the rationale for this panel as follows:

Quantitative estimation of fecal fat is essential for determination of steatorrhea while the D-Xylose absorption test reflects adequacy of carbohydrate absorption. Serum carotene is used as a screening test for fat soluble vitamin absorption and protein electrophoresis is valuable in identifying exudative enteropathy. Serum folate levels are decreased in many patients although not all have megaloblastic anemia.

Interpretive Reports. The laboratory can report the test results of the strategy to the attending physician in the form of an interpretive report.

REFERENCES

Gastric Analysis and Acid-Peptic Disease of the Stomach and Duodenum

Beeler MF: Gastric analysis. In Beeler MF: Interpretations in Clinical Chemistry. Chicago, American Society of Clinical Pathologists, 1978, pp 45–59.

Cannon DC: Examination of gastric and duodenal contents. In Henry JB (ed): Clinical Diagnosis and Management by Laboratory Methods, ed 16. Philadelphia, WB Saunders Company, 1979, pp 759–778.

Grossman MI, Kurata JH, Rotter JI et al: Peptic ulcer: New therapies, new diseases. Ann Intern Med 95:609–627, 1981.

Malagelada J-R, Davis CS, O'Fallon WM, et al: Laboratory disagnosis of gastrinoma: I. A prospective evaluation of gastric analysis and fasting serum gastrin levels. Mayo Clin Proc 57:211–218, 1982.

Wallach J: Gastric and duodenal fluids. In Wallach J: Interpretation of Diagnostic Tests ed 3. Boston, Little, Brown & Company, 1978, pp 143–144.

Walsh JH: Peptic ulcer: Clinical and endocrine aspects. In Beeson PB, McDermott W, Wyngaarden JB (eds): Cecil Textbook of Medicine, ed 15. Philadelphia, WB Saunders Company, 1979, pp 1507–1509.

Zollinger-Ellison Syndrome

Clain JE: Diagnosis and management of gastrinoma (Zollinger-Ellison syndrome), editorial. Mayo Clin Proc 57:265–268, 1982.

Deveney CW, Deveney KS, Jaffe BM, et al: Use of calcium and secretin in the diagnosis of gastrinoma (Zollinger-Ellison syndrome). Ann Intern Med 87:680–686, 1977.

Ippoliti AF: Zollinger-Ellison syndrome: Provocative diagnostic tests, editorial. Ann Intern Med 87:788–789, 1977.

Kahn CR, Rosen SW, Weintraub BD, et al: Ectopic production of chorionic gonadotropin and its subunits by islet-cell tumors. N Engl J Med 297:565–569, 1977.

Malagelada J-R, Davis CS, O'Fallon WM, et al: Laboratory diagnosis of gastrinoma: I. A prospective evaluation of gastric analysis and fasting serum gastrin levels. Mayo Clin Proc 57:211–218, 1982a.

Malagelada J-R, Glanzman SL, Go VLW: Laboratory diagnosis of gastrinoma: II. A prospective study of gastrin challenge tests. Mayo Clin Proc 57:219–226, 1982b.

McGuigan JE, Trudeau WL: Immunochemical measurement of elevated levels of gastrin in the serum of patients with pancreatic tumors of the Zollinger-Ellison variety. N Engl J Med 278:1308–1313, 1968.

McGuigan JE, Wolfe MM: Secretin injection test in the diagnosis of gastrinoma. Gastroenterology 79:1324–1331, 1980.

Robbins SL, Cotran RS: The pancreas. In Robbins SL, Cotran RS (eds): Pathologic Basis of Disease, ed 2. Philadelphia, WB Saunders Company, 1979, pp 1092–1114.

Stabile BE, Braunstein GD, Passaro E: Serum gastrin and human chorionic gonadotropin in the Zollinger-Ellison syndrome. Arch Surg 115:1090–1095, 1980.

Wallach J: Gastric and duodenal fluids. In Wallach J: Interpretation of Diagnostic Tests ed 3. Boston, Little, Brown & Company, 1978, pp 143–144.

Walsh JH: Peptic ulcer: Clinical and endocrine aspects. In Beeson PB, McDermott W, Wyngaarden JB (eds): Cecil Textbook of Medicine, ed 15. Philadelphia, WB Saunders Company, 1979, pp 1507–1509.

Zollinger RM, Ellison EH: Primary peptic ulcers of the jejunum associated with islet cell tumors of the pancreas. Ann Surg 142:709–728, 1955.

Malabsorption Syndrome

Beeler MF: Laboratory diagnosis of malabsorption. In Beeler MF: Interpretations in Clinical Chemistry. Chicago, American Society of Clinical Pathologists, 1978, pp 77–93.

Brooks FP: Testing pancreatic function. N Engl J Med 286:300–302, 1972.

Gambino R: Fecal fat. Lab Report For Physicians 3:57–58, 1981.

Glickman RM: Malabsorption. In Wyngaarden JB, Smith LH (eds): Cecil Textbook of Medicine, ed 16. Philadelphia, WB Saunders Company, 1982, pp 678–703.

Gray GM: Diseases producing malabsorption and maldigestion. In Rubenstein E, Federman DD (eds): Scientific American Medicine. New York, Scientific American, Inc, 1982, pp 4X1–1 to 4X1–15.

Henry JB, Howanitz PJ: Organ panels and the relationship of the laboratory to the physician. In Jones RJ, Palulonis RM (eds): Laboratory Tests in Medical Practice. Chicago, American Medical Association, 1980, p 31.

Perera DR, Weinstein WM, Rubin CE: Small intestinal biopsy. Hum Pathol 6:157–217, 1975.

Rosenberg IH, Hardison WG, Bull DM: Abnormal bile-salt patterns and intestinal bacterial overgrowth associated with malabsorption. N Engl J Med 276:1391–1397, 1967.

Rosenberg IH, Sitnin MD: Screening for fat malabsorption, editorial. Ann Intern Med 95:776–777, 1981.

Simko V: Fecal fat microscopy. Acceptable predictive value in screening for steatorrhea. Am J Gastroenterol 75:204–208, 1981.

Spivak JL, Barnes HV: Malabsorption. In Spivak JL, Barnes HV (eds): Manual of Clinical Problems in Internal Medicine, ed 2. Boston, Little, Brown & Company, 1978, pp 252–255.

CHAPTER 14

PANCREATIC SUBPROBLEMS

PANCREATIC INFLAMMATION
  Acute Pancreatitis
  Chronic Pancreatitis

PANCREATIC INFLAMMATION

ACUTE PANCREATITIS

Definition and Significance

Acute pancreatitis is a sudden, diffuse enzymatic destruction of the pancreas, presumably caused by the escape of active lytic pancreatic enzymes into the glandular parenchyma. It is thought that there may be leakage of a toxic substance into the blood, the peritoneal cavity, or both and that this may cause shock, circulatory collapse, and even death (Ranson, 1980).

Acute pancreatitis occurs about once in every 500 to 600 hospital admissions. It is most common in middle life and is frequently associated with biliary tract disease and alcoholism. Pancreatitis associated with biliary tract disease is seen more commonly in women; the association with alcoholism is seen more commonly in men.

Acute pancreatitis related to gallstones carries a significant mortality, but the prognosis is excellent if freedom from subsequent attacks can be achieved by surgical therapy. Alcoholic pancreatitis carries a lower mortality but a discouragingly high incidence of recurrence of acute attacks or progression to chronic pancreatitis. The overall mortality of acute pancreatitis is around 10 per cent.

Other less common causes of acute pancreatitis are trauma, extension of inflammation from adjacent peptic ulcers or abdominal infections, blood-borne bacterial infections, viral infections such as mumps, vascular thrombosis and embolism, polyarteritis nodosa, hypothermia, certain drugs, hyperlipoproteinemia (Chapter 10), hyperparathyroidism, and hypercalcemic states (Chapter 9). In about 10 to 50 per cent of cases, the cause is obscure (Table 14–1).

Pathophysiology

Proteolysis, lipolysis, and hemorrhage are the major morphologic features of acute pancreatitis. These processes are undoubtedly secondary to autodigestion by pancreatic enzymes. The active form of trypsin is clearly one of the major factors in acute pancreatitis, and it has been demonstrated in the pancreatic fluid in patients with acute pancreatitis (Fedail et al., 1979).

Table 14–1. CAUSES OF ACUTE
PANCREATITIS*

Alcohol ingestion (acute and chronic alcoholism)
Biliary tract disease (gallstones)
Postoperative (abdominal, non-abdominal)
Postendoscopic retrograde cholangiopancreatography
  (ERCP)
Trauma (especially blunt abdominal type)
Metabolic
  Hyperlipidemia
  Hyperparathyroidism
  Renal failure
  After renal transplantation†
  Acute fatty liver of pregnancy‡
Hereditary pancreatitis
Infections
  Mumps
  Viral hepatitis
  Other viral infections (coxsackievirus, echovirus)
  Ascariasis
  Mycoplasma
Drug associated
  Diuretics and antihypertensive drugs
    Thiazides
    Furosemide
    Ethacrynic acid
    Clonidine§
  Anti-inflammatory and immunosuppressive agents
    Azathioprine
    6-Mercaptopurine
    Sulfasalazine
    Corticosteroids
    L-Asparaginase
    Acetaminophen§
  Antimicrobials
    Isoniazid§
    Tetracycline
    Rifampin§
  Miscellaneous
    Oral contraceptives
    Phenformin
    Propoxyphene§
Connective tissue disorders with vasculitis
  Systemic lupus erythematosus
  Necrotizing angiitis
  Thrombotic thrombocytopenic purpura
Penetrating duodenal ulcer
Obstruction of the ampulla of Vater
  Regional enteritis
  Duodenal diverticulum
Other

*Adapted from Greenberger NJ, Toskes PP, Isselbacher
KJ: Disease of the pancreas. In Harrison's Principles of
Internal Medicine, ed 9. Copyright © 1980 by McGraw-
Hill, Inc. Used by permission of McGraw-Hill Book
Company, New York, p 1503.
†Pancreatitis occurs in 3 per cent of renal transplant
patients and is due to many factors including surgery,
hypercalcemia, drugs (corticosteroids, azathioprine, L-as-
paraginase, diuretics), and viral infections.
‡Pancreatitis also occurs in otherwise uncomplicated
pregnancy and is most often associated with cholelithiasis.
§Isolated case reports only.

The key issue is: which factors initiate this
autodigestion? The suspected factors are related to bile reflux, duodenal reflux, hyper-
secretion-obstruction, and alcohol-induced
changes. The first two factors are postulated
to be due to reflux of bile or duodenal contents
and activation of pancreatic enzymes; the third
factor, to rupture of pancreatic ducts secondary to hypersecretion. The mechanism by
which excessive alcohol intake causes acute
pancreatitis is unclear (Balart and Ferrante,
1982; Robbins and Cotran, 1979).

Serum and urine amylase levels typically rise
within a few hours of onset in patients with
acute pancreatitis and return to normal within
10 days (Gambill, 1976). Serum lipase levels,
though tending to parallel serum amylase levels in acute pancreatitis, can rise more slowly
(Beeler, 1970; Lifton et al., 1974a). However,
serum lipase levels can rise before serum amylase levels, and the elevation can persist for
a longer period of time (Patt et al., 1966; Song
and Tietz, 1970). Lipase is absent from the
urine (Tietz and Repique, 1973).

Clinical Contexts

Diagnosis. The clinical features of acute
pancreatitis include the following:

1. More than 95 per cent of patients develop
excruciating midepigastric pain that radiates in
minutes or hours through to the back.

2. Approximately 75 to 85 per cent of patients develop nausea and vomiting.

3. More than 50 per cent of patients develop
fever.

4. Nearly 50 per cent of patients develop
shock and obtundation if the episode lasts
more than several hours.

5. An ileus usually develops in patients who
show signs of hypovolemia (Gray, 1980).

Additional features that may be seen are
tachycardia; pleural effusion, often left-sided
(see Chapter 11); an abdominal mass, abscess,
or cyst; acute renal failure (see Chapter 12);
respiratory failure; jaundice (see Chapter 15);
hematemesis; mental confusion; mania; and
diabetic coma. Uncommon events include tetany, cutaneous fat necrosis resembling erythema nodosum, and polyarthritis.

Other disorders to be ruled out include
perforated viscus, mesenteric vascular disease,
volvulus, ruptured spleen, acute appendicitis,
acute calculous cholecystitis, small-bowel obstruction, dissecting aneurysm, acute myocar-

dial infarction (see Chapter 10), nephrolithiasis, and acute porphyria.

Management. Laboratory studies can be useful as a prognostic guide and as a means of monitoring the patient's response to therapy.

Screening. Screening for acute pancreatitis by laboratory studies in the absence of clinical features of disease is not indicated.

Strategy

Test Sequence. The best test sequence for diagnosing acute pancreatitis is parallel and serial measurements of serum amylase and lipase and urine amylase levels. These measurements should be obtained when the patient is initially encountered and periodically thereafter until the process is resolved. Based on experience, we believe that measuring serum amylase and lipase and urine amylase levels every 24 hours is adequate for detecting elevations of either enzyme.

The amylase-creatinine clearance ratio may be calculated if random, simultaneously collected serum and urine samples are analyzed for both creatinine and amylase. An advantage of the formula for this calculation is that urine volumes cancel out, thus obviating the need for a timed urine collection. Unfortunately, because of methodologic problems, together with poor diagnostic sensitivity and specificity, the amylase-creatinine clearance ratio has not proven to be as effective as early reports suggested (Gambino, 1980).

The formula follows (Salt and Schenker, 1976):

$$\frac{C_{am}}{C_{cr}}\% = \frac{\text{amylase, urine}}{\text{amylase, serum}} \times \frac{\text{creatinine, serum}}{\text{creatinine, urine}} \times 100$$

Measurement of serum amylase isoenzymes should be considered. However, the results of this study can vary significantly according to methodology. Furthermore, it is not widely available.

Measurement of methemalbumin in serum, ascites, or pleural fluid has been reported to be useful in differentiating acute edematous from acute hemorrhagic pancreatitis (Geokas et al., 1974). This test sequence should be supplemented by an appropriate serum biochemical profile, a complete blood count, and a urinalysis.

Gauthier and co-workers (1981) recommend the following tests for monitoring acute pancreatitis:

1. Daily determinations:
   a. Serum amylase, calcium, phosphorus, electrolytes, urea nitrogen, creatinine, LDH, transaminase, bilirubin, albumin, and glucose.
   b. Complete blood count.
   c. Blood gases.
   d. Urinary amylase.
   e. Electrolytes.
   f. Urea.
2. Determinations less often than daily:
   a. A coagulation profile every second day.
   b. Lipid studies on admission and occasionally during parenteral hyperalimentation, if the latter is used.

Upper gastrointestinal roentgenographs can demonstrate distortion of the duodenal loop by the pancreas. An ultrasonic study can demonstrate edema or pseudocyst formation, and computed tomographic (CT) x-ray scan can be useful for estimating the size and shape of the pancreas (Gray, 1980).

Patient Preparation. It may be important to obtain the urine specimen for the amylase-creatinine clearance after the patient has been given intravenous fluids to promote urinary output of at least 30 ml/hr (Gray, 1980). (See Part 3 for chemistry and hematology tests.)

Specimen Collection and Handling. Amylase in serum and urine is quite stable, with negligible loss of activity at room temperature in the course of a week or at refrigerator temperature over a 2-month period. Heparin is the only common anticoagulant that does not inhibit amylase activity. Serum lipase is stable at room temperature for a week and at refrigerator temperature for 3 weeks; it can be frozen for several months (Kachmar and Moss, 1976). (See Part 3.)

Methodology. Consult the laboratory for its methodologies, reference intervals, accuracy and precision, and potential sources of interferences. Amylase may be measured by saccharogenic, amyloclastic, or chromolytic (dyed-starch) methods. Each of these procedures is satisfactory if properly standardized and controlled. We measure serum amylase on the DuPont ACA using maltopentose as the substrate (DuPont Co, Instrument Products, ACA Division, Wilmington, Del.). Our reference intervals are as follows: serum amylase, 25 to 100 IU/100 ml; urine amylase, up to 400 IU/24 hours.

Many of the limitations on the use of lipase determinations are related to technical problems. Compared with methods of determining levels of amylase, manual lipase measurements are more difficult and take longer. We measure serum lipase on the DuPont ACA using triolein as the substrate. Our reference interval is as follows: serum lipase, 4 to 24 IU/100 ml. (See Part 3.)

Interpretation

Diagnosis. Serum and urine amylase levels tend to become elevated during the first 2 to 3 hours after the onset of pancreatitis, and, in mild to moderately severe attacks, they return to normal after 2 to 10 days. The urine amylase level is the last to return to normal. More prolonged elevation is encountered with more severe pancreatitis or when there has been recrudescence of the acute process during recovery. Elevations beyond 3 or 4 weeks are not uncommonly caused by pancreatic pseudocyst or pancreatic cancer (Gambill, 1976).

Reported sensitivities of serum amylase as a test for acute pancreatitis vary from 45 to 95 per cent (Stefanini et al., 1965). An elevated serum amylase level above 1000 Somogyi units/ 100 ml usually means acute pancreatitis that is often associated with biliary tract disease. Cases of acute pancreatitis related to excessive alcohol intake often have serum amylase values from 250 to 500 Somogyi units/100 ml. It is unfortunate but true that fatal acute pancreatitis can occur even when serum amylase values are not elevated.

The specificity of serum amylase as a test for acute pancreatitis is also low, especially with values from 250 to 500 Somogyi units/100 ml. A number of other acute abdominal disorders can be associated with elevations of serum amylase to these levels, such as cholecystitis, peptic ulcer, postgastric resection, intestinal obstruction, mesenteric thrombosis, and peritonitis. Stefanini and colleagues (1965) stated that the triad of elevated serum amylase, serum glucose, and blood leukocytes adds greater credence to the diagnosis of acute pancreatitis than elevation of serum amylase alone. Table 14–2 presents common laboratory test results that can be elevated or depressed in acute pancreatitis.

The elevation of serum lipase is less sensitive but more specific as a test for acute pancreatitis than elevated serum amylase. Lifton (1974a) found that 63 per cent of patients with pancreatitis had an elevated serum lipase level, compared with 73 per cent of patients with elevated serum amylase and with 83 per cent having an increase in one or the other or both enzymes. There were two patients whose serum lipase level increased before their serum amylase level increased. Absence of elevation of either enzyme permits us to exclude acute pancreatitis with greater confidence because the combined sensitivity is greater than that for serum amylase alone (increased sensitivity of parallel tests).

The specificity of serum lipase as a test for acute pancreatitis can be useful in distinguishing whether an elevated serum amylase is due to acute inflammation of the parotid glands or acute pancreatitis. Serum amylase can be elevated in both of these disorders, whereas serum lipase is not elevated in inflammation of the parotid glands.

An elevated amylase-creatinine clearance ratio (reference interval: 1.0 to 4.0 per cent), as a result of defective proximal tubular reabsorption of amylase (Johnson et al., 1976), occurs in many patients with clear-cut acute pancreatitis. Dürr and associates (1977), however, reported that 29 of 79 patients with proven acute pancreatitis had amylase-creatinine ratios that were not increased during the acute course of the illness. An elevated amylase-creatine clearance ratio is not specific for acute pancreatitis and can occur in patients with burns, diabetic ketoacidosis, and acute defective tubular function (Levitt, 1979). An increased ratio has also been reported in severe renal insufficiency (Morton et al., 1975), duodenal perforation (Berger et al., 1976), and pancreatic cancer (Levine et al., 1975). The early enthusiasm for the amylase-creatinine ratio in the diagnosis of acute pancreatitis appears to have waned (Levitt and Johnson, 1978).

An elevated serum amylase level in the presence of a urine amylase that is not elevated suggests macroamylasemia (amylase bound to IgG or IgA). Persons with macroamylasemia are usually well and do not have acute pancreatitis. The diagnosis may be confirmed by a low amylase-creatinine clearance ratio (lower reference limit: less than 1.0 per cent).

Normal serum amylase is composed of one third pancreatic type and two thirds salivary type isoenzymes. Measurement of serum amylase isoenzymes can be useful in determining whether an elevated serum amylase level is of pancreatic origin (Lehrner, 1976). However,

Table 14–2. COMMON LABORATORY TEST RESULTS IN ACUTE PANCREATITIS*

Laboratory Test	Value	Pathophysiologic Factors
Chemistry (Serum)		
Bilirubin, total	↑	Swollen pancreas can cause obstructive jaundice; gallstones?
Calcium, total	↑ ↓	When pancreatitis is related to hyperparathyroidism. Related to decreased albumin as well as possible hypoparathyroidism, increased thyrocalcitonin, and combination with fatty acids in the peritoneal cavity
Carbon dioxide	—	
Chloride	—	
Cholesterol	↑	Related to coexisting liver disease; turbid serum with elevated triglycerides
	↓	In about 40 per cent of patients at initial hospitalization
Creatine phosphokinase	↑	With more severe or prolonged disease, but of little diagnostic value
Creatinine	↑	In about 40 per cent of patients at initial hospitalization
Glucose	↑	Often found; related to islet-cell involvement and stress
Lactic dehydrogenase	↑	From necrotic pancreatic tissue
Phosphatase, alkaline	↑	Swollen pancreas can cause obstructive jaundice; gallstones?
Phosphorus, inorganic	↓	Low or low normal in about 40 per cent of patients at initial hospitalization
Potassium	↓	Usually normal or only slightly depressed
Proteins, total	↓	Related to loss into the peritoneal cavity
Proteins, albumin	↓	Related to loss into the peritoneal cavity; synthesis can be decreased with coexisting liver disease
Sodium	—	
Transaminase, aspartate amino	↑	From necrotic pancreatic tissue
Urea nitrogen	↑	With more severe cases with shock and oliguria
Uric acid	↑	From necrotic pancreatic tissue
Hematology (Blood)		
Hemoglobin	↑ ↓	Related to hemoconcentration
Hematocrit	↑	Related to hemoconcentration
Leukocyte count, total	↑	Usually elevated, slightly to moderately
Platelet count	↓	Disseminated intravascular coagulation

Key:
— = No change; ↑ = can be increased; ↓ = can be decreased.
*Information from Friedman RB, Anderson RE, Entine SM, et al: Effects of diseases on clinical laboratory tests. Clin Chem 26:1D–476D, 1980; Wolf PL: Interpretation of Biochemical Multitest Profiles: An analysis of 100 Important Conditions. New York, Masson Publishing USA, Inc. 1977; Balart LA, Ferrante WA: Pathophysiology of acute and chronic pancreatitis. Arch Intern Med 142:113-117, 1982.

these measurements are not helpful for determining whether patients without elevation of serum amylase have pancreatitis (Levitt, 1979).

Management. There is poor correlation between the degree of elevation of serum amylase and lipase levels and the severity of the pancreatitis (Gullick, 1973). Gambill (1976) related the case of a man who, during one of several attacks of pain, with jaundice and fever, had a serum amylase level of 1600 units/100 ml and a urine amylase excretion of 29,000 units per hour. These values, observed prior to the use of opiates, returned to essentially healthy levels by the third day, at which time the surgeon found a stone wedged in the ampulla of Vater and only minimal pancreatic edema. Table 14–3 gives laboratory studies indicative of a severe disease.

Geokas and associates (1974) consistently found methemalbumin in the sera of 18 patients with acute hemorrhagic pancreatitis but not in the sera of 20 patients with acute edematous pancreatitis, in five with gastrointestinal

Table 14–3. LABORATORY STUDIES INDICATING SEVERE PANCREATITIS*

Laboratory Test	Value
HGB/HCT–Initial	– > 14g per dl/50%
HGB/HCT–After hydration	– < 8g per dl/30%
WBC	– > 20,000/μl
Urine volume	– < 20 ml/hr
Urine sp. gr.	– > 1.025
Blood glucose	– > 200 mg%
Serum Ca++	– < 7.5 mg%
Pulmonary function	
PaO$_2$	– < 60 mm Hg
PaCO$_2$	– > 45 mm Hg
pH	– < 7.4
Renal function	
BUN	– > 30 mg%
Creatinine	– > 2.0 mg%
Hepatic function	
Bilirubin	– > 4.0 mg%
Albumin	– < 3.0 g%
Prothrombin time	– > 14.0 sec
SGOT	– > 250 U/ml
LDH	– > 350 IU
Coagulation	
Platelets	– ↓
Fibrinogen	– ↓
Fibrin split products	– ↑

*Adapted from Conn HF, Conn RB: Current Diagnosis. Philadelphia, WB Saunders Company, 1980, p 646.

bleeding, and in two with intra-abdominal hemorrhage.

Test Requests and Reports

Test Requests. The execution of the test sequence for acute pancreatitis (i.e., parallel and serial measurements of serum amylase and lipase and of urine amylase; and measurements

of serum and urine amylase and creatinine, and calculation of the amylase-creatinine clearance ratio) may be offered by the laboratory as a problem-solving service. Figure 14–1 illustrates a pancreatic organ panel. Henry and Howanitz (1980) gave the rationale for this panel as follows:

Serum amylase is most valuable in the diagnosis of acute pancreatitis in the first 24 hours. Urine amylase and serum lipase are more sensitive than serum amylase two or more days after the onset of pancreatitis or in cases of relapsing pancreatitis. Recent literature has indicated that the ratio of amylase clearance to creatinine clearance is the most sensitive indicator of pancreatitis. This amylase/creatinine ratio can be calculated using a spot urine for the determination of urine amylase and creatinine. Since a spot urine avoids a timed or interval collection period, it is often more practical and accurate.

Interpretive Reports. The test results from the execution of the strategy, including the calculation of the amylase-creatinine clearance ratio, may be collated and returned to the attending physician in the form of an interpretive report.

CHRONIC PANCREATITIS

Definition and Significance

Chronic pancreatitis is an inflammatory destructive process of the pancreas often characterized by repeated flareups of a mild or subclinical type of acute pancreatitis. There is

PANCREATIC					
Amylase, Serum Somogyi Units/dl	50–150				
Amylase, Urinary units/min	1–5				
Lipase, Serum units/ml	0.5–1.8				
Calcium mEq/L	4.5–5.4				
Creatinine Serum mg/dl	0.6–1.2				
Urine Creatinine mg/dl					
Amylase/Creatinine Clearance	1–3.5				

Figure 14–1. Organ panel for the pancreas. (From Henry JB, Murphy J: Effective utilization of clinical laboratories. In Henry JB (ed): Clinical Diagnosis and Management by Laboratory Methods, ed 16. Philadelphia, WB Saunders Company, 1979, p 2042.)

relative preservation of the islets. The disease occurs in the same type of patient who develops acute pancreatitis, particularly the patient with excessive alcoholic intake or biliary tract disease. Its exact etiology is unclear. Although not a common disease, chronic pancreatitis is important because it can cause debilitating pain and terminate in pancreatic insufficiency and the malabsorption syndrome (Sarles, 1974; Strum and Spiro, 1971). (See the discussion of malabsorption in Chapter 13.)

Pathophysiology

The pathogenesis of chronic pancreatitis is obscure. As the secretions of lipase and proteolytic enzymes decrease, there is progressive impairment of fat and protein digestion with increased amounts of fat and protein nitrogen in the stool (Balart and Ferrante, 1982). There must be a 90 per cent reduction in secretion of pancreatic lipase and trypsin before azotorrhea and steatorrhea occur (DiMagno, 1979). Glucose intolerance with insulin-dependent diabetes mellitus is a late manifestation (see Chapter 16 for a discussion of diabetes mellitus) (Cooperman, 1981).

Clinical Contexts

Diagnosis. Patients with chronic pancreatitis present with either abdominal pain, malabsorption, or both and tend to fall into three groups (Brooks, 1979):

1. Those who sustain repeated attacks of mild abdominal pain.
2. Those who have actual acute pancreatitis followed by gradual development of pancreatic insufficiency.
3. Those who have a steady progression of pancreatic insufficiency with or without pain.

The pain is generally less severe than in acute pancreatitis and can be associated with nausea and vomiting. A history of alcoholism, biliary tract disease, or blunt trauma is often present. Steatorrhea, jaundice, abdominal mass (pancreatic inflammation or pseudocyst), and gastrointestinal bleeding can occur. Two thirds of patients have glucose intolerance late in the disease. Males are affected five to ten times more frequently than females, and the average age of onset is in the fourth decade. Table 14–4 presents common laboratory results in chronic pancreatitis.

Management. Laboratory studies may be used to follow the course of chronic pancreatitis and to document the presence of end-stage disease.

Screening. Laboratory studies are not used to screen for chronic pancreatitis in the absence of clinical features of disease.

Strategy

Test Sequence. During acute exacerbations, a strategy identical to that for acute pancreatitis may be used as described earlier in this chapter. However, as a result of a decreased mass of pancreatic tissue, serum amylase levels and renal clearance of amylase are frequently normal in chronic pancreatitis.

As the disease progresses, a reduced pancreatic exocrine mass may be documented by measuring pancreatic secretion of bicarbonate in the duodenal contents after stimulation by secretin or by measuring trypsin concentration in the duodenal contents after a liquid test meal (the Lundh meal). Serum trypsin by radioimmunoassay (RIA) has been proposed as a test for chronic pancreatitis (Andriulli et al., 1981).

Patient Preparation. The patient should be fasting. Recommended procedures are as follows (Brooks, 1972; Gray, 1980):

1. Conduct a secretin test.
   a. Perform a duodenal intubation under fluoroscopic guidance with a double-lumen tube allowing gastric and duodenal aspiration.
   b. After 20 minutes for basal conditions to be established, give 0.1 unit secretin intravenously to test for allergic reaction.
   c. If there is no allergic reaction, give 1.0 unit of secretin per kg of body weight in 10 ml saline intravenously.
   d. Take four separate 20-minute collections from the distal duodenum to be analyzed for bicarbonate.
2. Give the Lundh meal.
   a. Perform intubation as in the secretin test.
   b. Administer a liquid meal.
   c. Analyze the duodenal contents for trypsin at 20-minute intervals.
3. Conduct a therapeutic trial (Meyer, 1977).
   a. If the fecal fat excretion is markedly reduced by pancreatic enzyme supplements, a diagnosis of pancreatic maldigestion is very likely.

Table 14–4.   COMMON LABORATORY TEST RESULTS IN CHRONIC PANCREATITIS*

Laboratory Test	Value†‡	Pathophysiologic Factors
Chemistry (Serum)		
Bilirubin, total	↑	Concomitant liver disease
Calcium, total	↓	Related to decreased albumin, malabsorption, or both
Carbon dioxide	—	
Chloride	—	
Cholesterol	↑	In some cases
Creatine phosphokinase	—	
Creatinine	—	
Glucose	↑	Related to stress, islet-cell destruction, or both
Lactic dehydrogenase	—	
Phosphatase, alkaline	↑	Concomitant liver disease
Phosphorus, inorganic	—	
Potassium	—	
Proteins, total	↓	In some cases
Proteins, albumin	↓	In about 25 per cent of patients at initial hospitalization; may be related to liver disease
Sodium	—	
Transaminase, aspartate amino	↑	In about 50 per cent of patients at initial hospitalization; may be related to liver disease
Urea nitrogen	—	
Uric acid	—	
Hematology (Blood)		
Hemoglobin	—	
Hematocrit	—	
Leukocyte count, total	↑	In about 25 per cent of patients at initial hospitalization
Platelet count	↑	

Key:
— = no change; ↑ = can be increased; ↓ = can be decreased.
*Based on information from Friedman RB, Anderson RE, Entine SM, et al: Effects of diseases on clinical laboratory tests. Clin Chem 26:1D–476D, 1980; Beeler MF: Interpretations in Clinical Chemistry. Chicago, American Society of Clinical Pathologists, 1978.
†These test results can occur in addition to the test results for acute pancreatitis (Table 14–2) if an episode of acute pancreatitis occurs in a patient who has chronic pancreatitis.
‡See test results for malabsorption (Table 13–10) which may also be present.

Ultrasonography can be useful for revealing an enlarged pancreatic head or a dilated duct system. It can also identify fluid-filled pseudocysts. Endoscopic retrograde pancreatography can identify discrete lesions that are blocking pancreatic ducts (Gray, 1980).

Specimen Collection and Handling. The specimens should be collected in chemically clean containers and promptly analyzed.

Methodology. Consult the laboratory for its methodologies, reference intervals, accuracy and precision, and potential sources of interference. See McNeely (1980).

Interpretation

Diagnosis. If the patient's duodenal contents after secretin stimulation show values below the lower reference limits for a healthy population for volume, bicarbonate, and amylase, the test results confirm insufficiency of the exocrine pancreas, i.e., chronic pancreatitis. Normal secretory levels are greater than 2 ml of fluid per kg of body weight over the 80-minute period, and this fluid should contain at least 6 units of amylase per kg of body weight. The incremental increase in bicarbonate should be 85 mEq/liter (Gray, 1980). Dreiling (1970) reported 5 per cent false-positive and 5 per cent false-negative secretin test results for pancreatic disease. Hansky (1971) found 23 per cent false-negative results in chronic pancreatitis, and Crozier (1970) reported 17 per cent false-negative results in detecting pancreatic disease.

For the Lundh meal, healthy patients had concentrations of 161 to 212 µg/ml of trypsin in the first 20-minute specimen (Brooks, 1972). Lower values are consistent with insufficiency of the exocrine pancreas.

Management. Laboratory studies obtained at the time the patient is first seen can serve as a baseline against which the course of the disease may be evaluated.

Test Requests and Reports

Test Requests. If the clinical features suggest an episode of acute pancreatitis, the test sequence for the problem of acute pancreatitis may be ordered. In addition, the test sequence for chronic pancreatitis (e.g., the secretin test), available at the medical facility, may also be ordered.

Interpretive Report. The results of the execution of the test sequences for acute and chronic pancreatitis may be returned to the attending physician in the form of an interpretive report.

REFERENCES

Acute Pancreatitis

Balart LA, Ferrante WA: Pathophysiology of acute and chronic pancreatitis. Arch Intern Med 142:113–117, 1982.

Beeler MF: Amylase and lipase. Clinical chemistry No CC-61 (1970).Commission on Continuing Education, American Society of Clinical Pathologists, 1970.

Berger GMB, Cowlin J, Turner TJ: Amylase:creatinine clearance ratio and urinary excretion of lysozyme in acute pancreatitis and acute duodenal perforation. S Afr Med J 50:1559–1561, 1976.

Dürr HK, Bode JC, Lankisch PG, et al: Amylase-creatinine clearance ratio in pancreatitis; letter. N Engl J Med 296:635, 1977.

Fedail SS, Harvey RF, Salmon RR, et al: Trypsin and lactoferrin levels in pure pancreatic juice with pancreatic disease. Gut 20:983–986, 1979.

Gambill EA: Pancreatitis and the acute abdomen: Clinical and laboratory approaches to diagnosis. In Clearfield HR, Dinoso VP (eds): Gastrointestinal Emergencies. New York, Grune & Stratton, 1976, pp 231–243.

Gambino R: Amylase/creatinine clearance ratios. Lab Report for Physicians 2:1–2, 1980.

Gauthier A, Escoffier JM, Camatte R, et al: Severe acute pancreatitis. Clin Gastroenterology 10:209–224, 1981.

Geokas MC, Rinderknecht H, Walberg CB, et al: Methemalbumin in the diagnosis of acute hemorrhagic pancreatitis. Ann Intern Med 81:483–486, 1974.

Gray GM: Diseases of the Pancreas. In Rubenstein E, Federman DD (eds): Scientific American Medicine. New York, Scientific American, Inc., 1980, 4V–1 to 4V–8.

Gullick HD: Relation of the magnitude of blood enzyme elevation to severity of exocrine pancreatic disease. Am J Dig Dis 18:375–383, 1973.

Henry JB, Howanitz PJ: Organ panels and the relationship of the laboratory to the physician. In Jones RJ, Palulonis RM (eds): Laboratory Tests in Medical Practice. Chicago, American Medical Association, 1980, p 30.

Johnson SG, Ellis CJ, Levitt MD: Mechanism of increased clearance of amylase/creatinine in acute pancreatitis. N Engl J Med 295:1214–1217, 1976.

Kachmar JF, Moss DM: Enzymes. In Tietz NW (ed): Fundamentals of Clinical Chemistry, ed 2. Philadelphia, WB Saunders Company, 1976, pp 565–698.

Lehrner LM, Ward JC, Karn RC, et al: An evaluation of the usefulness of amylase isozyme differentiation in patients with hyperamylasemia. Am J Clin Pathol 66:576–587, 1976.

Levine RI, Glauser FL, Berk JE: Enhancement of the amylase-creatinine clearance ratio in disorders other than pancreatitis. N Engl J Med 292:329–332, 1975.

Levitt MD: Clinical use of amylase clearance and isoamylase measurements. Mayo Clin Proc 54:428–431, 1979.

Levitt MD, Johnson SG: Is the C_{Am}/C_{Cr} ratio of value for the diagnosis of pancreatitis? Gastroenterology 75:118–119, 1978.

Lifton LJ, Slickers KA, Katz DA, et al: Amylase vs lipase in the diagnosis of acute pancreatitis. Clin Chem 20:880, 1974a.

Lifton LJ, Slickers KA, Pragay DA, et al: Pancreatitis and lipase: A reevaluation with a five-minute turbidimetric lipase determination. JAMA 229:47–50, 1974b.

Morton WJ, Alpers DH, Tedesco FJ: Serum amylase measurements in patients with renal insufficiency. Gastroenterology 68:961, 1975.

Patt HH, Kramer SP, Woel G, et al: Serum lipase determination in acute pancreatitis. Arch Surg 92:718–723, 1966.

Ranson JHC: Surgical treatment of acute pancreatitis. Dig Dis Sci 25:453–459, 1980.

Robbins SL, Cotran RS: The pancreas. In Robbins SL, Cotran RS (eds): Pathologic Basis of Disease. Philadelphia, WB Saunders Company, 1979, pp 1092–1114.

Salt WB, Schenker S: Amylase—Its clinical significance: A review of the literature. Medicine 55:269–289, 1976.

Song H, Tietz NW, Tan C: Usefulness of serum lipase, esterase and amylase estimation in the diagnosis of pancreatitis—A comparison. Clin Chem 16:264–268, 1970.

Stefanini P, Ermini M, Carboni M: Diagnosis and management of acute pancreatitis. Am J Surg 110:866–875, 1965.

Tietz NW, Repique EV: Proposed standard method for measuring serum lipase activity in serum by a continuous sampling technique. Clin Chem 19:1268–1275, 1973.

Chronic Pancreatitis

Andriulli A, Masoero G, Felder M, et al: Circulating trypsin-like immunoreactivity in chronic pancreatitis. Dig Dis Sci 26:532–537, 1981.

Balart LA, Ferrante WA: Pathophysiology of acute and chronic pancreatitis. Arch Intern Med 142:113–117, 1982.

Brooks FP: Testing pancreatic function. N Engl J Med 286:300–303, 1972.

Brooks FP: Chronic pancreatitis. In Beeson PB,

McDermott W, Wyngaarden JB: Cecil Textbook of Medicine, ed 15. Philadelphia, WB Saunders Company, 1979, pp 1554–1557.

Cooperman AM: Chronic pancreatitis. In Cooperman AM (ed): Symposium on Liver, Spleen, and Pancreas. Surg Clin North Am, 61:71–83, 1981.

Crozier RE: The secretin test. Its shortcomings as a practical clinical diagnostic procedure. Lahey Clinic Foundation Bull 19:17–21, 1970.

DiMagno EP: Medical treatment of pancreatic insufficiency. Mayo Clin Proc 54:435–442, 1979.

Dreiling DA: The early diagnosis of pancreatic cancer. Scand J Gastroenterol 5:Suppl 6:115–122, 1970.

Gray GM: Diseases of the pancreas. In Rubenstein E, Federman DD (eds): Scientific American Medicine. New York, Scientific American, Inc, 1980, pp 4V–1 to 4V–8.

Hansky J: Pancreatic function tests: Comparison of standard and augmented secretin. Aust NZ J Med 1:109–113, 1971.

Meyer JH: The ins and outs of oral pancreatic enzymes, editorial. N Engl J Med 296:1347–1348, 1977.

McNeely MDD: Gastrointestinal function. In Sonnenwirth AC, Jarett L (eds): Gradwohl's Clinical Laboratory Methods and Diagnosis, ed 8. St. Louis, The CV Mosby Company, 1980.

Sarles H: Chronic calcifying pancreatitis: Chronic alcoholic pancreatitis. Gastroenterology 66:604–616, 1974.

Strum WB, Spiro HM: Chronic pancreatitis. Ann Intern Med 74:264–277, 1971.

CHAPTER 15

HEPATOBILIARY SUBPROBLEMS

LABORATORY STUDIES IN LIVER DISEASE

LIVER FUNCTION TESTS

Even though only a few laboratory tests actually measure liver function, we follow the convention of using the term *liver function tests* synonymously with *liver chemistry tests*.

Laboratory tests of liver function usually do not establish an exact etiology of liver disease. They merely indicate whether the liver is normal or diseased, and if diseased, the extent or severity. Taken together with the history and physical examination, these tests are sometimes suggestive of one specific liver disease.

Other studies, such as scintigraphy, sonography, angiography, laparoscopy, and liver biopsy, are often necessary for confirming the diagnosis.

Liver function tests are easier to understand and interpret if we view them according to the pathophysiologic derangements that cause the test results to become abnormal. There are four pathophysiologic questions that are useful to ask.

1. Is there ongoing liver cell injury, and what is its severity? (Liver Cell Injury?)

2. Is there hyperbilirubinemia and/or cholestasis? (Hyperbilirubinemia or Cholestasis?)

3. Are the metabolic functions of the liver compromised? (Metabolic Derangement?)

4. Is the disease process acute or chronic? (Acute versus Chronic Disease?)

Question 1 (Liver Cell Injury?) can be answered by the following serum tests:

1. Gamma glutamyl transferase (GGT).

2. Glutamic oxaloacetic transaminase (SGOT)—also known as aspartate amino transferase (AST).

3. Glutamic pyruvic transaminase (SGPT) —also known as alanine aminotransferase (ALT).

4. Lactic dehydrogenase (LDH)—not a very sensitive or specific test for liver disease.

There are at least three situations in which a SGPT test can provide information not given by a SGOT test alone:

1. In heart disease, an elevation of SGPT is sensitive to heart failure. Although this elevation has been attributed to congestion of the liver, Gambino (1979*b*) believes it correlates better with poor perfusion of the liver secondary to low cardiac output. Cohen and Kaplan (1978) suggest that liver dysfunction secondary to left-sided ventricular failure is not uncommon and can be seen in the absence of right-sided heart failure. The transaminase level (SGOT and SGPT) can be high enough to cause confusion with viral hepatitis (up to 2000 Karmen units) and is due to centrilobular ischemia and necrosis.

2. In viral hepatitis, the SGPT-SGOT ratio is greater than 1. It is less than 1 in alcoholic hepatitis.

3. In viral hepatitis, the SGPT elevation is higher and persists longer than the SGOT elevation (Koff, 1978).

In Question 2 (Hyperbilirubinemia and/or Cholestasis?), *hyperbilirubinemia* refers to an elevated bilirubin; the literal meaning of *cholestasis* is stoppage of bile. In this question we use cholestasis to refer to elevated serum bile acids, alkaline phosphatase (ALP), GGT, and 5′-nucleotidase with or without hyperbilirubinemia. Although not commonly measured, elevation of bile acids is invariably present in cholestasis (Kaplowitz, 1978). Question 2 can be answered by means of the following tests:

1. ALP.

2. GGT.

3. 5′-Nucleotidase.

4. Bile acids.

5. Total bilirubin.

6. Direct bilirubin.

Serum GGT testing tends to be underused.

It has the following benefits (Gambino, 1979*a;* Noll, 1978):

1. It is a sensitive indicator for detecting cholestasis.

2. It is a sensitive indicator of liver metastases.

3. It is a sensitive screening test for alcohol abuse.

4. It is useful for discriminating between an elevation of serum ALP of liver disease and an elevation of serum ALP of bone disease.

5. It is more specific than serum ALP or SGOT for liver disease.

After the first 3 months of age (when it is elevated), the serum GGT level falls into the adult range. Unlike the ALP level, GGT concentrations are not elevated during the period of bone growth. This suggests that measurement of serum GGT may be of value in the evaluation of hepatobiliary disease in children (Shore et al., 1975).

Serum GGT elevation can occur in the absence of any other pathologic findings or test results. In this situation, a history of ethanol ingestion or medications, particularly anticonvulsants, phenobarbital, or phenytoin, should be searched for. Statland (1982) uses the presence of an elevated serum ALP to distinguish an elevated GGT level secondary to hepatobiliary disease from an elevated GGT secondary to drug ingestion. An elevation of serum ALP is not as sensitive a test as an elevation of GGT for hepatobiliary disease, but it is more specific. A patient with an unexplained isolated elevation of serum GGT should be followed with serial determinations. If the elevation persists after 6 months, further studies should be considered (e.g., evaluation for "silent" gallstones). Serum GGT can be elevated in pancreatic disease, myocardial infarction, diabetes mellitus, and hypertriglyceridemia (Noll, 1978).

Serum from healthy individuals contains no conjugated bilirubin whatsoever. Routine measurements of serum conjugated bilirubin give an upper reference limit, (e.g., 0.2 mg/ 100 ml). This is due to technical problems with routine measurements that remain to be solved. Elevation of serum conjugated bilirubin, even in the presence of a normal total bilirubin, is a sensitive indicator of liver disease (Blanckaert, 1980; Blanckaert et al., 1980; Gambino, 1980).

As a general principle, if the serum liver

ALP or direct bilirubin, or both are elevated secondary to cholestasis, the serum GGT, and bile acids will be elevated.

Question 3 (Metabolic Derangement?) can be answered by the following serum and plasma tests:

1. Total protein.
2. Albumin.
3. Serum protein electrophoresis (SPE).
4. Prothrombin time (PT).
5. Partial thromboplastin time (PTT).
6. Glucose.
7. Cholinesterase.
8. Serum urea nitrogen (SUN).
9. Ammonia.

Serum albumin, cholinesterase, the PT, and PTT measure the liver's ability to synthesize proteins. Glucose measures its ability to store glycogen, whereas SUN and ammonia measure its excretory functions (an elevated cerebrospinal fluid glutamine has the same significance as an elevated plasma ammonia).

Question 4 (Acute versus Chronic Disease?) can be answered by the following serum tests:

1. Globulins (total protein minus albumin).
2. SPE.
3. Quantitative measurement of individual immunoglobulins.

Chronic disease is often manifested by elevation of gamma globulins and depression of albumin. Prolongation of the PT and PTT may also occur in chronic disease.

We prefer to measure serum albumin and globulins by electrophoresis. This not only overcomes the problem of overestimation of serum albumin by dye-binding methods (Speicher et al., 1978) but also increases the information content of the globulins by differentiating them into individual fractions. For instance, the beta-gamma bridging of cirrhosis would be detected only by electrophoresis. The serum flocculation tests (thymol turbidity and cephalin flocculation) are obsolete, non-specific indicators of liver injury (Burke, 1975) and should be discarded.

Measuring excretion of foreign dyes, such as rose bengal, Bromsulphalein (BSP), and indocyanine green, has been used to detect liver disease (Brody and Leichter, 1979). BSP has been the most widely used. Measurement of BSP excretion is an extremely sensitive test of liver disease because most kinds of liver disease, with few exceptions, are characterized by compromised excretion of BSP. Adverse

reactions (local slough at the site of dye extravasation and anaphylaxis) as well as the ability to detect liver disease by other tests have decreased the use of the BSP excretion test.

A practical set of liver function tests using a hepatic panel or profile follows:

1. SGOT.
2. ALP.
3. Total bilirurin.
4. Direct bilirubin.
5. SPE. Total protein and albumin can be substituted, but the information content is not as complete.
6. PT.

Sensitivity for liver disease can be further increased by performance of GGT. SGPT determinations are useful in heart failure with poor cardiac output, in discriminating between alcoholic and viral hepatitis, and in following viral hepatitis. Measuring the PTT can increase the sensitivity for detecting hepatic impairment for synthesizing proteins.

Elevation of serum bile acids is a very sensitive test for liver disease of any kind (Kaplowitz, 1978) and is said to be a more sensitive indicator than standard liver function tests (Demers, 1978; Douglas et al., 1981; *Lancet* editorial, 1982). Two-hour postprandial bile acids may be more sensitive than fasting bile acids. However, SGPT was shown to be a more sensitive indicator than serum bile acids for the detection of carriers of hepatitis virus, non-A, non-B (Mishler et al., 1981).

Patient Preparation. Except for the 2-hour postprandial bile acids test, there are no special preparation requirments for liver function tests. Prolonged fasting (24 to 48 hours) can elevate serum bilirubin one to two times. Consult the laboratory for procedures regarding the 2-hour postprandial bile acids test. (See Part 3 for chemistry and hematology tests.)

Specimen Collection and Handling. A clot tube of blood will suffice for most liver function tests (i.e., tests performed on serum). Blood drawn in a tube containing sodium citrate is necessary for the PT and PTT (i.e., tests performed on plasma). The tube should be completely filled, thoroughly mixed, and promptly delivered to the laboratory. If the patient's hematocrit is over 70 per cent, the PT should be drawn in a tube containing 15 to 20 per cent less anticoagulant than normal (Starr et al., 1977).

Hemolyzed specimens should not be used

for serum SGOT and SGPT measurements because the activities of these enzymes are 15 and 7 times higher, respectively, in erythrocytes than in serum. Serum for bilirubin measurements should be free of lipemia and hemolysis, and it should be shielded from light. (See Part 3.)

Methodology. Serum bile acids are usually measured by radioimmunoassay (RIA). Consult the laboratory for its methodologies, accuracy and precision, reference intervals, and sources of inteference. (See Part 3.)

TEST REQUESTS AND REPORTS

Test Requests

Figure 15–1 shows an example of a hepatic panel, by which tests may be ordered as a group instead of individually. This profile is designed to determine whether or not the liver is diseased, and if it is, to offer clues concerning which particular variety of disease is present. Henry and Howanitz (1980) described the rationale for this panel as follows:

The SGOT is the most sensitive single enzyme assay for assessing hepatic cellular injury. Alkaline phosphatase is useful in determining the degree of hepatobiliary obstruction or interference with bile flow as is gamma glutamyl transpeptidase. Since alcoholism and its related effects constitute the third leading cause of death in the United States today, a special feature of serum gamma glutamyl transpeptidase is its elevation with only mild alcohol intake. Partial thromboplastin time and prothrombin time are both quite useful as a liver function test especially for chronic liver disease, but also valuable as a prerequisite for liver biopsy to assess hemostasis.

Interpretive Reports

Liver function test results may be reported in the form of an interpretive report. This report may contain an interpretive comment, which can increase the relevance of the raw data to the patient's clinical problem; i.e., it can reduce the raw data to information.

HEPATITIS

ACUTE VIRAL HEPATITIS

Definition and Significance

Acute viral hepatitis refers to a clinical episode having begun less than 6 months from the time of diagnosis. It is a systemic viral infection of the body, with primary manifes-

HEPATIC					
SGO Transaminase IU/L	1–39				
Alkaline Phosphatase IU/L	Adult 4–13 Child 13–20				
Bilirubin Total mg/dl	0.1–1.2				
Bilirubin Direct mg/dl	0.0–0.2				
Prothrombin time, sec	9.2–11.2				
Gamma Glutamyl Transpeptidase IU/L	Female 3–55 Male 15–85				
Partial Thrombo- plastin time, sec	15–38				
Total Proteins gm/dl	6.7–8.3				
Albumin gm/dl	3.7–4.9				

Figure 15–1. Hepatic panel. (From Henry JB, Murphy J: Effective utilization of clinical laboratories. In Henry JB (ed): Clinical Diagnosis and Management by Laboratory Methods, ed 16. Philadelphia, WB Saunders Company, 1979, p 2044.)

tations in the liver that can be caused by one of several agents:

1. Hepatitis virus A.
2. Hepatitis virus B.
3. Hepatitis virus non-A, non-B.

It is difficult to distinguish these three varieties of hepatitis from one another on the basis of liver histology because they all show a similar picture of liver cell necrosis and mononuclear inflammation (Bianchi et al., 1971; Phillips and Poucell, 1981).

Acute viral hepatitis is a frequently encountered disease that is significant not only for the morbidity and mortality it causes for individuals but also for the epidemics it causes as it spreads from one patient to another through direct contact or through infected materials. (It should be distinguished from the other varieties of acute hepatitis shown in Table 15–1.) The disease often causes enough morbidity because of fatigue and jaundice to prevent the patient from carrying on at work or at the usual state of activity. A small percentage of cases can be fatal, either in the acute stage as a result of liver failure or in the chronic stage as a result of chronic active hepatitis, cirrhosis, and hepatoma (Fig. 15–2).

Hepatitis A is spread primarily by the fecal-oral route; hepatitis B, by the parenteral route.

Table 15–1. TYPES OF ACUTE HEPATITIS*

Acute Viral Hepatitis
Acute viral hepatitis, type A
Acute viral hepatitis, type B
Acute viral hepatitis, not specifiable as type A or type B

Hepatitis Associated With Systemic Viral and Virus-like Infection
Yellow fever hepatitis
Infectious mononucleosis hepatitis
Cytomegalovirus hepatitis
Human herpesvirus 1 hepatitis
Congenital rubella hepatitis
Coxsackie virus hepatitis
Mumps hepatitis

Alcoholic Hepatitis

Drug-Induced Hepatitis
From toxicity, predictable
From idiosyncrasy, not predictable

Toxic Hepatitis
From chemicals and poisons
From radiation

*Information from Leevy CM, Popper H, Sherlock S (eds): Diseases of the Liver and Biliary Tract. DHEW Publication No. (NIH) 76-725. Washington, DC, US Government Printing Office, 1976, pp 1–9.

Hepatitis B is also a venereal disease, particularly prevalent in male homosexuals. The spread of hepatitis non-A, non-B, is similar to hepatitis B.

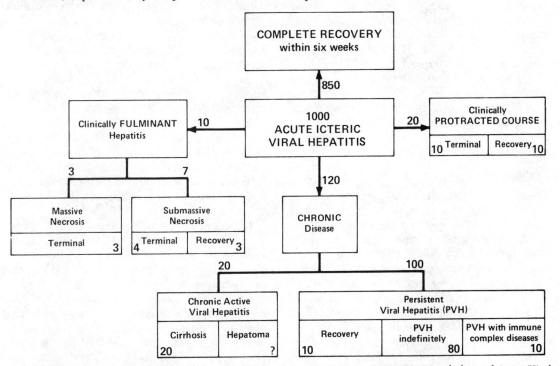

Figure 15–2. Prognosis of acute viral hepatitis in icteric patients. (From Peters RL: Morphology of Acute Viral Hepatitis, Chicago, American Society of Clinical Pathologists, Professional Education Series, 1975, p 11.)

The prevalence of *hepatitis B virus* is approximately 0.5 per cent, as indicated by the presence of hepatitis B surface antigen in the serum of blood donors in the United States. The carrier rate for hepatitis B virus is much higher for patients with a past history of hepatitis, multiple transfusions, parenteral drug abuse, chronic liver disease, chronic renal failure, leukemia, Hodgkin's disease, polyarteritis nodosa, Down's syndrome, leprosy, and male homosexuality.

Acute hepatitis secondary to *hepatitis A virus* is usually a milder disease than that secondary to hepatitis B virus. An antibody to hepatitis A virus is present in the sera of 40 per cent of urban populations and 80 per cent of individuals older than 50 years. Although the presence of this antibody can signal an acute infection, it usually indicates an infection at some time during the past.

Most cases of hepatitis following blood transfusions in the United States are usually, but not necessarily, *hepatitis virus non-A, non-B* in origin (Aach and Kahn, 1980). Other causes of post-transfusion hepatitis include drugs and viral hepatitis not related to transfusions (Schmidt, 1980).

There is no curative therapy for viral hepatitis. Medical care is supportive or preventive. Amelioration of the disease in an exposed person can be obtained through passive immunization, pooled gamma globulin for type A and type non-A, non-B hepatitis, and hepatitis B immune globulin for type B hepatitis. The Food and Drug Administration has licensed a hepatitis B vaccine that was more than 90 per cent effective in preventing infection in a large clinical trial (Szmuness et al., 1980).

Pathophysiology

Acute viral hepatitis is a severe inflammation of the liver that causes necrosis of hepatic cells. It varies in severity depending on the number of liver cells destroyed; i.e., the range extends from a few cells (focal or spotty necrosis) to all cells (massive necrosis). The dying and necrotic cells release their contents into the bloodstream and the serum concentrations of SGOT and SGPT become elevated. The ability to synthesize proteins, as measured by decreased serum albumin and prolonged plasma PT, is only mildly compromised in acute viral hepatitis. A mild, but occasionally severe, cholestatic component (cholestatic hepatitis) can cause elevation of serum bilirubin and ALP. This elevation of serum bilirubin can be further aggravated by impairment of hepatic uptake, conjugation, and excretion of bilirubin as well a mild degree of hemolysis. (See the discussion of cholestasis and hyperbilirubinemia later in this chapter.)

Clinical Contexts

Diagnosis. Clinical features of acute viral hepatitis vary according to several ways in which the disease manifests itself (Jeffries, 1979).

Anicteric Hepatitis. This condition is distinguished by the absence of jaundice. (Levels of serum bilirubin below 2.5 mg/100 ml usually do not produce jaundice.) The symptoms are similar to those of many other viral infections. The diagnosis can be suspected in an epidemic, in patients exposed to known infection, or in patients with tender enlargement of the liver.

Icteric Hepatitis. There are three phases:

1. Patients in the *preicteric phase* show nonspecific constitutional and gastrointestinal symptoms; fever; anorexia; weakness; headache; myalgia; arthralgia; loss of taste for cigarettes; urticarial or erythematous maculopapular rash; enlarged, tender liver; and dark urine (bilirubin).

2. In the *icteric phase,* signs and symptoms include fever, subsiding after onset of jaundice; jaundice maximal in 2 weeks, subsiding to normal in 6 weeks; anorexia, nausea, and vomiting, subsiding after bed rest; increasing right upper-quadrant discomfort; enlarged, tender liver; and palpable spleen.

3. In the *convalescent phase,* recovery takes place as follows: Normal health is regained in weeks to months; variable tiredness and malaise occur; mild hepatic tenderness is present; and symptoms are precipitated by unaccustomed activity.

Cholestatic Hepatitis. Jaundice is more severe and prolonged than in the icteric form. Pruritus is present, and liver enlargement persists during the period of jaundice. Diarrhea may occur.

Fulminant Hepatitis. Features include high fever; severe abdominal pain; vomiting persisting after bed rest; sudden decrease in liver size; hepatic encephalopathy with drowsiness, irritability, insomnia, and confusion; and ascites appearing during the acute illness.

Complications include hypoglycemia, bleeding, pneumonia, septicemia, and renal failure (Blitzer, 1980).

Management. Repeated liver function tests are useful for gauging response to therapy as well as for making a prognosis. In fulminant hepatitis, other laboratory studies may be required to diagnosis and manage hepatic failure, hepatic encephalopathy, bleeding, infection, and renal failure.

Screening. Anicteric hepatitis can be discovered by screening for the presence of serum HBs Ag., e.g., blood donor screening, and by biochemical profiles involving elevated serum transaminases (see Chapter 8).

There is lack of agreement about the usefulness of screening for hepatitis B in populations in which the frequency of hepatitis B is high. These would include patients with a history of parenteral drug abuse, chronic renal failure, leukemia, Hodgkin's disease, polyarteritis nodosa, Down's syndrome, leprosy, and male homosexuality. Screening for the presence of hepatitis B surface antibody is now practiced to determine who should be immunized with hepatitis B vaccine. It is unnecessary to immunize individuals who already have antibody.

Strategy

Test Sequence. Perform liver function tests as described earlier in this chapter, namely SGOT, SGPT, ALP, GGT, bilirubin, SPE, and PT measurements. Viral hepatitis A and B can be confirmed or excluded by measuring appropriate serologic markers. There are no serologic markers available for viral hepatitis non-A, non-B (Overby, 1979).

If viral hepatitis A is clinically suspected, measure hepatitis A antibody (anti-HAV). If anti-HAV is present, it should be fractionated into IgG and IgM components.

If viral hepatitis B is clinically suspected, measure hepatitis B surface antigen (HBsAg), hepatitis B surface antibody (anti-HBs), and hepatitis B core antibody (anti-HBc). Measurements of hepatitis Be antigen (HBeAg) and hepatitis Be antibody (anti-HBe) can provide additional useful information about infectivity and prognosis in patients with acute viral hepatitis B.

Patient Preparation. No special preparation is required. See the discussion of liver function tests early in this chapter and Part 3 for chemistry and hematology tests.

Specimen Collection and Handling. Liver function tests are discussed earlier in this chapter. Specimens for viral markers are collected in a plain clot tube. If the tests are not performed right away, the serum should be separated from the cells and refrigerated. Strict safety precautions should be practiced. (See Part 3.)

Methodology. The most sensitive methods for viral serologic markers employ either RIA or enzyme immunoassay techniques.

Consult the laboratory for methodologies, accuracy and precision, reference intervals, and sources of interference. (See Part 3.)

Interpretation

Diagnosis. Table 15–2 presents liver function test findings and other common laboratory test results in acute hepatitis. These results tend to show transaminase elevations during the end of the preicteric phase, which peak in the icteric phase, and then subside.

Figure 15–3 shows the times of appearance and disappearance of various markers for hepatitis B. Figure 15–4 shows similar data for hepatitis A. Because HBsAg, anti-HBc, and anti-HBs are present at different times, it is necessary to study all three markers to confirm or exclude hepatitis B with confidence.

Because only anti-HAV can be studied in hepatitis A, it is necessary to demonstrate either a rise in titer of IgM-HAV or a rising titer of IgG-HAV to establish a diagnosis of acute hepatitis A. Presence of anti-HAV alone does not establish such a diagnosis because 40 per cent of urban populations and 80 per cent of individuals over 50 years of age have anti-HAV in their sera from a previous infection (Soloway, 1980). Therefore, the predictive value of anti-HAV for acute infection is very low (Bryan, 1980).

Table 15–3 serves as a guide for the interpretation of serologic markers for viral hepatitis (Miller, 1980).

Drugs can cause a hepatitis similar to viral hepatitis and should always be considered in the differential diagnosis (Zimmerman, 1978) (see Part 3).

Hepatitis non-A, non-B is a diagnosis of exclusion for which the various other causes of acute hepatitis listed in Table 15–1 must be ruled out.

Management. In acute viral hepatitis, SGPT levels rise higher than and the elevation persists longer than SGOT levels. Therefore,

Table 15–2. LIVER FUNCTION TESTS IN ACUTE VIRAL HEPATITIS

Question	Test	Result*†
Liver cell injury?	Glutamic oxaloacetic transaminase (SGOT)	500–5000 U/liter (essentially 100%)
	Glutamic pyruvic transaminase (SGPT)	500–5000 U/liter (>SGOT usually) (essentially 100%)
Cholestasis?	Alkaline phosphatase (ALP)	80–240 U/liter (>90%)
	Gamma glutamyl transferase (GGT)	Elevated, 5–10× normal
	Total bilirubin	5–20 mg/100 ml
	Direct bilirubin	Elevated
Metabolic derangement?	Albumin	Normal to slightly depressed
	Prothrombin time (PT)	Normal to slightly prolonged
Chronic disease?	Globulins (total protein minus albumin)	Normal to slightly elevated

In addition, the following common laboratory test results can be outside the reference intervals.
  ↓ Cholesterol (depressed liver synthesis)
  ↓ Glucose (can occur with various types of liver disease)
  ↑ Lactic dehydrogenase (some elevation, but not a very good test for liver disease)
  ↑ Uric acid (can occur. Cause?)
  ↓ Hemoglobin (mild transient anemia can occur)
  ↓ Leukocyte count (mild transient decrease can occur); ↑ in fulminant disease
  ↓ Platelet count (can occur in fulminant disease and be accompanied by anemia and leukocytosis)

*Information from Friedman RB, Anderson RE, Entine SM, et al: Effects of diseases on clinical laboratory tests. Clin Chem 26:1D–476D, 1980; Koff RS: Viral Hepatitis. New York, John Wiley & Sons, 1978; Shearman DJC, Finlayson NDC: Diseases of the Gastrointestinal Tract and Liver. New York, Churchill Livingstone, 1982; Wallach J: Interpretation of Diagnostic Tests: A Handbook Synopsis of Laboratory Medicine, ed 3. Boston, Little, Brown & Company, 1978; and Wallnöfer H, Schmidt E, Schmidt FW (eds): Diagnosis of Liver Disease: An Illustrated Textbook. Stuttgart, Georg Thieme Publishers, 1977.
†Results vary with course and severity.

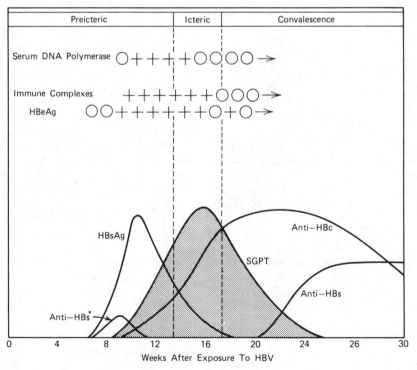

Figure 15–3. Acute hepatitis B, pattern of seroimmunologic alterations in relation to SGPT and presence of serum DNA polymerase and immune complexes. Anti-HBs is present but not detectable as free antibody. (From Koff RS: Viral Hepatitis. New York, John Wiley & Sons, Inc, 1978, p 137. Reprinted by permission.)

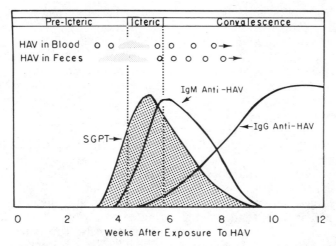

Figure 15–4. Acute hepatitis A, pattern of seroimmunologic alterations in relation to SGPT and presence of virus in blood and feces. (From Koff RS: Viral Hepatitis. New York, John Wiley & Sons, Inc, 1978, p 136. Reprinted by permission.)

SGPT theoretically is a better indicator than SGOT for following the convalescence of patients with acute hepatitis. In practice, however, SGOT measurements are quite adequate as an indicator (Koff, 1978). Isolated unconjugated hyperbilirubinemia without hemolysis is occasionally seen after acute viral hepatitis. Most cases probably represent a previously unrecognized Gilbert's syndrome, although there is a possibility this syndrome may be caused by viral hepatitis (Shearman and Finlayson, 1982).

Clinical findings, liver function tests results, and histologic evidence as to the severity, evolution, and prognosis of viral hepatitis are usually consistent. There may be conflict, however. For example, on occasion the morphologic findings in the liver biopsy indicate disease that is more severe than the clinical and liver function tests show, and vice versa (Bian-

Table 15–3. PRACTICAL GUIDE FOR THE INTERPRETATION OF SEROLOGIC MARKERS OF VIRAL HEPATITIS*

Clinical Interpretation	IgM Anti-HA†	HBsAg	HBeAg	Anti-HBe	Anti-HBc	Anti-HBs
Acute HA	+	−	−	−	−	−
Incubation period or early acute HB	−	+	+	−	−	−
Acute HB	−	+	+	−	+	−
Fulminant HB	−	+	−	−	+	+/−
Convalescence from acute HB	−	−	−	+	+	+/−
Chronic HB	−	+	+/−	+/−	+	+/−
Persistent HB carrier state	−	+	−	+	+	−
Past infection with HB virus	−	−	−	−	+	+
Infection with HB virus without detectable (excess) HBsAg	−	−	−	−	+	−
Immunization without infection	−	−	−	−	−	+
Non-A/non-B hepatitis by exclusion of markers for HA and HB	−	−	−	−	−	−

Key:

Anti-HA = hepatitis A antibody; HBsAg = hepatitis B surface antigen; HBeAg = hepatitis B "e" antigen; anti-HBe = hepatitis B "e" antibody; anti-HBc = hepatitis B core antibody; anti-HBs = hepatitis B surface antibody.

*From Vyas GN, Schmid R: Immunodiagnosis of viral hepatitis. West J Med 133:241–242, 1980.

†Clinically unrecognized infection occurring in childhood accounts for the high incidence of IgG anti-HA antibodies in 80 to 90 per cent of adults in underdeveloped countries as compared with 25 to 50 per cent of adults in Europe and the United States.

chi et al., 1971). The following laboratory findings indicate a poor prognosis:

1. Falling serum transaminases in the face of clinical deterioration.

2. Severely prolonged plasma PT (over 20 seconds with a control of 12 seconds).

3. Serum bilirubin over 20 mg/100 ml in the absence of hemolysis extending and persisting late into the course of the disease. (Bilirubin over 30 mg/100 ml can be seen in hemolytic anemia, such as sickle cell anemia, and in glucose 6-phosphate deficiency and does not necessarily indicate a poorer prognosis.)

4. Marked depression of serum glucose (under 40 mg/100 ml) and/or SUN (under 5 mg/100 ml).

5. Elevated plasma ammonia. See Tygstrup and Ranek (1981) for a discussion of fulminant hepatic failure.

Test Requests and Reports

See the discussion of liver function tests earlier in this chapter for methods of requesting tests and interpretive reporting of test results. Interpretive reports of viral serologic markers may also be accomplished (Soloway, 1980). Figure 15–5 shows an example of an interpretive report for viral markers that was developed by Neff (1981) using an Apple II microcomputer (Apple Computer, Inc., Cupertino, Cal.).

CHRONIC HEPATITIS AND PRIMARY BILIARY CIRRHOSIS

Definition and Significance

Chronic Hepatitis. This is an inflammation of the liver that persists longer than 6 months; i.e., there is deep concern about progression to cirrhosis or liver failure (Czaja and Summerskill, 1978). Liver function test results are outside the reference intervals, and liver histology shows pathologic changes. The patient often shows no clear-cut beginning of the hepatic inflammation as manifested by signs or symptoms of liver disease. Test results that provide the best clue to the presence of chronic hepatitis are elevations of SGOT and SGPT. The pathologic findings in the liver biopsy consist of portal and periportal mononuclear inflammation (lymphocytes, plasma cells, and monocytes) with or without fibrosis and peri-

portal necrosis (piecemeal necrosis) (Phillips and Poucell, 1981).

Chronic hepatitis is of two kinds:

1. *Chronic persistent hepatitis* occurs when chronic inflammation of the liver persists longer than 6 months. Liver function test results are outside the reference intervals, and there is chronic inflammation of the liver portal triads. The portal triads are minimally expanded and scarred, and the chronic inflammation is sharply confined to the portal triads, spilling over little, if at all, into the parenchyma of the liver lobules. Few, if any, liver cells surrounding the portal triad are undergoing necrosis; i.e., there is little, if any, piecemeal necrosis. This is usually a benign condition with a good prognosis.

2. *Chronic active hepatitis* is marked by prolonged inflammation of the liver lasting longer than 6 months. Liver function test results fall outside the reference intervals. The liver shows chronically inflamed portal triads that are expanded and scarred. The chronic inflammation spills out of the portal triads, causing necrosis of adjacent liver cells (piecemeal necrosis). The necrotic liver cells undergo replacement by scar tissue. Chronic active hepatitis can develop into cirrhosis that is usually of the macronodular variety in which nodules can be up to 5 cm in diameter (Bianchi et al., 1977; De Groote, et al., 1968). Hepatoma can be an additional complication.

Chronic active hepatitis has a variety of etiologies:

1. Association with hepatitis B virus.

2. No association with hepatitis B virus (non-A, non-B, and lupoid type).

3. Association with drugs (oxyphenisatin, methyldopa, and isoniazid).

4. Wilson's disease.

5. Deficiency of alpha$_1$-antitrypsin.

Hepatitis A virus is not a cause of chronic active hepatitis.

The histologic appearance of the liver in chronic active hepatitis is sometimes similar to that in primary biliary cirrhosis (Christoffersen et al., 1972). When histologic appearance does not permit differentiation between these two conditions, the discrimination can sometimes be made by a combination of clinical features, liver function test results, and response to corticosteroid therapy.

Primary Biliary Cirrhosis. This is a destructive disease of the larger hepatic ducts. Its cause is unknown. It typically occurs in

General Consultation Request

The Ohio State University Hospitals

To _____IMMUNOLOGY_____ Date _____   DOE, JANE
    (Physician and/or service)   900-01-9109

        ☐ Outpatient   ☐ Inpatient

Provisional Diagnosis:

Reason for Referral:

                HEPATITIS PROFILE TESTING

_____(Use reverse side if necessary)_____**M.D.**

Report and Opinion of Consultant

                                                    Date ____9/10/82_____

        HEPATITIS PROFILE 1.   (DIAGNOSTIC)

        PATIENT I.D.

        NAME DOE, JANE   DATE
        HOSPITAL #   900-01-9109   SPECIMEN # U 2 W

        TEST: TEST RESULTS:

        HBAG (HB-S-AG)   POSITIVE *
        HBCB (HB-C-AB)   POSITIVE *
        HAMB (HA-IGM-AB)   NEGATIVE

        INTERPRETATION:

        SEROLOGICAL EVIDENCE FOR RECENT HEPATITIS-B INFECTION, SUGGEST
        RETEST SPECIMEN IN 10-12 WEEKS FOR ANTIBODY TO HEPATITIS-B
        SURFACE ANTIGEN (HBAB).

_____(Use reverse side if necessary)_____**M.D.**

The Ohio State University
Form 3352-Rev. 6/78
(461001)

1-4 \ \ \ \ \ \ \ \ \ \ \ \ \ \ \ \ \ \ \   **Consults**

Figure 15–5.   Interpretive report. (Courtesy of Ohio State University Hospitals.)

middle-aged women in whom liver function test results indicate cholestasis. (See the discussion of cholestasis and hyperbilirubinemia later in this chapter.) The liver histology shows large intrahepatic ducts undergoing necrosis with granulomatous inflammation. These large liver ducts are best discovered in a wedge biopsy of the liver. They are frequently missed in needle biopsies, and the chronic inflammation in the smaller portal triads can be confused with chronic active hepatitis (Koff, 1978). Patients with primary biliary cirrhosis have altered immunologic responsiveness, which is often associated with various collagen diseases (Schaffner, 1979).

Pathophysiology

Chronic persistent hepatitis is the most common long-term sequela of acute icteric viral hepatitis (Fig. 15–2). It can be associated with a chronic hepatitis B carrier state and is HBsAg-positive in from 20 to 60 per cent of cases. Evidence of chronic hepatitis can remain for months to years, but the condition hardly ever progresses to cirrhosis and requires no treatment.

Chronic active hepatitis results in progressive destruction of periportal liver parenchyma through destruction of liver tissue by mononuclear inflammation originating in the portal triads. This piecemeal necrosis is considered to be the pathogenetic mechanism whereby liver cells are destroyed and replaced by scar tissue. This is a serious disease that can ultimately result in cirrhosis and hepatic failure. The rate of destruction of liver cells is mirrored by elevations of SGOT and SGPT, but quantitative correlations between the number of liver cells undergoing destruction and the level of elevation of the serum transaminases are poor. Depression of serum albumin and prolongation of the plasma PT reflect decreased protein synthesis by the liver. Increased levels of serum globulins indicate chronic inflammation.

Primary biliary cirrhosis can be associated with diseases of immunologic origin (scleroderma, Sjögren's syndrome). Patients have high titers of serum autoantibodies (Schaffner, 1979). Recurrence of primary biliary cirrhosis after liver transplantation has been reported (Neuberger et al., 1982). Septal and interlobular bile ducts are destroyed by a granulomatous inflammatory process.

Four histopathologic stages are recognized:

1. Stage I: Portal hepatitis (destruction of large ducts).
2. Stage II: periportal hepatitis (proliferation of small ducts proximal to the destroyed large ducts).
3. Stage III: Septal fibrosis, bridging necrosis, or both (scarring).
4. Stage IV: Cirrhosis (biliary cirrhosis) (Ludwig et al., 1978).

The destruction of bile ducts causes intrahepatic obstruction with cholestasis and marked elevations of serum ALP, bilirubin, and cholesterol. (See the discussion of cholestasis and hyperbilirubinemia later in this chapter.) Elevated levels of serum autoantibodies are present.

The course of the patient is one of gradual deterioration. Portal hypertension can develop early. The patient usually dies of progressive liver failure with gastrointestinal bleeding and hepatic coma.

Clinical Contexts

Diagnosis

Chronic Active Hepatitis. The clinical spectrum of this disease extends from asymptomatic illness at one end to fatal hepatic failure at the other. It affects all age groups but is more common in young adults and adolescents. Often the onset is insidious over a period of several weeks to months. The disease can be discovered incidentally, in which case the duration of illness is uncertain.

Clinical features include fatigue, jaundice, malaise, anorexia, low-grade fever, and the complications of cirrhosis (Wands, et al., 1980). Extrahepatic findings (more common in women without serologic evidence of hepatitis B) include amenorrhea, bloody diarrhea, abdominal pain, arthralgia and arthritis, macular and papular eruptions, acne, erythema nodosum, pleurisy, pericarditis, anemia, azotemia, and sicca syndrome (keratoconjunctivitis and xerostomia).

Chronic active hepatitis can progress slowly, rapidly, or intermittently. It can also regress. In severe cases, the fatality rate can be high. Death occurs secondary to liver failure and hepatic coma or to other complications of cirrhosis.

The definitive diagnosis is made by histologic findings in the liver. In addition to making the diagnosis, it is imperative to establish its cause if possible.

Chronic Persistent Hepatitis. Patients can

be well or symptomatic. When they are symptomatic, clinical features include malaise, fatigue, decrease of performance, lack of appetite, alcohol intolerance, sensation of pressure and fullness in the abdomen, and rare vascular spiders and palmar erythema (Wallnofer, 1977). The definitive diagnosis is made by liver histology. Table 15–4 contrasts the features of chronic active and chronic persistent hepatitis.

Primary Biliary Cirrhosis. This is a disease of women ranging from 40 to 60 years of age. Symptoms and signs include pruritus, jaundice with dark urine and pale stools, cutaneous xanthomas, often a firm enlarged liver, palpable spleen, weight loss, diarrhea, bleeding, pathologic fractures, and terminal hepatocellular failure (Jeffries, 1979).

In addition to differentiation from chronic active hepatitis, primary biliary cirrhosis must be distinguished from stenosing cholangitis and from bile duct obstruction resulting from stone, stricture, or carcinoma. The definitive diagnosis is made by liver histology if possible. Otherwise, it is made by a combination of clinical features, laboratory studies, and response to corticosteroid therapy.

Management. Although the progress of chronic hepatitis and primary biliary cirrhosis

Table 15–4. DISTINGUISHING FEATURES OF CHRONIC ACTIVE AND CHRONIC PERSISTENT HEPATITIS*

Features	Chronic Active Hepatitis	Chronic Persistent Hepatitis
Clinical		
Onset like acute viral hepatitis	30%	70%
Recurrent acute episodes	Common	Infrequent
Extrahepatic involvement (e.g., arthralgias, pleuritis, colitis)	Common	Rare
Prognosis	Variable	Good
Liver histology		
Piecemeal necrosis	Characteristic	Inconstant
Site of inflammation	Portal, extending into lobule	Portal
Lobular architecture	Distorted	Preserved
Fibrosis	Common	Slight
Progression to cirrhosis	Common	Rare

*From Wands JR, Koff RS, Isselbacher KJ: Chronic active hepatitis. In Harrison's Principles of Internal Medicine, ed 9. Copyright © 1980 by McGraw-Hill, Inc. Used by permission of McGraw-Hill Book Company, New York, p 1470.

can be followed by liver function tests, serial liver biopsies are the best method of evaluating the evolution of these diseases.

Screening. Screening programs for chronic hepatitis and primary biliary cirrhosis are not indicated in the absence of clinical features. Clues to the presence of these diseases can be obtained, however, during screening for other purposes, such as hepatitis B screening or biochemical profiles.

Strategy

Test Sequence. Perform liver function tests using serum as described previously, namely, SGOT, SGPT, ALP, GGT, bilirubin, SPE, and PT measurements. When considering primary biliary cirrhosis, study the following autoantibodies: antismooth muscle, antimitochondrial, and antinuclear antibody (ANA). In chronic active hepatitis not due to hepatitis B, consider laboratory studies for Wilson's disease and alpha$_1$-antitrypsin deficiency. (See Chapter 17 for a discussion of alpha$_1$-antitrypsin deficiency and Wilson's disease.)

Patient Preparation. No special preparation is required. (See the discussion of liver function tests early in this chapter and Part 3 for chemistry and hematology tests.)

Specimen Collection and Handling. Collect specimens for autoantibody studies in a plain clot tube. Promptly separate the serum and refrigerate it immediately. (See the first part of this chapter for comments regarding liver function tests and Part 3.)

Methodology. Consult the laboratory for its methodologies, accuracy and precision, reference intervals, and sources of interference. Autoantibody studies are measured using tissue antigens and fluorescent markers. In testing for antimitochondrial antibodies, reagent variables can lead to diagnostic error (Winter et al., 1979). (See Part 3.)

Interpretation

Diagnosis. Table 15–5 gives the pattern of liver function test findings and other common laboratory results in chronic persistent hepatitis, Table 15–6 in chronic active hepatitis, and Table 15–7 in primary biliary cirrhosis. Table 15–8 contrasts the prevalence of autoantibodies for these three varieties of chronic liver disease. The presence of antimitochondrial antibodies is especially confirmatory in the diagnosis of primary biliary cirrhosis. About 90 per

Table 15–5. LIVER FUNCTION TESTS IN CHRONIC PERSISTENT HEPATITIS

Question	Test	Result*†
Liver cell injury?	Glutamic oxaloacetic transaminase (SGOT)	Normal to moderatly elevated
	Glutamic pyruvic transaminase (SGPT)	Normal to moderately elevated
Cholestasis?	Alkaline phosphatase (ALP)	Normal to slightly elevated
	Gamma glutamyl transferase (GGT)	Normal to moderately elevated
	Total bilirubin	Normal to slightly elevated
	Direct bilirubin	Normal to slightly elevated
Metabolic derangement?	Albumin	Usually normal
	Prothrombin time (PT)	Usually normal
Chronic disease?	Globulins (total protein minus albumin)	Normal to slightly increased

*Information from Koff RS: Viral hepatitis. New York, John Wiley & Sons, 1978; Shearman DJC, Finlayson NDC: Diseases of the Gastrointestinal Tract and Liver. New York, Churchill Livingstone, 1982; Wallach J: Interpretation of Diagnostic Tests: A Handbook Synopsis of Laboratory Medicine, ed. 3. Boston, Little, Brown & Company, 1978; and Wallnöfer H, Schmidt E, Schmidt FW (eds): Diagnosis of Liver Disease: An Illustrated Textbook. Stuttgart, Georg Thieme Publishers, 1977.
†Results vary with course and severity.

cent of patients with primary biliary cirrhosis will have positive reactions; therefore, the absence of these antibodies helps exclude the diagnosis. Titers over 1:160 are generally limited to primary biliary cirrhosis; titers are rarely greater than 1:40 in chronic active hepatitis (Czaja, 1981).

A needle biopsy of the liver is diagnostic for chronic active and chronic persistent hepatitis, but a single needle biopsy can miss the classic granulomatous inflammation of the larger bile ducts in primary biliary cirrhosis because of sampling error. A therapeutic trial for 6

months with corticosteroids can be helpful in distinguishing chronic active hepatitis from primary biliary cirrhosis; chronic active hepatitis responds, but primary biliary cirrhosis does not (Czaja, 1981).

If a diagnosis of chronic persistent hepatitis is made, serologic markers for hepatitis B should be studied. (See the subproblem of acute hepatitis earlier in this chapter for interpretation of these markers.) If a diagnosis of chronic active hepatitis is made, an etiology should be sought, namely, hepatitis B, non-A, non-B-hepatitis, or lupoid hepatitis; drug-as-

Table 15–6. LIVER FUNCTION TESTS IN CHRONIC ACTIVE HEPATITIS

Question	Test	Result*†
Liver cell injury?	Glutamic oxaloacetic transaminase (SGOT)	100–1000 U/liter (95–100%)
	Glutamic pyruvic transaminase (SGPT)	100–1000 U/liter (95–100%)
Cholestasis?	Alkaline phosphatase (ALP)	Slightly elevated (90%)
	Gamma glutamyl transferase (GGT)	Invariably elevated
	Total bilirubin	Elevated, 3–10 mg/100 mg (90%)
	Direct bilirubin	Elevated
Metabolic derangement	Albumin	Depressed (50%)
	Prothrombin time (PT)	Prolonged (50%)
Chronic disease?	Globulins (total protein minus albumin)	Elevated, commonly

In addition, the following common laboratory test results can be outside the reference intervals.*
↓ Glucose (related to destruction of functioning hepatic tissue)
↓ Hemoglobin (mild to moderate anemia common)
↓ Hematocrit (mild to moderate anemia common)
↓ Leukopenia, common
↓ Platelets, common

*Information from Friedman RB, Anderson RE, Entine SM, et al: Effects of diseases on clinical laboratory tests. Clin Chem 26:1D-476D, 1980; Koff RS: Viral Hepatitis. New York, John Wiley & Sons, 1978; Shearman, DJC, Finlayson NDC: Diseases of the Gastrointestinal Tract and Liver. Churchill Livingstone, 1982; Wallach J: Interpretation of Diagnostic Tests: A Handbook Synopsis of Laboratory Medicine, ed. 3. Boston, Little, Brown & Company, 1978; and Wallnöfer H, Schmidt E, Schmidt FW (eds): Diagnosis of Liver Disease: An Illustrated Textbook. Stuttgart, Georg Thieme Publishers, 1977.
†Results vary with course and severity.

Table 15–7. LIVER FUNCTION TESTS IN PRIMARY BILIARY CIRRHOSIS

Question	Test	Result*†
Liver cell injury?	Glutamic oxaloacetic transaminase (SGOT)	Normal to slightly elevated (<200 U/liter)
	Glutamic pyruvic transaminase (SGPT)	Normal to slightly elevated (<200 U/liter)
Cholestasis?	Alkaline phosphatase (ALP)	Markedly elevated as disease progresses (to 20 × normal)
	Gamma glutamyl transferase (GGT)	Markedly elevated
	Total bilirubin	Markedly elevated as disease progresses (to 30 mg/100 ml)
	Direct bilirubin	Elevated
Metabolic derangement?	Albumin	Normal to depressed as disease progresses
	Prothrombin time (PT)	Normal to elevated as disease progresses
Chronic disease?	Globulin (total protein minus albumin)	Normal to elevated as disease progresses

In addition, the following common laboratory test results can be outside the reference intervals:*
↑ Cholesterol (moderate to marked increase of cholesterol and phospholipids with normal triglycerides)
↓ Glucose (related to destruction of functioning liver tissue)
↓ Sodium (frequently found, especially in patients with ascites)
↓ Uric acid (cause?)

*Information from Friedman RB, Anderson RE, Entine SM, et al: Effects of diseases on clinical laboratory tests. Clin Chem 26:1D–476D, 1980; Shearman DJC, Finalyson NDC: Diseases of the Gastrointestinal Tract and Liver. New York, Churchill Livingstone, 1982; Wallach J: Interpretation of Diagnostic Tests: A Handbook Synopsis of Laboratory Medicine, ed. 3. Boston, Little, Brown & Company, 1978; Wallnöffer H, Schmidt E, Schmidt FW (eds): Diagnosis of Liver Disease: An Illustrated Textbook. Stuttgart, Georg Thieme Publishers, 1977; and Wolf PL: V Clinical significance of an increased or decreased serum alkaline phosphatase level. Arch Pathol Lab Med 102:497–501, 1978.
†Results vary with course and severity.

sociated hepatitis (Zimmerman, 1978); alpha₁-antitrypsin deficiency; or Wilson's disease. (See Chapter 17.)

Management. Liver function tests and serologic studies are not completely reliable for following the course and prognosis of chronic liver disease but can be useful in following response to therapy. Liver biopsy is the definitive yardstick by which the course of these diseases is measured. Serum levels of bile acids provide a more sensitive indication of active hepatitis than conventional liver function tests (Czaja, 1981; Korman et al., 1974).

In a review of chronic active hepatitis by Czaja et al., (1981), SGOT values were more predictive of histologic findings than gamma globulin levels, correctly reflecting morphologic status in 67 per cent of patients during treatment and 80 per cent after treatment. SGOT elevations of more than twice normal during and after therapy were reliably associated with chronic active liver disease. However, after therapy only 56 per cent of patients with recurring histologic activity had SGOT levels greater than twice normal and 19 per cent had normal levels. Patients who had sustained elevation of SGOT to at least ten-fold normal or five-fold increases in conjunction with at least twice-normal serum globulin concentrations usually died within 3 years if left untreated (Czaja, 1981).

The usefulness of certain physical and labo-

Table 15–8. PREVALENCE OF AUTOANTIBODIES IN CHRONIC PERSISTENT HEPATITIS, CHRONIC ACTIVE HEPATITIS, AND PRIMARY BILIARY CIRRHOSIS*

	Antismooth Muscle Antibody†	Antimitochondrial Antibody†	Antinuclear Antibody†
Chronic persistent hepatitis	Negative	Negative	Negative
Chronic active hepatitis	60–90%	20–60%	20–60%
Primary biliary cirrhosis	10–50%	80–100%†	25%

*Information from Friedman RB, Anderson RE, Entine SM, et al: Effects of diseases on clinical laboratory tests. Clin Chem 26:1D–476D, 1980; Wallach J: Interpretation of Diagnostic Tests: A Handbook Synopsis of Laboratory Medicine. Boston, Little, Brown & Company, 1978; Wyngaarden JB, Smith LH (ed): Cecil Textbook of Medicine, ed 16. Philadelphia, WB Saunders Company, 1982.
†Autoantibodies are sometimes found in patients with acute viral hepatitis, extrahepatic obstruction, and cryptogenic cirrhosis. They are unusual in patients with alcoholic hepatitis and alcoholic cirrhosis.

ratory findings in predicting the morphologic diagnosis of cirrhosis in severe chronic active liver disease was determined in 101 patients, 39 of whom had cirrhosis (Czaja et al., 1980). Hypoalbuminemia (found in 69 per cent) and hypergammaglobulinemia (found in 67 per cent) had the greatest diagnostic sensitivity for cirrhosis, but they lacked specificity. The predictive value of thrombocytopenia with either hepatic encephalopathy, or ascites for cirrhosis is 85 per cent. However, only 56 per cent of cirrhotics have this combination of findings. Therefore, the definitive diagnosis of cirrhosis is by histologic features. Because of sampling variability, macronodular cirrhosis can be reliably excluded only after three successive liver biopsies (Czaja et al., 1980).

Test Requests and Reports. See the first part of this chapter for methods of requesting liver function tests and interpretive reporting of test results.

CIRRHOSIS

Definition and Significance

The term *cirrhosis*, as commonly used, means liver sclerosis or scarring. Cirrhosis is a diffuse process characterized by fibrosis and the conversion of normal liver architecture into structurally abnormal nodules. It causes significant morbidity and mortality by means of liver cell failure and portal hypertension. In the United States, cirrhosis is the fifth most common cause of death and the third leading cause of all deaths in the age group 25 to 65 years. Cirrhosis has a variety of etiologies (O'Brien and Gottlieb, 1979):

1. Association with alcohol abuse (Laennec's, portal, nutritional, alcoholic)—30 to 60 per cent.
2. Pigment (metabolic)
   a. Associated with hemochromatosis (pigment cirrhosis)—2 to 5 per cent.
   b. Associated with Wilson's disease—rare.
3. Postnecrotic—10 to 30 per cent.
4. Biliary (primary and secondary)—10 to 20 per cent.
5. Miscellaneous and cryptogenic forms—15 to 25 per cent.

A morphologic classification of cirrhosis that can serve as a preliminary step toward an etiologic classification follows (O'Brien, 1979):

1. Micronodular cirrhosis (nodules less than 1.0 cm in diameter).

2. Macronodular cirrhosis (nodules up to 5 cm in diameter).
3. Mixed micro- and macronodular cirrhosis as well as incomplete septal cirrhosis in which nodules are not well formed.

Cirrhosis associated with alcohol abuse is usually micronodular. Postnecrotic cirrhosis and the cirrhosis associated with Wilson's disease are usually macronodular. Postnecrotic cirrhosis often results from chronic hepatitis. Cryptogenic cirrhosis has no discernible cause.

A definitive diagnosis of cirrhosis is made by liver biopsy.

Pathophysiology

The pathophysiology of cirrhosis as it relates to liver function tests is concerned with several processes, namely, ongoing liver cell destruction, mild biliary tract obstruction, decreasing synthetic and metabolic function, and chronic inflammation and scarring with accompanying hemodynamic alterations (Galambos, 1979).

Ongoing liver cell destruction is secondary to the etiologic agent causing the cirrhosis. The rate of destruction can vary. For instance, the destruction in alcoholic cirrhosis can vary with alcohol intake and is reflected by elevations of SGOT and SGPT. Fatty liver and alcoholic hepatitis can be due to alcohol abuse, and the latter is related to the development of cirrhosis. Pressure on bile ducts and structural changes of the liver cells can be associated with slight to moderate elevations of serum ALP and bilirubin (Baptista et al., 1981).

As the functional mass of liver cells decreases, the ability to synthesize protein is diminished, resulting in a depressed serum albumin and a prolonged plasma PT. Terminal liver failure is marked by inability to eliminate ammonia with elevation of blood ammonia, low SUN, and hypoglycemia.

Chronic inflammation is usually accompanied by increased serum globulins. Scarring and regenerative nodules can result in portal hypertension with ascites, formation of collateral venous channels, and splenomegaly.

Clinical Contexts

Diagnosis. Cirrhosis can develop suddenly or insidiously. Signs and symptoms include anorexia, fatigue, weakness, jaundice, ascites, peripheral edema, enlarged or shrunken nontender liver, splenomegaly, spider angiomas, palmar erythema, bleeding esophageal varices, and coma. These clinical features, together with appropriate liver function tests, radiologic studies, liver biopsy, and other procedures, confirm or exclude a diagnosis of cirrhosis.

Management. The course of cirrhosis can be followed by liver function tests. Serum transaminases are not very helpful and vary from normal to slightly elevated. Progressive decompensation is often indicated by a falling serum albumin level, hyperbilirubinemia, and a lengthening plasma PT. Serial liver biopsies are the definitive measure of whether the cirrhosis is static or progressive.

Screening. In the absence of clinical findings, laboratory tests to screen for cirrhosis are not ordinarily used. However, a depressed serum albumin level detected by a biochemical profile can be the first clue to the presence of an unsuspected cirrhosis.

Strategy

Test Sequence. The strategy of using liver function tests for the diagnosis and manage-ment of micronodular and macronodular cirrhosis is similar to that for acute hepatitis, namely, SGOT, SGPT, ALP, GGT, bilirubin, SPE, and PT measurements. These tests may have to be supplemented by radiologic studies, liver biopsy, and other procedures.

Patient Preparation. No special preparation is required for liver function tests. (See the discussion of liver function tests early in this chapter and Part 3 for chemistry and hematology tests.)

Specimen Collection and Handling. See the first part of this chapter for comments regarding liver function tests. (See Part 3.)

Methodology. Consult the laboratory for its methodologies, accuracy and precision, reference intervals, and sources of interference. (See Part 3.)

Interpretation

Diagnosis. Table 15–9 gives the pattern of liver function tests in cirrhosis. The pattern is essentially the same for both micronodular and macronodular varieties. Liver function test re-

Table 15–9. LIVER FUNCTION TESTS IN CIRRHOSIS

Question	Test	Result*†
Liver cell injury?	Glutamic oxaloacetic transaminase (SGOT)	Normal to slightly elevated (< 300 U/liter (65–75%), but may be higher
	Glutamic pyruvic transaminase (SGPT)	Elevated (< SGOT, usually) (50%)
Cholestasis?	Alkaline phosphatase (ALP)	Normal to slightly elevated 3× upper limit, or (40–50%)
	Gamma glutamyl transferase (GGT)	Often elevated
	Total bilirubin	Normal to slightly elevated
	Direct bilirubin	Normal to slightly elevated (< 50% of total)
Metabolic derangement?	Albumin	Depressed
	Prothrombin time (PT)	Prolonged
Chronic disease?	Globulins (total protein minus albumin)	Elevated

In addition, the following common laboratory test results can be outside the reference intervals.*
  ↓ Calcium (related to decreased albumin)
  ↓ Cholesterol (can be significantly reduced)
  ↓ Glucose (related to destruction of functioning liver), or ↑ (increased prevalence of diabetes mellitus)
  ↑ Lactic dehydrogenase (slight increase can occur)
  ↓ Potassium (frequent in patients with ascites and edema)
  ↓ Sodium (especially in patients with ascites)
  ↑ Urea nitrogen (with gastrointestinal hemorrhage)
  ↓ Urea nitrogen (can occur with liver disease)
  ↑ Uric acid, or ↓ (cause?)
  ↓ Hemoglobin (approximately 75% of chronic liver disease patients have anemia, usually mild)
  ↓ Hematocrit (approximately 75% of chronic liver disease patients have anemia, usually mild)
  ↓ Leukocytes (related to hypersplenism), or ↑ (with necrosis or hemorrhage)
  ↓ Platelets (related to hypersplenism or may have findings compatible with intravascular coagulation), or ↑ (cause?)

*Information from Friedman RB, Anderson RE, Entine SM, et al: Effects of disease on clinical laboratory tests. Clin Chem 26:1D–476D, 1980; Shearman DJC, Finlayson NDC: Diseases of the Gastrointestinal Tract and Liver. New York, Churchill Livingstone, 1982; Wallach J: Interpretation of Diagnostic Tests: A Handbook Synopsis of Laboratory Medicine, ed 3. Boston, Little, Brown & Company, 1978; and Wallnöfer H, Schmidt E, Schmidt FW (eds): Diagnosis of Liver Disease: An Illustrated Textbook. Stuttgart, Georg Thieme Publishers, 1977.
  †Results vary with course and severity.

sults in fatty liver may be normal except for an elevated serum GGT and minor increases of serum transaminases and alkaline phosphatase. Liver function test results in alcoholic hepatitis may be similar to those in cirrhosis. In more acute instances of alcoholic hepatitis the evidence for metabolic derangement and chronic disease may be slight, and alcoholic hepatitis must be distuiguished from acute viral hepatitis. In alcoholic hepatitis the transaminases are usually below 200 U/l, and only rarely above 500 U/l, and the SGOT is higher than the SGPT (Shearman and Finlayson, 1982).

A needle biopsy of the liver is diagnostic for micronodular cirrhosis. Because a single needle biopsy can miss the morphologic diagnosis of macronodular cirrhosis, three separate biopsies may be necessary to rule out macronodular cirrhosis with confidence (Czaja et al., 1980). This is because the needle can puncture the center of a large macronodule in which the histology does not show cirrhosis.

The diagnosis of *micronodular cirrhosis* by needle biopsy does not necessarily establish the etiology. For example, a history of alcoholism is necessary to establish a diagnosis of alcoholic micronodular cirrhosis, and the finding of alcoholic hyaline on histologic examination is helpful. Similarly, excessive iron storage in liver cells is suggestive of cirrhosis associated with hemochromatosis.

The diagnosis of *macronodular cirrhosis* by needle biopsy does not establish the etiology, which can be any of those diseases that cause chronic active hepatitis:

1. Association with hepatitis B (Phillips and Poucell, 1981).

2. No association with hepatitis B, e.g., lupoid type.

3. Association with drugs (oxyphenisatin, methyldopa, and isoniazid) (Zimmerman, 1978).

4. Alpha$_1$-antitrypsin deficiency. (See Chapter 17.)

5. Wilson's disease. (See Chapter 17.)

Management. Liver function tests can be useful in following the natural course and occurrence of complications in cirrhosis. An acute severe impairment of the blood supply of the liver in a cirrhotic patient, such as that which occurs in portal vein thrombosis, is associated with the following findings:

1. A dramatic rise in serum transaminases and LDH (up to several thousand units per liter).

2. A rise in serum ALP and GGT, but not as high as transaminases.

3. Lengthening of plasma PT.

4. Leukocytosis.

With portal hypertension, portal vein thrombosis, and decreased clotting factors, the risk of upper gastrointestinal tract hemorrhage is great.

Other studies that indicate metabolic failure of the liver include the following:

1. Elevated plasma ammonia ($>$ 120 μg/100 ml or 67 μmol/liter).

2. Depressed serum glucose ($<$ 40 mg/100 ml).

3. Depressed SUN ($<$ 5 mg/100 ml). (Gastrointestinal hemorrhage or renal failure can elevate SUN.)

Test Requests and Reports

See the first part of this chapter for methods of requesting liver function tests and interpretive reporting of test results.

OBSTRUCTIVE LIVER DISEASE

CHOLESTASIS AND HYPERBILIRUBINEMIA

Definition and Significance

Cholestasis refers to disorders that impair bile formation or bile flow. Various products that are usually excreted in the bile accumulate, and serum levels of bile acids, GGT, ALP, and 5'-nucleotidase become elevated. Hyperbilirubinemia and jaundice may also occur. Cholestasis does not include prehepatic (hemolytic) jaundice, nor does it include jaundice resulting from disorders of bilirubin uptake, conjugation, storage, and excretion, i.e., Gilbert's syndrome, Crigler-Najjar syndrome, Rotor's syndrome, Dubin-Johnson syndrome (Javitt, 1979; Kaplowitz, 1978). Not all patients with cholestasis are jaundiced, and not all jaundiced patients have cholestasis.

Cholestasis can provide a clue to the following types of conditions (Fig. 15–6):

1. Intrahepatic diseases that are mainly hepatocellular (e.g., acute viral hepatitis).

2. Intrahepatic diseases that are cholestatic and hepatocellular (e.g., cirrhosis).

3. Intrahepatic diseases that are mainly cholestatic (e.g., drug effect).

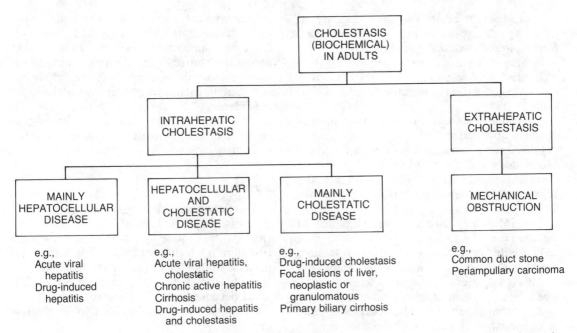

Figure 15–6. Profile of cholestasis. This condition is manifested by elevated serum bile acids, gamma glutamyl transferase, alkaline phosphatase, and 5'-nucleotidase.

4. Extrahepatic diseases that are due to mechanical obstruction (e.g., common duct stone).

Cholestasis is a common and often serious problem. The decision for surgical therapy depends on the correct diagnosis of an extrahepatic cause. Frequently, a clear-cut diagnosis cannot be made on the basis of history, physical, and laboratory studies but must take advantage of other techniques, such as ultrasonography, computed tomographic (CT) scan, and endoscopic retrograde cholangiography (ERCP) (Cello, 1982). Some varieties of cholestasis, such as intrahepatic obstruction resulting from cholestatic viral hepatitis, respond poorly to surgery (Kaplowitz, 1978).

Pathophysiology

The pathophysiology of cholestasis is complex and not completely understood (Erlinger, 1978). Although serum bile acids are elevated in virtually all liver diseases, they are always elevated in cholestasis (Kaplowitz, 1978). Primary cholestasis, such as primary biliary cirrhosis, is characterized by a cholic acid–chenodeoxycholic acid ratio of greater than 1; in

hepatocellular diseases such as cirrhosis and chronic hepatitis, the ratio is less than 1 (Demers, 1978). Although jaundice is not an essential component of cholestasis, an elevation of serum GGT and ALP usually is.

Clinical Contexts

Diagnosis. Disorders characterized by clinical cholestasis can be suggested by pruritus with or without jaundice. Xanthoma, xanthelasma, and hyperpigmentation can also be observed but usually only after cholestasis has persisted for some time. Cholestasis can exist without any of these symptoms and signs, but if it does, it is much less likely to become clinically apparent (Kaplowitz, 1978).

These diseases and disorders may be accompanied by evidence of chemical cholestasis, such as elevated levels of bile acids, ALP, and GGT. Cholestasis can be present in the absence of jaundice or pruritus, e.g., detection of an elevated level of serum ALP (see Chapter 9) or serum GGT by a biochemical profile. Though measurements are not frequently performed, elevation of serum bile acids is an essential component of chemical cholestasis.

Cholestasis in adults can be secondary to either an *intrahepatic* or *extrahepatic* etiology. *Intrahepatic cholestasis* is of three kinds:

1. Mainly hepatocellular.
2. Mainly cholestatic.
3. A combination of hepatocellular and cholestatic.

Extrahepatic cholestasis is secondary to mechanical obstruction.

Drugs are a common cause of intrahepatic cholestasis, and a meticulous history of drug ingestion should be obtained whenever the possibility of cholestasis exists (Bianchi et al., 1974).

The following disorders are examples of intrahepatic cholestasis:

1. Acute viral hepatitis—which is mainly hepatocellular but may have a significant cholestatic component. Its clinical features have been described earlier in this chapter.
2. Chronic hepatitis and cirrhosis—both have hepatocellular and cholestatic components. Their clinical features have been described.
3. Primary biliary cirrhosis—mainly cholestatic. Its clinical features have been described.
4. Metastatic malignancy—mainly cholestatic. Clinical features include symptoms of a primary tumor with asymptomatic hepatic involvement; non-specific symptoms of weakness, weight loss, fever, sweating, and loss of appetite; and evidence of widespread clinical cancer with features of active hepatic disease, such as abdominal pain, hepatomegaly, ascites, jaundice, portal hypertension, friction rub, and tenderness of the liver.
5. Infiltration of the liver by a granulomatous process or other space-occupying lesions—mainly cholestatic. It is often not accompanied by dramatic features of liver disease. The findings can be limited to hepatomegaly and abnormal liver function tests. Needle biopsy of the liver is helpful. In patients with sarcoidosis who have no clinical or laboratory evidence of liver disease, the biopsy is positive in about 80 per cent of cases. Some patients with other focal lesions of the liver, such as hemangioma or adenoma, can be entirely asymptomatic.

Extrahepatic cholestasis can be virtually asymptomatic, such as periampullary carcinoma, or it can present with dramatic symptoms, such as excruciating pain caused by a stone in the common bile duct.

Management. Liver function tests, especially determinations of serum ALP, bile acids GGT, and sometimes bilirubin, can be used to follow the course of intrahepatic and extrahepatic cholestasis. Occasionally, these studies will contain useful prognostic information.

Screening. Screening for cholestasis by laboratory studies in the absence of clinical features of disease (pruritus or jaundice) is not ordinarily indicated.

Strategy

Test Sequence. Perform liver function tests by measuring SGOT, SGPT, ALP, GGT, bilirubin, SPE, and PT. Cholestasis presents a situation in which a serum GGT is very useful because of its greater sensitivity for cholestatic liver disease. If possible, measure serum bile acids because their elevation is the most sensitive single test available for cholestatic liver disease.

Fischer and colleagues (1981) described an algorithmic approach to cholestatic jaundice in adults. The point of departure was a patient who has cholestatic jaundice as evidenced by conjugated hyperbilirubinemia, a serum ALP greater than three times the upper reference limit, pruritus, and a serum bilirubin greater than 3.0 mg/100 ml that is persistent or rising.

Cello (1982) outlined a diagnostic approach to the jaundiced patient. In addition to laboratory tests, the algorithmic approach uses plain film of the abdomen, ultrasonography or CT scan, radionuclide scan, ERCP, oral cholecystography, liver biopsy, transhepatic cholangiography, surgery, and intraoperative cholangiography.

Patient Preparation. No special preparation is required for liver function tests. (See the discussion earlier in this chapter and Part 3 for chemistry and hematology tests.) Consult the laboratory for details of a 2-hour postprandial bile acids measurement. Some laboratories prescribe a fast of 8 hours followed by a test meal of specific composition.

Specimen Collection and Handling. Serum for measurement of bile acids should be promptly separated and refrigerated until the test is performed. (See the discussion of laboratory studies in liver disease earlier in this chapter.)

Methodology. Consult the laboratory for its methodologies, accuracy and precision, ref-

Table 15–10. LIVER FUNCTION TESTS IN CHOLESTASIS
(NO SIGNIFICANT HEPATOCELLULAR COMPONENT)

Question	Test	Result*† (varies with course and severity)
Liver cell injury?	Glutamic oxaloacetic transaminase (SGOT)	Normal to elevated (to 10× normal)
	Glutamic pyruvic transaminase (SGPT)	Normal to elevated (to 10× normal)
Cholestasis?	Alkaline phosphatase (ALP)	Elevated (to 20× normal)
	Gamma glutamyl transferase (GGT)	Elevated
	Total bilirubin	Usually elevated (to 20× normal)
	Direct bilirubin	Elevated
Metabolic derangement?	Albumin	Normal to depressed
	Prothrombin time (PT)	Normal to prolonged
Chronic disease?	Globulins	Normal to increased
In addition, serum cholesterol can be increased in relation to decreased excretion.		

*Information from Cello JP: Diagnostic approaches to jaundice. Hospital Practice, February, 1982, Wolf, PL: Clinical significance of an increased or decreased alkaline phosphatase level. Arch Pathol Lab Med 102:497–501, 1978.
†Results vary with course and severity.

erence intervals, and sources of interference. The measurement of bile acids is usually performed by RIA.

Interpretation

Diagnosis. Table 15–10 gives the general pattern of liver function test results in cholestasis. This pattern is similar for both intrahepatic and extrahepatic causes of cholestasis. It is critically important to distinguish those causes requiring surgical therapy from those requiring medical therapy. Hyperbilirubinemia can exist in the absence of cholestasis, such as occurs in Gilbert's syndrome, Crigler-Najjar syndrome, Rotor's syndrome, and the Dubin-Johnson syndrome. Table 15–11 gives the findings for the five most common causes of cholestasis with jaundice. Intrahepatic or extrahepatic cholestasis can cause the problem of the malabsorption syndrome secondary to a deficiency of bile salts in the duodenum (see Chapter 13).

Serum GGT had a sensitivity of 97 per cent

Table 15–11. LABORATORY DIAGNOSIS OF JAUNDICE*

Parameter	Common Bile Duct Stone	Periampullar Carcinoma	Acute Viral Hepatitis	Drug-Induced Cholestasis	Alcoholic Liver Disease
Bilirubin (mg/dl)	0 to >10	>5 to 20	0 to >20	5 to 10	0 to >20
Alkaline phosphatase	Normal to >10 times normal	2 to 10 times normal	Normal to 3 times normal	2 to 10 times normal	<5 times normal
SGOT	Normal to >10 times normal	Normal	10 to 50 times normal	Normal to 5 times normal	<10 times normal
SGPT	Normal to >10 times normal	Normal	10 to 50 times normal	Normal to 5 times normal	<2 times normal
Amylase	Normal to >10 times normal	Normal	Normal	Normal	Normal to slightly increased
Cholesterol	Normal	Normal	Normal	Increased	Normal
White blood cell count	Increased	Normal	Normal	Normal	Increased
Gram-negative sepsis	Common	Rare	No evidence	None	Occasional

*Adapted from Cello JP: Diagnostic approaches to jaundice. Hospital Practice, February 1982, p 53.

for detecting liver metastases and serum ALP a sensitivity of 77 per cent (Kim et al., 1977). Liver function tests should be used to exclude liver metastases (Tempero et al., 1982) and other focal liver lesions, e.g., granulomata.

Drugs can be a cause of cholestasis and should always be considered in the differential diagnosis (Zimmerman, 1978) (see Part 3).

Management. Repeated liver function tests can be helpful in evaluating the severity of cholestasis, in following its natural evolution, and in evaluating its response to therapy.

Test Requests and Reports

See the first portion of this chapter for methods of requesting liver function tests and interpretive reporting of test results. Catrou and associates (1980) developed and evaluated an algorithm for interpreting biochemical profiles showing hyperbilirubinemia to aid in the generation of interpretive comments to accompany the laboratory report.

REFERENCES

Liver Function Tests

Blanckaert N: Analysis of bilirubin mono- and diconjugates. Determination of their relative amounts in biological samples. Biochem 185:115–128, 1980.

Blanckaert N, Kabra PM, Farina FA, et al: Measurement of bilirubin and its monoconjugates and diconjugates in human serum by methanolysis and high-performance liquid chromatography. J Lab Clin Med 96:198–212, 1980.

Brody DH, Leichter L: Clearance tests of liver function. Med Clin North Am 63:621–630, 1979.

Burke MD: Liver function. Hum Pathol 6:273–286, 1975.

Cohen JA, Kaplan MM: Left-sided heart failure presenting as hepatitis. Gastroenterology 74:583–587, 1978.

Demers LM: Serum bile acids in health and hepatobiliary disease. In Demers LM, Shaw LM (eds): Evaluation of Liver Function: A Multifaceted Approach to Clinical Diagnosis. In Demers LM, Shaw LM (eds): Baltimore, Urban and Schwarzenberg, 1978.

Douglas JG, Beckett GJ, Nimmo IA, et al: Clinical value of bile salts in anicteric liver disease. Gut 22:141–148, 1981.

Gambino R: Gamma glutamyl transpeptidase—An underused test. Lab Report for Physicians 1:2–4, 1979a.

Gambino R: Lab rounds. An unexpected elevation of SGPT. Lab Report for Physicians 1:5, 1979b.

Gambino R: Serum bilirubin—II. Elevated conjugated and normal total. Lab Report for Physicians 2:19–22, 1980.

Henry JB, Howanitz PJ: Organ panels and the relationship of the laboratory to the physician. In Jones RJ, Palulonis RM (eds): Laboratory Tests in Medical

Practice. Chicago American Medical Association, 1980, p 42.

Kaplowitz N: Cholestatic liver disease. Hospital Practice, August 1978, pp 83–92.

Koff RS: Viral Hepatitis. New York, John Wiley & Sons, 1978, p 139.

Mishler JM, Barbosa L, Mihalko LJ, et al: Serum bile acids and alanine aminotransferase concentrations: Comparison of efficacy as indirect means of identifying carriers of non-A, non-B hepatitis agents and of onset, severity, and duration of posttransfusion non-A, non-B hepatitis in recipients. JAMA 246:2340–2344, 1981.

Noll WW: Gamma-glutamyl transferase. Clinical Chemistry No. CC-109, Chicago, American Society of Clinical Pathology, 1978.

Serum bile acids in hepatobiliary disease, editorial Lancet 2:1136–1138, 1982.

Shore GM, Hoberman L, Dowdey ABC, et al: Serum gamma-glutamyl transpeptidase activity in normal children. Am J Clin Pathol 63:245–250, 1975.

Speicher CE, Widish JR, Gaudot FJ, et al: An evaluation of the overestimation of serum albumin by bromcresol green. Am J Clin Pathol 69:347–350, 1978.

Starr AV, Schmidt PJ, Dede D: Proper handling of specimens for coagulation studies. Laboratory Medicine 8:26–27, November, 1977.

Statland BE: The γ-glutamyl transferase test. JAMA 247:2716, 1982.

Acute Viral Hepatitis

Aach RD, Kahn RA: Post-transfusion hepatitis: Current perspectives. Ann Intern Med 92:539–546, 1980.

Bianchi L, DeGroote J, Desmet VJ, et al: Morphological criteria in viral hepatitis. Lancet 1:333–337, 1971.

Blitzer BL: Fulminant hepatic failure: A rare but often lethal coma syndrome. Postgrad Med 68:153–162, 1980.

Bryan JA: Viral hepatitis. 1. Clinical and laboratory aspects and epidemiology. Postgrad Med 68:66–76, 1980.

Jeffries GH: Acute viral hepatitis. In Beeson PB, McDermott W, Wyngaarden JB (eds): Cecil Textbook of Medicine, ed 15. Philadelphia, WB Saunders Company, 1979, pp 1650–1656.

Koff RS: Viral Hepatitis. New York, John Wiley & Sons, 1978, p 139.

Miller DJ: Seroepidemiology of viral hepatitis: Correlation with clinical findings. Postgrad Med 68:137–148, 1980.

Neff JC: Personal communication, 1981.

Overby LR: The new serology of liver disease. In Gitnick GL (ed): Current Gastroenterology and Hepatology. Boston, Houghton-Mifflin Professional Publishers, Medical Division, 1979, pp 276–309.

Phillips MJ, Poucell S: Modern aspects of the morphology of viral hepatitis. Hum Pathol 12:1060–1084, 1981.

Schmidt P: Don't jump to conclusions about posttransfusion hepatitis. Diagnostic Medicine November–December 1980, pp 23–24.

Shearman DJC, Finlayson NDC: Diseases of the Gastrointestinal Tract and Liver. New York, Churchill Livingstone, 1982, 476–500.

Soloway HB: Interpreting hepatitis profiles. Diagnostic Medicine, January–February 1980, pp 29–34.

Szmuness WF, Stevens CE, Harley EJ, et al: Hepatitis B vaccine: Demonstration of efficacy in a controlled trial in a high-risk population in the United States. N Engl J Med 303:833–841, 1980.

Tygstrup N, Ranek L: Fulminant hepatic failure. Clin in Gastroenterol 10:191–208, 1981.

Zimmerman H-J: Hepatotoxicity. The Adverse Effects of Drugs and other Chemicals on the Liver. New York, Appelton-Century Crofts, 1978.

Chronic Hepatitis and Primary Biliary Cirrhosis

Bianchi L, DeGroote J, Desmet VJ, et al: Acute and chronic hepatitis revisited. Lancet 2:914–919, 1977.

Christoffersen, P, Poulsen H, Scheuer PJ: Abnormal bile duct epithelium in chronic aggressive hepatitis and primary biliary cirrhosis. Hum Pathol 3:227–235, 1972.

Czaja AJ: Current problems in the diagnosis and management of chronic active hepatitis. Mayo Clin Proc 56:311–323, 1981.

Czaja AJ, Summerskill WHJ: Chronic hepatitis: To treat or not to treat? Med Clin North Am 62:71–85, 1978.

Czaja AJ, Wolf AM, Baggenstoss AH: Clinical assessment of cirrhosis in severe chronic active liver disease: Specificity and sensitivity of physical and laboratory findings. Mayo Clin Proc 55:360–364, 1980.

Czaja AJ, Wolf AM, Baggenstoss AH: Laboratory assessment of severe chronic active liver disease during and after corticosteroid therapy: Correlation of serum transaminase and gamma globulin levels with histologic features. Gastroenterology 80:687–692, 1981.

DeGroote J, Desmet VJ, Gedigk P, et al: A classification of chronic hepatitis. Lancet 2:626–628, 1968.

Jeffries GH: Biliary cirrhosis: In Beeson PB, McDermott W, Wyngaarden JB (eds): Cecil Textbook of Medicine, ed. 15. Philadelphia, WB Saunders Company, 1979, pp 1666–1667.

Koff RS: Viral Hepatitis. New York. John Wiley & Sons, 1978, p. 223.

Korman MG, Hoffman AF, Summerskill WHJ: Assessment of activity in chronic liver disease: Serum bile acids compared with conventional tests and histology. N Engl J Med 290:1399–1402, 1974.

Ludwig J, Dickson ER, McDonald GSA: Staging of chronic nonsuppurative destructive cholangitis (syndrome of primary biliary cirrhosis). Virchows Arch [Pathol Anat] 379:103–112, 1978.

Neuberger J, Portmann B, Macdougall BRD, et al: Recurrence of primary biliary cirrhosis after liver transplantation. N Engl J Med 306:1–4, 1982.

Phillips MJ, Poucell S: Modern aspects of the morphology of viral hepatitis. Hum Pathol 12:1060–1084, 1981.

Schaffner F: Primary biliary cirrhosis as a collagen disease. Postgrad Med 65:97–102, 1979.

Sherlock S: Chronic hepatitis. Postgrad Med 65:81–88, 1979.

Wallnöfer H, Schmidt E, Schmidt RF (eds): Diagnosis of Liver Disease. An Illustrated Textbook. Stuttgart, Georg Thieme Publishers, 1977, p 117.

Wands JR, Koff RS, Isselbacher KJ: Chronic active hepatitis. In Isselbacher KJ, Adams RD, Braunwald E, et al (eds.): Harrison's Principles of Internal Medicine, ed 9. New York, McGraw-Hill Book Company, 1980, pp 1470–1473.

Winter SL, Kraft SC, Boyer JL: Antimitochondrial antibodies: Reagent variables may lead to diagnostic error. Dig Dis Sci 24:15–20, 1979.

Zimmerman H-J: Hepatotoxicity. The Adverse Effects of Drugs and other Chemicals on the Liver. New York, Appleton-Century Crofts, 1978.

Cirrhosis

Baptista A, Bianchi L, DeGroote J, et al: Alcoholic liver disease: Morphological manifestations. Lancet 1:707–711, 1981.

Czaja A, Wolf AM, Baggenstoss AH: Clinical assessment of cirrhosis in severe chronic active liver disease. Specificity and sensitivity of physical and laboratory findings. Mayo Clin Proc 55:360–364, 1980.

Galambos JT: Cirrhosis: Major Problems in Internal Medicine, vol 17. Philadelphia, WB Saunders Company, 1979, pp 128–182.

O'Brien MJ, Gottlieb LS: Cirrhosis. In Robbins SL, Cotran RS (eds): Pathologic Basis of Disease, ed 2. Philadelphia, WB Saunders Company, 1979, pp 1045–1047.

Phillips MJ, Poucell S: Modern aspects to the morphology of viral hepatitis. Hum Pathol 12:1060–1084, 1981.

Shearman DJC, Finlayson, NDC: Diseases of the Gastrointestinal Tract and Liver. New York, Churchill Livingstone, 1982.

Zimmerman H-J: Hepatotoxicity. The Adverse Effects of Drugs and other Chemicals on the Liver. New York, Appleton-Century Crofts, 1978.

Cholestasis and Hyperbilirubinemia

Bianchi L, DeGroote J, Desmet V, et al: Guidelines for diagnosis of therapeutic drug-induced injury in liver biopsies. Lancet 1:854–857, 1974.

Catrou PG, Crawford BE, Beeler MF: Clinical evaluation of an algorithm for interpreting biochemical profiles showing hyperbilirubinemia. Am J Clin Pathol 74:61–63, 1980.

Cello JP: Diagnostic approaches to jaundice. Hospital Practice, February 1982, pp 49–60.

Demers LM: Serum bile acids in health and hepatobiliary disease. In Demers LM, Shaw LM (eds): Evaluation of Liver Function. A Multifaceted Approach to Clinical Diagnosis. Baltimore, Urban & Schwarzenberg, 1978, pp 33–50.

Erlinger S: Cholestasis: Pump failure, microvilli defect, or both? Lancet 1:533–534, 1978.

Fischer MG, Gelb AM, Weingarten LA: Cholestatic jaundice in adults. Algorithms for diagnosis. JAMA 245:1945–1948, 1981.

Javitt NB: Hyperbilirubinemic and cholestatic syndromes. Postgrad Med 65:120–130, 1979.

Kaplowitz N: Cholestatic liver disease. Hospital Practice, August 1978, pp 83–92.

Kim NK, Yasmineh WG, Freier EF, et al: Value of alkaline phosphatase, 5'-nucleotidase, γ-glutamyl transferase, and glutamate dehydrogenase activity, measurements (single and combined) in serum in diagnosis of metastasis to the liver. Clin Chem 23:2034–2038, 1977.

Tempero MA, Petersen RJ, Zetterman RK, et al: Detection of metastatic liver disease. Use of liver scans and biochemical tests. JAMA 248:1329–1332, 1982.

Zimmerman HJ: Hepatotoxicity. The Adverse Effects of Drugs and Other Chemicals on the Liver. New York. Appleton-Century Crofts, 1978

CHAPTER 16

ENDOCRINE SUBPROBLEMS

ADRENAL DISEASE
  Cushing's Syndrome
  Pheochromocytoma
DISORDERS OF PANCREATIC
  ISLETS
  Diabetes Mellitus

ADRENAL DISEASE

CUSHING'S SYNDROME

Definition and Significance

Cushing's syndrome is a clinical and metabolic disorder caused by an excess of glucocorticoids. The effect of this excess induces a distinctive clinical picture and places the patient at risk for a large number of pathologic processes, including hypertension and diabetes mellitus. Because Cushing's syndrome is potentially curable, it is important to consider it whenever hypertension, diabetes mellitus, or other features of this condition are present. The term *Cushing's syndrome* refers to the disorder resulting from the variety of causes given in Table 16–1. In addition, it can be iatrogenic, secondary to the administration of glucocorticoids.

The term *Cushing's disease* refers to an excess of glucocorticoids secondary to overproduction of adrenocorticotropic hormone (ACTH) by the pituitary. The most common cause, overall, of Cushing's syndrome is a pituitary-dependent corticotropin-induced bilateral adrenal hyperplasia, i.e., Cushing's disease (*Lancet* editorial, 1981). If the presence of Cushing's syndrome is confirmed, another subproblem—its etiology—should be addressed.

Pathophysiology

Cortisol is the end product of glucocorticoid synthesis by the cortex of the adrenal glands. Figure 16–1 presents the synthesis, metabolism, and excretion of glucocorticoids. The effects of elevated glucocorticoid levels are profound and widespread (Table 16–2).

In individuals without congenital deficiencies of the dehydrogenase and hydroxylase enzymes (almost all persons) tetrahydrocortisol is the main urinary product. However, of the total plasma cortisol there is a small amount of plasma free cortisol, which is cleared by the

Table 16–1. ORIGIN OF THE CUSHING
SYNDROMES: FREQUENCY OF
PATHOLOGIC LESIONS*†

	%	
Pituitary Cushing's syndrome‡		68
Pituitary tumor§¶	40	
No pituitary tumor	28	
Adrenal Cushing's syndrome		17
Adenoma	9	
Carcinoma	8	
Nodular hyperplasia	(?)	
Ectopic Cushing's syndrome‡		15

*From Gold EM: The Cushing syndromes: Changing
views of diagnosis and treatment. Ann Intern Med 90:830,
1979.

†Per cent of total cases taken from sources cited.

‡Huff TA: Clinical syndromes related to disorders of
adrenocorticotrophic hormone, in The Pituitary: A Current Review, edited by Allen MB Jr, Mahesh VB. New
York, Academic Press, Inc., 1977, pp. 153–168.

§Plotz CM, Knowlton AI, Ragan C: The natural history
of Cushing's syndrome. Am J Med 13:597–614, 1952.

¶Burke CW, Beardwell CG: Cushing's syndrome. Q J
Med 42:175–204, 1973.

kidneys and excreted in the urine. This urinary
free cortisol can be measured by radioimmunoassay.

Clinical Contexts

Diagnosis. Cushing's syndrome should be
considered when a patient presents with a
cushingoid habitus (moon facies and truncal
obesity), diabetes mellitus, and/or hypertension. Additional features that make the diagnosis more likely include ecchymoses, muscle
weakness, hypokalemia, and osteoporosis (Table 16–3).

Distinguishing between simple obesity and
mild Cushing's syndrome is often difficult.
Many obese patients are hypertensive, have
fine skin, develop amenorrhea, and are prone
to develop psychiatric disorders. Diabetes mellitus may also occur in such patients. Obesity
of the arms or legs is not consistent with a
diagnosis of Cushing's syndrome (Liddle,
1982).

Management. After therapy, e.g., surgical
excision of an adrenal cortical tumor, periodic
measurements of glucocorticoid levels are necessary to evaluate whether these levels have
returned to normal and to determine the existence of hormonal deficiencies resulting from
therapy.

Screening. Targeted screening for Cushing's syndrome in the absence of clinical manifestations of the disease is not indicated. In
the appropriate clinical setting, impaired glucose tolerance (sensitivity 94 per cent), central
obesity (sensitivity 88 per cent), and hypertension (sensitivity 82 per cent) can indicate the
presence of Cushing's syndrome (Liddle,
1982).

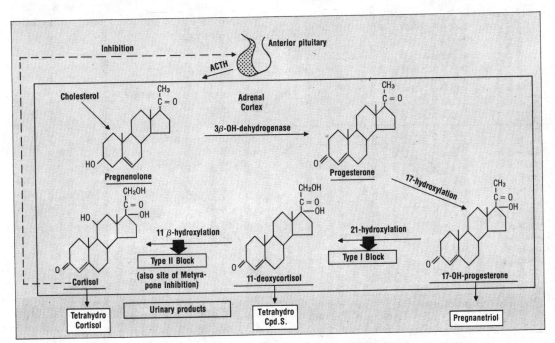

Figure 16–1. Schematic presentation of metabolic pathway of glucocorticoids and excretory products. In addition
to tetrahydrocortisol a very small amount of cortisol is excreted in the urine (From the Bio-Science Handbook, 12th
ed., Van Nuys, Calif, Bio-Science Laboratories, 1979, p 80.)

Table 16–2. CLINICAL–METABOLIC CORRELATES IN CUSHING SYNDROME

I. Metabolic Effects
  A. Fat metabolism
    Truncal obesity, widening of mediastinum
    Hypercholesterolemia, accelerated
      atherosclerosis
  B. Protein metabolism
    Muscle wasting with proximal myopathy
    Fragility of skin—ecchymoses, striae
    Growth hormone unresponsiveness
  C. Carbohydrate metabolism
    Latent or overt diabetes mellitus
  D. Electrolyte balance
    Aldosterone or DOC excess with hypertension, hypokalemic alkalosis

II. Endocrine Effects
  A. 1,25 Dihydroxycholecalciferol antagonism—
    secondary PTH excess and osteopenia
  B. Growth hormone suppression—growth failure
  C. MSH excess—hyperpigmentation
  D. Androgen excess—hirsutism, amenorrhea, and
    infertility

III. Neurologic Effects
  A. Psychosis or emotional lability

*From Bledsoe T: Disorders of the adrenal glands. In Harvey AM, Johns RJ, McKusick VA et al (eds): The Principles and Practice of Medicine, ed 20, 1980, p 781. Courtesy of Appleton-Century-Crofts, Publishing Division of Prentice-Hall, Inc, Englewood Cliffs, NJ.

Strategy

Test Sequence. The diagnosis of Cushing's syndrome can be confirmed or excluded in several different ways (Melby, 1971):

1. Overnight dexamethasone suppression of the morning plasma cortisol.

2. Random elevation of plasma cortisol.

Table 16–3. FREQUENCY OF CLINICAL MANIFESTATIONS IN CUSHING'S SYNDROME*

	Per Cent
Impaired glucose tolerance	94
Central obesity	88
Hypertension	82
Oligomenorrhea	72
Osteoporosis	58
Purpura and striae	42
Muscle atrophy	36
Hirsutism	30
Edema	20
Hypokalemia (unprovoked)	18
Kidney stones	12
Psychotic mentation	6

*From Liddle GW: Cushing's syndrome. In Wyngaarden JB, Smith LH (eds): Cecil Textbook of Medicine, ed 16. Philadelphia, WB Saunders Company 1982, p 1233.

3. Loss of diurnal variation of plasma cortisol.

4. Elevation of urinary free cortisol.

5. Elevation of urinary 17-hydroxycorticosteroids (17-OHCS).

6. Elevation of urinary 17-ketogenic steroids.

We believe the overnight dexamethasone suppression test is the best initial study to rule out the presence of Cushing's syndrome because its diagnostic sensitivity is essentially 100 per cent. Since false-positive suppression tests occasionally occur (Gold, 1979), diagnostic specificity is somewhat less than 100 per cent (Watts and Keffer, 1982).

If the overnight dexamethasone test is negative, a diagnosis of Cushing's syndrome is ruled out. If the overnight dexamethasone test is positive, the presence of Cushing's syndrome must be confirmed by another test, of which determination of the 24-hour urinary free cortisol may be the most specific (Gold, 1979; Watts and Keffer, 1982). Ashcraft and colleagues (1982) demonstrated that a low-dose dexamethasone test (0.5 mg every 6 hours) could be used in outpatients as an alternative study. Cushing's syndrome was diagnosed if the serum value on day 2 at 4 P.M. was greater than 5 μg/100 ml.

Patient Preparation. The dexamethasone suppression test is carried out as follows:

1. Dexamethasone, 1.0 mg, and a sedative are given orally at bedtime. The patient's sleep should not be disturbed.

2. A fasting blood specimen is drawn the next morning for measurement of plasma cortisol.

No special preparation is required for the 24-hour urine collection.

Specimen Collection and Handling. Heparinized plasma is the usual choice for collecting plasma cortisol for radioimmunoassay (RIA). A 24-hour urine sample is collected without preservative for urinary free cortisol by RIA. If there is any delay in analysis, the urinary volume should be measured and an aliquot frozen. A 10-ml sample is usually adequate for the urinary assay.

Methodology. Consult the laboratory for its methodologies, reference intervals, accuracy and precision, and potential sources of interference. We believe that plasma cortisol and urinary free cortisol determinations by RIA are the methods of choice (Apter et al.,

1975; Juselius and Barnhart, 1974). Some investigators have measured salivary cortisol as a reflection of plasma free cortisol levels. Plasma cortisol by RIA measures the total level, only 10 per cent of which is free (Walker et al., 1978).

Measurement of urinary glucocorticoids by the Porter-Silber method or the 17-ketogenic steroid method is outmoded (Nelson and Keffer, 1982).

Interpretation

Diagnosis. The combination of a positive dexamethasone suppression test followed by an elevated 24-hour urinary free cortisol is diagnostic for Cushing's syndrome. Stress, failure to take medication, or diphenylhydantoin treatment can cause a false-positive dexamethasone suppression test (Watts and Keffer, 1982).

Table 16–4 gives reference intervals and decision levels for Cushing's syndrome. Total reliance upon a single set of laboratory values is not recommended. For example, high levels of estrogen, such as those encountered in pregnancy or during treatment with contraceptives, lead to elevation of plasma cortisol by raising the concentration of cortisol-binding globulin; however, there is no increase in cortisol secretion rate or in urinary 17-OHCS. Conversely, hyperthyroidism can increase urinary 17-OHCS, but there is no increase in plasma cortisol. To avoid misinterpretations, the laboratory values should always be interpreted in the context of the clinical picture (Liddle, 1982).

Additional disorders can *increase* the levels of plasma cortisol, such as diabetic acidosis, carcinoid syndrome, acute alcoholic intoxication, alcoholism, acute myocardial infarction, acute or chronic renal failure, and stress. The following disorders can *decrease* plasma cortisol: anterior pituitary hypofunction, myotonia atrophica, asthma, respiratory distress syndrome, and exercise (Friedman et al., 1980). The effect of interference by drugs and other agents (e.g., estrogens, spironolactone, phenytoin, and alcohol) should always be considered when estimating cortisol. In depression that is not due to Cushing's syndrome, cortisol production can be increased in association with loss of diurnal rhythm and occasionally with increased urinary free cortisol (*Lancet* editorial, 1981). Once Cushing's syndrome has been confirmed, its specific etiology should be pursued (Cook et al., 1980), i.e., the subproblem, etiology of Cushing's syndrome.

In 1964, Nugent and colleagues reported partial success with the application of Bayes' theorem in the diagnosis of Cushing's syndrome using only clinical signs and basic nonsteroidal laboratory data. They were able to successfully confirm or exclude the diagnosis of Cushing's syndrome in half of a group of patients suspected of having the disease. They suggested that weakness, fragile skin, and red or purple striae more than 1 cm wide might be additional valuable signs to confirm or exclude Cushing's syndrome.

Common laboratory test results for Cushing's syndrome are given in Table 16–5.

Management. Follow-up studies of plasma and urinary cortisol levels should be conducted

Table 16–4. REFERENCE INTERVALS AND DECISION LEVELS FOR CUSHING'S SYNDROME*

	Healthy Subjects	Subjects with Cushing's Syndrome
Overnight dexamethasone suppression†	<5 μg/100 ml (usually)	>10 μg/100 ml
Random plasma cortisol	8–25 μg/100 ml (8 A.M.)	>15 μg/100 ml
Loss of diurnal variation of plasma cortisol	<8 μg/100 ml (4 P.M.)	usually at all times
Urinary free cortisol	10–80 μg/24 hr	>80 μg/24 hrs
Urinary 17-hydroxycorticosteroids	3–7 mg/g creatinine	>10 mg/gm creatinine
Male	3–10 mg/24 hrs	
Female	2–8 mg/24 hrs	
Urinary 17-ketogenic steroids		
Male	5–23 mg/24 hrs	
Female	3–15 mg/24 hrs	

*Information from Wyngaarden JB, Smith LH (eds): Cecil Textbook of Medicine, ed 16. Philadelphia, WB Saunders Company, 1982; Watts NB, Keffer JH: Practical Endocrine Diagnosis, ed 3. Philadelphia, Lea & Febiger, 1982.

†Values between 5 and 10 μg/100 ml must be considered non-diagnostic and the study repeated or a different parameter measured.

Table 16–5. COMMON LABORATORY TEST RESULTS IN CUSHING'S SYNDROME

Laboratory Test	Value	Pathophysiologic Factors
Chemistry (Serum)		
Bilirubin, total	—	
Calcium, total	↓	Related to decreased albumin
Carbon dioxide	↑	Related to metabolic alkalosis
Chloride	↓	Increased renal tubular loss
Cholesterol	↑	Related to altered carbohydrate metabolism
Creatinine phosphokinase	—	
Creatinine	—	
Glucose	↑	Glucose intolerance caused by glucocorticoids
Lactic dehydrogenase	—	
Phosphatase, alkaline	↑	Related to bone disease
Phosphorus, inorganic	↓	Related to diuresis from hypoglycemia
		Occasionally due to high glucocorticoid concentration
Potassium	↓	Increased renal tubular loss
Proteins, total	↓	Related to negative protein balance
Proteins, albumin	↓	Related to negative protein balance
Sodium	↑	Renal conservation of sodium
Transaminase, aspartate amino	—	
Urea nitrogen	↑	Associated with excessive protein catabolism
Uric acid	↓	Adrenal steroids are uricosuric
Hematology (Blood)		
Hemoglobin	↑	Occasionally found
	↓	Related to malignancy
Hematocrit	↑	Occasionally found
	↓	Related to malignancy
Leukocyte count, total	↑	Caused by glucocorticoids
Platelet count	—	

Key: — = No change; ↑ = can be increased; ↓ = can be decreased.
*Information from Friedman RB, Anderson RE, Entine SM et al: Effects of diseases on clinical laboratory tests. Clin Chem 26:1D–476D, 1980; Wolf PL: Interpretation of Biochemical Multitest Profiles: An Analysis of 100 Important Conditions. New York, Masson Publishing, Inc, 1977.

for patients who have received "definitive" therapy for Cushing's syndrome. Flint and Jacobs (1974) reported that 6 of 34 patients after adrenalectomy for Cushing's syndrome had excess mineralocorticoids secondary to ACTH-producing tumors outside the pituitary adrenal axis—some tumors not manifesting themselves until 9 years after adrenalectomy. Appropriate follow-up studies, initially at 6 months and then at yearly intervals, seem adequate to exclude development of new tumors or metastases unless clinical symptoms dictate an earlier evaluation.

Test Requests and Reports

Test Requests. Henry and Murphy (1979) include the measurement of urinary free cortisol per 24 hours in the organ panel for hypertension (see Fig. 10–9). This strategy uses hypertension as a clue to the presence of Cushing's syndrome. Execution of the test sequence for the diagnosis of Cushing's syndrome, as outlined in this chapter, can be

offered by the laboratory as a problem-solving service.

Interpretive Reports. The results of the strategy may be collated and returned to the attending physician in the form of an interpretive report. Of the laboratories that we surveyed in the United States, 2 per cent used interpretive reports for disorders of steroid metabolism (Speicher and Smith, 1980).

PHEOCHROMOCYTOMA

Definition and Significance

Pheochromocytoma is an uncommon neoplasm that originates from chromaffin cells. Over 90 per cent of these tumors are situated between the diaphragm and the pelvic floor, most commonly in the adrenal glands and sometimes bilaterally. Pheochromocytomas are multiple in 3 to 5 per cent of cases and malignant (with the ability to metastasize) in 5 to 10 per cent of cases (Robbins and Cotran, 1979). About 80 per cent of pheochromocyto-

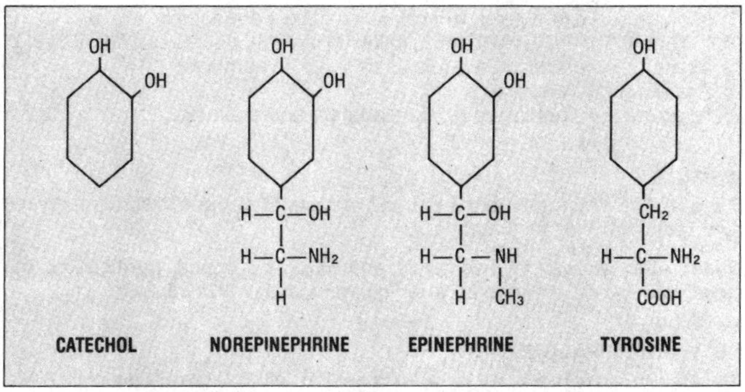

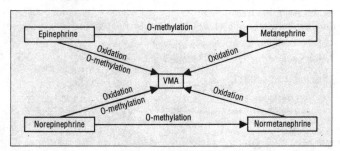

Figure 16–2. Metabolism of catecholamines. (From the Bio-Science Handbook, 12th ed., Van Nuys, Calif, Bio-Science Laboratories, 1979, pp 86.)

mas occur sporadically in adults. Most of those occurring sporadically in adults are solitary and arise within the adrenal medulla. Others are familial and may be associated with multiple endocrine neoplasia syndromes (Table 13–3). Some occur in children (Markel and Johnson, 1975).

Pheochromocytoma is of clinical interest because of its role in causing hypertension. Even though this tumor is responsible for less than 1 per cent of cases of hypertension, it is of great diagnostic importance because it represents a surgically curable cause of hypertension.

Pathophysiology

Each adrenal gland is composed of a cortex and a medulla. The medulla secretes the hormones epinephrine and norepinephrine. Pheochromocytoma is a tumor that is functionally similar to the adrenal medulla. It secretes increased amounts of epinephrine and norepinephrine into the blood. These hormones are chemically related to catechol and amines and, therefore, are referred to as *catecholamines*.

They are synthesized from tyrosine. Figures 16–2 and 16–3 depict the chemical formulas, primary pathways, and products of the metabolism of catecholamines. Epinephrine and norepinephrine have profound effects on many organs and systems of the body (Table 16–6).

Clinical Indications

Diagnosis. The clinical features and differential diagnosis of pheochromocytoma are listed in Table 16–7. Patients can present with hypertension and symptoms secondary to hypertension without any of the other distinguishing features found in groups I through IV. Suspicion of pheochromocytoma should be aroused by the following features:

1. Intermittent hypertension.
2. Elevation of blood pressure during induction of anesthesia or on abdominal palpation.
3. Unexplained tendency to cardiac arrhythmias.
4. Orthostatic hypotension.
5. Rarely, hypotension (by an epinephrine-producing tumor).

Figure 16–3. Metabolism of epinephrine and norepinephrine. (From the Bio-Science Handbook, 12th ed., Van Nuys, Calif, Bio-Science Laboratories, 1979, pp 87.)

Table 16–6.   ACTIONS OF EPINEPHRINE AND NOREPINEPHRINE ON BODY SYSTEMS*

System or Organ	Function	Effect	
		Epinephrine	*Norepinephrine*
Cardiovascular	Peripheral resistance	Decrease	Increase
	Systolic blood pressure	Increase	Increase
	Diastolic blood pressure	No effect	Increase
	Heart rate	Increase	Slight increase
	Cardiac output	Increase	No change
	Blood vessels in denervated limb	Vasodilation	Vasoconstriction
	Coronary vessels	Vasodilation	Vasodilation
	Pulse rate	Increase	Decrease
	Eosinophil count	Increase	No effect
	Net peripheral vascular effect	Vasodilation	Limited vasodilator actions; overall vasoconstriction
Skeletal muscle	Blood flow through individual	100% increase	No change or decrease
Kidney	organs	40% increase	20% increase
Liver		100% increase	No material effect
Brain		20% increase	Slight decrease
Respiratory system	Bronchial muscle activity	Inhibition	Inhibition
Endocrine	Blood sugar level	Increase	Increase
Eye	Pupillary dilators	Excitation	Excitation
Intestines	Motility	Inhibition	Inhibition
Genital system (rat, cat)	Nonpregnant uterine muscle contraction	Inhibition	Inhibition
Central nervous system (human)	Mental state effect	Anxiety	No effect

*From Stewart TC, Freeman JA: Vanilmandelic Acid and Catecholamine Determinations. Chicago, American Society of Clinical Pathologists, 1976, p 13.

6. Elevated hematocrit (true polycythemia being rare).

7. Spells of anxiety with a feeling of impending doom. Similar episodes occur in individuals taking monoamine oxidase (MAO) inhibitors with attacks provoked by cheese and other substances.

8. Café-au-lait spots, neurofibromas, and hemangioma (von Recklinghausen's disease).

9. Beefy red hands.

10. Presence of multiple endocrine adenomatosis.

Patients with diabetes mellitus and thyrotoxicosis can have a clinical presentation similar to that of pheochromocytoma, and pheochromocytoma should be ruled out (Bledsoe, 1980).

Gifford and colleagues (1964) found that headache was the most common presenting complaint in patients with pheochromocytoma (20 of 37 patients with paroxysmal hypertension and 17 of 39 with persistently functioning tumors). A system review revealed that the majority of patients suffered from headache, excessive perspiration, and palpitation with or without tachycardia; nervousness and weight loss were also common.

Management. Laboratory studies should be repeated after surgery to demonstrate that all tumor tissue has been removed and that test results have shown a return to normal.

Screening. It is difficult to select patients to be screened for pheochromocytoma. The Mayo Clinic study places the prevalence of pheochromocytoma as a cause of hypertension at 0.25 per cent (1 in 400) (Tucker and Labarthe, 1977). This means that if we screen every hypertensive patient for pheochromocytoma, we would be screening 399 patients with hypertension who do not have a pheochromocytoma to find one patient with hypertension who does.

Weinstein and Feinberg (1978) discussed five basic screening options (Fig. 16–4) in terms of their cost-effectiveness, i.e., the amount it costs to detect each true-positive result when the costs of all false-positive results also are considered, and whether the cost would be offset by the therapeutic savings of earlier detection. It is becoming increasingly clear that

Table 16–7. PHEOCHROMOCYTOMA: PRESENTING FEATURES AND DIFFERENTIAL DIAGNOSIS*

Presenting Features	Differential Diagnosis
Group I. Hypertension	
Episodic	Essential hypertension
Headache	Renal hypertension
Paroxysmal	Other causes of endocrine
dyspnea	hypertension
Persistent	
cerebrovascular	
episodes	
Group II. Spells	
Excessive perspiration	Other causes of
Palpitations	catecholamine release,
Pain (headache, angina,	e.g., hypoglycemia
abdominal pain)	5-hydroxy-tryptamine
Nervousness and	over-production
apprehension	Carcinoid
Paresthesia	Mastocytosis
Pallor	Menopausal symptoms
	Cervical spondylosis
	Horton's headaches
	Associated with use of
	monoamine oxidase
	inhibitors
Group III. Metabolic Diabetes	
Loss of weight	Diabetes mellitus
Fever	Hyperthyroidism
Group IV. Hypotension (rare)	
Hypovolemia	Other causes of shock
Shock	
Polycythemia	

*From Bledsoe T: Disorders of the adrenal glands. In Harvey AM, Johns RJ, McKusick VA et al (eds): The Principles and Practice of Medicine, ed 20. 1980, p. 793. Courtesy of Appleton-Century-Crofts, Publishing Division of Prentice-Hall; Inc, Englewood Cliffs, NJ.

health resources are limited and will have to be applied in a manner that achieves the greatest good for the greatest number of people. This socioeconomic ideal, however, may not always be consistent with the ideal for the individual patient. The option that achieves the greatest and earliest detection, regardless of cost, is the ideal.

Strategy

Test Sequence. Pharmacologic procedures are no longer commonly used for evaluation of patients suspected of having pheochromocytomas. Such tests yield as high as 30 per cent false-positive and negative responses, and they are associated with serious or life-threatening side effects (Engelman, 1982). The diagnosis of pheochromocytoma is best confirmed by demonstrating increases in catecholamines, vanillylmandelic acid (VMA), and metanephrines in blood, urine, or both. The measurements are usually performed on 24-hour urine samples, but random, timed urine samples can be used. Most patients with pheochromocytoma will have elevated urinary catecholamines, VMA, and metanephrines. In some patients, however, one or more of these determinations will be within the reference intervals for patients without pheochromocytomas (Howanitz and Howanitz, 1979). Obviously, the highest detection rate is achieved by conducting all three studies for every patient because parallel testing increases diagnostic sensitivity (Galen and Gambino, 1975). Since this is not always practical, the study with the highest detection rate, or diagnostic sensitivity (i.e., determination of urinary metanephrines), should be chosen. All patients with an elevated level of urinary metanephrines should have the diagnosis of pheochromocytoma confirmed by urinary VMA. Although some false-negative results do occur, determination of urinary metanephrines has been recommended as the most sensitive screening method for diagnosing pheochromocytoma (Remine et al., 1974). If the clinical features of pheochromocytoma are present and the results for urinary metanephrines are negative, additional studies are needed. If the episodes of hypertension are intermittent, timed urine specimens collected during periods of hypertension are necessary to document the increase in catecholamine excretion.

Galen and Gambino (1975) reviewed the strategy for the laboratory diagnosis of pheochromocytoma and pointed out that repeat measurements of urinary metanephrines can help to decrease false positives. This repetition helps to eliminate false positives due to transient pathophysiological conditions and analytical errors and is similar to the repeated testing for diabetes mellitus discussed later in this chapter.

Determination of plasma catecholamine (a technically demanding procedure) is not a suitable screening test for pheochromocytoma because plasma catecholamine values can vary widely under a variety of circumstances even in patients without the tumor (Engelman, 1982). Although it is agreed that plasma catecholamines are not an appropriate screening test for pheochromocytoma (Bravo et al., 1979; McCarthy et al., 1980); it is suggested

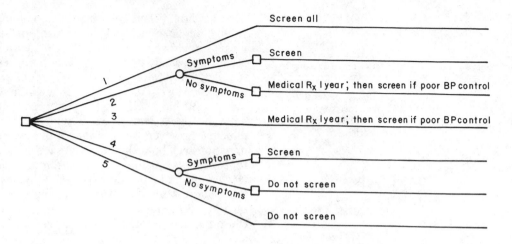

Alternative strategies for the detection of Pheochromocytoma

Figure 16–4. Alternative strategies for the detection of pheochromocytoma. (From Benson ES, Rubin M (eds): Logic and Economics of Clinical Laboratory Use. New York and Amsterdam, Elsevier North-Holland, 1978, p 15.)

that in patients with a clinical picture of pheochromocytoma, plasma catecholamines may be better predictors of the presence of pheochromocytoma than either urinary VMA or metanephrines. Preliminary data suggest that clonidine will depress the plasma catecholamine concentration in non-pheochromocytoma patients but will have no effect in patients with pheochromocytoma (Bravo et al., 1981).

Patient Preparation. Avoid drugs and foods that interfere with the chemical measurements in use at the laboratory.

Specimen Collection and Handling. Urinary specimens for catecholamine, VMA, and metanephrines are usually collected in acid. Consult the laboratory for details. It is essential that the urine be kept acidic during the entire collection. The addition of 25 ml 6 normal hydrochloric acid to a 24-hour urine collection is adequate.

Urine samples collected for 24 hours are preferable. The bladder should be emptied at the beginning of the collection, and the urine discarded. The bladder should again be emptied at the end of 24 hours, and the urine saved. In a similar manner, for timed urinary samples of less than 24 hours duration, discard the specimen at the beginning of the collection and save the specimen at the end of the timed interval.

Methodology. Consult the laboratory concerning its methods for measuring urinary and plasma catecholamines, VMA, and metaneph-

rines; reference intervals; accuracy and precision; and potential sources of interference.

Colorimetric techniques for measuring VMA are obsolete and should be abandoned because the results are affected adversely by phenolic acids of dietary origin, such as those that occur in coffee, vanilla, and certain vegetables and fruits. Measurement of urinary metanephrines is usually reliable and easy to perform. Measurement of urinary free catecholamines is more discriminating than that of urinary total catecholamines. In patients with intermittent attacks due to pheochromocytoma it may be useful to collect timed urinary samples and to fractionate urinary catecholamines into norepinephrine and epinephrine (Howanitz and Howanitz, 1979).

The best method for measuring urinary metanephrines is by high-voltage electrophoresis (100 per cent sensitive). Alternatively, a method using ion exchange columns with chromatography has been useful. The traditional column chromatography method has been adequate but not outstanding (Watts and Keffer, 1982).

Interpretation

Diagnosis. Gitlow and associates (1970) found that a level of urinary metanephrines greater than 2.2 μg/mg creatinine has a diagnostic sensitivity of 100 per cent and a diagnostic specificity of 98 per cent for pheochromocytoma. The data of Engelman (1982) support this (Fig. 16–5). Any positive result for urinary metanephrines should be confirmed by measurement of urinary VMA. According to Gitlow and co-workers (1970), the diagnostic sensitivity of urinary VMA is 96 per cent and its diagnostic specificity is 100 per cent. Gitlow's group preferred to express values in terms of urinary creatinine and found that adult subjects without pheochromocytoma have a mean urinary value of 0.42 μg metanephrines/mg creatinine and a mean urinary value of 1.4 μg VMA/mg creatinine.

Children's values differ from those of adults. Levels of urinary metanephrines and VMA tend to be higher and more variable in children, not reaching adult levels until about 15 years of age (Gitlow, 1968).

If the urinary values of metanephrines, VMA, and catecholamines are not expressed in terms of urinary creatinine, the following amounts of catecholamines and their metabolites are usually excreted under normal circumstances in a 24-hour period: less than 1.3 mg metanephrines, less than 6.8 mg VMA, and less than 0.1 mg free catecholamines (Engelman, 1982). Table 16–8 gives common laboratory test results in pheochromocytoma.

With the patient at rest in the supine position a plasma catecholamine level of 1000 ng/liter or less rules out pheochromocytoma (Bravo et al., 1979).

Once a tumor is diagnosed it needs to be localized using radiographic techniques (Sisson et al., 1981).

Management. Patients who have undergone surgery for removal of a pheochromocytoma should have additional studies to determine the adequacy of the surgery before they are discharged from the hospital. Because most patients normally excrete increased quantities of catecholamines for 4 to 5 days after surgery, the urinary collections should be delayed until after the end of the first postoperative week so that the results of the test are interpretable. Follow-up determinations, initially at 6 months

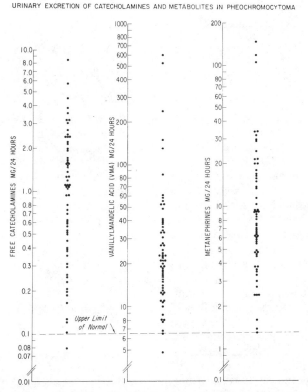

URINARY EXCRETION OF CATECHOLAMINES AND METABOLITES IN PHEOCHROMOCYTOMA

Figure 16–5. Distribution of excretion values for catecholamines and metabolites determined on single 24-hour urine collections in 64 patients with pheochromocytoma. The vertical axis depicts values on a logarithmic scale. (From Engelman, K: The adrenal medulla and the sympathetic nervous system. In Wyngaarden JB, Smith LH (eds): Cecil Textbook of Medicine, ed. 16, Philadelphia, WB Saunders Company, 1982, p 1309.)

Table 16–8. COMMON LABORATORY TEST RESULTS IN PHEOCHROMOCYTOMA*

Laboratory Test	Value	Pathophysiologic Factors
Chemistry (Serum)		
Bilirubin, total	—	
Calcium, total	↑	May be caused by ectopic parathyroid hormone production or associated parathyroid hyperplasia in familial cases
Carbon dioxide	—	
Chloride	—	
Cholesterol	—	
Creatinine phosphokinase	—	
Creatinine	—	
Glucose	↑	Caused by catecholamines
Lactic dehydrogenase	—	
Phosphatase, alkaline	—	
Phosphorus, inorganic	↓	Related to ectopic parathyroid hormone production or associated parathyroid hyperplasia in familial cases
Potassium	↓	Probable result of high plasma renin activity
Proteins, total	↑	Related to hemoconcentration
Proteins, albumin	—	
Sodium	—	
Transaminase, aspartate amino	—	
Urea nitrogen	—	
Uric acid	—	
Hematology (Blood)		
Hemoglobin	↑	Hemoconcentration not uncommon—increased erythropoietin
Hematocrit	↑	May be due to decreased plasma volume, increased erythrocyte mass, or both—increased erythropoietin.
Leukocyte count, total	—	
Platelet count	—	

Key: — = No change; ↑ = can be increased; ↓ = can be decreased.

*Information from Friedman RB, Anderson RE, Entine SM et al: Effects of diseases on clinical laboratory tests. Clin Chem 26:1D–476D, 1980; Engelman K: Pheochromocytoma. In Wyngaarden JB, Smith LH (eds): Cecil Textbook of Medicine, ed 16. Philadelphia, WB Saunders Company, 1982, pp 1302–1312.

and then at yearly intervals, seem adequate to exclude development of new tumors or metastases unless clinical symptoms dictate an earlier evaluation (Engelman, 1982). Histologic criteria for determining the malignancy of a pheochromocytoma are not always reliable.

Drugs can affect the analytic sensitivity and analytic specificity of the assays, and these effects are method dependent. In vivo effects of drugs include the following:

1. MAO inhibitors may increase urinary metanephrines and VMA.

2. Alpha-methyldopa may increase urinary metanephrines, VMA, and catecholamines by some techniques.

3. Urinary VMA may be either increased or decreased by alpha-methyldopa, depending on technique (Howanitz and Howanitz, 1979).

Severe stress of any kind can elevate urinary metanephrines, VMA, and catecholamines.

Test Requests and Reports

Test Requests. Henry and Murphy (1979) included the measurement of urinary meta-

nephrines (μg/mg creatinine) in the organ panel for hypertension (Fig. 10–9). This strategy uses hypertension as a clue to the presence of pheochromocytoma. Execution of the test sequence for the diagnosis of pheochromocytoma can be offered by the laboratory as a problem-solving service.

Interpretive Reports. The results of the strategy can be collated and returned to the attending physician in the form of an interpretive report.

DISORDERS OF PANCREATIC ISLETS

DIABETES MELLITUS

Definition and Significance

Diabetes mellitus is a disease characterized by hyperglycemia and by either a relative or absolute deficiency of insulin. It exhibits a constellation of pathophysiologic changes that are related to a disturbance in glucose homeostasis. Clinical features vary from none to a wide variety of serious complications. It tends to be familial.

Surveys in the United States have revealed that 2 to 4 per cent of the population has documented diabetes and that a similar percentage has compromised glucose tolerance that had been previously undetected. With advancing age, a greater proportion of the population, as high as 40 to 60 per cent in the ninth decade, has compromised glucose tolerance (Cahill, 1982). Shabo (1980) states:

Diabetes is increasing at an alarming rate. It is estimated by the National Commission on Diabetes that diabetes is increasing at a rate of about 6 per cent per year. The progression may seem familiar in this time of economic turmoil, when we think about interest rates and compounded rates of interest. Within 12 to 15 years the incidence of diabetes will double in this country. Within 25 years the incidence will quadruple.

We are dealing with a very major public health problem. In an American born today there is a one in five chance of diabetes developing in his lifetime. Diabetes is the third leading cause of death in this country, taking approximately 300,000 lives a year. A diabetic patient is 17 times more prone to kidney disease, 5 times more prone to gangrene (which often leads to amputation), and twice as likely to have a heart attack or stroke than a person without diabetes. This disorder decreases life expectancy by a third. And the economic toll of the disease in the United States today, excluding complications of diabetes, is approximately $5.3 billion annually.

Within the last few years, a new classification of diabetes mellitus and other categories of glucose intolerance has been devised, based on contemporary knowledge of this heterogeneous syndrome, by the National Diabetes Data Group (1979). This new system includes the following classes:

1. Insulin-dependent diabetes mellitus (IDDM): Insulin-dependent, ketosis-prone type of diabetes, associated with increased or decreased frequency of certain histocompatibility antigens (HLA) on chromosome 6 and with islet-cell antibodies. Formerly called *juvenile diabetes,* the term should be abandoned since it can occur at any age.
2. Non-insulin–dependent diabetes (NIDDM) and non-ketosis–prone types of diabetes, not secondary to other conditions: Further subdivided according to whether the patient is obese (obese NIDDM) or not obese (non-obese NIDDM).
3. Diabetes associated with other conditions and syndromes: Further subdivided according to the known or suspected etiologic factors listed as follows:
   a. Pancreatic disease.
   b. Hormonal.
   c. Drug or chemical induced.
   d. Insulin receptor antibodies.
   e. Certain genetic syndromes of other types.
4. Gestational diabetes (GDM): Limited to individuals in whom glucose intolerance develops or in whom it is discovered during pregnancy.
5. Impaired glucose tolerance (IGT): Serum glucose levels intermediate between those considered healthy and those considered diabetic.
6. Previous abnormality of glucose tolerance (Prev AGT): Individuals with non-compromised glucose tolerance who have experienced transient hyperglycemia either spontaneously or in response to identifiable stimuli. The terms *latent diabetes* and *prediabetes* should be abandoned. Individuals in this class include the following:
   a. Persons with GDM whose glucose tolerance has returned to normal after parturition.
   b. Obese diabetics whose glucose tolerance has returned to normal after losing weight.
   c. Persons who exhibit compromised glucose tolerance as a result of metabolic stress secondary to trauma or injury.
7. Potential for compromised glucose tolerance (Pot AGT): Individuals at risk for IDDM include the following, in decreasing order of risk:
   a. Persons with islet-cell antibodies.
   b. A monozygotic twin of an IDDM diabetic.
   c. A sibling of an IDDM diabetic.
   Individuals at risk for NIDDM include the following, in decreasing order of risk:
   a. A monozygotic twin of a NIDDM diabetic.
   b. A first-degree relative of a NIDDM diabetic (siblings, parents, and offspring).
   c. A mother of a neonate weighing more than 9 pounds.
   d. Obese individuals.
   e. Members of racial or ethnic groups with a high prevalence of diabetes, e.g., American Indian tribes.

Pathophysiology

The pathophysiologic derangements of diabetes mellitus are related to the body's inability to metabolize glucose, secondary to a relative or absolute deficiency of insulin (Watts and Keffer, 1982). The acute effects can range from mild hyperglycemia to severe ketoacidosis, a condition in which the body's metabolism has switched almost entirely to using ketone bodies as an energy source. Hyperosmolar coma can be a complication. Other chronic complications include atherosclerosis, myocardial infarction, ocular disease, kidney disease, nervous system disease, skin disease, and infection.

New knowledge about the pathophysiology of diabetes was a major reason for the new more standardized and comprehensive classification (National Diabetes Data Group, 1979). The classification is based on contemporary knowledge and is adaptable to future advances.

Additional new knowledge relates to hemoglobin A_{1C}, which is a glycosylated hemoglobin, or glycohemoglobin, that differs from normal adult hemoglobin A by having a carbohydrate moiety attached to the N-terminal valine of the beta chain. Its utility in the management of diabetes mellitus is that its level reflects the mean glucose level, not merely on the date it is measured, but over the preceding several weeks. Hemoglobin A_{1C} levels are not affected by meals, insulin, or exercise on the day of sampling. These levels have been correlated with cholesterol and triglyceride levels as well as abnormalities of erythrocyte, leukocyte, and platelet function. Research is under way to determine whether levels of hemoglobin A_{1C} correlate with the occurrence of chronic complications (Watts and Keffer, 1982).

Clinical Contexts

Diagnosis. The clinical features of IDDM include the following: polydipsia, polyuria, weight loss, lassitude, blurred vision, leg cramps, inattentiveness, irritability, craving for sweets, nausea, vomiting, dehydration, stupor, and coma leading to death.

The clinical features of NIDDM are milder and include the following: glycosuria, hyperglycemia, glucose intolerance, or some complication of diabetes such as premature myocardial infarction, premature peripheral vascular insufficiency, and diabetic neuropathy or diabetic nephropathy.

Management. Measurements of serum and urine glucose, as well as of hemoglobin A_{1C}

are useful. This discussion does not address the management of complications such as diabetic ketoacidosis.

Screening. Screening for diabetes mellitus, in the absence of clinical features of disease, is practiced in certain settings, e.g., the Armed Forces, where the goal is to identify individuals who have long-term physical liabilities.

Strategy

Test Sequence. Perform the serum glucose tests as indicated in Figure 16–6 (Burke, 1979; National Diabetes Data Group, 1979). Measurement of hemoglobin A_{1C} has been proposed as a strategy for assessing the adequacy of control of a given case of diabetes mellitus over a period of time (Boden et al., 1980). Some investigators (Dunn et al., 1979) propose that since an increased blood level of hemoglobin A_{1C} is more specific than the glucose tolerance test for diabetes mellitus, its measurement may have a role in diagnosis. However, it does not seem to be sensitive enough for the diagnosis of diabetes mellitus (Watts and Keffer, 1982).

Patient Preparation. Glucose measurements should be taken after the following conditions are met:

1. The patient should be otherwise in good health and ambulatory.

2. The patient should not be exposed to drugs that interfere with results (Table 16–9).

3. The diet should be unrestricted for at least 3 days in carbohydrate, greater than 150 gm/day.

4. Physical activity should be unrestricted.

5. A 10- to 16-hour fast should be undertaken (water only) before the morning of the test.

6. The subject should remain seated and should refrain from smoking during the test.

7. The test should be performed in the morning.

Specimen Collection and Handling. Perform measurements on serum or plasma promptly. If a delay in measurements is anticipated, use fluoride tubes to preserve glucose.

Methodology. Consult the laboratory for its methodologies, reference intervals, accuracy and precision, and sources of interference. Use enzymatic methods, i.e., glucose oxidase or hexokinase. Patients taking vitamin C have depressed serum glucose levels with glucose oxidase methods. Methods using hexokinase

Table 16–9. DRUGS AND CHEMICAL AGENTS ASSOCIATED WITH DIABETES MELLITUS AND IMPAIRED GLUCOSE TOLERANCE*

Diuretics and Antihypertensive Agents†
Chlorthalidone (Hygroton, Combipres, Regroton)
Clonidine (Catapres, Combipres)
Diazoxide (Hyperstat, Proglycem)
Furosemide (Lasix)
Metalazone
Thiazides (several forms, many trade names)
Bumetamide‡
Clopamide‡
Clorexolone‡
Ethacrynic acid‡ (Edecrin)
(Note: Hyperglycemic response to diuretics may be independent of K+ fluctuations)

Hormonally Active Agents†
Adrenocorticotropin (Acthar)
Tetracosactrin‡
Glucagon
Glucocorticoids (natural and synthetic)
Oral contraceptives
Somatotropin
Thyroid hormones (thyrotoxic doses)
Dextrothyroxine (Choloxin)
Calcitonin‡ (Calcimar)
Medroxyprogesterone (AMEN, Depo-Provera, Provera)‡
Prolactin‡

Psychoactive Agents†
Chlorprothixene (Teractan)
Haloperidol (Haldol)
Lithium carbonate (Eskalith, Lithane, others)
Phenothiazines
Chlorpromazine (Thorazine)
Perphenazine (Trilafon, Etrafon, Triavil)
Clopenthixol‡
Tricyclic Antidepressants
Amitriptyline (Elavil, Endep, Etrafon, Triavil)
Desipramine (Norpramin, Pertofrane)
Doxepin (Adapin, Sinequan)
Imipramine (Presamine, Tofranil, Imavate)
Nortriptylene (Aventyl)
Marijuana‡

Catecholamines and Other Neurologically Active Agents†
Diphenylhydantoin (Dilantin)
Epinephrine (Adrenalin chloride, Asthma-Meter, Sus-Prine)
Isoproterenol (Isuprel)
Levadopa (Bendopa, Dopar, Larodopa, Sinemet)
Norepinephrine (Levarterenol, Levophed)
Buphenine‡ (Nylidrin)
Fenoterol‡
Propranolol‡ (Inderal)

Analgesic, Antipyretic, and Anti-Inflammatory Agents†
Indomethacin (Indocin)
Acetaminophen‡ (overdose amounts) (Tylenol, Nebs, others)
Aspirin‡ (overdose amounts)
Morphine‡

Antineoplastic Agents†
Alloxan
L-Asparaginase
Streptozotocin
Cyclophosphamide‡ (Cytoxan)
Megestrol Acetate‡ (Megace)

Miscellaneous Agents†
Isoniazid (INAH, Nydrazid, others)
Nicotinic acid (Cerebro-Nicin, Nicobid, others)
Carbon disulfide‡
Cimetidine‡
Edetic acid‡ (EDTA)
Ethanol‡
Heparin‡
Mannoheptulose‡
Nalidixic acid‡ (NegGram)
Nickel chloride‡
Niridazole‡
Pentamidine‡ (Lomidine)
Phenolphthalein‡ (Ex-Lax)
Rodenticide‡ (Vacor)
Thiabendazole‡

*Adapted from the National Diabetes Data Group. Diabetes 28:1979, p 1045. Used with permission from the American Diabetes Association, Inc.

†For many of these agents, it cannot be determined whether the hyperglycemic response represents solely a pharmacologic action or an interaction between a predisposition for abnormal glucose tolerance and the pharmacologic effects of the agent. Drugs exacerbating pre-existing diabetes and a number of agents shown to cause hyperglycemia in animals but with no reported effect in humans have not been listed.

‡Association not clearly established for one of the following reasons: (1) confounded by the simultaneous administration of other drugs; (2) limited to a single case report; (3) conflicting or contradictory evidence; (4) drug reported to cause interference with laboratory test for serum glucose.

have fewer potential interferences than those using glucose oxidase. Reduction methods are obsolete and can overestimate serum glucose, e.g., 40 mg/100 ml higher than the enzymatic methods in the presence of uremia (uric acid and creatinine are reducing substances) (Howanitz and Howanitz, 1979). (See Part 3 for serum glucose studies, including drug interferences, and for lists of differential diagnoses for high and low serum glucose levels.) Table 16–9 lists drugs and other agents some of which may interfere with non-specific methods.

Hemoglobin A_{1C} can be measured by column chromatography.

Interpretation

Diagnosis. Criteria for the diagnosis of diabetes mellitus are presented in Figure 16–6 and Table 16–10. See Table 16–11 for common laboratory test results in diabetes mellitus.

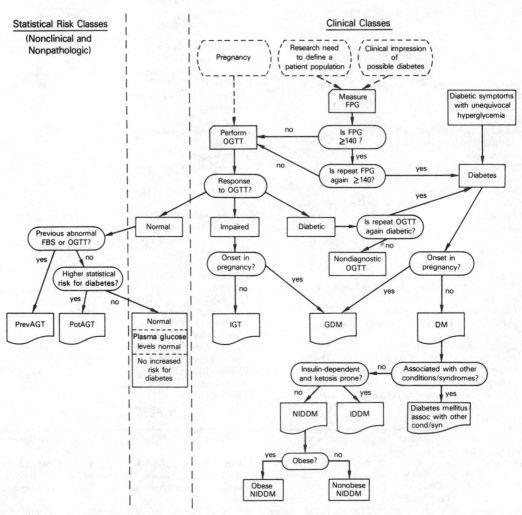

Figure 16–6.   Procedure for classifying adult research subjects or clinical patients. (From National Diabetes Data Group: Classification and diagnosis of diabetes mellitus and other categories of glucose intolerance. Diabetes 28:1979, p. 1047. Reproduced with permission from the American Diabetes Association, Inc.)

Table 16–10. DIAGNOSTIC CRITERIA FOR DIABETES MELLITUS AND IMPAIRED GLUCOSE TOLERANCE*

Diabetes Mellitus

Unequivocal elevation of serum and plasma glucose ($\geq$200 mg/100 ml) and classic symptoms

Fasting serum and plasma glucose $\geq$140 mg/100 ml, more than once

Oral glucose tolerance test (challenge dose 75 gm†) $\geq$200 mg/100 ml at ½, 1, or 1½ and at 2 hours, more than once

Impaired Glucose Tolerance

Fasting plasma glucose >115 mg/100 ml but <140 mg/100 ml

Oral glucose tolerance test (challenge 75 gm) $\geq$200 mg/100 ml at ½, 1, or 1½ hours and 140–200 mg/100 ml at 2 hours, only once

Gestational Diabetes Mellitus

Oral glucose tolerance test (challenge 100 gm) two of the following levels must be met or exceeded:

Fasting 105 mg/100 ml
1 hour 190 mg/100 ml
2 hours 165 mg/100 ml
3 hours 145 mg/100 ml

---

*National Diabetes Data Group. Diabetes 28:1039, 1979.

†Challenge dose for children is 1.75 gm/kg of ideal body weight, up to 75 gm.

Management. Blood hemoglobin A_{1C} should not be elevated. The reference interval is approximately 3 to 6 per cent of total blood hemoglobin in well-managed patients with diabetes mellitus.

Test Requests and Reports

Test Requests. The test sequence for the diagnosis of diabetes mellitus can be offered by the laboratory as a clinical problem-solving service.

Interpretive Reports. The results of the strategy can be collated and returned to the attending physician in the form of an interpretive report. In using the new criteria for diagnosis of diabetes mellitus (National Diabetes Data Group, 1979), we have found it helpful to keep a record in the laboratory of each patient's studies. This is particularly helpful when the interpretation of a given study is dependent on the results of a previous study, for instance, in determining whether this is the first or second pathologic glucose tolerance test. This is an ideal area for computer-assisted interpretive reporting.

Table 16–11. COMMON LABORATORY TEST RESULTS IN DIABETES MELLITUS

Laboratory Test	Value	Pathophysiologic Factors
Chemistry (Serum)		
Bilirubin, total	—	
Calcium, total	↓	Related to osmotic diuresis secondary to hyperglycemia
Carbon dioxide	↓	Related to ketoacidosis
Chloride	↓	Related to osmotic diuresis secondary to hyperglycemia
Cholesterol	↑	Related to disturbed carbohydrate metabolism, triglyceride levels may be elevated also
Creatinine phosphokinase	↑	Related to ketoacidosis
Creatinine	↑	High levels of glucose and acetone can interfere with methodology
Glucose	↑	Essential component of diabetes mellitus
Lactic dehydrogenase	↑	In 20 per cent of patients
Phosphatase, alkaline	↑	In 10 to 45 per cent of patients
Phosphorus, inorganic	↑	Related to glucose intolerance
	↓	Osmotic diuresis secondary to hyperglycemia
Potassium	↑	Related to low insulin levels
	↓	Related to osmotic diuresis secondary to hyperglycemia
Proteins, total	—	
Proteins, albumin	↓	Tends to be low
Sodium	↓	Osmotic diuresis secondary to hyperglycemia
Transaminase, aspartate amino	↑	In 10 per cent of patients at initial hospitalization
Urea nitrogen	↑	Related to protein catabolism
Uric acid	↑	In 30 per cent of patients at initial hospitalization
Hematology (Blood)		
Hemoglobin	—	
Hematocrit	—	
Leukocyte count, total	—	
Platelet count	↑	In 25 per cent of patients at initial hospitalization

Key: — = No change; ↑ = can be increased; ↓ = can be decreased.

*Information from Friedman RB, Anderson RE, Entine SM et al: Effects of diseases on clinical laboratory tests. Clin Chem 26:1D–476D, 1980; Wolf PL: Interpretation of Biochemical Multitest Profiles: An Analysis of 100 Important Conditions. New York, Masson Publishing, Inc, 1977.

CLINICAL LABORATORY
Memorial Hospital of Union County

Criteria (National Diabetes Data Group—Diabetes 28: 1039, 1979):
1. Fasting A.M. blood sugar (FBS): Less than 115 mg/100 ml considered within normal limits; diabetes mellius excluded, and GTT not necessary.

2. FBS greater than 115 mg/100 ml but less than 140 mg/100 ml: Schedule for GTT.

3. FBS greater than 140 mg/100 ml on more than one (1) occasion: Diagnosis of diabetes mellitus confirmed, and GTT not indicated.

Patient should meet the following criteria for a valid oral glucose tolerance test:
1. Normal activity
2. Carbohydrate intake greater than 150 g/day
3. Patient not ill or taking medications
4. Patient not smoking
5. GTT done in A.M.

Adult Challenge Dose—75 gm	Gestational Dose—100 gm
Fasting _____	Fasting _____
½ hr _____	1 hr _____
1 hr _____	2 hr _____
1½ hr _____	3 hr _____
2 hr _____	

Comment:

_____

Signature

_____

Date

Figure 16–7. Interpretive report for the oral glucose tolerance test (GTT). (Courtesy of Rebecca S. Craig, M. T., Marysville, Ohio.)

Of the laboratories that we surveyed in the United States (Speicher and Smith, 1980), 21 per cent used interpretive reports for the problem of diabetes mellitus (Fig. 16–7).

REFERENCES

Cushing's Syndrome

Apter D, Jänne O, Vihko R: Sephadex chromatography in the radioimmunoassay of serum and urinary cortisol. Clin Chim Acta 63:139–148, 1975.

Ashcraft MW, Van Herle AJ, Vener SL et al: Serum cortisol levels in Cushing's syndrome after low- and high-dose dexamethasone suppression. Ann Intern Med 97:21–26, 1982.

Cook DM, Kendall JW, Jordan R: Cushing's syndrome: Current concepts of diagnosis and therapy. West J Med 132:111–122, 1980.

Cushing's disease: Clinical features and diagnostic problems, editorial. Lancet 1:1034–1035, 1981.

Flint LD, Jacobs EC: Belated recognition of adrenocorticotrophic hormone-producing tumors in post-adrenalectomized Cushing's syndrome. J Urol 112:688–692, 1974.

Friedman RB, Anderson RE, Entine SM et al: Effects of diseases on clinical laboratory tests. Clin Chem 26:1D–476D, 1980.

Gold EM: The Cushing syndromes: Changing views of diagnosis and treatment. Ann Intern Med 90:829–844, 1979.

Henry JB, Murphy J: Effective utilization of clinical laboratories. In Henry JB (ed): Clinical Diagnosis and Management of Laboratory Methods, ed 16. Philadelphia, WB Saunders Company, 1979, pp 2039–2048.

Juselius RE, Barnhart F: Competitive protein-binding radioassay of urinary cortisol. Clin Chem 20:1470–1474, 1974.

Liddle GW: Cushing's syndrome. In Wyngaarden JB, Smith LH (eds): Cecil Textbook of Medicine, ed 16. Philadelphia, WB Saunders Company, 1982, pp 1232–1237.

Melby JC: Assessment of adrenocortical function. N Engl J Med 285:735–739, 1971.

Nugent CA, Warner HR, Dunn JT et al: Probability theory in the diagnosis of Cushing's syndrome. J Clin Endocrinol 24:621–627, 1964.

Speicher CE, Smith JW: Interpretive reporting in clinical pathology. JAMA 243:1556–1560, 1980.

Walker RF, Fahmy DR, Read GF: Adrenal status assessed by direct radioimmunoassay of cortisol in whole saliva or parotid saliva. Clin Chem 24:1460–1463, 1978.

Watts NB, Keffer JH: Practical Endocrine Diagnosis ed 3. Philadelphia, Lea & Febiger, 1982.

Pheochromocytoma

Bledsoe T: Disorders of the adrenal glands. In Harvey AM, Johns RJ, McKusick VA et al (eds): The Principles and Practice of Medicine, ed 20. New York, Appleton-Century-Crofts, 1980, pp 776–794.

Bravo EL, Tarazi RC, Fouad FM et al: Clonidine-suppression test: A useful aid in the diagnosis of pheochromocytoma. N Engl J Med 305:623–626, 1981.

Bravo EL, Tarazi RC, Gifford RW Jr et al: Circulating and urinary catecholamines in pheochromocytoma: Diagnostic and pathophysiologic implications. N Engl J Med 301:682–686, 1979.

Engelman K: Pheochromocytoma. In Wyngaarden JB, Smith LH (eds): Cecil Textbook of Medicine, ed 16. Philadelphia, WB Saunders Company, 1982, pp 1307–1312.

Galen RS, Gambino SR: Beyond Normality: The Predictive Value and Efficiency of Medical Diagnoses. New York, John Wiley & Sons, Inc, 1975.

Gifford RW, Kvale WF, Maher FT et al: Clinical features, diagnosis and treatment of pheochromocytoma: A review of 76 cases. Mayo Clin Proc 39:281–302, 1964.

Gitlow SE, Mendlowitz M, Bertain LM: The biochemical techniques for detecting and establishing the presence of pheochromocytoma. A review of ten years' experience. Am J Cardiol 26:270–279, 1970.

Gitlow SE, Mendlowitz M, Wilk EK et al: Excretion of catecholamine catabolites by normal children. J Lab Clin Med 72:612–620, 1968.

Henry JB, Murphy J: Effective utilization of clinical laboratories. In Henry JB (ed): Clinical Diagnosis and Management by Laboratory Methods, ed 16. Philadelphia, WB Saunders Company, 1979, pp 2039–2048.

Howanitz PJ, Howanitz JH: Evaluation of endocrine function. In Henry JB (ed): Clinical Diagnosis and Management by Laboratory Methods, ed 16. Philadelpha, WB Saunders Company, 1979, pp 402–476.

Markel SF, Johnson RM: The clinical features and laboratory diagnosis of functional paraganglioma (pheochromocytoma). Laboratory Medicine 6:39–65, 1975.

McCarthy D, Bravo EL, Tarazi RC et al: Value of predictive value, letters. N Engl J Med 302:1479–1480, 1980.

Remine WH, Chong GC, Van Heerdan JA et al: Current management of pheochromocytoma. Ann Surg 179:740–748, 1974.

Robbins SL, Cotran SR: Pathologic Basis of Disease, ed 2. Philadelphia, WB Saunders Company, 1979, pp 1402–1407.

Sisson JC, Frager MS, Valk TW, et al: Scintigraphic localization of pheochromocytoma. N Engl J Med 305:12–17, 1981.

Tucker RM, Labarthe DR: Frequency of surgical treatment for hypertension in adults at the Mayo Clinic from 1973 through 1975. Mayo Clin Proc 52:549–555, 1977.

Watts NB, Keffer JH: Practical Endocrine Diagnosis, ed 3. Philadelphia, Lea & Febiger, 1982.

Weinstein MC, Fineberg HV: Cost-effectiveness analysis for medical practices: Appropriate laboratory utilization. In Benson ES, Rubin M (eds): Logic and Economics of Clinical Laboratory Use. New York, Elsevier North-Holland, Inc, 1978, pp 3–32.

Diabetes Mellitus

Boden G, Master RW, Gordon SS et al: Monitoring metabolic control in diabetic outpatients with glycosylated hemoglobin. Ann Intern Med 92:357–360, 1980.

Burke DM: Diabetes mellitus: Test strategies for diagnosis and management. Postgrad Med 66:213–219, 1979.

Cahill GF: Diabetes mellitus. In Wyngaarden JB, Smith LH (eds): Cecil Textbook of Medicine, ed 16. Philadelphia, WB Saunders Company, 1982, pp 1053–1072.

Dunn PJ, Cole RA, Soeldner JS et al: Reproducibility of hemoglobin A_{IC} and sensitivity to various degrees of glucose intolerance. Ann Intern Med 91:390–396, 1979.

Howanitz PJ, Howanitz JH: Carbohydrates. In Henry JB (ed): Clinical Diagnosis and Management by Laboratory Methods, ed 16. Philadelphia, WB Saunders Company, 1979, pp 153–188.

National Diabetes Data Group: Classification and diagnosis of diabetes mellitus and other categories of glucose intolerance. Diabetes 28:1039–1057, 1979.

Shabo AL: Increased incidence of diabetes. Extracted from Audio-Digest Ophthalmology, Vol 18, No 11, in the Audio Digest Foundation series: 1577 East Chevy Chase Drive, Glendale, Cal. West J Med 133:94, 1980.

Speicher CE, Smith JW: Interpretive reporting in clinical pathology. JAMA 243:1556–1560, 1980.

Watts NB, Keffer JH: Practical Endocrine Diagnosis, ed 3. Philadelphia, Lea & Febiger, 1982.

CHAPTER 17

METABOLIC SUBPROBLEMS

INBORN ERRORS OF
   METABOLISM
   Alpha$_1$-Antitrypsin Deficiency
   Cystic Fibrosis
   Wilson's Disease

INBORN ERRORS OF METABOLISM

ALPHA$_1$-ANTITRYPSIN DEFICIENCY

Definition and Significance

Alpha$_1$-antitrypsin deficiency is a rare but important inherited disorder characterized by a deficiency of the serum glycoprotein alpha$_1$-antitrypsin, which is synthesized by liver cells and is able to inhibit the activity of a variety of proteolytic enzymes. In 1963 Laurell and Eriksson discovered this genetically determined deficiency of alpha$_1$-antitrypsin and noted its association with early onset of severe emphysema. Five years later, the relationship between the deficiency and childhood cirrhosis was observed (Sharp, 1976). This disease can present in a variety of ways:
1. Hepatic disease
   a. Neonatal hepatitis.
   b. Chronic active hepatitis and cirrhosis of children, adolescents, or adults.
   c. Hepatocellular carcinoma.

2. Pulmonary disease.
   a. Chronic obstructive pulmonary disease (COPD).

Homozygous alpha$_1$-antitrypsin deficiency has a prevalence of 0.025 per cent and heterozygous alpha$_1$-antitrypsin deficiency, a prevalence of 2 to 8 per cent. There is no therapy, short of liver transplantation. Phenobarbital, a most efficient inducer of hepatic enzyme activity, does nothing to raise serum alpha$_1$-antitrypsin levels or clear the precursor material from hepatocytes. Environmental lung irritants, such as tobacco smoke, appear to aggravate the severity of the pulmonary disease process (Morse, 1978).

Parenteral replacement therapy with an alpha$_1$-antitrypsin concentrate of normal plasma has been recently evaluated (Gadek et al., 1981).

Pathophysiology

The various phenotypes of alpha$_1$-antitrypsin in an individual may be characterized by the *Pi system*. Pi stands for protease inhibitor. The molecular variants of alpha$_1$-antitrypsin can be separated by acid-starch gel electrophoresis and are genetically determined by two codominant alleles. Therefore, each individual has two codominant alleles.

The most common phenotype in persons with normal levels of serum alpha$_1$-antitrypsin is PiMM, found in 80 to 95 per cent of the population. PiZZ is a rare homozygous phenotype in which the serum levels of alpha$_1$-antitrypsin are very low. Heterozygotes (i.e., phenotype PiMZ) have intermediate levels of alpha$_1$-antitrypsin. Besides PiZZ, another phenotype—PiSZ—is also associated with low serum levels of alpha$_1$-antitrypsin. Levels of alpha$_1$-antitrypsin observed with the common phenotypes are given in Table 17–1. Patients of the phenotype PiZZ are at risk of developing hepatic and/or pulmonary disease (Morse, 1978). Heterozygotes are at risk for disease, but the extent of risk needs further study (Campra et al., 1973; Cockroft et al., 1981; Kueppers et al., 1976).

Patients with the deficiency can synthesize alpha$_1$-antitrypsin in the liver, but they lack a releasing factor; as a result, alpha$_1$-antitrypsin accumulates in the liver.

Healthy persons maintain serum levels of alpha$_1$-antitrypsin at around 200 to 400 mg/100 ml. The serum levels of this acute-phase protein in a healthy population can be doubled or tripled by inflammation, neoplastic disease, pregnancy, or estrogen therapy. In patients with a severe deficiency, levels can increase only slightly despite such stimuli, and in those with a moderate deficiency, basal values can usually be doubled. (See Chapter 8 for a discussion of inflammation and acute-phase proteins.)

The pathogenesis of these hepatic and pulmonary diseases is not well understood. It appears that uninhibited proteolytic enzymes in the liver and lung are probably responsible for continual tissue damage (Gadek et al., 1981).

Ongoing damage to liver cells is reflected by elevated levels of serum glutamic oxaloacetic transaminase (SGOT) and serum pyruvic transaminase (SGPT). The histologic picture is consistent with chronic active hepatitis (see

Chapter 15). As chronic active hepatitis progresses to macronodular cirrhosis and hepatocellular function decreases, serum albumin may become depressed, serum gamma globulins may be increased, and plasma prothrombin time (PT) may be prolonged (see Chapter 15).

COPD is associated with changes in pulmonary function tests and blood gas studies. These are discussed in Chapter 11.

Clinical Contexts

Diagnosis. The clinical features of hepatic alpha$_1$-antitrypsin deficiency are those of either chronic active hepatitis or cirrhosis, or both. These features are described in Chapter 15.

A finding of periodic-acid Schiff (PAS)–positive, diastase-resistant globules in the cytoplasm of liver cells found on liver biopsy is diagnostic of alpha$_1$-antitrypsin deficiency until proved otherwise. These globules are visible in hematoxylin- and eosin-stained sections. However, recent reports indicate that these globules may not be completely specific for the disease (Roggli et al., 1981; Pariente et al., 1981; Cox et al., 1982). A few cases have been discovered which show no circulating alpha$_1$-antitrypsin and no liver globules (Morse, 1978).

The clinical features of pulmonary alpha$_1$-antitrypsin deficiency are those of COPD (see Chapter 11).

Management. Management of the hepatic and pulmonary diseases of alpha$_1$-antitrypsin deficiency is the same as that for subproblems of chronic active hepatitis, cirrhosis, and COPD.

Screening. In the absence of a family history of clinical features of chronic liver and lung disease, screening for alpha$_1$-antitrypsin deficiency is not ordinarily indicated. In a report by Sveger (1976), screening of 200,000 newborns found 120 with PiZ, 48 PiSZ, two PiZ$^-$, and one PiS$^-$. The PiZ and PiSZ phenotypes were associated with covert or readily apparent hepatic dysfunction in the first 3 months of life. An argument can be made for preemployment testing for workers who might be exposed to occupational air pollution (Morse, 1978).

Strategy

Test Sequence. The test sequence for the diagnosis of alpha$_1$-antitrypsin deficiency re-

Table 17–1. LEVELS OF ALPHA$_1$-ANTITRYPSIN OBSERVED WITH COMMON PHENOTYPES*

Phenotype	Serum Total Alpha$_1$-Antitrypsin Level†
PiZZ	5 to 15%
PiSZ	31%
PiSS	63%
PiMZ	61%
PiMS	83%
PiMM	Normal

*Information from Alper CA: Deficiency of alpha-1-antitrypsin, editorial. Ann Intern Med 78:298–299, 1973.

†Per cent mean serum level in a healthy reference population.

quires assessment of the serum level of the glycoprotein. It is also necessary to use a technique that can ascertain the patient's phenotype. Determining the phenotype will eliminate the false-negative results that can occur when patients with the deficiency present with serum levels of total alpha$_1$-antitrypsin that are not depressed, such as heterozygotes with acute inflammation. Measurement of serum total alpha$_1$-antitrypsin cannot be expected to detect Pi types MZ or MS reliably. Therefore, quantitative screening methods must be accompanied by Pi phenotyping for detection of type MZ or MS (Talamo et al., 1972).

The strategy for the diagnosis and management of the hepatic disease of alpha$_1$-antitrypsin deficiency is the same as that for chronic active hepatitis and cirrhosis (see Chapter 15); diagnosis and management of the pulmonary disease are the same as for COPD (see Chapter 11).

Patient Preparation. No special preparation is required.

Specimen Collection and Handling. A serum specimen is required. Hemolyzed specimens can interfere with measurement of alpha$_1$-antitrypsin by nephelometry but not by radial immunodiffusion.

Methodology. Consult the laboratory for its methodologies, reference intervals, accuracy and precision, and potential sources of interference. The following techniques can be used:

1. Serum protein electrophoresis (SPE).

2. Measurement of alpha$_1$-antitrypsin by radial immunodiffusion, electroimmunodiffusion, or nephelometry.

3. Functional assay for total serum trypsin inhibitory capacity.

4. Phenotyping of alpha$_1$-antitrypsin by acid-starch gel electrophoresis followed by crossed antigen-antibody electrophoresis, immunofixation, or isoelectric focusing in poly-

Table 17–2. COMMON LABORATORY TEST RESULTS IN ALPHA$_1$-ANTITRYPSIN DEFICIENCY*

Laboratory Test	Value	Pathophysiologic Factors
Chemistry (Serum)		
Bilirubin, total	↑	Related to liver disease
Calcium, total	↓	Related to decreased albumin
Carbon dioxide	↑	Related to chronic obstructive pulmonary disease (COPD)
Chloride	↓	Suggests chronic hypoventilation
Cholesterol	↓	Related to liver disease
Creatine phosphokinase	—	
Creatinine	—	
Glucose	—	
Lactic dehydrogenase	↑	Related to liver disease
Phosphatase, alkaline	↑	Related to liver disease
Phosphorus, inorganic	—	
Potassium	↑	With acidosis
	↓	With coexisting metabolic alkalosis
Proteins, total	↑	Polyclonal gammopathy with cirrhosis
Proteins, albumin	↓	Decreased synthesis with liver disease
Sodium	—	
Transaminase, aspartate amino	↑	Related to liver disease
Urea nitrogen	—	
Uric acid	—	
Hematology (Blood)		
Hemoglobin	↑	Polycythemia secondary to hypoxemia
	↓	Hypersplenism and/or high incidence of peptic ulcer with COPD
Hematocrit	↑	Polycythemia secondary to hypoxemia
	↓	Hypersplenism and/or high incidence of peptic ulcer with COPD
Leukocyte count, total	↑	Related to inflammation, especially of lungs
	↓	Hypersplenism
Platelet count	↓	Hypersplenism

Key:
— = No change; ↑ = can be increased; ↓ = can be decreased.
*Information from Friedman RB, Anderson RE, Entine SM et al: Effects of diseases on clinical laboratory tests. Clin Chem 26:1D–476D, 1980; Morse JO: Alpha-1-antitrypsin deficiency. N Engl J Med 299:1045–1048, 1099–1105, 1978.

acrylamide gel (Creason et al., 1980; Morse, 1978).

Functional assays for total trypsin inhibitory activity of serum correlate well with immunologic assays of serum alpha$_1$-antitrypsin because 80 to 90 per cent of the total inhibitory activity of serum is accounted for by alpha$_1$-antitrypsin. Immunologic measurement is preferable to functional assay.

Interpretation

Diagnosis. For homozygotes, the diagnosis of alpha$_1$-antitrypsin deficiency can be made by demonstrating a decreased serum level of this protease inhibitor. Since 90 per cent of the total alpha$_1$-globulin fraction on SPE is composed of alpha$_1$-antitrypsin, a conspicuous absence or deficiency of this fraction is presumptive evidence of deficiency. A 6-month survey of sera from hospitalized patients by SPE found this deficiency in 5 of 1500 specimens examined (Laurell and Eriksson, 1963). Sera having decreased or absent alpha$_1$-globulin fractions should be subjected to quantitative immunologic measurement of alpha$_1$-antitrypsin and determination of the phenotype.

As mentioned earlier in this chapter, the reference interval for a healthy population for serum alpha$_1$-antitrypsin is 200 to 400 mg/100 ml. The presence of inflammation, neoplastic disease, pregnancy, or estrogen therapy can elevate the serum levels in patients with the disease and cause it to be within the reference intervals for healthy people. This is a common reason for not diagnosing alpha$_1$-antitrypsin deficiency in emphysematous patients who are initially admitted to the hospital, inasmuch as they are likely to harbor acute infections as the precipitating event for their admission (Daniels, 1975).

Patients homozygous for alpha$_1$-antitrypsin deficiency (phenotype PiZZ) have serum levels of 5 to 15 per cent of those for healthy people. Heterozygotes of varying phenotypes have serum levels intermediate between phenotype PiZZ and healthy people of phenotype PiMM and can be missed if only SPE is used. Thus it is desirable, although technically difficult to determine the phenotype of patients suspected of having the disease. Some investigators have commented on the inadequacy of immunochemical determination of serum levels alone for detection of heterozygotes of phenotypes PiMZ or PiMS (Talamo et al., 1972).

Diagnoses of chronic active hepatitis, cirrhosis, and COPD are described in Chapters 11 and 15 in these particular subproblems.

Table 17–2 gives the results of common laboratory tests in alpha$_1$-antitrypsin deficiency. Figure 17–1 gives an overview of the diagnostic reasoning.

Management. Once a diagnosis of alpha$_1$-antitrypsin deficiency has been established, there is no merit in following the serum levels as either a prognostic or therapeutic guide. Chronic active liver disease, cirrhosis, and COPD are managed as described in these particular subproblems.

Test Requests and Reports

Test Requests. The execution of the test sequence for alpha$_1$-antitrypsin deficiency may be offered as a problem-solving service. Figure 17–2 shows an example of such a request form.

Interpretive Reports. The test results can be entered on the same form used to request the test sequence (Fig. 17–2), and the collated information can be returned to the attending physician in the form of an interpretive report. Of the laboratories we surveyed in the United States, 1 per cent used interpretive reports for the subproblem of alpha$_1$-antitrypsin deficiency (Speicher and Smith, 1980).

CYSTIC FIBROSIS

Definition and Significance

Cystic fibrosis (CF) is a hereditary disease of children and young adults that can affect many organ systems, such as the pancreas, liver, sweat glands, lungs, and gastrointestinal tract. The exact etiology is unknown. No serum factor has been identified biochemically, and no biologic test for a serum factor has been sufficiently accurate to allow confident identification of heterozygotes or homozygotes (Gibson, 1980); however, developments in the identification of a specific pathologic lesion suggest that progress may be forthcoming (Manson, 1980). Clinical manifestations are related to disturbances in the function of exocrine glands, causing their secretions to be unusually thick and tenacious.

Cystic fibrosis is the most common semilethal genetic abnormality in the United States (Wood et al., 1976). It is perpetuated as an autosomal recessive trait with a carrier rate of

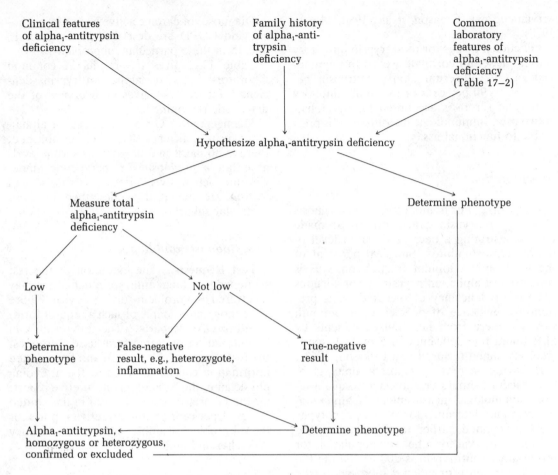

Figure 17-1.   Diagnostic reasoning for alpha$_1$-antitrypsin deficiency.

approximately 5 per cent in the white population in the United States. The prevalence of this disorder is 1 per 1600 to 2000 live white births; this is greater than the prevalence for neonatal hypothyroidism and phenylketonuria, for which screening programs have already been established (Scully et al., 1981). Cystic fibrosis is less frequent in blacks (1 in 17,000) and has never been found in Orientals. Correct diagnosis is essential, not only to detect those patients who require life-saving therapy but also to avoid the psychologic and economic trauma of incorrectly assigning the disease to a normal person.

A testimony to the benefits of modern medical care is the report of Shwachman and associates (1977), which documented 70 patients with cystic fibrosis above 25 years of age. In 1958, Shwachman's group had reported on 105 patients, of whom only ten were over the age of 15, the oldest being only 23 years old (Shwachman and Kulczycki, 1958).

The number of adults receiving care from the United States Cystic Fibrosis Centers has been increasing at an average rate of about 200 patients each year. It has been predicted that almost 4000 adults would be receiving care at the centers by the end of 1985 (Warwick and Pogue, 1977).

Pathophysiology

Because the exact cause of cystic fibrosis is unclear, there are no laboratory studies that are capable of detecting the basic genetic defect. Most methods of laboratory diagnosis emphasize the demonstration of abnormalities of exocrine glands or the secondary effects of these abnormalities.

In the 1930s it was discovered that pancreatic exocrine function was diminished as a result of obstruction of pancreatic ducts by thick, tenacious secretions of mucus. This decreased the amount of pancreatic enzymes in the intes-

UNIVERSITY HEALTH CENTER OF PITTSBURGH	α_1 ANTITRYPSIN EVALUATION	Patient Name: Address or Location:
Marks or Special Instructions:		Patient No: Patient Age: Date:

1. Agarose Gel Electrophoresis pH 8.6 — depressed α_1 globulins (electrophoretic strip may be attached)

2. Serum Trypsin Inhibitory Capacity ___0.32___ mg Trypsin inhibited/ml (STIC)

Normal Range:	0.60 to 1.17 mg/ml
Heterozygous Deficiency:	0.20 to 0.49 mg/ml
Homozygous Deficiency:	0.02 to 0.15 mg/ml

3. α_1 Antitrypsin by Radial Immunodiffusion: ___79___ mg/dl

Normal Range:	160 to 350 mg/dl
Heterozygous Deficiency:	75 to 180 mg/dl
Homozygous Deficiency:	0 to 40 mg/dl

4. Phenotyping Result (If indicated)

PiSS

COMMENTS:

α_1 antitrypsin results in the heterozygous deficiency range. Further studies reveal phenotype consistent with PiSS. Family members should be typed for further information.

Figure 17–2.   Interpretive report for alpha$_1$-antitrypsin evaluation. (Courtesy of WI Smith, M.D., Pittsburgh, Pa.)

tinal tract, and measurement of pancreatic enzymes such as trypsin and chymotrypsin in the stool and duodenal tract was used as a method of diagnosis. The albumin concentration in meconium is increased, and this increased albumin has been used as a screening test.

Later it was discovered that patients with cystic fibrosis suffered salt depletion shock in hot weather and that the sweat sodium and chloride in these patients were decreased. Measurement of these electrolytes in sweat offered a better method for diagnosis than measurement of pancreatic enzymes in the duodenum and stool. It is postulated that an abnormality of the sweat glands prevents the reabsorption of sodium and chloride so that levels of these electrolytes become elevated

(Dann and Blau, 1978; Robbins and Cotran, 1979).

Clinical Contexts

Diagnosis. The main clinical features of cystic fibrosis are related to dysfunction of the lungs and pancreas. Obstruction of the pancreatic ducts with secondary pancreatic insufficiency can lead to meconium ileus in 10 to 15 per cent of newborns with cystic fibrosis. Meconium ileus presents with evidence of intestinal obstruction and abdominal distention caused by inspissated meconium in the intestine. This is because the meconium, which is normally present in the intestine, is not digested and softened by pancreatic enzymes. In older children pancreatic insufficiency can present with a malabsorption syndrome and failure to thrive. (See Chapter 13 for a discussion of malabsorption and Chapter 14 for a discussion of pancreatitis and pancreatic insufficiency.)

According to Gottlieb and associates (1980) and Wood and co-workers (1976), some gastrointestinal presentations that suggest CF are as follows:

1. Cirrhosis of the liver.
2. Portal hypertension.
3. Deficiency of vitamins A, D, E, and K.
4. Duodenal ulcer.
5. Rectal prolapse.
6. Acute or recurrent pancreatitis.

COPD can develop secondary to thick plugs of mucus secreted in the bronchial tree (see Chapter 11). Chronic coughing and wheezing characterize the patient's clinical picture, and there is a propensity to persistent pulmonary infections that are responsible for 80 to 90 per cent of deaths.

Some of the pulmonary presentations that suggest CF are as follows (Gottlieb et al., 1980; Wood et al., 1976):

1. COPD: Bronchitis or emphysema.
2. Characteristic chest roentgenogram.
3. Recurrent pulmonary infections.
4. Bronchiectasis.
5. Hemoptysis.
6. Atelectasis.
7. Staphylococcal or pseudomonas pulmonary infection.
8. Pneumothorax.
9. Cor pulmonale.
10. Recurrent polyposis of the nasal passages (chronic pansinusitis) and minor lung infections in 10 to 15 per cent of older children and young adults.

Additional symptoms include the following (Gottlieb et al., 1980; Wood et al., 1976):

1. Clubbing.
2. Diabetes mellitus (see Chapter 16).
3. Salty taste of sweat.
4. Hyponatremia.
5. Hypochloremic dehydration in warm weather.
6. Male infertility.
7. A family history of cystic fibrosis.

In the past, 50 per cent of cystic fibrosis patients died before the age of 10 and almost all by 30 years of age. Improved diagnosis and management, particularly of the pulmonary complications, have increased the survival to 77 per cent at 20 years of age (Shwachman et

al., 1977). Stern and co-workers (1977) reviewed the adolescent and adult presentation of CF.

Management. The use of laboratory studies for the management of cystic fibrosis is based on the therapy of pulmonary and gastrointestinal complications. (See Chapter 11 for a discussion of COPD, and see Chapter 13 for a discussion of malabsorption.)

Screening. Although the prevalence of cystic fibrosis is about 1 per 2000 white births, which is greater than that for neonatal hypothyroidism, screening of all newborns is not possible. This is because the sweat test, the only reliable method of diagnosing cystic fibrosis, is too time consuming and costly to perform on every infant. Therefore, in the absence of clinical features, targeted screening of newborns for cystic fibrosis is indicated only when there is a family history of the disease. Continuing education of physicians about the clinical features of CF is important, since only 17 per cent of CF patients are asymptomatic during their first year of life (Gibson, 1980; *Lancet* editorial, 1980).

Strategy

Test Sequence. The Gibson-Cooke sweat test is the best laboratory tool for the diagnosis of cystic fibrosis (Gibson and Cooke, 1959; *Lancet* editorial, 1982). The large number of false-positive and false-negative results with other techniques, such as the direct measurement of chloride on the skin (Kopito and Shwachman, 1969) and sweat conductivity (Shwachman et al., 1965), has rendered them unacceptable. Most of the errors from other tests have been due to false-positive results (David and Phillips, 1982; Rosenstein et al., 1978; Smalley et al., 1978). In 1976, the Committee for Evaluation of Testing for Cystic Fibrosis of the National Academy of Sciences recommended the Gibson-Cooke technique as the method of choice for diagnosis ("Evaluation of Testing," 1976). The Gibson-Cooke sweat test requires a skilled technologist and meticulous quality control. As with any procedure, it is usually done best in centers where it is performed often. Although the sweat defect is present at birth, testing should be delayed for 2 to 3 months to obtain the most accurate readings. The sweat test must be performed twice.

There are several screening tests for cystic

fibrosis, the effectiveness of which is not very high; i.e., there is no really good method for screening (*Lancet* editorial, 1982):

1. Stool specimens
   a. *BMC test strip* (Berry, 1980; Gibson, 1980): Widely used in Western European countries, it contains an indicator to detect an increased concentration of albumin in meconium. In a collaborative study, 102,159 infants were tested according to instructions: 216 had positive test results, of which 18 were found to have sweat test–confirmed CF (92 per cent false-positive results). The data suggest a false-negative rate of 59 per cent. Berry and associates (1980) were able to refine the test strip technique by confirming all positive test strip results in 20,490 specimens with a more quantitative test for albumin, radial immunodiffusion. This refined technique helped to decrease the false-positive result rate.
   b. *Lactase test strip* (Berry et al., 1980; Gibson, 1980): This is used to screen for CF by measuring increased lactase activity detected by glucose production after incubation of meconium with lactose. Screening with the lactase test strip in 44,816 specimens and confirming positive test results using a quantitative test for albumin had a false-positive result rate of 68 per cent. The data also suggest a false-negative result rate of 68 per cent.
   c. *Stool trypsin method* (Forrest et al., 1981): A trypsin assay of stool dried on filter paper was evaluated in 20,000 5-day-old babies. Sweat tests were required in only seven babies. Three of them had cystic fibrosis. The test gave a false-negative result in at least two babies.
2. Finger tip specimen.
   a. *Chloride plate test* (Shwachman and Mahmoodian, 1981): An agar plate test was used to determine the concentration of chloride on the finger tips. Readings of 2+ or less excluded cystic fibrosis in 1589 cases with only two doubtful instances, whereas 4+ readings were recorded in 198 cases of CF and 3+ readings in 15 cases of CF. In doubtful cases, four individuals had 4+ readings and 11 had 3+ readings.
3. Serum specimen
   a. *Serum immunoreactive trypsin (IRT)*: The serum IRT is very high in newborns with CF (Crossley et al, 1979) and depressed in an overwhelming majority of older patients with CF.

Patient Preparation. The Gibson-Cooke sweat test is the same for infants, children, or adults and is performed as follows (Gibson and Cooke, 1959; "Evaluation of Testing," 1976):

1. Wash the skin site with distilled water.
2. Stimulate sweating using pilocarpine by iontophoresis.
3. Wash the skin rapidly five times with distilled water and dry thoroughly.
4. Collect sweat for at least 30 minutes on a 2 × 2-inch gauze pad taken from a pre-weighed, closed vial (handle with forceps only) that is placed on the skin, covered with polyethylene, and secured with tape. Warwick, Viela and Hansen (1979) compared the errors resulting from the use of gauze and the use of filter paper in the gravimetric chloride titration test.
5. After collection, place the gauze in the vial, then weigh the vial. The vial must be sealed to prevent errors caused by evaporation. At least 50 mg of sweat is required, even in newborns.
6. Elute the sweat from the gauze with 5 ml of distilled water.
7. Measure the concentration of sodium and chloride in the diluted sweat and calculate their concentration in the sweat.

The sweat test must be performed twice. If duplicate results are not acceptable, the entire procedure should be repeated at a later date (Warwick, Hansen, Viela et al., 1979). Salinity of sweat increases with age in normal subjects, and a modified test has been proposed for adults (*Lancet* editorial, 1982).

Specimen Collection and Handling. The main hazard of the Gibson-Cooke sweat test is evaporative loss of water from the specimen after the vial has been weighed. This will cause the concentrations of serum sodium and chloride to be falsely elevated and to give a false-positive test result.

Methodology. Consult the laboratory for methodology, reference intervals, accuracy and precision, and potential sources of interference. Sweat sodium can be measured by flame photometry or an ion specific electrode. We prefer a chloridometer to measure sweat chloride.

Interpretation

Diagnosis. In most laboratories, a sweat chloride concentration greater than 60 mEq/liter is diagnostic. However, the vast majority of CF patients have levels of about 90 to 100 mEq/liter. Marginal sweat chloride concentrations in the 30- to 60-mEq/liter range usually indicate allergic lung disease and not cystic fibrosis. The mean sweat chloride concentration during childhood is about 20 mEq/liter and in adults about 35 mEq/liter, with some increase in variation from the mean with age. Sweat sodium concentrations are usually about 10 to 20 mEq/liter higher than those of chloride.

For a reliable diagnosis, the Gibson-Cooke sweat test should be performed more than once, and the patient should have appropriate clinical features of the disease. The sweat test is normal in obligate heterozygotes (parents) and siblings. It cannot be used as a test for the carrier state.

In some patients with adrenal insufficiency, ectodermal dysplasia, nephrogenic diabetes insipidus, hypothyroidism, and mucopolysaccharidosis (Wood et al., 1976), a positive sweat test has been reported. It should be possible to exclude these diseases by their clinical features.

See Table 17–3 for the results of common laboratory tests in cystic fibrosis. Figure 17–3 gives an overview of the diagnostic reasoning.

Management. The level of sweat chloride does not correlate with the severity of disease. A given patient tends to have a very constant level of chloride in the sweat on repeated testings.

Scoring systems have been developed to follow CF patients. The National Institutes of

Table 17–3. COMMON LABORATORY TEST RESULTS IN CYSTIC FIBROSIS*

Laboratory Test	Value	Pathophysiologic Factors
Chemistry (Serum)		
Bilirubin, total	—	
Calcium, total	↓	Related to decreased albumin
Carbon dioxide	—	
Chloride	↓	With massive salt loss due to sweating
Cholesterol	↑	In 90 per cent of patients at initial hospitalization
Creatine phosphokinase	—	
Creatinine	—	
Glucose	↑	In 8 to 45 per cent of patients; related to pancreatic disease?
Lactic dehydrogenase	—	
Phosphatase, alkaline	↑	In 40 to 65 per cent of children; causes include liver disease and/or vitamin D deficiency secondary to malabsorption with bone disease
Phosphorus, inorganic	—	
Potassium	—	
Proteins, total	—	
Proteins, albumin	↓	With advanced lung disease, suggests expansion of plasma volume secondary to cor pulmonale
Sodium	↓	With complications, such as massive salt loss due to sweating
Transaminase, aspartate amino	↑	In 55 per cent of patients at hospitalization; related to liver disease
Urea nitrogen	↓	In 45 per cent of patients at initial hospitalization
Uric acid	—	
Hematology (Blood)		
Hemoglobin	↓	In late stage of lung disease; may reflect hemodilution
Hematocrit	↓	In late stage of lung disease; may reflect hemodilution
Leukocyte count, total	↑	Reflects inflammation, often pulmonary
Platelet count	—	

Key:
— = No change; ↑ = can be increased; ↓ = can be decreased.

*Information from Friedman RB, Anderson RE, Entine SM et al: Effects of diseases on clinical laboratory tests. Clin Chem 26:1D–476D, 1980; Wallach J: Interpretation of Diagnostic Tests: A Handbook Synopsis of Laboratory Medicine, ed 3. Boston, Little, Brown & Company, 1978.

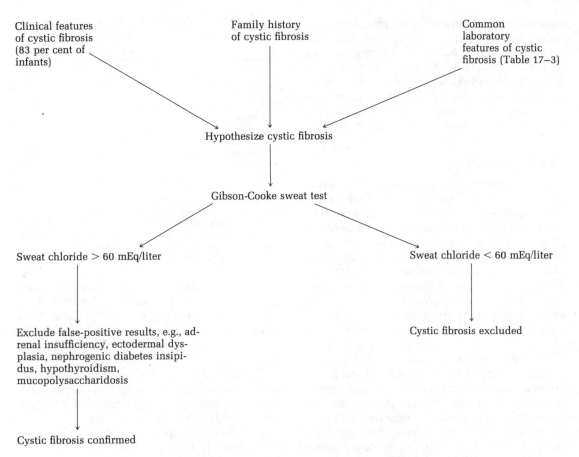

Figure 17–3. Diagnostic reasoning for cystic fibrosis.

Health (NIH) scoring system places 75 per cent of the evaluation score on the pulmonary system. Total lung capacity, vital capacity, functional residual capacity, and ratio of residual volume to total lung capacity are all gradually compromised. The maximal expiratory flow rate declines 8 to 10 per cent per year in females and less in males, which parallels the increased longevity of CF males.

Test Requests and Reports

Test Requests. The execution of the Gibson-Cooke sweat test may be offered as a problem-solving service.

Interpretive Reports. The results of the testing may be returned to the attending physician in the form of an interpretive report. Of the laboratories we surveyed in the United States, 2 per cent used interpretive reports for cystic fibrosis (Speicher and Smith, 1980).

WILSON'S DISEASE

Definition and Significance

In 1912, Wilson described four young adults afflicted with a neurologic disorder that now bears his name (Wilson, 1912). This condition is also known as hepatolenticular degeneration. It is a rare but important autosomal recessively inherited disease caused by a decrease in the biliary excretion of copper, with secondary accumulation of copper in the brain, liver, kidney, Descemet's membrane of the cornea, and other tissues. The gene is not common, and only homozygotes are affected. Tourian (1982) estimates that the disease has a gene frequency of 0.006 and a prevalence of 0.01 per cent. On the average, 25 per cent of the children of two heterozygotes can be expected to have the disease; 50 per cent will be carriers and 25 per cent will be normal. The disease can simulate several different neurologic disorders, many different psychiatric disorders, viral hepatitis, chronic active hepatitis, cirrhosis, acquired hemolytic anemia, or even renal osteodystrophy. It can be treated beneficially by the administration of penicillamine, which binds and then eliminates copper from the body. In the absence of treatment, the disease is invariably fatal (Cartwright, 1978).

Pathophysiology

Approximately 95 per cent of the serum copper in normal persons is bound to the alpha$_2$-globulin known as ceruloplasmin. The remaining 5 per cent is loosely bound to serum albumin. Tissue copper is present as the prosthetic element of copper proteins such as cytochrome oxidase, tyrosinase, and superoxide dismutase. In Wilson's disease, there is defective synthesis of ceruloplasmin, with low levels of ceruloplasmin in the serum. This is associated with a decrease in serum concentration of copper and an increase in the easily dissociable albumin-bound copper with increased copper excretion in the urine. There is decreased biliary excretion of copper, and copper accumulates in the tissues, particularly the brain, liver, and corneas. Increased free copper is as toxic as excess iron, zinc, mercury, or lead. In the brain it causes degenerative changes, especially of the basal ganglia. In the liver it causes degenerative changes manifested as acute hepatitis, chronic active hepatitis, and macronodular cirrhosis (Robbins and Cotran, 1979). The pathophysiologic changes in the liver are as described in the subproblems chronic hepatitis and primary biliary cirrhosis and cirrhosis (see Chapter 15). Hemolysis secondary to oxidative damage to the erythrocytes by copper, as well as acute intravascular hemolysis associated with acute liver failure, has been described in Wilson's disease (Roche-Sicot and Benhamou, 1977).

Clinical Contexts

Diagnosis. The signs and symptoms of Wilson's disease appear as early as 4 years of age or as late as the sixth decade, but most commonly in the second and third decades (Fitzgerald et al., 1975). Patients can be asymptomatic, or they can present with any combination of the features described next. They may or may not have Kayser-Fleischer rings, which are green or golden deposits from

Table 17–4. GENERAL SYMPTOMS AND SIGNS IN 40 PATIENTS WITH WILSON'S DISEASE*

Kayser-Fleischer rings	37
Splenomegaly	21
Hyperpigmentation of legs	20
Bleeding and easy bruising	17
Edema	12
Arthralgias	11
Jaundice	11
Palpable liver	9
Ascites	9
Fever	5
Bone deformities	4
Hematemesis and melena	4

*From Strickland GT, Leu M: Wilson's disease: Clinical and laboratory manifestations in 40 patients. Medicine 54:113–137, 1975. Used by permission of The Williams & Wilkins Co., Baltimore.

copper accumulation in Descemet's membrane of the cornea. They are best detected by a trained observer using a slit-lamp. Table 17–4 gives general symptoms and signs, and Table 17–5 neurologic symptoms and signs in 40 patients with Wilson's disease.

The clinical features of Wilson's disease secondary to central nervous system degenerative changes often begin insidiously but can progress rapidly. They are as follows:

1. Difficulty in speech and handwriting.
2. Dysphagia.
3. Ataxia and muscular rigidity.
4. Choreoathetoid movements.
5. Muscular contractures.

Table 17–5. NEUROLOGICAL SYMPTOMS AND SIGNS IN 40 PATIENTS WITH WILSON'S DISEASE*

Coordination poor	28
Psychological impairment	27
Tremor	26
Dysarthria	26
Dysphagia	26
Masked facies	25
Walking disturbed	25
Rigidity	24
Dementia	23
Dystonia and hypertonia	23
Drooling	22
Choreoathetosis	12
Coma	12
Blurred vision	6
Headache	5
Convulsions	3

*From Strickland GT, Leu M: Wilson's disease: Clinical and laboratory manifestations in 40 patients. Medicine 54:113–137, 1975. Used by permission of The Williams & Wilkins Co., Baltimore.

6. Mental deterioration.

The hepatic manifestations of Wilson's disease (Scott et al., 1978) can precede neurologic dysfunction and include the following:

1. Acute hepatitis.
2. "Infectious mononucleosis."
3. Chronic hepatitis.
4. "Juvenile cirrhosis."
5. Fulminant hepatitis.

The features of chronic active hepatitis and cirrhosis are described under these particular subproblems (see Chapter 15).

Copper accumulation in the kidneys can cause the Fanconi syndrome and renal tubular acidosis. Proximal renal tubular reabsorption is impaired in most patients, as manifested by aminoaciduria, peptiduria, glucosuria, uricosuria (low serum urate), and phosphaturia (low serum phosphate). An occasional patient with Wilson's disease may present with symptoms related to bone disease (Cartwright, 1978).

Copper released from tissues to plasma can cause hemolytic anemia that can be acute or intermittent. Hemolysis can also be intravascular and associated with acute liver failure (Cartwright, 1978; Roche-Sicot and Benhamou, 1977). Deiss and colleagues (1971) developed a staging classification for patients with Wilson's disease:

1. *Stage I:* Asymptomatic Wilson's disease.
2. *Stage II:* Symptomatic Wilson's disease.
3. *Stage III and IV:* Advanced Wilson's disease.

Management.   Therapy of Wilson's disease with penicillamine can be monitored by measuring the urinary excretion of copper. Hepatic disease can be monitored by liver function tests and liver biopsies. The patient should be carefully followed to detect any sensitivity to penicillamine.

Screening.   Screening for Wilson's disease in the absence of clinical features of the disease is not indicated, except in persons who are blood relatives of patients with a confirmed diagnosis of Wilson's disease (Sternlieb, 1978). The diagnosis should be pursued, however, in any young adult with unexplained disease of the liver or central nervous system; a negative Coombs' test, non-spherocytic hemolytic anemia; or low serum urate (Cartwright, 1978).

Strategy

Test Sequence.   The test sequence for the diagnosis of Wilson's disease is to confirm the diagnosis by either one or both of the following (Sternlieb, 1978; Sternlieb and Scheinberg, 1979):

1. Low serum ceruloplasmin in the presence of Kayser-Fleischer rings by slit-lamp examination.
2. Low serum ceruloplasmin in the presence of a liver biopsy sample having increased copper.

The daily excretion of urinary copper should be measured because most patients with Wilson's disease excrete greater than 100 μg of copper per 24 hours in the urine. The interpretation of this test sequence can result in a small number of both false-negative and false-positive results.

Wilson's disease can be excluded by an elevated level of serum ceruloplasmin.

If the diagnosis cannot be confirmed as just described and if the clinical features suggest Wilson's disease, evaluate the patient's ability to incorporate radioactive copper into ceruloplasmin (Sternlieb and Scheinberg, 1979). This is the most sensitive and specific laboratory study available. Even patients with Wilson's disease who have a serum level of ceruloplasmin within the reference interval for a healthy population will incorporate little or no radiocopper into ceruloplasmin, whereas patients with other liver disorders and elevated hepatic copper level secondary to biliary tract disease incorporate the radiocopper in a normal manner.

The radioactive copper test is of special value in resolving diagnostic dilemmas in a patient with chronic liver disease and one or more of the following:

1. An elevated hepatic copper concentration.
2. Kayser-Fleischer rings.
3. An increased urinary excretion of copper. Although the radiation to which this test exposes patients is within acceptable limits (Chervu and Sternlieb, 1974), the test should not be used as a substitute for initial quantitative copper analysis and histologic examination of a liver biopsy specimen, unless biopsy is contraindicated (Sternlieb and Scheinberg, 1979).

Consider the following additional studies:

1. Liver function tests to diagnose and follow liver disease.
2. Urinary copper measurements and complete blood count to manage penicillamine therapy.

Patient Preparation. Serum ceruloplasmin and serum, liver, and urine copper measurements require no special patient preparation. Of course, there should be no contraindications to liver biopsy, such as bleeding diathesis.

The radioactive copper test is performed as follows (Sternlieb and Scheinberg, 1979):

1. Have the patient fast for at least 8 hours.
2. Administer 0.3 mCi ^{64}Cu in 150 to 200 ml of milk.
3. Obtain blood samples at 1, 2, 4, 24, and 48 hours after administration of the radiocopper for assay for radioactivity in a scintillation counter.
4. Allow the patient to eat 2 hours after drinking the milk.

(See Part 3 for chemistry and hematology tests.)

Specimen Collection and Handling. Serum for ceruloplasmin measurements should be quickly separated from cells and refrigerated. Serum, body fluids, and tissues for quantitative copper determinations should be collected in syringes and glassware free of contamination, and reagents should be made up with chemicals of the highest purity. (See Part 3.)

Methodology. Consult the laboratory for methodologies, reference intervals, accuracy and precision, and potential sources of interference. Be careful about using the decision levels of Sternlieb and Scheinberg (1979) unless you are confident that a measurement of ceruloplasmin in your laboratory is equivalent to the measurement used in their laboratory. Protein measurements are notoriously difficult to standardize.

Serum ceruloplasmin can be measured by:

1. Immunochemical methods such as radial immunodiffusion, electroimmunodiffusion, and nephelometry.
2. Enzymatic methods, such as measuring ceruloplasmin's enzymatic action on paraphenylene diamine and other substrates.

Atomic absorption spectrometry is a good method for measurement of copper in serum, urine, plasma, or liver. However, spectrophotometry, neutron activation, and radioisotopic dilution techniques can also be used (Sunderman, 1973). Unfortunately, histochemical demonstration of hepatic copper by rubeanic acid or rhodanine staining is unreliable (*Lancet* editorial, 1981). (See Part 3.)

Interpretation

Diagnosis. In the appropriate clinical setting, a serum ceruloplasmin concentration less than 20 mg/100 ml, when accompanied by either Kayser-Fleischer rings or an elevated hepatic copper concentration, confirms the diagnosis of Wilson's disease. A serum copper concentration greater than 30 mg/100 ml essentially excludes the diagnosis, since it was found in only two of 500 determinations of serum ceruloplasmin in the combined series of patients of Walshe and of Sternlieb and Scheinberg (1979). In most patients with Wilson's disease, the copper content of the liver is greater than 250 μg/gm of dry weight. In some patients, the copper content can reach a level of 2000 μg/gm. The upper reference limit for hepatic copper concentration in a healthy reference population is 50 μg/gm of dry weight.

A decrease in serum ceruloplasmin below 20 mg/100 ml is not specific for Wilson's disease and can be found in malnutrition, sprue, the nephrotic syndrome, and heterozygotes. An increase in hepatic copper is not specific for Wilson's disease and can be found in the normal fetus and newborn baby and in patients with prolonged cholestasis, Indian childhood cirrhosis, and chronic copper poisoning (*Lancet* editorial, 1981). Kayser-Fleischer rings are not specific for Wilson's disease and can occur in chronic liver disease other than Wilson's disease (Flemming et al., 1977; Frommer et al., 1977). An increase in urinary copper excretion is not specific for patients with Wilson's disease and can be found in patients with

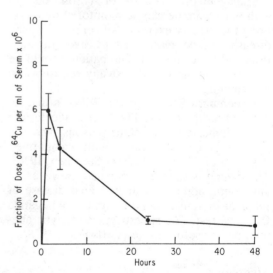

Figure 17–4.   Mean (± SEM) concentrations of ^{64}Cu in sera of 11 patients with Wilson's disease at various times after the ingestion of a 2-mg dose of radiocopper. (From Sternlieb I, Scheinberg IH: The role of radiocopper in the diagnosis of Wilson's disease. Gastroenterology 77:141, 1979.)

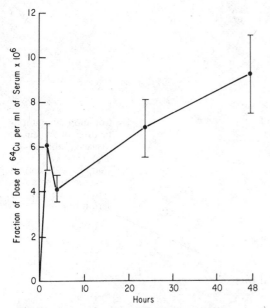

Figure 17–5. Mean (± SEM) concentrations of ^{64}Cu in sera of 11 patients with miscellaneous liver diseases at various times after the ingestion of a 2-mg dose of radiocopper. (From Sternlieb I, Scheinberg IH: The role of radiocopper in the diagnosis of Wilson's disease. Gastroenterology 77:141, 1979.)

cholestasis, hepatitis, and cirrhosis (Frommer, 1981).

Approximately 5 per cent of patients with Wilson's disease can have false-negative laboratory measurements of ceruloplasmin, in that the levels are greater than 20 mg/100 ml. Ceruloplasmin is an acute-phase protein, and patients with Wilson's disease can have levels of ceruloplasmin that are not depressed (greater than 20 mg/100 ml) in the presence of inflammation, pregnancy, and estrogen therapy. (See Chapter 8 for a discussion of acute-phase proteins in inflammation.)

If after all of these considerations, the clinical features of the patient's disease are not consistent with the laboratory test results, the patient's ability to incorporate radioactive copper into ceruloplasmin should be evaluated. This is the most sensitive and specific laboratory study available. Figures 17–4 and 17–5 give the results of the radioactive copper test in patients with Wilson's disease and in patients with miscellaneous liver diseases, respectively.

Table 17–6. COMMON LABORATORY TEST RESULTS IN WILSON'S DISEASE*

Laboratory Test	Value	Pathophysiologic Factors
Chemistry (Serum)		
Bilirubin, total	↑	Related to liver disease
Calcium, total	↓	Related to decreased albumin
Carbon dioxide	↓	Related to Fanconi syndrome
Chloride	↓	Found in 40 per cent of patients
Cholesterol	↓	Related to liver disease
Creatinine phosphokinase	—	
Creatinine	↑	Elevated in 15 per cent of patients
Glucose	↓	In 5 per cent, related to malnourishment
Lactic dehydrogenase	—	Related to liver disease
Phosphatase, alkaline	↑	Related to liver disease, occasionally bone disease
Phosphorus, inorganic	↓	Increased clearance by kidneys
Potassium	↓	Related to Fanconi syndrome
Proteins, total	↑	Related to cirrhosis with polyclonal gammopathy
	↓	Related to decreased albumin
Proteins, albumin	↓	Decreased synthesis by the liver
Sodium	—	
Transaminase, aspartate amino	↑	Related to liver disease
Urea nitrogen	↑	Mildly elevated in 15 per cent of patients
	↓	In 5 per cent, related to malnourishment
Uric acid	↓	Increased clearance by kidneys; may be a clue to the presence of Wilson's disease
Hematology (Blood)		
Hemoglobin	↓	May have hemolytic anemia or hypersplenism
Hematocrit	↓	May have hemolytic anemia or hypersplenism
Leukocyte count, total	↓	May have hypersplenism
Platelet count	↓	May have hypersplenism

Key:
— = No change; ↑ = can be increased; ↓ = can be decreased.
 *Information from Friedman RB, Anderson RE, Entine SM et al: Effects of diseases on clinical laboratory tests. Clin Chem 26:1D–476D, 1980. Wolf PL: Interpretation of Biochemical Multitest Profiles: An Analysis of 100 Important Conditions. New York, Masson Publishing, Inc, 1977. Strickland GT, Leu M: Wilson's disease: Clinical and laboratory manifestations in 40 patients. Medicine 54:113–137, 1975.

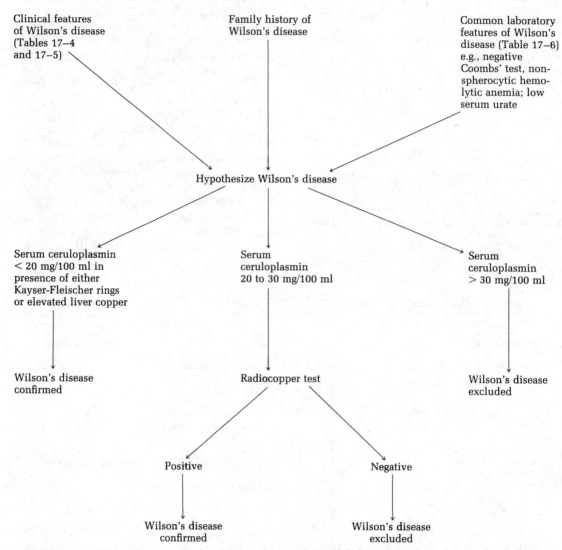

Figure 17–6. Diagnostic reasoning for Wilson's disease. Be careful about using these decision levels regarding ceruloplasmin of Sternlieb and Scheinberg (1979) unless you are confident that a measurement of ceruloplasmin performed in your laboratory is equivalent to the measurement in their laboratory.

Stromeyer and Ishak (1980) studied the histology of the liver in 34 cases of Wilson's disease. Seven patients had early changes ranging from slight pleomorphism of hepatocytes to fatty metamorphosis, vacuolated nuclei, and focal necrosis. Seven other specimens showed chronic active hepatitis in addition to changes similar to those of the first group. The 20 cirrhotic specimens showed macronodular or mixed micronodular-macronodular patterns, and eight contained Mallory bodies. Copper was demonstrated in 13 of 15 specimens with adequate stains. Some of the findings were suggestive of Wilson's disease, but none were considered specific. Table 17–6 gives the results of common laboratory tests in Wilson's disease. Figure 17–6 gives an overview of the diagnostic reasoning.

Management. Penicillamine therapy should be monitored by:

1. *Urine copper*: Initially, the patient's 24-hour urinary copper level should increase five times or more over pretreatment levels, and 1 to 3 mg per day can be excreted during the first months of therapy.
2. Tests to detect the following conditions, which may indicate penicillamine sensitivity:
   a. Leukopenia.
   b. Thrombocytopenia.
   c. Proteinuria.

Rash, fever, and lymphadenopathy may be additional features of sensitivity to penicillamine. Chronic active hepatitis and cirrhosis of Wilson's disease can be managed as outlined in Chapter 15.

Test Requests and Reports

Test Requests. The execution of the test sequence for the diagnosis of Wilson's disease can be offered as a problem-solving service.

Interpretive Reports. The test results from the execution of the strategy can be collated and returned to the attending physician in the form of an interpretive report.

REFERENCES

Alpha₁-antitrypsin Deficiency

Campra JL, Craig JR, Peters RL, et al: Cirrhosis associated with partial deficiency of alpha-1-antitrypsin in an adult. Ann Intern Med 78:233–238, 1973.

Cockroft DW, Tennent RK, Horne SL: Pulmonary emphysema associated with the FZ alpha-1-antitrypsin phenotype. Can Med Assoc J 124:737–742, 1981.

Cox DW, Pariente EA, Benhamou J, et al: Hepatocyte PAS-positive diastase-resistant inclusions in alcoholic cirrhosis, letters. Am J Clin Pathol 78:135–136, 1982.

Creason PL, Creason MJ, Bader PI: Isoelectric focusing and alpha-1-antitrypsin globulin phenotyping. Laboratory Medicine 11:673–678, 1980.

Daniels JC: Abnormalities of protease inhibitors. In Ritzmann SE, Daniels JC (eds): Serum Protein Abnormalities. Diagnostic and Clinical Aspects. Boston, Little, Brown & Company, 1975, pp 243–263.

Gadek JE, Klein HG, Holland PV, et al: Replacement therapy of alpha-1-antitrypsin deficiency. Reversal of protease-antiprotease imbalance within the alveolar structures of PiZ subjects. Clin Invest 68:1158–1165, 1981.

Kueppers F, Dickson ER, Summerskill WHJ: Alpha-1-antitrypsin phenotypes in chronic liver disease and primary biliary cirrhosis. Mayo Clin Proc 51:286–288, 1976.

Laurell CB, Eriksson S: The electrophoretic alpha-1-globulin pattern of serum in alpha-1-antitrypsin deficiency. Scand J Clin Lab Invest 15:132–140, 1963.

Morse JO: Alpha-1-antitrypsin deficiency. New Engl J Med 299:1045–1048, 1099–1105, 1978.

Pariente EA, Degott C, Martin JP, et al: Hepatocyte PAS-positive diastase-resistant inclusions in the absence of alpha-1-antitrypsin deficiency-high prevalence in alcoholic cirrhosis. Am J Clin Pathol 76:299–302, 1981.

Roggli V, Hausner R, Askew JB: Alpha-1-antitrypsin globules in hepatocytes of elderly persons with liver disease. Am J Clin Pathol 75:538–542, 1981.

Sharp HL: The current states of alpha-1-antitrypsin, a protease inhibitor, in gastrointestinal disease. Gastroenterology 70:611–621, 1976.

Speicher CE, Smith JW: Interpretive reporting in clinical pathology. JAMA 243:1556–1560, 1980.

Sveger T: Liver disease in alpha-1-antitrypsin deficiency detected by screening of 200,000 infants. N Engl J Med 294:1316–1321, 1976.

Talamo RC, Laughley CE, Levine BW et al: Genetic vs. quantitative analysis of serum alpha-1-antitrypsin. N Engl J Med 287:1067–1069, 1972.

Cystic Fibrosis

Berry HK, Kellogg FW, Lichstein SR, et al: Elevated meconium lactase activity: Its use as a screening test for cystic fibrosis. Am J Dis Child 134:930–934, 1980.

Crossley JR, Elliott RB, Smith PA: Dried-blood spot screening for cystic fibrosis in the newborn. Lancet 1:472–474, 1979.

Dann LG, Blau K: Exocrine-gland function and the basic biochemical defect in cystic fibrosis. Lancet 2:405–407, 1978.

Diagnosis of cystic fibrosis, editorial. Lancet 2:1196–1197, 1982.

David TJ, Phillips BM: Overdiagnosis of cystic fibrosis. Lancet 2:1204–1206, 1982.

Evaluation of Testing for Cystic Fibrosis: Report of the Committee for a Study for Evaluation of Testing for Cystic Fibrosis. J. Pediatr 88(Pt 2): 711–750, 1976.

Forrest DC, Wilcken B, Turner G: Screening for cystic fibrosis by a stool trypsin method. Arch Dis Child 56:151–155, 1981.

Gibson LE: Screening of newborns for cystic fibrosis, editorial. Am J Dis Child 134:925–926, 1980.

Gibson LE, Cooke RE: A test for concentration of electrolytes in sweat in cystic fibrosis of the pancreas utilizing pilocarpine by iontophoresis. Pediatrics 23:545–549, 1959.

Gottlieb AJ, Zamkoff KW, Jastremski MS, et al: The Whole Internist Catalog. Philadelphia, WB Saunders Company, 1980, pp 213–214.

Kopito L, Shwachman H: Studies in cystic fibrosis: Determination of sweat electrolytes in situ with direct reading electrode. Pediatrics 43:794–798, 1969.

Manson JC, Brock DJH: Development of a quantitative immunoassay for the cystic fibrosis gene. Lancet 1:330–331, 1980.

Population screening for carriers of recessively inherited disorders, editorial. Lancet 2:679–680, 1980.

Robbins SL, Cotran RS: Cystic fibrosis. In Robbins SL, Cotran PS (eds): Pathologic Basis of Disease, ed 2. Philadelphia, WB Saunders Company, 1979, pp 583–586.

Rosenstein BJ, Langbaum TS, Gordes E, et al: Cystic fibrosis: Problems encountered with sweat testing. JAMA 240:1987–1988, 1978.

Scully RE, Galdabini JJ, McNeely BU (eds): Case records of the Massachusetts General Hospital: Case 14–1981. N Engl J Med 304:831–836, 1981.

Shwachman H, Kowalski M, Khaw KT: Cystic fibrosis: A new outlook. 70 patients above 25 years of age. Medicine 56:129–149, 1977.

Shwachman H, Kulczycki LL: Long-term study of one hundred five patients with cystic fibrosis. Am J Dis Child 96:6–15, 1958.

Shwachman H, Mahmoodian A: Reappraisal of the chloride plate test as screening test for cystic fibrosis. Arch Dis Child 56:137–139, 1981.

Shwachman H, Mahmoodian A, Kopito L et al: A standard procedure for measuring conductivity of sweat as a diagnostic test for cystic fibrosis. J Pediatr 66:432–434, 1965.

Smalley CA, Addy DP, Anderson CM: Does that child really have cystic fibrosis? Lancet 2:415–417, 1978.

Speicher CE, Smith JW: Interpretive reporting in clinical pathology. JAMA 243:1556–1560, 1980.

Stern RC, Boat TF, Doershuk CF et al: Cystic fibrosis diagnosed after age 13. Twenty-five teenage and adult patients including three asymptomatic men. Ann Intern Med 87:188–191, 1977.

Warwick WJ, Hansen L, Viela I, et al: Comparison of the chloride electrode and gravimetric chloride titration sweat tests. Am J Clin Pathol 72:142–145, 1979.

Warwick WJ, Pogue RE: Cystic fibrosis: An expanding challenge for internal medicine. JAMA 238:2159–2162, 1977.

Warwick WJ, Viela I, Hansen LG: Comparison of the errors due to the use of gauze and the use of filter paper in the gravimetric chloride titration test. Am J Clin Pathol 72:211–215, 1979.

Wood RE, Boat TF, Doershuk CF: Cystic fibrosis. Am Rev Respir Dis 113:833–878, 1976.

Wilson's Disease

Cartwright GE: Diagnosis of treatable Wilson's disease. N Engl J Med 24:1347–1350, 1978.

Chervu LR, Sternlieb I: Dosimetry of copper radionuclides. J Nucl Med 15:1011–1013, 1974.

Deiss A, Lynch RE, Lee GR et al: Long-term therapy of Wilson's disease. Ann Intern Med 75:57–65, 1971.

Fitzgerald MA, Gross JB, Goldstein NP et al: Wilson's disease (hepatolenticular degeneration) of late adult onset: Report of case. Mayo Clin Proc 50:438–442, 1975.

Flemming CR, Dickson ER, Wahner HV et al: Pigmented corneal rings in non-Wilsonian liver disease. Ann Intern Med 86:285–288, 1977.

Frommer DJ: Urinary copper excretion and hepatic copper concentrations in liver disease. Digestion 21:169–178, 1981.

Frommer DJ, Morris J, Sherlock S et al: Kayser–Fleischer-like rings in patients without Wilson's disease. Gastroenterology 72:1331–1335, 1977.

Robbins SL, Cotran RS: Wilson's disease. In Robbins SL, Cotran RS: Pathologic Basis of Disease, ed 2. Philadelphia, WB Saunders Company, 1979, pp 241–243.

Roche-Sicot J, Benhamou J: Acute intravascular hemolysis and acute liver failure associated as a first manifestation of Wilson's disease. Ann Intern Med 86:301–303, 1977.

Scott J, Gollan JL, Samourian S, et al: Wilson's disease presenting as chronic hepatitis. Gastroenterology 74:645–651, 1978.

Sternlieb I: Diagnosis of Wilson's disease, editorial. Gastroenterology 74:787–793, 1978.

Sternlieb I, Scheinberg IH: The role of radiocopper in the diagnosis of Wilson's disease. Gastroenterology 77:138–142, 1979.

Stromeyer FW, Ishak KG: Histology of the liver in Wilson's disease: A study of 34 cases. Am J Clin Pathol 73:12–24, 1980.

Sunderman FW: Atomic absorption spectrometry of trace metals in clinical pathology. Hum Pathol 4:549–582, 1973.

Tourian A: Wilson's disease. In Wyngaarden, JB, Smith LH (eds): Cecil Textbook of Medicine, ed 16. Philadelphia, WB Saunders Company, 1982, pp 1126–1128.

Wilson SAK: Progressive lenticular degeneration: A familial nervous disease associated with cirrhosis of the liver. Brain 34:295–509, 1912.

Wilson's disease and copper-associated protein, editorial. Lancet 1:644–646, 1981.

PART 3

UNEXPECTED TEST RESULTS

This part contains information that will be helpful in determining the cause of an unexpected test result, whether normal or abnormal. For example, if the SGOT is not elevated in a patient with acute myocardial infarction, it is an unexpected *normal* result; if the SGOT is elevated in a person who appears healthy, it is an unexpected *abnormal* result. Chapter 9 discusses a generic approach to the unexpected test result.

Basically, the approach is as follows:

1. Repeat the test while making certain that the patient is properly prepared, the specimen collection and handling are correct, the methodology is good, and the correct reference interval is used.

2. Determine whether the patient is taking a drug, which can potentially affect the test result (pharmacologic, allergic, idiosyncratic, or toxic effect).

3. If the repeated test result(s) is still unexplained and there are no drug effects, consider the differential diagnosis for the test result(s).

Our emphasis is clearly on the approach to unexpected test result(s). We acknowledge that the lists of drug and disease effects are incomplete and that many effects are uncorroborated. They represent a simple compilation from the references. Some occur only in certain disease states. We would appreciate your comments concerning errors of commission or omission. Address correspondence to Dr. Speicher.

The majority of drug and disease effects were found in Young et al., 1975, and Friedman et al., 1980. These are invaluable references, and everyone using laboratory tests should have ready access to them. We hope a mechanism can be found to continuously update their data bases—a monumental yet vital task.

Unexpected test results can be a clue to disease. Several test results may form a pattern; for example, elevated serum bilirubin, alkaline, phosphatase, and transaminase levels suggest hepatitis. See the pattern for each subproblem in Chapters 8 through 17.

A characteristic pattern of test results does not, of course, make the diagnosis, but merely serves to trigger the hypothesis for a particular disease, as shown in Figure 1–2 and as illustrated in the overviews of diagnostic reasoning for alpha$_1$-antitrypsin deficiency, cystic fibrosis, and Wilson's disease (Figures 17–1, 17–3, and 17–6). Once a particular hypothesis or clinical subproblem is triggered, an effective strategy can be used to confirm or exclude it.

Caution: The lists of drugs are sensitive (they include many drugs) but are quite nonspecific (the drug effects may occur only rarely and some are unproven). Therefore, if abnormal test results occur in a patient who is taking a drug for these test results, the reader should do the following:

1. Consult the references for information on the mechanism of the drug effect: Is it a pharmacologic, allergic, idiosyncratic, or toxic effect and what is its expected prevalence?

2. Interpret the potential drug effect in the context of the patient's clinical findings including coexisting disease and other drugs. Look for findings that might support a drug allergy (e.g., fever, rash, eosinophilia).

3. Confirm the drug effect by discontinuing the drug and observing whether the affected test results(s) return to or toward normal. This usually occurs within several days but sometimes takes longer. A drug effect can be proved only by challenging the patient with the drug to determine whether the test result(s) can be reproduced. However, challenging the patient with a drug that can produce dangerous side effects is inadvisable and unwise.

299

Serum Bilirubin, Total

Patient Preparation. A fasting specimen is preferable because lipemia can interfere with some procedures. However, prolonged fasting can increase the serum bilirubin 1.3 times after 24 hours and 2.2 times after 48 hours.

Specimen Collection and Handling. Serum or heparinized plasma may be used. Hemolysis should be avoided because it can depress results when the diazo method is used. Direct sunlight can cause up to 50 per cent decrease in serum bilirubin within 1 hour. Therefore, serum should be kept in the dark, and the measurement should be carried out within 2 to 3 hours of collecting the blood. Bilirubin will keep for up to a week in a darkened refrigerator; it will keep for 3 months in a darkened freezer.

Methodology. Although the direct spectrophotometric method for total serum bilirubin is accept- able for infants, the best methods for total conjugated bilirubin in adults are the classic methods of Malloy and Evelyn or Jendrassik and Grof (Tietz, 1976). Because there is no stable standard for conjugated bilirubin, unproven methods should be approached with caution. Consult the laboratory for its methodology, including in vitro drug interference.

Reference Interval. The best methods have an upper reference limit for conjugated bilirubin of less than 0.2 mg/100 ml. Any method with an upper reference limit of greater than 0.4 mg/100 ml is unacceptable. The reference interval for unconjugated bilirubin is 0.1 to 1.0 mg/100 ml; for total bilirubin, 0.1 to 1.2 mg/100 ml. Consult the laboratory for its reference intervals.

Agents Associated With Increased Levels of Serum Bilirubin in Vivo

Acetaminophen	Chlorothiazide	Ethacrynic acid	Mefenamic acid
Acetazolamide	Chlorpromazine	Ethanol	Melphalan
Acetohexamide	Chlorpropamide	Ethchlorvynol	Meprobamate
Acetophenazine	Chlorprothixene	Ether	Mercaptopurine
Allopurinol	Chlorthalidone	Ethionamide	Mesoridazine
Aluminum nicotinate	Chlorzoxazone	Ethosuximide	Metaxalone
Amiloride	Cholinergics	Ethyl chloride	Methandrostenolone
Aminosalicylic acid	Cinoxacin	Factor IX complex, human	Methdilazine
Amitriptyline	Clindamycin	Fenoprofen	Methimazole
Amodiaquine	Clofibrate	Floxuridine	Methotrexate
Amphotericin B	Clomiphene	Flucytosine	Methoxsalen
Amyl nitrite	Clonidine	Fluorouracil	Methoxyflurane
Anabolic steroids	Colchicine	Fluoxymesterone	Methyclothiazide
Androgens	Contrast media, iodine-	Fluphenazine	Methyldopa
Anisindione	containing	Flurazepam	Methyltestosterone
Anticonvulsants	Copper	Fructose infusions	Metolazone
Antifungal agents	Coumarin derivatives	Furazolidone	Monoamine oxidase
Antimalarials	Cyclizine	Gentamicin	inhibitors
Antimony compounds	Cyclobenzaprine	Glucose infusions	Morphine
Antipyretics	Cyclophosphamide	Glycopyrrolate	Nalidixic acid
Asparaginase	Cyclopropane	Gold	Naproxen
Azathioprine	Cycloserine	Haloperidol	Niacin
Barbiturates	Cyclothiazide	Halothane	Niacinamide
Benzodiazepines	Cytarabine	Hycanthone	Nicotinyl alcohol
Benzthiazide	Dantrolene	Hydantoins	Nitrofurantoin
Bethanechol chloride	Dapsone	Hydrazines	Nitrofurazone
Bismuth salts	Demeclocycline	Hydrochlorothiazide	Norethindrone
Busulfan	Desipramine	Hydroflumethiazide	Nortriptyline
Butaperazine	Dextrothyroxine	Idoxuridine	Oral contraceptives
Carbamazepine	Diazepam	Imipramine	Oxacillin
Carbarsone	Dienestrol	Indanediones	Oxazepam
Carbenoxolone	Diethylstilbestrol	Indomethacin	Oxymetholone
Carmustine	Dimercaprol	Iodine solution	Oxyphenbutazone
Cephalosporins	Disulfiram	Iron compounds	Oxytocic agents
Chlorambucil	Doxepin	Isocarboxazid	Papaverine
Chloramphenicol	Erythromycin	Isoniazid	Paraldehyde
Chlordiazepoxide	Estradiol	Kanamycin	Pargyline
Chlormezanone	Estrogens	Levodopa	Pemoline
Chloroquine	Estrone	Lincomycin	Penicillins

300

Perphenazine
Phenazopyridine
Phenelzine
Phenindione
Phenobarbital
Phenothiazines
Phenylbutazone
Phytonadione
Piperacetazine
Piperazine
Polythiazide
Primaquine
Probenecid
Procainamide
Procarbazine
Prochlorperazine
Progesterones

Promazine
Promethazine
Propoxyphene
Propylthiouracil
Protein hydrolysate
Protriptyline
Quinacrine
Quinethazone
Quinidine
Quinine
Radiographic agents
Rifampin
Salicylates
Sorbitol infusions
Stanozolol
Streptomycin
Sulfacetamide

Sulfachlorpyridazine
Sulfadiazine
Sulfameter
Sulfamethizole
Sulfamethoxazole
Sulfamethoxypyridine
Sulfapyridine
Sulfinpyrazone
Sulfisoxazole
Sulfonamides
Sulfones
Sulfoxone
Sulindac
Testosterones
Tetracycline
Thiazides
Thiethylperazine

Thioguanine
Thiosemicarbazones
Thiothixene
Tolazamide
Tolbutamide
Trichlormethiazide
Trifluoperazine
Triflupromazine
Trimeprazine
Trimethadione
Trimethobenzamide
Trimethoprim
Trimipramine
Trioxsalen
Vidarabine
Vitamin K

Differential Diagnosis for Elevated Serum Bilirubin

Cardiovascular
Congestive heart failure

Respiratory
Bacterial pneumonia
Influenza
Mycoplasmal pneumonia
Pulmonary embolism and infarction
Respiratory distress syndrome

Genitourinary
Usually no effect

Gastrointestinal
Ulcerative colitis

Pancreatic
Pancreatitis: Acute, chronic
Pancreatic cyst and pseudocyst

Hepatobiliary
Biliary cirrhosis
Cholangitis
Cholecystitis: Acute
Cholestasis
Chronic active hepatitis
Cirrhosis of liver: Cause unspecified
Extrahepatic biliary obstruction
Granulomatous hepatitis
Hemochromatosis
Hepatic failure
Hereditary defects in bilirubin metabolism: Dubin-Johnson syndrome, Gilbert's disease, Rotor's syndrome, Crigler-Najjar syndrome
Idiopathic jaundice of pregnancy
Jaundice in newborn due to hepatocellular damage
Laennec's or alcoholic cirrhosis
Liver abscess
Necrosis of liver: Acute, subacute
Postcholecystectomy syndrome
Reye's syndrome
Toxic hepatitis
Viral hepatitis

Hematologic
Acquired hemolytic anemia
Disorder of glutathione metabolism
Erythroleukemia

Hemoglobin C disease
Hereditary elliptocytosis, spherocytosis
Hemolytic disease
Infectious mononucleosis
Lymphocytic leukemia
Paroxysmal nocturnal hemoglobinuria
Pernicious anemia
Polycythemia: Vera, secondary
Sickle cell anemia
Thalassemia major
Thrombotic thrombocytopenic purpura

Endocrine
Diabetes mellitus
Hyperthyroidism

Metabolic
A-betalipoproteinemia
Carcinoid syndrome
Glycogen-storage disease
Hepatolenticular degeneration
Hereditary fructose intolerance
Mucopolysaccharidoses

Infectious
Infections associated with hemolysis:
Aspergillosis, cytomegalic inclusion disease, influenza, leishmaniasis, malaria
Other infections, especially involving liver:
Amebiasis, ascariasis, bartonellosis, brucellosis, chickenpox, disseminated tuberculosis, echinococciasis, herpes simplex, histoplasmosis, hydatidosis, leptospirosis, lymphogranuloma venereum, measles, relapsing fever, schistosomiasis, *Toxocara canis*, toxoplasmosis, typhoid fever, yellow fever

Immunologic
Polyarteritis nodosa
Systemic lupus erythematosus

Musculoskeletal
Usually no effect

Neuropsychiatric
Hepatic encephalopathy

Neoplastic
Histiocytosis X

Lymphoma: Hodgkin's disease, lymphosarcoma, reticulum cell sarcoma
Malignant neoplasm: Intrahepatic bile ducts, liver, pancreas
Secondary malignant neoplasm: Liver

Miscellaneous
Alcoholism

Amyloidosis
Eclampsia
Effect of x-ray irradiation
Heat stroke
Large hematoma
Physiologic jaundice of newborn
Toxic effects: Lead and its compounds, other non-medicinal metals

Agents Associated With Decreased Levels of Serum Bilirubin in Vivo

Barbiturates
Chlorophenothane
Corticosteroids

Ethanol
Penicillin

Phenobarbital
Sulfisoxazole

Sulfonamides
Thioridazine

Differential Diagnosis for Decreased Serum Bilirubin

Cardiovascular
Usually no effect

Respiratory
Usually no effect

Genitourinary
Usually no effect

Gastrointestinal
Celiac disease

Pancreatic
Usually no effect

Hepatobiliary
Usually no effect

Hematologic
Anemia

Endocrine
Usually no effect

Metabolic
Usually no effect

Infectious
Usually no effect

Immunologic
Usually no effect

Musculoskeletal
Usually no effect

Neuropsychiatric
Usually no effect

Neoplastic
Usually no effect

Miscellaneous
Decreased albumin

Serum Calcium, Total

Patient Preparation. Posture affects serum proteins, ambulatory patients having slightly higher (approximately 10 per cent) serum calcium (bound to protein) than recumbent patients. It is preferable to draw a fasting specimen.

Specimen Collection and Handling. Serum or heparinized plasma may be used. Blood should be drawn in the absence of venous stasis because stasis can cause hemoconcentration (e.g., increase of serum calcium of 0.2 to 0.3 mEq/liter or 0.4 to 0.6 mg/100 ml). Cork stoppers should never be used, because they may contain calcium. Serum or plasma should not remain in prolonged contact with erythrocytes, because the cells become permeable to calcium with time.

Methodology. Atomic absorption is the method of choice. However, many modern automated methods give results that agree reasonably well with atomic absorption. Consult the laboratory for its methodology, including in vitro drug interference.

Reference Interval. The reference interval for plasma or serum is as follows: 9.2 to 11.0 mg/100 ml or 4.6 to 5.5 mEq/liter. The serum total calcium should always be interpreted with knowledge of the serum albumin level and should be adjusted up or down 0.8 mg/100 ml for every gram of deviation of serum albumin up or down from a mean value of around 4.5 gm/100 ml. Consult the laboratory for its reference intervals.

Agents Associated With Increased Levels of Serum Calcium in Vivo

Alkaline antacids	Chlorothiazide	Estradiol	Nandrolone	Secretin
Anabolic steroids	Chlorthalidone	Estrogens	Oral contraceptives	Testolactone
Androgens	Dienestrol	Fluoxymesterone	Oxymetholone	Testosterone
Bendroflumethiazide	Diethylstilbestrol	Hydrochlorothiazide	Parathyroid extract	Thiazides
Calcium gluconate	Dihydrotachysterol	Methandrostenolone	Polythiazide	Trichlormethiazide
Calcium salts	Dromostanolone	Methyltestosterone	Progesterone	Vitamin D

Differential Diagnosis for Elevated Serum Calcium
(see page 147)

Cardiovascular
  Usually no effect

Respiratory
  Berylliosis

Genitourinary
  Renal tubular acidosis
  Renal dwarfism

Gastrointesintal
  Peptic ulcer: Site unspecified

Pancreatic
  Acute pancreatitis

Hepatobiliary
  Usually no effect

Hematologic
  Lymphocytic leukemia: Acute, chronic
  Multiple myeloma
  Myelocytic leukemia: Acute, chronic
  Polycythemia vera

Endocrine
  Acromegaly
  Adrenal cortical hyperfunction
  Adrenal cortical hypofunction
  Anterior pituitary hypofunction
  Hyperparathyroidism
  Hyperthyroidism
  Hypothyroidism
  Ovarian hyperfunction
  Pheochromocytoma

Metabolic
  Hyperlipoproteinemia: Types IIA, IIB
  Hypophosphatasia
  Milk-alkali syndrome

Infectious
  Granulomatous disease

Immunologic
  Usually no effect

Musculoskeletal
  Osteitis deformans
  Osteomalacia
  Osteoporosis
  Rheumatoid arthritis

Neuropsychiatric
  Usually no effect

Neoplastic
  Lymphoma: Hodgkin's disease, lymphosarcoma, reticulum cell sarcoma
  Malignant neoplasm: Bladder, bone, breast, bronchus and lung, esophagus, kidney, liver, pancreas; some tumors secrete parathyroid hormone
  Secondary malignant neoplasm: Bone, respiratory system

Miscellaneous
  Acute alcohol intoxication
  Alcoholism
  Dehydration
  Epilepsy
  Exercise

High serum albumin
Hypervitaminosis D
Idiopathic hypercalcemia of infancy
Sarcoidosis
Toxic effect: Non-medicinal metals

Agents Associated With Decreased Levels of Serum Calcium in Vivo

Acetazolamide	Cortisone	Furosemide	Mercurial compounds	Phosphates
Anticonvulsants	Dactinomycin	Gastrin	Mercurial diuretics	Prednisone
Asparaginase	Diuretics	Glucagon	Methicillin	Saline
Calcitonin	Dromostanolone	Glucocorticoids	Methoxyflurane	Sodium sulfate
Carbenoxolone	Edetate	Glucose	Mithramycin	Streptozocin
Chlorothiazide	Enflurane	Insulin	Oral contraceptives	Sulfates
Citrates	Ethinyl estradiol	Laxatives	Phenobarbital	Tetracycline
Corticosteroids	Fluorides	Magnesium salts	Phenytoin	

Agents Associated With Decreased Levels of Serum Calcium in Vivo

Cardiovascular
  Fat embolism

Respiratory
  Hyperventilation syndrome (only ionized fraction low)

Genitourinary
  Glomerulonephritis: Focal, rapidly progressive
  Kidney calculus
  Medullary cystic disease
  Nephrotic syndrome
  Renal dwarfism
  Renal failure: Acute, chronic
  Renal tubular acidosis

Gastrointestinal
  Celiac disease
  Malabsorption: Cause unspecified
  Protein-losing enteropathy
  Regional enteritis
  Ulcerative colitis
  Whipple's disease
  Zollinger-Ellison syndrome

Pancreatic
  Pancreatitis: Acute, chronic

Hepatobiliary
  Cirrhosis of liver: Cause unspecified
  Laennec's or alcoholic cirrhosis

Hematologic
  Acute lymphocytic leukemia
  Heavy-chain disease: Alpha, gamma
  Pernicious anemia

Endocrine
  Anterior pituitary hypofunction

Diabetes mellitus
Hypoparathyroidism
Ovarian hypofunction
Pseudohypoparathyroidism

Metabolic
  Analbuminemia
  Cystic fibrosis
  Cystinosis
  Lactosuria

Infectious
  Leprosy

Immunologic
  Usually no effect

Musculoskeletal
  Osteomalacia
  Osteopetrosis
  Osteoporosis
  Vitamin D deficiency rickets

Neuropsychiatric
  Epilepsy

Neoplastic
  Usually no effect

Miscellaneous
  Acute alcohol intoxication
  Alcoholism
  Heat stroke
  Low serum albumin
  Overhydration
  Pemphigus
  Pregnancy
  Protein malnutrition

Serum Carbon Dioxide, Total

Patient Preparation. Physical activity and respiratory rate should be reasonably stable; i.e., the patient should refrain from heavy exercise immediately prior to giving the blood sample.

Specimen Collection and Handling. Serum or heparinized plasma may be used. Specimens used for the measurement of total CO_2 should be handled anaerobically at all times. If the specimen is collected in a Vacutainer,* the top of the container should not be removed until the specimen is to be withdrawn and analyzed.

Methodology. If the sample is exposed to air, as in the standard AutoAnalyzer† procedure, the result may be low by as much as 6 mEq/liter for a 1-hour exposure. This can be prevented by covering the AutoAnalyzer cup with parafilm. The microgasometer method protects the sample from air and therefore does not have the open-sample cup problem. Consult the laboratory for its methodology, including in vitro drug interference.

Reference Interval. The reference interval for plasma or serum is as follows: arterial blood, 21 to 28 mM/liter; venous blood 24 to 30 mM/liter. Consult the laboratory for its reference intervals.

---

*Becton Dickinson and Company, Rutherford, N.J.
†Technicon Instruments Corporation, Tarrytown, N.Y.

Agents Associated With Increased Levels of Serum Carbon Dioxide in Vivo

Bendroflumethiazide	Cephalexin	Ethacrynic acid	Methychlothiazide	Prednisolone
Betamethasone	Chlorthalidone	Fludrocortisone	Methylprednisolone	Prednisone
Bicarbonates	Corticosteroids	Gentamicin	Metolazone	Probucol
Carbenicillin	Dexamethasone	Hydrocortisone	Paramethasone	Salicylates
Carbenoxolone	Enflurane	Hydroflumethiazide	Polythiazide	Thiazides

Differential Diagnosis for Elevated Serum Carbon Dioxide

Cardiovascular
Arteriosclerosis
Chronic ischemic heart disease
Congestive heart failure
Essential hypertension
Malignant hypertension

Respiratory
Anthracosis
Asbestosis
Asthma
Berylliosis
Chronic bronchitis
Chronic obstructive pulmonary disease
Pulmonary emphysema
Pulmonary tuberculosis
Respiratory acidosis
Silicosis
Viral pneumonia

Genitourinary
Renal tubular acidosis

Gastrointestinal
Intestinal obstruction
Peptic ulcer: Site unspecified
Pyloric stenosis: Acquired

Pancreatic
Usually no effect

Hepatobiliary
Hepatic failure

Hematologic
Usually no effect

Endocrine
Adrenal cortical hyperfunction
Ectopic ACTH production
Hypothyroidism

Metabolic
Acute intermittent porphyria
Metabolic alkalosis

Infectious
Tetanus

Immunologic
Usually no effect

Musculoskeletal
Usually no effect

Neuropsychiatric
Acute poliomyelitis
Guillaine-Barré syndrome
Myasthenia gravis
Transient cerebral ischemia

Neoplastic
Benign neoplasm: Brain, breast, central nervous system
Lymphoma: Hodgkin's disease
Malignant neoplasm: Brain, lung
Secondary malignant neoplasm: Respiratory system

Miscellaneous
Gangrene
Sarcoidosis

Agents Associated With Decreased Levels of Serum Carbon Dioxide in Vivo

Acetazolamide	Fructose	Nitrofurantoin	Streptozocin
Ammonium chloride	Lipomul	Paraldehyde	Tetracycline
Dimercaprol	Mercury compounds	Phenformin	Triamterene
Edetate	Methicillin	Salicylates	Trimethadione
Ethanol			

Differential Diagnosis for Decreased Serum Carbon Dioxide

Cardiovascular
Congestive heart failure
Shock

Respiratory
Asthma
Pulmonary collapse
Pulmonary congestion and hypostasis
Resolving pneumonia
Respiratory alkalosis

Genitourinary
Renal failure: Acute, chronic
Renal tubular acidosis

Gastrointestinal
Celiac disease
Diarrhea
Fistula of stomach and duodenum
Gastroenteritis and colitis
Malabsorption: Cause unspecified

Pancreatic
Usually no effect

Hepatobiliary
Usually no effect

Hematologic
Sickle cell crisis

Endocrine
Adrenal cortical hypofunction
Diabetes mellitus
Hyperparathyroidism
Hyperthyroidism

Metabolic
Cystinosis
Diabetic acidosis
Hepatolenticular degeneration
Metabolic acidosis
Thiamine deficiency

Infectious
Gram-negative sepsis
Tetanus

Immunologic
Usually no effect

Musculoskeletal
Usually no effect

Neuropsychiatric
Hepatic encephalopathy

Neoplastic
Usually no effect

Miscellaneous
Acute alcohol intoxication
Dehydration
Delirium tremens
Eclampsia
Exercise
Hypothermia
Obstetrical labor
Overhydration
Pregnancy
Starvation
Toxic effects: Non-medicinal metals

Serum Chloride

Patient Preparation. There is a slight decrease in serum chloride after meals because of the chloride required for the formation of gastric hydrochloric acid (HCl). Vigorous exercise for 30 minutes can increase the serum chloride concentration by 2 mEq/liter.

Specimen Collection and Handling. Serum or heparinized plasma may be used. Hemolysis can decrease serum chloride secondary to a dilutional effect because the concentration of chloride in red blood cell fluid is less than in serum. In addition, if a clotted sample is exposed to air, there can be a water shift from the red blood cells to the serum with a decrease in serum chloride.

Methodology. The coulometric-amperometric titration of chloride is probably the most accurate method available for determining chloride in routine clinical chemistry laboratories. Iodide or bromide in the patient's serum can interfere with some colorimetric methods, causing erroneously high values. Consult the laboratory for its methodology, including in vitro drug interference.

Reference Interval. The reference interval for plasma or serum is 95 to 103/mEq/liter. Consult the laboratory for its reference interval.

Agents Associated With Increased Levels of Serum Chloride in Vivo

Acetazolamide	Corticosteroids	Intra-amniotic saline	Phenylbutazone
Ammonium chloride	Diazoxide	Ion exchange resins	Potassium chloride
Androgens	Estrogens	Methoxyflurane	Salicylates
Chloride salts	Guanethidine	Methyldopa	Saline
Chlorothiazide	Hydrochlorothiazide	Oxyphenbutazone	Triamterene
Cholestyramine	Hydrocortisone		

Differential Diagnosis for Elevated Serum Chloride

Cardiovascular
Usually no effect

Respiratory
Respiratory alkalosis

Genitourinary
Acute renal failure
Chronic pyelonephritis
Membranoproliferative glomerulonephritis
Renal tubular acidosis
Renovascular hypertension
Ureterosigmoidoscopy

Gastrointestinal
Bacillary dysentery
Cholera
Diarrhea
Fistula of stomach and duodenum
Gastroenteritis and colitis
Intestinal obstruction

Pancreatic
Usually no effect

Hepatobiliary
Usually no effect

Hematologic
Multiple myeloma

Endocrine
Adrenal cortical hyperfunction
Adrenal cortical hypofunction

Diabetes insipidus
Hyperparathyroidism
Hypothalamic lesion
Ovarian hypofunction

Metabolic
Cystic fibrosis
Cystinosis
Galactosemia
Metabolic acidosis
Vitamin D deficiency rickets

Infectious
Usually no effect

Immunologic
Usually no effect

Musculoskeletal
Usually no effect

Neuropsychiatric
Usually no effect

Neoplastic
Malignant neoplasm: Stomach

Miscellaneous
Dehydration
Excessive sweating
Exercise
Heat stroke
Obstetrical labor

Agents Associated With Decreased Levels of Serum Chloride in Vivo

Bicarbonates	Diuretics	Hydroflumethiazide	Polythiazide
Bromides	Ethacrynic acid	Laxatives	Prednisolone
Carbenoxolone	Furosemide	Mannitol	Silver
Corticosteroids	Glucose	Mercurial diuretics	Thiazides
Corticotropin	Hydrochlorothiazide	Metolazone	Triamterene
Cortisone	Hydrocortisone		

Differential Diagnosis for Decreased Serum Chloride

Cardiovascular
   Congestive heart failure

Respiratory
   Chronic obstructive pulmonary disease
   Pulmonary emphysema
   Respiratory acidosis

Genitourinary
   Chronic renal failure

Gastrointestinal
   Bacillary dysentery
   Celiac disease
   Diarrhea
   Fistula of stomach and duodenum
   Gastroenteritis and colitis
   Intestinal obstruction
   Peptic ulcer: Site unspecified
   Pyloric stenosis: Acquired
   Ulcerative colitis
   Vomiting

Pancreatic
   Usually no effect

Hepatobiliary
   Usually no effect

Hematologic
   Usually no effect

Endocrine
   Adrenal cortical hyperfunction
   Adrenal cortical hypofunction
   Diabetes mellitus
   Ectopic ACTH production
   Inappropriate antidiuretic hormone
   Ovarian hyperfunction

Metabolic
   Acute intermittent porphyria
   Cystic fibrosis
   Hepatolenticular degeneration
   Hyperlipemia
   Metabolic alkalosis

Infectious
   Usually no effect

Immunologic
   Usually no effect

Musculoskeletal
   Usually no effect

Neuropsychiatric
   Meningitis: Bacterial, tuberculous

Neoplastic
   Carcinoma of lung

Miscellaneous
   Eclampsia
   Excessive sweating
   Gangrene
   Overhydration
   Pemphigus
   Sarcoidosis

Serum Cholesterol

Patient Preparation. In most persons, the serum cholesterol is affected very little by a recent meal. In some persons, however, the postprandial cholesterol concentration may be elevated up to 100 mg/100 ml. Cholesterol is bound to protein, with ambulatory patients having slightly higher (approximately 10 per cent) serum cholesterol than recumbent patients.

Specimen Collection and Handling. Serum or heparinized plasma may be used. Blood should be drawn in the absence of venous stasis because stasis can cause an increase in the cholesterol concentration (e.g., a 5 to 20 per cent increase when a tourniquet is applied for 5 minutes). Hemolysis should be avoided because hemoglobin can cause falsely elevated values in direct colorimetric procedures. Total serum cholesterol is stable at room temperature for up to 7 days. At $-20°C$ it is stable for 5 years.

Methodology. The method of Abell, which is an extraction procedure utilizing the Liebermann-Burchard reagent for color development (Tietz, 1976), is satisfactory. However, if colorimetric methods are used without extraction, serious errors can occur that result in a falsely elevated cholesterol concentration. The more recently developed enzymatic method for measuring serum cholesterol is the most accurate means for determination of cholesterol in routine clinical chemistry laboratories. Consult the laboratory for its methodology, including in vitro drug interference.

Reference Interval. The reference intervals for healthy persons may not represent the ideal reference intervals for prevention of atherosclerosis. These reference intervals are age and sex dependent. An approximate upper reference limit is 200 plus the patient's age in mg/100 ml. See Chapter 10 for further information. Consult the laboratory for its reference intervals.

Agents Associated With Increased Levels of Serum Cholesterol in Vivo

Acetohexamide	Cortisone	Imipramine	Prochlorperazine
Acetophenazine	Cyclizine	Levarterenol	Promazine
Anabolic steroids	Cylcophosphamide	Levodopa	Quinethazone
Androgens	Dantrolene	Lithium	Sucrose
Anticonvulsants	Dapsone	Meprobamate	Sulfadiazine
Ascorbic acid	Disopyramide	Methandrostenolone	Sulfonamides
Asparaginase	Disulfiram	Methimazole	Sulindac
Bile salts	Epinephrine	Methyltestosterone	Testosterone
Calcitriol	Estrogens	Miconazole	Thiabendazole
Chlormezanone	Ethchlorvynol	Niacin	Thiazides
Chlorpromazine	Ether	Oral contraceptives	Tolazamide
Chlorpropamide	Fluoxymesterone	Oxymetholone	Trifluoperazine
Clofibrate	Furosemide	Penicillamine	Trimethadione
Corticosteroids	Gold	Phenothiazines	Trimipramine
Corticotropin	Heparin	Phenytoin	Vitamin D

Differential Diagnosis for Elevated Serum Cholesterol

Cardiovascular
  Acute myocardial infarction
  Arteriosclerosis
  Chronic ischemic heart disease
  Essential hypertension
  Malignant hypertension

Respiratory
  Usually no effect

Genitourinary
  Benign prostatic hypertrophy
  Chronic renal failure
  Glomerulonephritis: Acute poststreptococcal, membranous, minimal change
  Nephrotic syndrome
  Renovascular hypertension

Gastrointestinal
  Usually no effect

Pancreatic
  Chronic pancreatitis
  Total pancreatectomy

Hepatobiliary
  Biliary cirrhosis
  Cholestasis
  Extrahepatic biliary obstruction
  Laennec's or alcoholic cirrhosis
  Necrosis of liver: Acute, subacute
  Toxic hepatitis

Hematologic
  Chronic myelocytic leukemia
  Multiple myeloma

Endocrine
  Adrenal cortical hyperfunction
  Anterior pituitary hypofunction
  Diabetes mellitus
  Hyperlipoproteinemia: Types I, IIA, IIB, III, IV, V
  Hypothyroidism
  Ovarian hypofunction
  Thyroiditis: Subacute

Metabolic
  Analbuminemia
  Anderson's disease
  Cystic fibrosis
  Forbes' disease
  Gout
  McArdle's disease
  von Gierke's disease

Infectious
  Ancylostomiasis

Immunologic
  Polyarteritis nodosa
  Systemic lupus erythematosus

Musculoskeletal
  Usually no effect

Neuropsychiatric
  Friedreich's ataxia

Neoplastic
  Malignant neoplasm: Intrahepatic bile ducts, pancreas, prostate

Miscellaneous
  Amyloidosis
  Dehydration
  Exercise
  Klinefelter's syndrome
  Pregnancy
  Stress
  Toxic effects: Non-medicinal metals

Agents Associated With Decreased Levels of Serum Cholesterol in Vivo

Allopurinol	Colchicine	Isoniazid	Oxandrolone
Aluminum nicotinate	Colestipol	Kanamycin	Oxymetholone
Aminosalicylic acid	Corticotropin	Levothyroxine	Paromomycin
Androgens	Dextrothyroxine	Lincomycin	Pentylenetetrazol
Antidiabetic drugs	Edetate	Liotrix	Phenformin
Antimony compounds	Erythromycin	Menotropins	Probucol
Ascorbic acid	Estradiol	Methandrostenolone	Progesterone
Asparaginase	Estrogens	Monoamine oxidase	Salicylates
Azathioprine	Ethanol	inhibitors	Sitosterols
Cellulose	Ethinyl estradiol	Nandrolone	Tetracycline
Cholestyramine	Glucagon	Neomycin	Thyroid hormones
Clofibrate	Haloperidol	Niacin	Tolbutamide
Clomiphene	Insulin	Nicotinyl alcohol	Triiodothyronine

Differential Diagnosis for Decreased Serum Cholesterol

Cardiovascular
  Congestive heart failure

Respiratory
  Bacterial pneumonia
  Chronic obstructive pulmonary disease
  Pulmonary tuberculosis
  Viral pneumonia

Genitourinary
  Usually no effect

Gastrointestinal
  Celiac disease
  Diarrhea
  Intestinal obstruction
  Malabsorption: Cause unspecified
  Mesenteric artery embolism
  Ulcerative colitis
  Whipple's disease

Pancreatic
  Acute pancreatitis

Hepatobiliary
  Chronic active hepatitis
  Cirrhosis of liver: Cause unspecified

  Hepatic failure
  Necrosis of liver: Acute, subacute
  Toxic hepatitis
  Viral hepatitis
  Yellow fever

Hematologic
  Acute myelocytic leukemia
  Anemia
  Folic acid deficiency anemia
  Hereditary spherocytosis
  Hemophilia
  Iron deficiency anemia
  Lymphocytic leukemia: Acute, chronic
  Monocytic leukemia
  Multiple myeloma
  Pernicious anemia
  Sickle cell anemia

Endocrine
  Acromegaly
  Hyperparathyroidism
  Hyperthyroidism
  Hypobeta- and abetalipoproteinemia
  Ovarian hyperfunction

Metabolic
Carcinoid syndrome
Tangier disease

Infectious
Herpes zoster
Leprosy
Leptospirosis
Multiple infections
Septicemia

Immunologic
Usually no effect

Musculoskeletal
Osteomyelitis

Rheumatoid arthritis

Neuropsychiatric
Brain infarction
Mental retardation

Neoplastic
Lymphoma: Hodgkin's disease, reticulum cell sarcoma
Malignant neoplasm: Liver, pancreas, prostate
Secondary malignant neoplasm: Disseminated, liver

Miscellaneous
Drug dependence: Opium and derivatives
Inanition
Protein malnutrition

Serum Creatine Phosphokinase (CPK)

Patient Preparation. A number of patient factors can increase serum CPK, usually by releasing CPK from muscle, (such as through coughing, electrocautery, intramuscular injections, muscle massage, and muscular exercise). The elevation due to muscular exercise is maximal on the day following the exercise. Low values have been observed with malnutrition.

Specimen Collection and Handling. Serum or heparinized plasma samples are preferred. The enzyme is inhibited by EDTA, citrate, and fluoride. There is rapid loss of CPK activity with storage; activity may persist at ambient temperature for 4 hours, at 4°C for 8 to 12 hours, and, when frozen, only 2 to 3 days. A small degree of hemolysis can be tolerated, but any significant hemolysis may interfere with the assay.

Methodology. Numerous procedures are available: colorimetric, fluorometric, and coupled enzyme methods. Kinetic methods are preferable, and the use of the reverse reaction has a number of chemical advantages. Consult your laboratory for its methodology, including in vitro drug interference.

Reference Interval. General reference intervals are 55 to 170 U/liter at 37°C for males and 30 to 135 U/liter at 37°C for females. However, there are also differences according to race, the enzyme level being higher in blacks than in whites. Consult the laboratory for its reference intervals.

Agents Associated With Increased Levels of Serum CPK in Vivo

Aminocaproic acid	Bromocriptine	Clonidine	Ethchlorvynol	Narcotic injections
Amphotericin B	Carbenicillin injections	Copper	Halothane	Oral contraceptives
Ampicillin injections	Carbenoxolone	Dantrolene	Insulin	Penicillin injections
Analgesic injections	Chlorpromazine	Digoxin injections	Lithium	Phenothiazine injections
Anesthetic agents	Clindamycin injections	Diuretic injections	Meperidine injections	Succinylcholine injections
Barbiturates	Clofibrate	Ethanol	Morphine injections	Tubocurarine injections

Differential Diagnosis for Elevated Serum CPK

Cardiovascular
Acute myocardial infarction
Acute myocarditis
Arterial embolism and thrombosis
Cardiac defibrillation
Cardiomyopathies

Respiratory
Asthma
Influenza
Pulmonary edema
Pulmonary embolism and infarction

Genitourinary
Usually no effect

Gastrointestinal
Usually no effect

Pancreatic
Acute pancreatitis

Hepatobiliary
Usually no effect

Hematologic
Christmas disease
Hemophilia

Endocrine
Acromegaly
Hypoparathyroidism
Hypothyroidism
Thyroiditis: Subacute

Metabolic
Diabetic acidosis
Hypokalemia
McArdle's disease

Infectious
Hydatidosis
Leptospirosis
Tetanus
Trichinosis
Typhoid fever

Immunologic
Dermatomyositis and polymyositis
Progressive systemic sclerosis
Systemic lupus erythematosus

Musculoskeletal
Crush injury following trauma
Familial progressive spinal muscular atrophy
Intramuscular injections
Muscle spasms
Myoglobinuria
Myotonia atrophica
Myotonia congenita
Progressive muscular dystrophy

Neuropsychiatric
Bacterial meningitis
Cerebral embolism and thrombosis
Cerebral infarction
Convulsions
Encephalomyelitis

Poliomyelitis: Acute
Status epilepticus

Neoplastic
Malignant neoplasm: Brain

Miscellaneous
Acute alcohol intoxication
Alcoholism
Delirium tremens
Drug dependence: Opium and derivatives

Effects of electric current
Exercise
Heat stroke
Hypothermia
Manic-depressive disorder
Paranoid states and other psychoses
Postoperative state
Postpartum
Toxic effects: Carbon monoxide, venom

Agents Associated With Decreased Levels of Serum CPK in Vivo

Ethanol
Phenothiazines

Differential Diagnosis for Decreased Serum CPK

Cardiovascular
Usually no effect

Respiratory
Usually no effect

Genitourinary
Usually no effect

Gastrointestinal
Usually no effect

Pancreatic
Usually no effect

Hepatobiliary
Usually no effect

Hematologic
Hereditary spherocytosis

Endocrine
Usually no effect

Metabolic
Usually no effect

Infectious
Usually no effect

Immunologic
Usually no effect

Musculoskeletal
Usually no effect

Neuropsychiatric
Usually no effect

Neoplastic
Usually no effect

Miscellaneous
Pregnancy: Early

Serum Creatinine

Patient Preparation. Patient factors do not usually interfere. This represents a significant advantage of using determinations of serum creatinine over serum urea nitrogen (SUN) for the assessment of renal function, since the SUN level is dependent on the amount of protein in the patient's diet.

Specimen Collection and Handling. A serum or heparinized plasma sample is preferred. If kept for a few days, specimens for creatinine analysis are best stored at refrigerator temperatures; if kept for longer periods of time, they should be frozen.

Methodology. Most of the methods used in clinical laboratories are not completely specific for creatinine but are adequate for clinical purposes. These methods commonly err in overestimating the serum creatinine by a small amount because of interference by creatinine-like compounds. Consult the laboratory for its methodology, including in vitro drug interference.

Reference Interval. A general reference interval is 0.6 to 1.2 mg/100 ml. However, there are differences due to sex (secondary to muscle mass). Using non-specific methods, serum or plasma levels for males are 0.9 to 1.5 mg/100 ml and for females, 0.8 to 1.3 mg/100 ml. Using more specific methods, the levels for males are 0.6 to 1.2 mg/100 ml and for females, 0.5 to 1.0 mg/100 ml. Consult the laboratory for its reference intervals.

Agents Associated With Increased Levels of Serum Creatinine in Vivo

Acetaminophen	Colistimethate	Mannitol	Penicillin
Alkaline antacids	Colistin	Meclofenamate	Phenacetin
Aminoglycosides	Demeclocycline	Mefenamic acid	Phenazopyridine
Amphotericin B	Dextran	Methicillin	Phenylbutazone
Barbiturates	Disopyramide	Methoxyflurane	Polymyxin
Capreomycin	Diuretics	Metolazone	Protein
Carmustine	Doxycycline	Minoxidil	Radiographic agents
Cefaclor	Edetate	Mithramycin	Streptokinase
Cefoxitin	Ethambutol	Mitomycin	Streptomycin
Cephaloridine	Flucytosine	Nalidixic acid	Tetracycline
Chlorthalidone	Gentamicin	Neomycin	Thiazides
Cinoxacin	Griseofulvin	Nitrofurantoin	Triamterene
Cisplatin	Hydroxyurea	Oxacillin	Trimethoprim
Cimetidine	Imipramine	Paraldehyde	Vancomycin
Clofibrate	Kanamycin	Paromomycin	Vitamin D
Clonidine	Lipomul	Penicillamine	Zomepirac

Differential Diagnosis for Elevated Serum Creatinine

Cardiovascular
Acute myocardial infarction
Angina pectoris
Arterial embolism and thrombosis
Arteriosclerosis
Bacterial endocarditis
Chronic ischemic heart disease
Congestive heart failure
Essential hypertension
Shock

Respiratory
Usually no effect

Genitourinary
Azotemia
Benign prostatic hypertrophy
Glomerulonephritis: Acute poststreptococcal, membranoproliferative, rapidly progressive
Hydronephrosis
Nephrotic syndrome
Pyelonephritis: Acute, chronic
Renal failure: Acute, chronic

Gastrointestinal
Diarrhea
Intestinal obstruction
Vomiting

Pancreatic
Acute pancreatitis

Hepatobiliary
Hepatic failure

Hematologic
Acquired hemolytic anemia: Autoimmune
Lymphocytic leukemia: Acute, chronic
Monocytic leukemia
Multiple myeloma
Myelocytic leukemia: Acute, chronic
Thrombotic thrombocytopenic purpura

Endocrine
Acromegaly
Adrenal cortical hypofunction
Diabetes mellitus
Hyperparathyroidism
Hyperthyroidism

314

Metabolic
Cystinosis
Gout
Hepatolenticular degeneration

Infectious
Bacterial meningitis
Epidemic typhus
Herpes zoster
Leptospirosis
Malaria
Psittacosis
Septicemia

Immunologic
Allergic purpura
Polyarteritis nodosa
Progressive systemic sclerosis
Systemic lupus erythematosus

Musculoskeletal
Amyotrophic lateral sclerosis

Myotonia atrophica

Neuropsychiatric
Bacterial meningitis

Neoplastic
Lymphoma: Hodgkin's disease, lymphosarcoma, reticulum cell carcoma
Malignant neoplasm: Bladder, corpus uteri, large intestine, prostate, testis

Miscellaneous
Amyloidosis
Dehydration
Diet: Roast meat
Eclampsia
Excessive sweating
Heat stroke
Sarcoidosis
Toxic effects: Non-medicinal metals

Agents Associated With Decreased Levels of Serum Creatinine in Vivo

None.

Differential Diagnosis for Decreased Serum Creatinine

Cardiovascular
Usually no effect

Respiratory
Usually no effect

Genitourinary
Usually no effect

Gastrointestinal
Usually no effect

Pancreatic
Usually no effect

Hepatobiliary
Usually no effect

Hematologic
Usually no effect

Endocrine
Usually no effect

Metabolic
Hepatolenticular degeneration

Infectious
Usually no effect

Immunologic
Usually no effect

Musculoskeletal
Usually no effect

Neuropsychiatric
Muscle wasting disease

Neoplastic
Usually no effect

Miscellaneous
Eclampsia
Pregnancy

Serum Glucose

Patient Preparation. A fasting specimen is a better method of evaluating the level of serum glucose. However, even after a meal, a serum glucose level can be diagnostic; i.e., a serum glucose level greater than 200 mg/100 ml in the presence of compatible clinical features can be diagnostic for diabetes mellitus.

Specimen Collection and Handling. Serum or heparinized plasma may be used. However, unless the serum or plasma is promptly separated from the blood cells and refrigerated, significant depression of serum glucose will occur secondary to its metabolism by the blood cells. This depression can be prevented by collecting the sample in a fluoride tube, which inhibits the blood cell enzymes.

Methodology. Many methods are available. The most accurate of these are the enzymatic methods. Of the enzymatic methods, the hexokinase method has fewer interferences (is more specific) than the glucose oxidase method, e.g., serum glucose by glucose oxidase is depressed by ascorbic acid. Nonspecific reduction methods should be avoided because they can significantly overestimate the serum glucose level. In uremia, for example, the reducing effect of serum non-protein nitrogenous products can cause overestimation of serum glucose by up to 40 mg/100 ml. Consult the laboratory for its methodology, including in vitro drug interference.

Reference Interval. A general reference interval for fasting serum glucose for enzymatic methods is approximately 70 to 110 mg/100 ml. However, small to moderate variations outside this reference interval do not necessarily indicate disease. See Chapter 17 for a discussion of diabetes mellitus. Consult the laboratory for its reference interval.

Agents Associated With Increased Levels of Serum Glucose
(see page 277)

Acetazolamide	Dexamethasone	Imipramine	Phenolphthalein
Aluminum nicotinate	Dextroamphetamine	Indomethacin	Phenothiazines
Amino acid solution	Dextrothyroxine	Isoniazid	Phenylbutazone
Aminosalicylic acid	Diazoxide	Isoproterenol	Phenylephrine
Amitriptyline	Dimercaprol	Levarterenol	Phenytoin
Androgens	Dopamine	Levodopa	Piperacetazine
Anesthetic agents	Enflurane	Lithium	Polythiazide
Arginine	Ephedrine	Medroxyprogesterone	Prednisolone
Asparaginase	Epinephrine	Meperidine	Prednisone
Baclofen	Estrogens	Meprednisone	Protriptyline
Benzodiazepines	Ethacrynic acid	Metolazone	Quinethazone
Benzthiazide	Ethanol	Morphine	Reserpine
Benzyl alcohol	Ether	Nalidixic acid	Salicylates
Beta-adrenergic drugs	Ethionamide	Narcotics	Secretin
Caffeine	Ferrous salts	Niacin	Sucrose
Chlorothiazide	Fludrocortisone	Nicotinic acid	Theophylline
Chlorpromazine	Fluoxymesterone	Nicotinyl alcohol	Thiabendazole
Chlorprothixene	Furosemide	Nitrofurantoin	Thiazides
Chlorthalidone	Glucagon	Nortriptyline	Thiothixene
Clonidine	Glucocorticoids	Oral contraceptives	Thyroid hormones
Clopamide	Glucose	Oxyphenbutazone	Triamcinolone
Corticosteroids	Haloperidol	Paraldehyde	Triamterene
Corticotropin	Halothane	Pentamidine	Trichlormethiazide
Cortisone	Heparin	Perphenazine	Tricyclic antidepressants
Cyclopropane	Hydrochlorothiazide	Phenelzine	Vinyl ether
Desipramine	Hydroflumethiazide		

Differential Diagnosis for Elevated Serum Glucose

Cardiovascular
  Acute myocardial infarction
  Congestive heart failure

Respiratory
  Asthma
  Bacterial pneumonia
  Pulmonary embolism and infarction

Genitourinary
  Membranous glomerulonephritis
  Renal failure: Acute, chronic
  Renovascular hypertension

Gastrointestinal
  Acute appendicitis
  Gastroenteritis and colitis
  Intestinal obstruction
  Postgastrectomy (dumping) syndrome

Pancreatic
 Pancreatitis: Acute, chronic
 Pancreatic cyst and pseudocyst

Hepatobiliary
 Hepatic disease

Hematologic
 Chronic myelocytic leukemia

Endocrine
 Acromegaly
 Adrenal cortical hyperfunction
 Diabetes mellitus
 Ectopic ACTH production
 Hyperthyroidism
 Hypothalamic lesion
 Pheochromocytoma

Metabolic
 Cystic fibrosis
 Diabetic acidosis
 Hemochromatosis
 Hyperlipoproteinemia: Types III, IV, V
 Thiamine deficiency

Infectious
 Phlebotomus fever

 Septicemia
 Syphilis
 Tularemia

Immunologic
 Usually no effect

Musculoskeletal
 Crush injury following trauma

Neuropsychiatric
 Bacterial meningitis
 Cerebral hemorrhage
 Wernicke's encephalopathy

Neoplastic
 Malignant neoplasm: Lung, pancreas, prostate

Miscellaneous
 Burns
 Eclampsia
 Exercise
 Hypothermia
 Klinefelter's syndrome
 Pregnancy
 Shock
 Stress

Agents Associated With Decreased Levels of Serum Glucose in Vivo

Acetaminophen
Acetohexamide
Allopurinol
Amino acids
Aminosalicylic acid
Amitriptyline
Amphetamines
Anabolic steroids
Androgens
Antihistamines
Antimony compounds
Atropine
Barbiturates
Calcium gluconate
Chloramphenicol
Chlorpropamide

Clofibrate
Cyproheptadine
Desipramine
Dextroamphetamine
Dicumarol
Dimercaprol
Erythromycin
Ethacrynic acid
Ethanol
Fenfluramine
Fluoxymesterone
Fructose infusions
Guanethidine
Haloperidol
Imipramine
Insulin

Isocarboxazid
Lincomycin
Marijuana
Methandrostenolone
Monoamine oxidase
 inhibitors
Nandrolone
Nifurtimox
Nortriptyline
Oxandrolone
Oxymetholone
Oxytetracycline
Pargyline
Pentamidine
Phenformin
Phentolamine

Piperacetazine
Potassium chloride
Probenecid
Progesterone
Promethazine
Propoxyphene
Propranolol
Protriptyline
Salicylates
Sulfonamides
Sulfonylureas
Thiothixene
Tolazamide
Tolbutamide
Tripelennamine
Tromethamine

Differential Diagnosis for Decreased Serum Glucose

Cardiovascular
 Congestive heart failure

Respiratory
 Usually no effect

Genitourinary
 Usually no effect

Gastrointestinal
 Gastroenteritis and colitis
 Gastroenterostomy
 Malabsorption
 Peptic ulcer: Site unspecified
 Postgastrectomy (dumping) syndrome

Pancreatic
 Pancreatitis

Hepatobiliary
 Biliary cirrhosis
 Cholangitis
 Chronic active hepatitis
 Cirrhosis: Cause unspecified
 Hepatic failure
 Laennec's or alcoholic cirrhosis
 Liver abscess
 Necrosis of liver: Acute, subacute
 Reye's syndrome
 Toxic hepatitis
 Viral hepatitis
 Yellow fever

Hematologic
 Chronic myelocytic leukemia
 Hemolytic disease of newborn

Endocrine
Adrenal cortical hypofunction
Adrenal medulla unresponsiveness
Anterior pituitary hypofunction
Early diabetes mellitus
Glucagon deficiency
Hypothalamic lesions
Hypothyroidism
Islet cell hyperplasia or tumor
Thyroiditis: Subacute

Metabolic
Anderson's disease
Carcinoid syndrome
Galactosemia
Hereditary fructose intolerance
Hypoglycemia: Cause unspecified
Idiopathic leucine sensitivity
Ketotic hypoglycemia
McArdle's disease
Maple syrup urine disease
von Gierke's disease

Infectious
Diphtheria
Mumps
Rabies

Immunologic
Usually no effect

Musculoskeletal
Acute arthritis: Pyogenic

Neuropsychiatric
Autonomic nervous system disorders
Forbes' disease

Neoplastic
Bulky neoplasms
Malignant neoplasm: Adrenal gland, bronchus and lung,
    fibrosarcoma, liver, pancreas, stomach
Secondary malignant neoplasm: Liver

Miscellaneous
Alcoholism
Deficiency state: Cause unspecified
Exercise
Factitious hypoglycemia
Heat stroke
Infant of diabetic mother
Pregnancy
Prematurity
Protein malnutrition
Toxic effects: Non-medicinal metals

Blood Hemoglobin

Patient Preparation. Patient factors do not generally interfere. Residing at an altitude greater than 4500 feet above sea level can increase blood hemoglobin by 7 to 8 per cent. Erect posture can cause a small increase in hemoglobin as a result of redistribution of body water, and muscular exercise has been reported to cause a small increase from a transient decrease in blood volume.

Specimen Collection and Handling. Satisfactory anticoagulants include EDTA, double oxalate, and heparin. Of these three, EDTA is preferable because it does not interfere with leukocyte and platelet counts and morphology. Venous stasis, secondary to a prolonged tourniquet application, can erroneously increase the blood hemoglobin level (2 to 6 per cent). Incorrect finger-stick sampling can cause errors in either direction. The level in ear lobe blood can be increased up to 15 per cent above finger-stick blood.

Methodology. Methods can be of four kinds: colorimetric, gasometric, specific gravity, and chemical. Of these, the colorimetric method (by which hemoglobin is converted to cyanmethemoglobin) is most widely used in clinical laboratories. Consult the laboratory for its methodology.

Reference Interval. Reference intervals are sex dependent: for females, 12.0 to 16.0 gm/100 ml; for males, 13.5 to 18.0 gm/100 ml. Consult the laboratory for its reference intervals.

Agents Associated With Increased Levels of Blood Hemoglobin in Vivo

Dromostanolone
Stanozolol

Differential Diagnosis for Elevated Blood Hemoglobin

Cardiovascular
  Usually no effect

Respiratory
  Anthracosis
  Asbestosis
  Asthma
  Berylliosis
  Chronic obstructive pulmonary disease
  Chronic sinusitis
  Pulmonary emphysema
  Silicosis

Genitourinary
  Usually no effect

Gastrointestinal
  Cholera
  Diarrhea
  Gastroenteritis and colitis
  Intestinal obstruction
  Peritonitis

Pancreatic
  Acute pancreatitis

Hepatobiliary
  Usually no effect

Hematologic
  Chronic myelocytic leukemia

Infectious mononucleosis
Polycythemia: Vera, secondary
Relative polycythemia

Endocrine
  Adrenal cortical hyperfunction
  Pheochromocytoma

Metabolic
  Usually no effect

Infectious
  Usually no effect

Immunologic
  Usually no effect

Musculoskeletal
  Usually no effect

Neuropsychiatric
  Transient cerebral ischemia

Neoplastic
  Benign neoplasm: Cardiovascular system, central nervous system

Miscellaneous
  Dehydration
  Exercise
  Heat stroke

Agents Associated With Decreased Levels of Blood Hemoglobin in Vivo

Acetaminophen	Adriamycin	Aminosalicylic acid	Ampicillin
Acetazolamide	Allopurinol	Amphetamine	Anticonvulsants
Acetohexamide	Aminoglutethimide	Amphotericin B	Antihistamines

Antimalarials
Antimony compounds
Antipyretics
Asparaginase
Barbiturates
Benzocaine
Benzodiazepines
Brompheniramine
Busulfan
Butaperazine
Carbenicillin
Carmustine
Cefoxitin
Cephalosporins
Chloramphenicol
Chloroquine
Chlorothiazide
Chlorpheniramine
Chlorpromazine
Chlorpropamide
Cholestyramine
Cimetidine
Clofibrate
Coal tar
Colchicine
Copper
Corticosteroids
Cromolyn
Cyclophosphamide
Cycloserine
Cytarabine
Dactinomycin
Dantrolene
Dapsone
Demeclocycline
Dehydrocholic acid
Dimercaprol

Dimethindene
Diphenhydramine
Disopyramide
Doxapram
Doxycycline
Edetate
Estrogens
Ethanol
Ethosuximide
Fenoprofen
Floxuridine
Flucytosine
Fluorides
Furazolidone
Furosemide
Gold
Hydralazine
Hydroflumethiazide
Hydroxyurea
Ibuprofen
Indomethacin
Isocarboxazid
Isoniazid
Levodopa
Lincomycin
Lipomul
Lomustine
Mechlorethamine
Meclofenamate
Mefenamic acid
Melphalan
Mercaptopurine
Metaxalone
Methadone
Methaqualone
Methotrexate
Methyldopa

Methylphenidate
Minocycline
Mithramycin
Monoamine oxidase
   inhibitors
Nalidixic acid
Neomycin
Niridazole
Nitrites
Nitrofurantoin
Nitrofurazone
Oral contraceptives
Oxyphenbutazone
Paramethadione
Penicillamine
Penicillins
Pentamidine
Phenazopyridine
Phenformin
Phenobarbital
Phenothiazines
Phenylbutazone
Phytonadione
Piperacetazine
Piperazine
Prilocaine
Primaquine
Primidone
Probenecid
Procainamide
Procarbazine
Pyrazinamide
Pyrimethamine
Quinacrine
Quinethazone
Quinidine
Quinine

Resorcinol
Rifampin
Salicylates
Spectinomycin
Stibophen
Streptomycin
Sulfacetamide
Sulfadiazine
Sulfamethizole
Sulfamethoxazole
Sulfapyridine
Sulfinpyrazone
Sulfisoxazole
Sulfonamides
Sulfones
Sulfoxone
Suramin
Tetracyclines
Thiazides
Thioguanine
Thioridazine
Thiosemicarbazones
Thiotepa
Ticarcillin
Tolazamide
Tolbutamide
Tolmetin
Triamterene
Trichlormethiazide
Trimethadione
Trimethoprim
Tripelennamine
Tripolidine
Vidarabine
Vitamin A
Vitamin K

Differential Diagnosis for Decreased Blood Hemoglobin

Cardiovascular
  Bacterial endocarditis
  Cardiomyopathies
  Fat embolism
  Malignant hypertension
  Pyelophlebitis
  Rheumatic fever

Respiratory
  Abscess of lung
  Anthracosis
  Asbestosis
  Berylliosis
  Bronchiectasis
  Chronic obstructive pulmonary disease
  Pneumonia: Bacterial, viral, mycoplasmal, resolving
  Pulmonary tuberculosis
  Silicosis

Genitourinary
  Benign prostatic hypertrophy
  Chronic pyelonephritis
  Glomerulonephritis: Acute poststreptococcal,
    membranoproliferative, rapidly progressive
  Hydronephrosis
  Medullary cystic disease
  Polycystic kidney disease
  Renal failure: Acute, chronic

Gastrointestinal
  Ancylostomiasis
  Celiac disease
  Diphyllobothriasis
  Diverticular disease of intestine
  Esophageal varices
  Fistula of stomach and duodenum
  Gastritis
  Malabsorption: Cause unspecified
  Peptic ulcer: Site unspecified
  Postgastrectomy (dumping) syndrome
  Protein-losing enteropathy
  Regional enteritis
  Strongyloidiasis
  Trichuriasis
  Ulcerative colitis
  Whipple's disease

Pancreatic
  Acute pancreatitis

Hepatobiliary
  Cirrhosis: Cause unspecified
  Laennec's or alcoholic cirrhosis
  Liver abscess
  Necrosis of liver: Acute, subacute
  Viral hepatitis

Hematologic
Anemia: Acquired autoimmune hemolytic anemia; aplastic anemia; folic acid deficiency; hemoglobin C, E, or H disease; hereditary elliptocytosis and spherocytosis; hereditary non-spherocytic hemolytic anemia; iron deficiency; paroxysmal nocturnal hemoglobinuria; pernicious anemia; Plummer-Vinson syndrome; sickle cell anemia; sideroblastic anemia; thalassemia major and minor; vitamin B_6 deficiency
Erythroleukemia
Heavy-chain disease, gamma
Hemolytic disease of newborn
Hemophilia
Hypersplenism
Idiopathic thrombocytopenic purpura
Lymphocytic leukemia: Acute, chronic
Monocytic leukemia
Myelocytic leukemia: Acute, chronic
Myelofibrosis
Multiple myeloma
Thrombotic thrombocytopenic purpura
Waldenström's macroglobulinemia

Endocrine
Adrenal cortical hyperfunction
Adrenal cortical hypofunction
Anterior pituitary hypofunction
Hyperthyroidism
Hypothyroidism
Hyperparathyroidism
Testicular hypofunction

Metabolic
A-betalipoproteinemia
Cystic fibrosis
Cystinosis
Gaucher's disease
Lesch-Nyhan syndrome
Niemann-Pick disease
Thiamine deficiency
Vitamin C deficiency
von Gierke's disease
Hepatolenticular degeneration

Infectious
Bacterial: Brucellosis, diphtheria, lymphogranuloma venereum, leprosy, leptospirosis, relapsing fever, syphilis, tuberculosis, typhoid fever
Fungal: Actinomycosis, aspergillosis, blastomycosis, histoplasmosis
Parasitic: Amebiasis, leishmaniasis, malaria, toxoplasmosis, trypanosomiasis

Rickettsial: Epidemic typhus, Rocky Mountain spotted fever, tick-borne fever
Septicemia
Viral: Cytomegalic inclusion disease, herpes zoster

Immunologic
Agammaglobulinemia
Allergic purpura
Cranial arteritis and related conditions
Dermatomyositis and polymyositis
Dysgammaglobulinemia
Immunodeficiency
Polyarteritis nodosa
Polymyalgia rheumatica
Progressive systemic sclerosis
Sjögren's syndrome
Systemic lupus erythematosus
Wegener's granulomatosis

Musculoskeletal
Fracture of bone
Juvenile rheumatoid arthritis
Osteomyolitis
Osteopetrosis
Rheumatoid arthritis
Rheumatoid (ankylosing) spondylitis

Neuropsychiatric
Usually no effect

Neoplastic
Benign neoplasm: Cardiovascular tissue, stomach
Histiocytosis X
Lymphoma: Hodgkin's disease, lymphosarcoma, reticulum cell sarcoma
Malignant neoplasm: Bladder, bone, corpus uteri, esophagus, gallbladder, kidney, large intestine, liver, pancreas, prostate, rectum, small intestine, stomach
Secondary malgnant neoplasm: Bone, respiratory system

Miscellaneous
Alcoholism
Amyloidosis
Diaphragmatic hernia
Effects of x-ray irradiation
Hemorrhage
Pemiphigus
Pregnancy
Protein malnutrition
Reiter's disease
Toxic effects: Lead and its compounds, non-medicinal metals

Blood Hematocrit

Patient Preparation. Patient factors do not generally interfere. Residing at an altitude greater then 4500 feet above sea level can increase the blood hematocrit by 7 to 8 per cent. Erect posture can cause a small increase in hematocrit as a result of redistribution of water, and muscular exercise has been reported to cause a small increase from a transient decrease in blood volume. After a meal the hematocrit tends to fall slightly.

Specimen Collection and Handling. Satisfactory anticoagulants include EDTA, double oxalate, and heparin. Of these three, EDTA is preferable because it does not interfere with leukocyte and platelet counts and morphology. Venous stasis, secondary to prolonged tourniquet application, can erroneously increase the blood hematocrit level (2 to 6 per cent). Incorrect finger-stick sampling can cause errors in either direction. The level in ear lobe blood can be increased up to 15 per cent above finger-stick blood.

Methodology. The hematocrit is usually determined by measuring the packed red blood cell volume after centrifugation. Because less time is required for centrifugation and because there is less error from trapping of plasma, the micromethod is preferred over the macromethod. Multichannel instruments sometimes use other methods; e.g., the Coulter Counter Model S* calculates the hematocrit from the MCV and the red blood count. Consult the laboratory for its methodology.

Reference Interval. Reference intervals are sex dependent: for females 38 to 47 per cent; for males, 40 to 54 per cent. Consult the laboratory for its reference intervals.

_____

*Coulter Diagnostics, Hialeah, Fla.

Agents Associated With Increased Blood Hematocrit Levels in Vivo

Androgens	Cobalt	Dromostanolone	Oral contraceptives
Atropine	Corticotropin	Fluoxymesterone	Vitamin B_{12}
Beta-adrenergic drugs	Cyclopropane	Nandrolone	

Differential Diagnosis for Elevated Blood Hematocrit

Cardiovascular
Acute myocardial infarction

Respiratory
Anthracosis
Asbestosis
Asthma
Berylliosis
Chronic obstructive pulmonary disease
Chronic sinusitis
Pulmonary emphysema
Silicosis

Genitourinary
Usually no effect

Gastrointestinal
Cholera
Diarrhea
Fistula of stomach and duodenum
Gastroenteritis and colitis
Intestinal obstruction
Mesenteric artery embolism
Peritonitis

Pancreatic
Acute pancreatitis

Hepatobiliary
Usually no effect

Hematologic
Chronic myelocytic leukemia
Infectious mononucleosis
Polycythemia: Vera, secondary
Relative polycythemia

Endocrine
Adrenal cortical hyperfunction
Adrenal cortical hypofunction
Pheochromocytoma

Metabolic
Diabetic acidosis

Infectious
Arthropod-borne hemorrhagic fever

Immunologic
Dermatomyositis and polymyositis

Musculoskeletal
Usually no effect

Neuropsychiatric
Transient cerebral ischemia

Neoplastic
Benign neoplasm: Central nervous system

Miscellaneous
Dehydration
Eclampsia
Effects of electric current
Exercise

Agents Associated With Decreased Blood Hematocrit Levels in Vivo

Acetohexamide
Adriamycin
Allopurinol
Aminoglutethimide
Aminosalicylic acid
Amphetamine
Amphotericin B
Ampicillin
Anticonvulsants
Antihistamines
Antimalarials
Antipyretics
Asparaginase
Barbiturates
Benzocaine
Benzodiazepines
Brompheniramine
Busulfan
Butaperazine
Carbenoxolone
Carmustine
Cefoxitin
Cephalosporins
Chloramphenicol
Chloroquine
Chlorothiazide
Chlorpheniramine
Chlorpromazine
Chlorpropamide
Cimetidine
Clofibrate
Colchicine
Copper
Corticosteroids
Cromolyn
Cycloserine
Cytarabine
Dactinomycin

Dantrolene
Dapsone
Demeclocycline
Dextran
Dimercaprol
Doxycycline
Diphenhydramine
Disopyramide
Doxapram
Edetate
Estrogens
Ethanol
Ethosuximide
Fenoprofen
Floxuridine
Flucytosine
Furazolidone
Furosemide
Gold
Hydralazine
Hydroflumethiazide
Hydroxyurea
Ibuprofen
Indomethacin
Isocarboxazid
Isoniazid
Levodopa
Lincomycin
Lomustine
Mechlorethamine
Meclofenamate
Mefenamic acid
Melphalan
Meprobamate
Mercaptopurine
Metaxalone
Methadone
Methaqualone

Methotrexate
Methyldopa
Methylphenidate
Minocycline
Monoamine oxidase
  inhibitors
Nalidixic acid
Neomycin
Niridazole
Nitrites
Nitrofurantoin
Nitrofurazone
Oral contraceptives
Oxyphenbutazone
Paramethadione
Pencillamine
Penicillins
Pentamidine
Phenazopyridine
Phenformin
Phenobarbital
Phenothiazines
Phenylbutazone
Phytonadione
Piperacetazine
Piperazine
Prilocaine
Primaquine
Primidone
Probenecid
Procainamide
Procarbazine
Propranolol
Pyrazinamide
Pyrimethamine
Quinacrine
Quinethazone
Quinidine

Quinine
Resorcinol
Salicylates
Spectinomycin
Stibophen
Streptomycin
Sulfacetamide
Sulfadiazine
Sulfamethizole
Sulfamethoxazole
Sulfapyridine
Sulfinpyrazone
Sulfisoxazole
Sulfonamides
Sulfones
Sulfoxone
Suramin
Tetracyclines
Thiazides
Thioguanine
Thioridazine
Thiosemicarbazones
Thiotepa
Ticarcillin
Tolazamide
Tolbutamide
Tolmetin
Triamterene
Trichlormethiazide
Trimethadione
Trimethoprim
Tripelennamine
Tripolidine
Vidarabine
Vitamin A
Vitamin K

Differential Diagnosis for Decreased Blood Hematocrit

Cardiovascular
  Acute myocardial infarction
  Bacterial endocarditis
  Cardiomyopathies
  Congestive heart failure
  Malignant hypertension
  Rheumatic fever

Respiratory
  Abscess of lung
  Anthracosis
  Asbestosis
  Berylliosis
  Bronchiectasis
  Chronic obstructive pulmonary disease
  Influenza
  Pneumonia: Bacterial, viral, mycoplasmal, resolving
  Pulmonary tuberculosis
  Silicosis

Genitourinary
  Benign prostatic hypertrophy
  Chronic pyelonephritis
  Glomerulonephritis: Acute poststreptococcal, mem-
    branoproliferative, rapidly progressive

  Hydronephrosis
  Medullary cystic disease
  Polycystic kidney disease
  Renal failure: Acute, chronic

Gastrointestinal
  Ancylostomiasis
  Celiac disease
  Diphyllobothriasis
  Diverticular disease of intestine
  Esophageal varices
  Fistula of stomach and duodenum
  Malabsorption: Cause unspecified
  Peptic ulcer: Site unspecified
  Postgastrectomy (dumping) syndrome
  Protein-losing enteropathy
  Regional enteritis
  Strongyloidiasis
  Trichuriasis
  Ulcerative colitis
  Whipple's disease

Pancreatic
  Acute pancreatitis

Hepatobiliary
Chronic active hepatitis
Cirrhosis: Cause unspecified
Laennec's or alcoholic cirrhosis
Liver abscess
Necrosis of liver: Acute, subacute
Viral hepatitis

Hematologic
Agranulocytosis
Anemia: Acquired hemolytic anemia; aplastic anemia;
   folic acid deficiency; hemoglobin C, E, or H disease;
   hereditary elliptocytosis and spherocytosis; hereditary
   non-spherocytic hemolytic anemia; iron deficiency;
   paroxysmal nocturnal hemoglobinuria; pernicious
   anemia; Plummer-Vinson syndrome; sickle cell ane-
   mia; sideroblastic anemia; thalassemia major and
   minor; vitamin B_6 deficiency
Erythroleukemia
Heavy-chain disease: Gamma
Hemolytic disease of newborn
Hypersplenism
Idiopathic thrombocytopenic purpura
Leukemic reticuloendotheliosis
Lymphocytic leukemia: Acute, chronic
Monocytic leukemia
Multiple myeloma
Myelocytic leukemia: Acute, chronic
Myelofibrosis
Thrombotic thrombocytopenic purpura

Endocrine
Adrenal cortical hyperfunction
Adrenal cortical hypofunction
Anterior pituitary hypofunction
Hyperparathyroidism
Hyperthyroidism
Hypothyroidism
Testicular hypofunction

Metabolic
A-betalipoproteinemia
Cystic fibrosis
Cystinosis
Gaucher's disease
Hepatolenticular degeneration
Niemann-Pick disease
Porphyria: Acute intermittent; congenital erythropoi-
   etic; erythropoietic protoporphyria or coproporphy-
   ria; hereditary coproporphyria; porphyria cutanea
   tarda
Thiamine deficiency
Vitamin C deficiency

Infectious
Bacterial: Bartonellosis, brucellosis, diphtheria, disseminated tuberculosis, leprosy, leptospirosis, lymphogranuloma venereum, syphilis, tuberculosis, typhoid
   fever

Fungal: Actinomycosis, aspergillosis, blastomycosis, histoplasmosis
Parasitic: Amebiasis, leishmaniasis, malaria, toxoplasmosis, trichinosis, trypanosomiasis
Rickettsial: Epidemic typhus, Rocky Mountain spotted
   fever, tick-borne fever
Septicemia
Viral: Chickenpox, cytomegalic inclusion disease,
   herpes simplex, herpes zoster

Immunologic
Agammaglobulinemia: Congenital sex-linked
Allergic purpura
Cranial arteritis and related conditions
Dysgammaglobulinemia (selective immunoglobulin de-
   ficiency)
Immunodeficiency: Common variable
Polymyalgia rheumatica
Polyarteritis nodosa
Polymyositis
Progressive systemic sclerosis
Systemic lupus erythematosus
Wegner's granulomatosis

Musculoskeletal
Juvenile rheumatoid arthritis
Osteomyelitis
Osteopetrosis
Rheumatoid arthritis
Rheumatoid (ankylosing) spondylitis

Neuropsychiatric
Bacterial meningitis
Myasthenia gravis

Neoplastic
Benign neoplasm: Cardiovascular system, stomach
Histiocytosis X
Lymphoma: Hodgkin's disease, lymphosarcoma, retic-
   ulum cell sarcoma
Malignant neoplasm: Bladder, bone, corpus uteri,
   esophagus, gallbladder, kidney, large intestine, liver,
   pancreas, prostate, rectum, small intestine, stomach
Secondary malignant neoplasm: Bone, respiratory sys-
   tem

Miscellaneous
Alcoholism
Amyloidosis
Depressive neurosis
Effects of x-ray irradiation
Diaphragmatic hernia
Hemorrhage
Pemphigus
Pregnancy
Protein malnutrition
Reiter's disease
Toxic effects: Lead and its compounds, non-medicinal
   metals, venom

Serum Lactic Dehydrogenase

Patient Preparation. A fasting specimen is preferable because patients may show some elevation of the serum LDH level after meals. An elevation has also been observed after muscular exercise.

Specimen Collection and Handling. A serum sample is satisfactory; it is best to separate the serum from the clot as soon as possible because red blood cells contain 150 times more LDH than serum. Heparinized plasma may be used, but plasma containing other anticoagulants, especially oxalate, should not be used. Hemolyzed serum or plasma should not be used. Specimens should be stored at room temperature, at which no loss of activity will occur for 2 or 3 days. If specimens are stored longer, they should be kept at 4°C with nicotinamide-adenine dinucleotide (NAD) or glutathione as preservative.

Methodology. A number of different methods are available: end-point colorimetric, end-point fluorometric, and kinetic. Kinetic methods, which monitor the oxidation of NADH (the reduced form of NAD) to NAD+, are preferable. Consult the laboratory for its methodology, including in vitro drug interference.

Reference Interval. Reference intervals differ according to methodology (e.g., 80 to 120 Wacker units, 150 to 450 Wroblewski units, 71 to 207 IU/liter, or 8 to 280 m IU). Consult the laboratory for its reference interval.

Agents Associated With Increased Levels of Serum LDH in Vivo

Anabolic steroids	Copper	Levodopa	Opiates
Anesthetic agents	Dicumarol	Meperidine	Pemoline
Anticonvulsants	Ethanol	Methotrexate	Propoxyphene
Carbenicillin	Fenoprofen	Methyltestosterone	Propranolol
Cefoxitin	Floxuridine	Metoprolol	Quinidine
Clindamycin	Fluorides	Mithramycin	Salicylates
Clofibrate	Halothane	Morphine	Sulfamethoxazole
Codeine	Imipramine	Nitrofurantoin	Sulfisoxazole

Differential Diagnosis for Elevated Serum LDH

Cardiovascular
Acute myocardial infarction
Acute myocarditis
Arterial embolism or thrombosis
Cardiomyopathies
Congestive heart failure
Intracardiac prosthetic valves causing chronic hemolysis
Rheumatic fever
Shock

Respiratory
Pneumonia: Bacterial, viral, mycoplasmal, resolving
Pulmonary alveolar proteinosis
Pulmonary embolism and infarction
Silicosis

Genitourinary
Nephrotic syndrome
Renal infarction
Renal failure: Acute, chronic

Gastrointestinal
Celiac disease
Intestinal obstruction
Mesenteric artery embolism
Regional enteritis
Ulcerative colitis

Pancreatic
Acute pancreatitis

Hepatobiliary
Cirrhosis: Cause unspecified
Dubin-Johnson syndrome
Extrahepatic biliary obstruction
Granulomatous hepatitis
Hepatic failure
Laennec's or alcoholic cirrhosis
Necrosis of liver: Acute, subacute
Toxic hepatitis
Viral hepatitis

Hematologic
Anemia:Acquired autoimmune hemolytic anemia; anemia due to disorder of glutathione metabolism; aplastic anemia; folic acid deficiency; hereditary elliptocytosis and spherocytosis; hereditary non-spherocytic hemolytic anemia; paroxysmal nocturnal hemoglobinuria; pernicious anemia; sickle cell anemia; thalassemia major
Erythroleukemia
Hemolytic disease of newborn
Infectious mononucleosis
Lymphocytic leukemia: Acute, chronic
Multiple myeloma
Myelocytic leukemia: Acute, chronic
Myelofibrosis

Endocrine
Diabetes mellitus
Hypoparathyroidism

Hypothyroidism
Thyroiditis: Subacute

Metabolic
Diabetic acidosis
Gaucher's disease
Hemochromatosis
Hepatolenticular degeneration
Hyperphosphatasia
McArdle's disease
Metabolic acidosis

Infectious
Actinomycosis
Amebiasis
Cytomegalic inclusion disease
Herpes zoster
Hydatidosis
Leptospirosis
Lymphogranuloma venereum
Psittacosis
Schistosomiasis
Septicemia
Trichinosis
Typhoid fever

Immunologic
Dermatomyositis and polymyositis
Progressive sytemic sclerosis

Musculoskeletal
Amyotrophic lateral sclerosis
Crush injury following trauma
Familial progressive spinal muscular atrophy
Muscle necrosis
Myositis

Myotonia atrophica
Myotonia congenita
Progressive muscular dystrophy
Rheumatoid arthritis

Neuropsychiatric
Bacterial meningitis
Cerebral hemorrhage and thrombosis

Neoplastic
Benign neoplasm: Cardiovascular tissue
Lymphoma: Hodgkin's disease, lymphosarcoma, reticulum cell sarcoma
Malignant neoplasm: Bone, breast, bronchus and lung, cervix, kidney, large intestine, liver, ovary, prostate, skin, small intestine, stomach, testis
Secondary malignant neoplasm: Bone, brain, digestive system, disseminated, liver

Miscellaneous
Alcoholism
Delirium tremens
Dermatitis herpetiformis
Drug dependence: Opium and derivatives
Ectopic pregnancy
Effects of electric current
Effects of x-ray irradiation
Exercise
Heat stroke
Hematoma
Hypothermia
Postoperative state
Pregnancy
Sarcoidosis
Toxic effects: Venom

Agents Associated With Decreased Levels of Serum LDH in Vivo

Clofibrate
Fluorides

Differential Diagnosis for Decreased Serum LDH

Cardiovascular
Usually no effect

Respiratory
Usually no effect

Genitourinary
Usually no effect

Gastrointestinal
Usually no effect

Pancreatic
Usually no effect

Hepatobiliary
Usually no effect

Hematologic
Usually no effect

Endocrine
Usually no effect

Metabolic
Usually no effect

Infectious
Usually no effect

Immunologic
Usually no effect

Musculoskeletal
Usually no effect

Neuropsychiatric
Usually no effect

Neoplastic
Usually no effect

Miscellaneous
Effects of x-ray irradiation

Blood Leukocyte Count, Total

Patient Preparation. Patient factors do not generally intefere. However, such things as cold exposure and muscular exercise can increase the blood leukocyte count.

Specimen Collection and Handling. EDTA or double oxalate should be used. Heparin is unsatisfactory.

Methodology. Blood leukocyte counts may be performed either by a manual hemacytometer method or by electronic counting. The electronic cell counter is better than the manual hemacytometer because of greater speed of performance, elimination of visual fatigue on the part of the technologist, and greater precision. Artifactual depression of the leukocyte count using electronic counters occurs with leukocyte fragility (immunosuppressive and antineoplastic drugs), lymphocytic fragility (lymphocytic leukemia), and clumping of leukocytes (monoclonal gammopathy, cryofibrinogenemia, cold agglutinins). Consult the laboratory for its methodology.

Reference Interval. The reference interval for the blood leukocyte count is 4500 to 11,000/μl. Consult the laboratory for its reference interval.

Agents Associated With Increased Blood Leukocyte Count in Vivo

Allopurinol	Desipramine	Isoniazid	Phenothiazines
Aminosalicylic acid	Digitalis	Kanamycin	Phenylbutazone
Amphetamine	Dydrogesterone	Levodopa	Pilocarpine
Amphotericin B	Enflurane	Lithium	Potassium iodide
Ampicillin	Epinephrine	Mercurial compounds	Prednisolone
Atropine	Erythromycin	Methicillin	Prednisone
Belladonna	Ether	Methyldopa	Quinine
Capreomycin	Gold	Methysergide	Radioactive iodine
Cephalothin	Haloperidol	Nalidixic acid	Streptokinase
Chloramphenicol	Halothane	Niacinamide	Sulfonamides
Chlorpropamide	Imipramine	Oral contraceptives	Tetracycline
Cloxacillin	Iodides	Oxyphenbutazone	Thiothixene
Colchicine	Iron dextran	Paraldehyde	Triamterene
Copper	Isoflurane	Phenindione	Vancomycin
Corticotropin			

Differential Diagnosis for Increased Blood Leukocyte Count

Cardiovascular
  Acute myocardial infarction
  Acute pericarditis
  Acute rheumatic fever
  Arterial embolism and thrombosis
  Bacterial endocarditis
  Dissecting aortic aneurysm
  Fat embolism
  Loeffler's endocarditis
  Phlebitis, thrombophlebitis
  Pulseless disease (aortic arch syndrome)
  Shock

Respiratory
  Abscess of lung
  Allergic alveolitis
  Anthracosis
  Asbestosis
  Asthma
  Berylliosis
  Bronchiectasis
  Chronic bronchitis
  Chronic obstructive pulmonary disease
  Disseminated tuberculosis
  Pneumonia: Bacterial, viral, mycoplasmal, resolving
  Pneumomediastinum
  Pulmonary collapse
  Pulmonary embolism and infarction
  Pulmonary tuberculosis

Genitourinary
  Hydronephrosis
  Nephrotic syndrome
  Poststreptococcal glomerulonephritis: Acute
  Pyelonephritis: Acute
  Renal infarction
  Renal failure: Acute, chronic

Gastrointestinal
  Ancylostomiasis
  Appendicitis: Acute
  Diverticulitis of colon
  Fistula of stomach and duodenum
  Gastritis
  Intestinal obstruction
  Mesenteric artery embolism
  Peptic ulcer: Site unspecified
  Peritonitis
  Regional enteritis
  Strongyloidiasis
  Trichuriasis

Ulcerative colitis
Whipple's disease
Bacillary dysentery

Pancreatic
Pancreatitis: Acute, chronic

Hepatobiliary
Cholangitis
Cholecystitis: Acute
Extrahepatic biliary obstruction
Laennec's or alcoholic cirrhosis
Liver abscess
Necrosis of liver: Acute, subacute
Postcholecystectomy syndrome

Hematologic
Acquired autoimmune hemolytic anemia
Erythroleukemia
Hemolytic disease of newborn
Hereditary non-spherocytic hemolytic anemia
Hereditary spherocytosis
Idiopathic thrombocytopenic purpura
Infectious mononucleosis
Leukemic reticuloendotheliosis
Lymphocytic leukemia: Acute, chronic
Myelocytic leukemia: Acute, chronic
Polycythemia: Vera, secondary
Sickle cell anemia
Thalassemia major
Thrombotic thrombocytopenic purpura
Waldenström's macroglobulinemia

Endocrine
Adrenal cortical hyperfunction
Adrenal cortical hypofunction
Thyroiditis: Subacute

Metabolic
Carcinoid syndrome
Cystic fibrosis
Diabetic acidosis
Familial periodic paralysis
Gout
Metabolic acidosis
Porphyria: Acute intermittent, hereditary coproporphyria, porphyria variegata

Infectious
Acute tonsillitis
Bacterial: Bartonellosis, brucellosis, chlamydia, diphtheria, disseminated tuberculosis, leprosy, leptospirosis, psittacosis, relapsing fever, syphilis, tetanus, tularemia, typhoid fever, whooping cough, etc.
Fungal: Actinomycosis, blastomycosis, coccidioidomycosis, histoplasmosis, moniliasis
Otitis externa and media
Parasitic: Amebiasis, schistosomiasis, toxoplasmosis, trichinosis, visceral larva migrans

Rickettsial: Epidemic typhus, Rocky Mountain spotted fever
Septicemia
Viral: Cytomegalic inclusion disease, eastern and western equine encephalitis, measles, mumps, rabies, smallpox

Immunologic
Agammaglobulinemia: Congenital sex-linked
Allergic purpura
Cranial arteritis and related conditions
Dermatomyositis and polymyositis
Polyarteritis nodosa

Musculoskeletal
Acute arthritis, pyogenic
Crush injury following trauma
Infantile cortical hyperostosis
Juvenile rheumatoid arthritis
Osteomyelitis
Rheumatoid arthritis

Neuropsychiatric
Acute poliomyelitis
Bacterial meningitis
Cerebral hemorrhage
Guillain-Barré syndrome
Familial periodic paralysis
Intracranial abscess
Polyneuritis

Neoplastic
Benign neoplasm: Cardiovascular tissue
Histiocytosis
Lymphoma: Hodgkin's disease, lymphosarcoma, reticulum cell sarcoma
Malignant neoplasm: Esophagus, kidney, large intestine, liver, pancreas, rectum, stomach
Secondary malignant neoplasm: Brain, respiratory system

Miscellaneous
Amyloidosis
Burns
Eclampsia
Ectopic pregnancy
Effects of electric current
Effects of x-ray irradiation
Emotional stress
Exercise
Gangrene
Heat stroke
Hemorrhage
Menstruation
Obstetrical labor
Pemphigus
Reiter's disease
Toxic effects: Carbon monoxide, non-medicinal metals, venom

Agents Associated With Decreased Blood Leukocyte Count in Vivo

Acetaminophen	Allopurinol	Amodiaquine	Antihistamines
Acetazolamide	Aminoglutethimide	Amphotericin B	Antineoplastic agents
Acetohexamide	Aminopyrine	Ampicillin	Antipyrine
Acetophenazine	Aminosalicylic acid	Anisindione	Asparaginase
Adriamycin	Amitriptyline	Anticonvulsants	Azathioprine

Barbiturates
Benzodiazepines
Benzthiazide
Beta-adrenergic blockers
Bismuth salts
Brompheniramine
Busulfan
Butaperazine
Capreomycin
Carbenicillin
Carbimazole
Carisoprodol
Carmustine
Cefoxitin
Cephalosporins
Chlorambucil
Chloramphenicol
Chlordiazepoxide
Chlorophenothane
Chloroquine
Chlorthalidone
Chlorothiazide
Chlorpheniramine
Chlorpromazine
Chlorpropamide
Chlorprothixene
Cholestyramine
Cimetidine
Cisplatin
Clindamycin
Clofibrate
Cloxacillin
Colchicine
Colistimethate
Colistin
Corticosteroids
Cyclobenzaprine
Cyclophosphamide
Cycloserine
Cyclothiazide
Cytarabine
Dactinomycin
Dapsone
Daunorubicin
Demeclocycline
Desipramine
Dextran
Diazepam
Diazoxide
Dibenzoxazepines
Dichlorphenamide
Dicumarol
Diethylpropion
Digitalis
Diiodohydroxyquin
Dimethindene

Diphenhydramine
Diphenylhydantoin
Dipyrone
Doxapram
Doxepin
Doxorubicin
Doxycycline
Edetate
Erythromycin
Ethacrynic acid
Ethanol
Ethopropazine
Ethosuximide
Ethoxzolamide
Fenoprofen
Flavoxate
Floxuridine
Flucytosine
Fluorides
Fluorouracil
Fluoxymesterone
Fluphenazine
Fumagillin
Furosemide
Gentamicin
Glutethimide
Gold
Griseofulvin
Haloperidol
Hetacillin
Hexamethylmelamine
Histamine
Hydralazine
Hydrochlorothiazide
Hydroflumethiazide
Hydroxychloroquine
Hydroxyurea
Ibuprofen
Idoxuridine
Imipramine
Indandione derivatives
Indomethacin
Isocarboxazid
Isoniazid
Levodopa
Lincomycin
Local anesthetics
Lomustine
Mafenide
Meclofenamate
Mechlorethamine
Mefenamic acid
Melphalan
Mephenytoin
Meprobamate
Mercaptopurine

Mercurial diuretics
Mesoridazine
Metaxolone
Methaqualone
Methazolamide
Methicillin
Methimazole
Methocarbamol
Methotrexate
Metoprolol
Methyldopa
Methylphenidate
Methylthiouracil
Methyprylon
Methysergide
Metolazone
Metronidazole
Minocycline
Minoxidil
Mithramycin
Mitomycin
Nafcillin
Naproxen
Nitrous oxide
Neomycin
Nutrofurantoin
Nortriptyline
Novobiocin
Orphenadrine
Oxacillin
Oxazepam
Oxyphenbutazone
Oxytetracycline
Paramethadione
Penicillamine
Penicillins
Pentazocine
Perphenazine
Phenacetin
Phenelzine
Phenindione
Phenobarbital
Phenothiazines
Phenylbutazone
Phenytoin
Piperacetazine
Polythiazide
Prednisolone
Prednisone
Primaquine
Primidone
Probenecid
Procainamide
Procarbazine
Prochlorperazine
Promazine

Promethazine
Propranolol
Propylthiouracil
Protriptyline
Pyrimethamine
Quinacrine
Quinethazone
Quinidine
Quinine
Radioactive compounds
Rifampin
Ristocetin
Salicylates
Sodium phosphate
Streptomycin
Sulfachlorpyridazine
Sulfadiazine
Sulfameter
Sulfamethizole
Sulfamethoxazole
Sulfinpyrazone
Sulfisoxazole
Sulfonamides
Sulfones
Sulfonylureas
Sulindac
Suramin
Tetracyclines
Thiabendazole
Thiacetazone
Thiazides
Thioguanine
Thioridazine
Thiosemicarbazones
Thiotepa
Thiothixene
Ticarcillin
Tolazamide
Tolazoline
Tolbutamide
Tranylcypromine
Trichlormethiazide
Triclofos
Trifluoperazine
Triflupromazine
Trimeprazine
Trimethadione
Trimethoprim
Trimipramine
Tripelennamine
Tripolidine
Vidarabine
Vinblastine
Vincristine
Vitamin A
Vitamin K
X-ray therapy

Differential Diagnosis for Decreased Blood Leukocyte Count

Cardiovascular
   Bacterial endocarditis
   Shock

Respiratory
   Bacterial pneumonia
   Influenza

Genitourinary
   Usually no effect

Gastrointestinal
   Bacillary dysentery
   Celiac disease

Pancreatic
  Usually no effect

Hepatobiliary
  Chronic active hepatitis
  Cirrhosis: Cause unspecified
  Laennec's or alcoholic cirrhosis
  Necrosis of liver: Acute, subacute
  Viral hepatitis
  Yellow fever

Hematologic
  Acquired autoimmune hemolytic anemia
  Agranulocytosis
  Aleukemic leukemia
  Aplastic anemia
  Congenital aplastic anemia
  Folic acid deficiency anemia
  Heavy-chain disease: Gamma
  Hemoglobin C disease
  Hereditary spherocytosis
  Hypersplenism
  Iron deficiency anemia
  Leukemic reticuloendotheliosis
  Lymphocytic leukemia: Acute, chronic
  Myelocytic leukemia: Acute, chronic
  Multiple myeloma
  Neutropenia
  Paroxysmal nocturnal hemoglobinuria
  Pernicious anemia
  Sideroblastic anemia
  Thalassemia major
  Vitamin B_6 deficiency anemia
  Waldenström's macroglobulinemia

Endocrine
  Anterior pituitary hypofunction
  Hyperparathyroidism
  Hyperthyroidism

Metabolic
  Gaucher's disease

Niemann-Pick disease
Hepatolenticular degeneration

Infectious
  Bacterial: Bartonellosis, brucellosis, chlamydial, diph-
    theria, disseminated tuberculosis, leptospirosis, phle-
    botomous fever, relapsing fever, tularemia, typhoid
    fever
  Fungal: Histoplasmosis
  Parasitic: Leishmaniasis, malaria, toxoplasmosis
  Rickettsial: Endemic and epidemic typhus, mite-borne
    typhus, rickettsialpox, Rocky Mountain spotted fever
  Septicemia
  Viral: Chickenpox, measles, rubella, smallpox

Immunologic
  Agammaglobulinemia: Congenital sex-linked
  Sjögren's syndrome
  Systemic lupus erythematosus

Musculoskeletal
  Felty's syndrome
  Osteopetrosis
  Rheumatoid arthritis

Neuropsychiatric
  Encephalitis: Eastern and western equine
  Encephalomyelitis
  Lymphocytic choriomeningitis

Neoplastic
  Lymphoma: Hodgkin's disease, lymphosarcoma, retic-
    ulum cell sarcoma
  Secondary malignant neoplasm: Bone

Miscellaneous
  Amyloidosis
  Cachexia
  Effects of x-ray irradiation
  Protein malnutrition
  Sarcoidosis
  Toxic effects: Lead and its compounds, non-medicinal
    metals

Serum Phosphatase, Alkaline (ALP)

Patient Preparation. Ideally, the patient should be fasting. This will eliminate the problem with those who show elevated serum alkaline phosphatase (ALP) after meals, such as patients of blood groups O or B who are secretors.

Specimen Collection and Handling. Use only serum or heparinized plasma. Avoid hemolysis because a small amount of ALP is present in erythrocytes. If possible, perform the analysis within 24 hours because serum ALP can increase with storage.

Methodology. A number of different methods are available, both end-point and kinetic. Kinetic methods are preferable. Consult the laboratory for its methodology, including in vitro drug interference.

Reference Interval. There are large differences in reference intervals secondary to methodology and the age and sex of the patient (see Chapter 9). Consult the laboratory for its reference intervals.

Agents Associated With Increased Levels of Serum ALP in Vivo

Acetaminophen	Chlorprothixene	Gold	Niacin	Quinacrine
Acetohexamide	Chlorzoxazone	Griseofulvin	Niacinamide	Quinethazone
Acetophenazine	Cinoxacin	Haloperidol	Nicotinyl alcohol	Quinidine
Albumin infusions	Clindamycin	Halothane	Nitrofurantoin	Rifampin
Allopurinol	Clofibrate	Hydantoins	Norethindrone	Salicylates
Amantadine	Clomiphene	Hydroflumethiazide	Nortriptyline	Spectinomycin
Aminosalicylic acid	Clonidine	Idoxuridine	Oral contraceptives	Stanozolol
Amitriptyline	Colchicine	Imipramine	Oxacillin	Streptokinase
Amodiaquine	Coumarin derivatives	Indomethacin	Oxazepam	Sulfadiazine
Amphotericin B	Cyclizine	Isocarboxazid	Oxymetholone	Sulfamethizole
Anabolic steroids	Cyclophosphamide	Isoniazid	Oxyphenbutazone	Sulfamethoxazole
Androgens	Cyclopropane	Kanamycin	Papaverine	Sulfapyridine
Anticonvulsants	Cycloserine	Levodopa	Paraldehyde	Sulfisoxazole
Antifungal agents	Cytarabine	Lincomycin	Pargyline	Sulfonamides
Antimony compounds	Dantrolene	Meclofenamate	Penicillamine	Sulfones
Asparaginase	Dapsone	Mechlorethamine	Phenacetin	Sulfonylureas
Azathioprine	Desipramine	Meprobamate	Phenazopyridine	Sulindac
Baclofen	Diazepam	Mercatopurine	Phenelzine	Testosterone
Barbiturates	Disulfiram	Methandrostenolone	Phenindione	Tetracycline
Bismuth salts	Erythromycin	Methimazole	Phenobarbital	Thiabendazole
Bromocriptine	Estradiol	Methotrexate	Phenothiazines	Thiazides
Capreomycin	Estriol	Methoxsalen	Phenylbutazone	Thioguanine
Carbenicillin	Estrogens	Methoxyflurane	Polythiazide	Thioridazine
Carmustine	Estrone	Methyldopa	Probenecid	Thiosemicarbazones
Cefaclor	Ethchlorvynol	Methyltestosterone	Prochlorperazine	Thiothixene
Cefoxitin	Ether	Metolazone	Progesterone	Tolazamide
Cephalosporins	Factor IX complex, human	Metoprolol	Promazine	Tolbutamide
Chenodeoxycholic acid	Fat emulsions	Minocycline	Promethazine	Tranylcypromine
Chloramphenicol	Fenoprofen	Minoxidil	Propoxyphene	Trichlormethiazide
Chlordiazepoxide	Fluoxymesterone	Mitotane	Propranolol	Trifluoperazine
Chlormezanone	Fluphenazine	Morphine	Propylthiouracil	Trimethadione
Chlorothiazide	Flurazepam	Nalidixic acid	Protein hydrolysate	Trimipramine
Chlorpromazine	Gentamicin	Nandrolone	Protriptyline	Trioxsalen
Chlorpropamide	Glycopyrrolate	Naproxen	Pyrazinamide	Vitamin D

Differential Diagnosis for Increased Serum ALP

Cardiovascular
Acute myocardial infarction
Congestive heart failure
Thrombophlebitis

Respiratory
Pulmonary embolism and infarction
Pulmonary tuberculosis
Viral pneumonia

Genitourinary
Acute pyelonephritis
Chronic renal failure
Nephrotic syndrome
Organization of renal infarct
Renal dwarfism
Renal tubular acidosis

Gastrointestinal
Acute infarction of small intestine

Celiac disease
Fistula of stomach and duodenum
Intestinal obstruction
Malabsorption: Cause unspecified
Mesenteric artery embolism
Peptic ulcer: Site unspecified
Regional enteritis
Ulcerative colitis
Whipple's disease

Pancreatic
Pancreatic cyst and pseudocyst
Pancreatitis: Acute, chronic

Hepatobiliary
Biliary cirrhosis
Cholangitis
Cholecystitis: Acute
Cholestasis
Chronic active hepatitis
Cirrhosis: Unspecified
Dubin-Johnson syndrome
Extrahepatic biliary obstruction
Granulomatous hepatitis
Hemochromatosis
Hepatic failure
Idiopathic jaundice of pregnancy
Laennec's or alcoholic cirrhosis
Liver abscess
Necrosis of liver: Acute, subacute
Postcholecystectomy syndrome
Toxic hepatitis
Viral hepatitis

Hematologic
Infectious mononucleosis
Lymphocytic leukemia: Acute, chronic
Monocytic leukemia
Myelocytic leukemia: Acute, chronic
Myelofibrosis
Sickle cell anemia

Endocrine
Acromegaly
Adrenal cortical hyperfunction
Diabetes mellitus
Hashimoto's thyroiditis
Hyperparathyroidism
Hyperthyroidism
Hypothyroidism
Thyroiditis: Subacute

Metabolic
Cystic fibrosis

Cystinosis
Familial hyperphosphatasemia
Gaucher's disease
Hepatolenticular degeneration
Niemann-Pick disease
Vitamin D deficiency rickets
Vitamin D resistant rickets

Infectious
Bacterial: Brucellosis, chlamydia, leptospirosis, typhoid fever
Fungal: Actinomycosis, blastomycosis, histoplasmosis
Parasitic: Amebiasis, hydatidosis, malaria, schistosomiasis
Septicemia
Viral: Cytomegalic inclusion disease, herpes zoster

Immunologic
Cranial arteritis and related conditions

Musculoskeletal
Fracture of bone
Osteitis deformans
Osteoblastic bone lesions
Osteogenesis imperfecta
Osteomalacia
Osteoporosis
Polyostotic fibrous dysplasia
Rheumatoid arthritis
Rheumatoid (ankylosing) spondylitis
Rickets

Neuropsychiatric
Friedreich's ataxia

Neoplastic
Lymphoma: Hodgkin's disease, lymphosarcoma, reticulum cell sarcoma
Malignant neoplasm: Bone, breast, bronchus and lung, esophagus, intrahepatic bile ducts, large intestine, liver, ovary, pancreas, prostate, stomach
Secondary malignant neoplasm: Bone, liver, respiratory system

Miscellaneous
Alcoholism
Amyloidosis
Childhood
Gangrene
Pregnancy: Late
Sarcoidosis
Unexplained elevation

Agents Associated With Decreased Levels of Serum ALP in Vivo

Azathioprine
Fluorides
Oral contraceptives
Trifluoperazine

Differential Diagnosis for Decreased Serum ALP

Cardiovascular
Usually no effect

Respiratory
Usually no effect

Genitourinary
Usually no effect

Gastrointestinal
Celiac disease
Whipple's disease
Zollinger-Ellison syndrome

Pancreatic
Usually no effect

Hepatobiliary
Usually no effect

Hematologic
Folic acid deficiency anemia
Pernicious anemia

Endocrine
Hypoparathyroidism
Hypothyroidism

Metabolic
Hypervitaminosis D

Hypophosphatasia
Lactosuria
Milk-alkali syndrome
Vitamin C deficiency

Infectious
Usually no effect

Immunologic
Usually no effect

Musculoskeletal
Chondrodystrophy

Neuropsychiatric
Usually no effect

Neoplastic
Usually no effect

Miscellaneous
Deficiency state: Type unspecified
Protein malnutrition

Serum Phosphorus, Inorganic

Patient Preparation. Ideally, the patient should be fasting because a postprandial depression of serum phosphorus is associated with phosphorylation of glucose. A depression has also been noted during the menstrual period.

Specimen Collection and Handling. Serum or heparinized plasma is preferred. Hemolysis and prolonged contact with the clot should be avoided because elevation of the serum phosphorus will occur. Once separated from the cells, the serum phosphorus is relatively stable and will keep for at least a week at refrigerator temperature.

Methodology. Serum phosphorus is usually measured colorimerically by reacting the phosphorus with molybdate reagent to form a blue color. Consult the laboratory for its methodology, including in vitro drug interference.

Reference Interval. The reference interval for serum phosphorus is 2.3 to 4.7 mg/100 ml. Remember that the interval is higher in children secondary to the effects of growth hormone, namely, 4.0 to 7.0 mg/100 ml. Consult the laboratory for its reference intervals.

Agents Associated With Increased Levels of Serum Inorganic Phosphorus in Vivo

Anabolic steroids	Hydrochlorothiazide	Minocycline	Phosphates
Androgens	Lipomul	Oral contraceptives	Tetracycline
Furosemide	Methicillin	Parathyroid extract	Vitamin D
Growth hormone			

Differential Diagnosis for Elevated Serum Inorganic Phosphorus

Cardiovascular
Usually no effect

Respiratory
Usually no effect

Genitourinary
Glomerulonephritis: Membranous, rapidly progressive
Nephrotic syndrome
Renal failure: Acute, chronic
Renal dwarfism
Renal rickets

Gastrointestinal
Intestinal obstruction
Mesenteric artery embolism

Pancreatic
Usually no effect

Hepatobiliary
Necrosis of liver: Acute, subacute

Hematologic
Acute lymphocytic leukemia
Acute myelocytic leukemia
Acquired autoimmune hemolytic anemia
Hereditary spherocytosis
Multiple myeloma

Endocrine
Acromegaly
Adrenal cortical hypofunction
Diabetes mellitus
Hypoparathyroidism: Idiopathic, surgical

Ovarian hyperfunction
Pseudohypoparathyroidism

Metabolic
Cystinosis
Diabetic acidosis
Hereditary fructose intolerance
Hypervitaminosis D
Metabolic acidosis
Milk-alkali syndrome

Infectious
Usually no effect

Immunologic
Usually no effect

Musculoskeletal
Fracture of bone
Osteitis deformans

Neuropsychiatric
Usually no effect

Neoplastic
Secondary malignant neoplasm: Bone

Miscellaneous
Acute alcoholic intoxication
Alcoholism
Childhood
Eclampsia
Exercise
Heat stroke
Sarcoidosis

Agents Associated With Decreased Levels of Serum Inorganic Phosphorus in Vivo

Acetazolamide
Alkaline antacids
Aluminum salts
Amino acids
Anabolic steroids
Androgens

Anesthetic agents
Anticonvulsants
Calcitonin
Epinephrine
Ether
Ethinyl estradiol

Ethylene
Fructose infusions
Glucagon
Glucose infusions
Hydrochlorothiazide
Insulin

Mithramycin
Oral contraceptives
Phenobarbital
Salicylates
Tetracycline

Differential Diagnosis for Decreased Serum Inorganic Phosphorus

Cardiovascular
Usually no effect

Respiratory
Asthma
Hyperventilation syndrome

Genitourinary
Renal tubular acidosis

Gastrointestinal
Celiac disease
Malabsorption: Cause unspecified
Vomiting
Whipple's disease
Zollinger-Ellison syndrome

Pancreatic
Acute pancreatitis

Hepatobiliary
Cirrhosis: Cause unspecified
Hepatic failure

Hematologic
Multiple myeloma
Pernicious anemia
Thalassemia: Major, minor

Endocrine
Adrenal cortical hyperfunction
Adrenal cortical hypofunction
Anterior pituitary hypofunction
Diabetes mellitus
Hyperparathyroidism
Hypoparathyroidism
Ovarian hypofunction
Pheochromocytoma

Metabolic
Cystinosis

Diabetic acidosis
Gout
Hepatolenticular degeneration
Hereditary fructose intolerance
Hypervitaminosis D
Hypophosphatemia, primary
Lactosuria
von Gierke's disease

Infectious
Septicemia

Immunologic
Usually no effect

Musculoskeletal
Osteomalacia
Osteomyelitis
Osteopetrosis
Vitamin D deficiency rickets
Vitamin D resistant rickets

Neuropsychiatric
Familial periodic paralysis

Neoplastic
Benign neoplasm: Breast, pancreas
Malignant neoplasm: Prostate, skin
Secondary malignant neoplasm: Respiratory system

Miscellaneous
Acute alcoholic intoxication
Alcoholism
Burns
Hyperalimentation
Hypokalemia
Nutritional recovery syndrome (rapid feeding after prolonged starvation)
Pregnancy
Protein malnutrition
Vomiting

Blood Platelets

Patient Preparation. Patient factors do not usually interfere. However, muscular exercise can increase the platelet count.

Specimen Collection and Handling. Venous blood should be collected in a siliconized glass tube with EDTA. Plastic tubes may be satisfactory but should be checked before use.

Methodology. Blood platelet counts can be performed either by a manual hemacytometer method or by electronic counting. The electronic cell counter is usually better than the manual hemacytometer because of less fatigue of the technologist, and greater precision. However, fragments of leukocytes, debris, and platelet clumping can interfere and suspicious or abnormal results should be confirmed using a freshly drawn sample and a phase contrast hemacytometer. Evaluate the peripheral smear. Consult the laboratory for its methodology.

Reference Interval. The reference interval for the blood platelets is 150,000 to 400,000/µl. Consult the laboratory for its reference interval.

Agents Associated With Increased Blood Platelets in Vivo

Epinephrine
Glucocorticoids
Oral contraceptives

Differential Diagnosis for Elevated Blood Platelets

Cardiovascular
Usually no effect

Respiratory
Pulmonary embolism and infarction
Pulmonary tuberculosis

Genitourinary
Chronic renal failure
Nephrotic syndrome

Gastrointestinal
Celiac disease
Regional enteritis
Ulcerative colitis

Pancreatic
Chronic pancreatitis

Hepatobiliary
Cirrhosis: Cause unspecified

Hematologic
Acute lymphocytic leukemia
Hemophilia
Hereditary non-spherocytic hemolytic anemia
Hereditary spherocytosis
Iron deficiency anemia
Myelocytic leukemia: Acute, chronic
Myelofibrosis
Polycythemia: Vera, secondary
Sideroblastic anemia
Sickle cell anemia

Thalassemia major
Vitamin B_6 deficiency anemia

Endocrine
Diabetes mellitus

Metabolic
Carcinoid syndrome

Infectious
Acute infection

Immunologic
Polyarteritis nodosa

Musculoskeletal
Crush injury following trauma
Rheumatoid arthritis

Neuropsychiatric
Usually no effect

Neoplastic
Lymphoma: Hodgkin's disease
Malignant neoplasm: Bronchus and lung, large intestine, liver, stomach, testis
Secondary malignant neoplasm: Bone, brain, digestive system, disseminated, liver, respiratory system

Miscellaneous
Amyloidosis
Burns
Exercise
Hemorrhage
Postsurgery: Especially splenectomy

Agents Associated With Decreased Blood Platelets in Vivo

Acetaminophen	Adriamycin	Amphotericin B	Antilymphocytic agents	Azathioprine
Acetazolamide	Allopurinol	Ampicillin	Antimony compounds	Barbiturates
Acetohexamide	Aminosalicylic acid	Anticonvulsants	Antineoplastic agents	Benzthiazide
Acetophenazine	Amitriptyline	Antihistamines	Asparaginase	Beta-adrenergic blockers

336

Bismuth salts
Bleomycin
Busulfan
Butaperazine
Carbenicillin
Carmustine
Cephalosporins
Chlorambucil
Chloramphenicol
Chlordiazepoxide
Chlorophenothane
Chloroquine
Chlorothiazide
Chlorpheniramine
Chlorpromazine
Chlorpropamide
Chlorprothixene
Cimetidine
Cisplatin
Clindamycin
Codeine
Colchicine
Cyclobenzaprine
Cyclophosphamide
Cycloserine
Cyclothiazide
Cytarabine
Dactinomycin
Demeclocycline
Deserpidine
Desipramine
Dextroamphetamine
Dextromethorphan
Diazoxide
Dichlorphenamide
Diethylpropion
Diethylstilbestrol
Digitalis

Digitoxin
Disulfiram
Doxepin
Doxorubicin
Doxycycline
Edetate
Erythromycin
Estrogens
Ethacrynic acid
Ethanol
Ethchlorvynol
Ethinamate
Ethopropazine
Ethozolamide
Fenoprofen
Floxuridine
Flucytosine
Fluorides
Fluorouracil
Fluphenazine
Furosemide
Glutethimide
Gold
Heparin
Hetacillin
Hexamethylmelamine
Hydantoins
Hydralazine
Hydrochlorothiazide
Hydroflumethiazide
Hydroxychloroquine
Hydroxyurea
Hypnotics
Imipramine
Immune serum globulin
Indomethacin
Iodine solution
Isoniazid

Levodopa
Lincomycin
Lomustine
Lipomul
Measles vaccine
Mechlorethamine
Meclofenamate
Mefenamic acid
Melphalan
Meprobamate
Mercaptopurine
Mercurial diuretics
Mesoridazine
Methacycline
Methaqualone
Methazolamide
Methicillin
Methimazole
Methotrexate
Methyldopa
Methylphenidate
Methyprylon
Metoprolol
Miconazole
Minocycline
Minoxidil
Mithramycin
Mitomycin
Mumps vaccine
Nalidixic acid
Naproxen
Neomycin
Nitrofurantoin
Nitroglycerin
Nortriptyline
Nystatin
Orphenadrine
Oxacillin

Oxyphenbutazone
Oxytetracycline
Paramethadione
Penicillamine
Penicillins
Pentamidine
Pertussis vaccine
Phenformin
Phenobarbital
Phenolphthalein
Phenothiazines
Phenylbutazone
Piperacetazine
Poliomyelitis vaccine
Polythiazide
Potassium iodide
Prednisone
Primidone
Probenecid
Procarbazine
Prochlorperazine
Promazine
Propranolol
Propylthiouracil
Protriptyline
Pyrazinamide
Pyrimethamine
Quinacrine
Quinethazone
Quinidine
Quinine
Reserpine
Rifampin
Ristocetin
Rubella virus vaccine
Salicylates
Sedatives
Smallpox vaccine

Sodium phosphate ^{32}P
Spironolactone
Streptomycin
Sulfachlorpyridazine
Sulfadiazine
Sulfameter
Sulfamethizole
Sulfinpyrazone
Sulfisoxazole
Sulindac
Sulfonamides
Sulfonylureas
Tetanus toxoid
Tetracyclines
Thiabendazole
Thiazides
Thioguanine
Thioridazine
Thiotepa
Thiothixene
Thiouracil
Ticarcillin
Tolazamide
Tolazoline
Tolbutamide
Trichlormethiazide
Trimethadione
Trimethoprim
Trimipramine
Tripelennamine
Tripolidine
Urea
Vidarabine
Vinblastine
Vincristine
Vitamin K
X-ray therapy

Differential Diagnosis for Decreased Blood Platelets

Cardiovascular
  Bacterial endocarditis
  Fat embolism

Respiratory
  Influenza
  Mycoplasmal pneumonia

Genitourinary
  Acute renal failure
  Rapidly progressive glomerulonephritis

Gastrointestinal
  Usually no effect

Pancreatic
  Usually no effect

Hepatobiliary
  Cholangitis
  Cirrhosis: Cause unspecified
  Chronic active hepatitis
  Hepatic failure
  Jaundice of newborn due to hepatocellular damage
  Laennec's or alcoholic cirrhosis
  Liver abscess

Necrosis of liver: Acute, subacute
Viral hepatitis

Hematologic
  Acquired autoimmune hemolytic anemia
  Agranulocytosis
  Aplastic anemia
  Congenital afibrinogenemia
  Disseminated intravascular coagulopathy
  Erythroleukemia
  Folic acid deficiency anemia
  Heavy-chain disease: Gamma
  Hemoglobin C disease
  Hemolytic disease of newborn
  Hereditary spherocytosis
  Hypersplenism
  Idiopathic thrombocytopenic purpura
  Iron deficiency anemia
  Lymphocytic leukemia: Acute, chronic
  Leukemic reticuloendotheliosis
  Monocytic leukemia
  Multiple myeloma
  Myelocytic leukemia: Acute, chronic
  Myelofibrosis

Paroxysmal nocturnal hemoglobulinuria
Pernicious anemia
Sickle cell anemia
Sideroblastic anemia
Thalassemia major
Thrombotic thrombocytopenic purpura
Vitamin B_6 deficiency anemia
von Willebrand's disease
Waldenström's macroglobulinemia

Endocrine
Usually no effect

Metabolic
Gaucher's disease
Haptolenticular degeneration
Neimann-Pick disease

Infectious
Bacterial: Bartonellosis, disseminated tuberculosis, leptospirosis
Fungal: Histoplasmosis
Parasitic: Malaria
Rickettsial: Arthropod-borne hemorrhagic fever, endemic typhus, Rocky Mountain spotted fever, tickborne fever
Septicemia
Viral: Cytomegalic inclusion disease, herpes simplex, rubella, smallpox

Immunologic
Allergic purpura
Immunodeficiency: Common variable
Progressive systemic sclerosis
Systemic lupus erythematosus

Musculoskeletal
Fracture of bone
Osteopetrosis

Neuropsychiatric
Usually no effect

Neoplastic
Benign neoplasm: Cardiovascular tissue
Histiocytosis X
Hydatidiform mole
Lymphoma: Hodgkin's disease, lymphosarcoma, reticulum cell sarcoma
Secondary malignant neoplasm: Bone, brain, digestive system, disseminated, respiratory system

Miscellaneous
Alcoholism
Burns
Eclampsia
Effects of x-ray irradiation
Heat stroke
Sarcoidosis
Toxic effects: Lead and its compounds, non-medicinal metals, venom

Serum Potassium

Patient Preparation. Patient factors do not generally interfere. A high blood platelet count will elevate serum but not plasma potassium.

Specimen Collection and Handling. Serum or heparinzed plasma should be used, but potassium salts of heparin should be avoided. Serum or plasma should be promptly separated from the clot, and hemolysis should be avoided. The serum potassium level is slightly higher than the plasma potassium level (0.1 to 0.7 mEq/liter) owing to release of platelet potassium during clotting. Opening and closing the fist prior to venous puncture should be avoided because the muscle action may result in an increase in serum or plasma potassium levels of 10 to 20 per cent.

Methodology. A variety of methods are available. Most modern laboratories measure serum potassium by emission flame photometry or by an ion-selective electrode. Consult the laboratory for its methodology, including in vitro drug interference.

Reference Interval. The reference interval for plasma potassium is 3.8 to 5.0 mEq/liter. The interval for serum potassium is slightly higher. Consult the laboratory for its reference interval.

Agents Associated With Increased Levels of Serum Potassium in Vivo

Amiloride	Glucagon	Lithium	Propranolol
Aminocaproic acid	Heparin	Mannitol infusions	Saline
Amphotericin B	Histamine	Methicillin	Salt substitutes
Antineoplastic agents	Indomethacin	Metolazone	Spironolactone
Arginine	Intra-amniotic saline	Penicillin	Succinylcholine
Cephaloridine	Isoniazid	Phenformin	Tetracycline
Epinephrine	Lipomul	Potassium salts	Triamterene

Differential Diagnosis for Elevated Serum Potassium

Cardiovascular
Congestive heart failure

Respiratory
Chronic obstructive pulmonary disease
Pulmonary emphysema
Respiratory distress syndrome

Genitourinary
Renal failure: Acute, chronic

Gastrointestinal
Usually no effect

Pancreatic
Usually no effect

Hepatobiliary
Usually no effect

Hematologic
Chronic myelocytic leukemia
Polycythemia vera
Thrombocythemia

Endocrine
Acromegaly
Adrenal cortical hypofunction
Diabetes mellitus
Hyperparathyroidism
Hypoaldosteronism

Metabolic
Carcinoid syndrome
Cystinosis
Diabetic acidosis
Metabolic acidosis

Neuropsychiatric
Hepatic encephalopathy

Infectious
Arthropod-borne hemorrhagic fever
Leptospirosis

Immunologic
Systemic lupus erythematosus

Musculoskeletal
Crush injury following trauma

Neuropsychiatric
Periodic paralysis
Status epilepticus

Neoplastic
Malignant neoplasm: Stomach

Miscellaneous
Dehydration
Heat stroke
Pemphigus

Agents Associated With Decreased Levels of Serum Potassium in Vivo

Acetazolamide	Aminosalicylic acid	Amphotericin B	Antibiotics
Aldosterone	Ammonium chloride	Ampicillin	Bendroflumethiazide

Benzthiazide
Betamethasone
Bisacodyl
Carbenicillin
Carbenoxolone
Cathartics
Cephalexin
Chlorothiazide
Chlorthalidone
Corticosteroids
Corticotropin

Ergot preparations
Estrogens
Edetate
Ethanol
Ethacrynic acid
Furosemide
Glucagon
Glucose infusions
Glutethimide
Griseofulvin
Hydantoins

Insulin
Laxatives
Levodopa
Licorice
Lithium
Meprobamate
Methyldopa
Methyprylon
Nikethamide
Oxytetracycline

Penicillin
Pentazocine
Polymyxin B
Progestins
Salicylates
Sodium infusions
Succinimide
Sulfonamides
Thiazides
Vitamin K

Differential Diagnosis for Decreased Serum Potassium

Cardiovascular
  Congestive heart failure
  Essential hypertension
  Malignant hypertension

Respiratory
  Asthma
  Chronic obstructive pulmonary disease

Genitourinary
  Chronic pyelonephritis
  Diuresis following relief of urinary tract ostruction
  Renal failure: Acute, chronic
  Renal tubular acidosis
  Salt losing nephropathy
  Ureterosigmoidostomy

Gastrointestinal
  Bacillary dysentery
  Celiac disease
  Diarrhea
  Fistula of stomach and duodenum
  Intestinal obstruction
  Malabsorption: Cause unspecified
  Peptic ulcer: Site unspecified
  Peritonitis
  Postgastrectomy (dumping) syndrome
  Pyloric stenosis, acquired
  Regional enteritis
  Ulcerative colitis
  Villous adenoma
  Vomiting
  Whipple's disease
  Zollinger-Ellison syndrome

Pancreatic
  Pancreatitis

Hepatobiliary
  Cirrhosis: Cause unspecified
  Laennec's or alcoholic cirrhosis
  Reye's syndrome

Hematologic
  Folic acid deficiency anemia
  Pernicous anemia
  Multiple myeloma
  Acute myelocytic leukemia

Endocrine
  Adrenal cortical hyperfunction
  Diabetes mellitus
  Ectopic ACTH production
  Hyperparathyroidism
  Hyperthyroidism
  Pseudoaldosteronism

Metabolic
  Acute intermittent porphyria
  Cystinosis
  Diabetic acidosis
  Hepatolenticular degeneration
  Metabolic alkalosis

Infectious
  Usually no effect

Immunologic
  Usually no effect

Musculoskeletal
  Usually no effect

Neuropsychiatric
  Familial periodic paralysis

Neoplastic
  Benign neoplasm: Anus, pancreas, rectum
  Malignant neoplasm: Large intestine, pancreas

Miscellaneous
  Alcoholism
  Chronic laxative abuse
  Effects of electric current
  Heat stroke
  Protein malnutrition

Serum Proteins, Total

Patient Preparation. The patient need not be fasting. However, ambulatory patients have slightly higher (approximately 10 per cent) serum protein levels than recumbent patients. An increase of 6 to 12 per cent occurs with vigorous exercise of short duration.

Specimen Collection and Handling. Serum is the preferred sample. The use of a tourniquet may lead to falsely elevated results. Hemolysis should be avoided because it adds protein to the serum and will falsely elevate the results.

Methodology. A variety of different methods are available. The Kjeldahl nitrogen procedure is the reference method, but the biuret and refractive index methods are the ones commonly employed by clinical laboratories. Consult the laboratory for its methodology, including in vitro drug interference.

Reference Interval. The reference interval is quite method dependent. A generally accepted interval for ambulatory persons is 6.0 to 7.8 gm/100 ml. Recumbent persons will have levels about 10 per cent lower. Consult the laboratory for its reference intervals.

Agents Associated With Increased Levels of Serum Total Proteins in Vivo

Anabolic steroids	Corticosteroids	Epinephrine	Oral contraceptives
Androgens	Corticotropin	Growth hormone	Progesterone
Angiotensin	Digitalis	Insulin	Thyroid hormone
Clofibrate			

Differential Diagnosis for Elevated Serum Total Proteins

Cardiovascular
  Rheumatic fever

Respiratory
  Bacterial pneumonia
  Pulmonary tuberculosis
  Respiratory distress syndrome

Genitourinary
  Usually no effect

Gastrointestinal
  Cholera

Pancreatic
  Usually no effect

Hepatobiliary
  Cirrhosis: Cause unspecified

Hematologic
  Multiple myeloma
  Waldenström's macroglobulinemia

Endocrine
  Adrenal cortical hypofunction
  Pheochromocytoma

Metabolic
  Carcinoid syndrome
  Diabetic acidosis

Infectious
  Chronic infection
  Leishmaniasis
  Lymphogranuloma venereum

Immunologic
  Collagen disease

Musculoskeletal
  Rheumatoid arthritis

Neuropsychiatric
  Cerebral embolism
  Huntington's chorea

Neoplastic
  Malignant neoplasm: Bronchus and lung
  Secondary malignant neoplasm: Respiratory system

Miscellaneous
  Dehydration
  Eclampsia
  Exercise
  Sarcoidosis
  Stress

Agents Associated With Decreased Levels of Serum Total Proteins in Vivo

Cathartics	Estrogens	Mercury compounds	Pyrazinamide
Dantrolene	Floxuridine	Nicotinyl alcohol	Rifampin
Dextran	Laxatives	Oral contraceptives	Trimethadione

Differential Diagnosis for Decreased Serum Total Proteins

Cardiovascular
  Congestive heart failure
  Constrictive pericarditis
  Essential hypertension

Respiratory
  Pulmonary tuberculosis

Genitourinary
  Chronic renal failure
  Glomerulonephritis: Acute poststreptococcal, membranous
  Nephrotic syndrome

Gastrointestinal
  Celiac disease
  Fistula of stomach and duodenum
  Gastritis
  Gastroenteritis and colitis
  Malabsorption
  Mesenteric artery embolism
  Peptic ulcer: Site unspecified
  Regional enteritis
  Ulcerative colitis
  Whipple's disease

Pancreatic
  Acute pancreatitis

Hepatobiliary
  Cholecystitis: Acute
  Cirrhosis of liver
  Toxic hepatitis

Hematologic
  Chronic lymphocytic leukemia
  Pernicious anemia

Endocrine
  Adrenal cortical hyperfunction
  Hyperthyroidism

Metabolic
  Hepatolenticular degeneration
  Thiamine deficiency

Infectious
  Disseminated tuberculosis
  Parasitic: Malaria, trichinosis
  Rickettsial: Epidemic typhus, Rocky Mountain spotted fever

Immunologic
  Immunodeficiency: Common variable

Musculoskeletal
  Usually no effect

Neuropsychiatric
  Friedreich's ataxia
  Meningitis: Tuberculous

Neoplastic
  Histiocytosis X
  Lymphoma: Hodgkin's disease, lymphosarcoma, reticulum cell sarcoma
  Malignant neoplasm: Large intestine, rectum, small intestine, stomach
  Secondary malignant neoplasm: Disseminated

Miscellaneous
  Amyloidosis
  Analbuminemia
  Burns
  Eclampsia
  Generalized dermatitis
  Heat stroke
  Overhydration
  Pemphigus
  Pregnancy
  Protein malnutrition

Serum Albumin

Patient Preparation. The patient need not be fasting. However, ambulatory patients have slightly higher (approximately 10 per cent) serum albumin levels than recumbent patients.

Specimen Collection and Handling. Serum is the preferred sample. The use of a tourniquet may lead to falsely elevated results. Hemolysis should be avoided because it adds protein to the serum and will falsely elevate the results with some commonly used methods, such as the bromcresol green method.

Methodology. A variety of different methods are available. Bromcresol green and serum protein electrophoresis (SPE) are the most commonly employed methods used in clinical laboratories. The bromcresol green method is not specific for albumin and may give falsely elevated results in the presence of alpha and beta globulins as well as hemoglobin. The bromcresol method may overestimate serum albumin by up to 1.0 gm/100 ml in patients with elevations of these globulins, such as in those with the nephrotic syndrome. Consult the laboratory for its methodology, including in vitro drug interference.

Reference Interval. The reference interval for serum albumin is 3.2 to 5.6 g/100 ml by electrophoresis and 3.8 to 5.0 g/100 ml by dye binding. Recumbent persons will have levels about 10 per cent lower than ambulatory persons. Consult the laboratory for its reference intervals.

Agents Associated With Increased Levels of Serum Albumin in Vivo

Albumin infusions
Gallamine
Progesterone

Differential Diagnosis for Elevated Serum Albumin

Cardiovascular
  Usually no effect

Respiratory
  Usually no effect

Genitourinary
  Usually no effect

Gastrointestinal
  Usually no effect

Pancreatic
  Usually no effect

Hepatobiliary
  Laennec's or alcoholic cirrhosis

Hematologic
  Usually no effect

Endocrine
  Hypothyroidism

Metabolic
  Usually no effect

Infectious
  Leishmaniasis

Immunologic
  Usually no effect

Musculoskeletal
  Usually no effect

Neuropsychiatric
  Multiple sclerosis

Neoplastic
  Usually no effect

Miscellaneous
  Dehydration
  Exercise
  Heat stroke
  Sarcoidosis

Agents Associated With Decreased Levels of Serum Albumin in Vivo

Acetaminophen	Cathartics	Dextran	Niacin
Anticonvulsants	Cyclophosphamide	Estrogens	Nicotinyl alcohol
Asparaginase	Dantrolene	Ethinyl estradiol	Oral contraceptives
Azathioprine	Dapsone	Halothane	Pyrazinamide

Differential Diagnosis for Decreased Serum Albumin

Cardiovascular
  Acute myocardial infarction
  Bacterial endocarditis
  Congestive heart failure
  Constrictive pericarditis

  Essential hypertension
  Rheumatic fever
Respiratory
  Bacterial pneumonia
  Pulmonary tuberculosis

Genitourinary
Chronic renal failure
Glomerulonephritis: Acute poststreptococcal, minimal change
Nephrotic syndrome

Gastrointestinal
Ancylostomiasis
Celiac disease
Gastritis
Gastroenteritis and colitis
Intestinal obstruction
Malabsorption: Cause unspecified
Mesenteric artery embolism
Peptic ulcer: Site unspecified
Peritonitis
Protein-losing enteropathy
Regional enteritis
Strongyloidiasis
Ulcerative colitis
Zollinger-Ellison syndrome

Pancreatic
Pancreatitis: Acute, chronic

Hepatobiliary
Biliary cirrhosis
Cholecystitis: Acute
Chronic active hepatitis
Cirrhosis: Cause unspecified
Hepatic failure
Laennec's or alcoholic cirrhosis
Liver abscess
Necrosis of liver: Acute, subacute
Viral hepatitis

Hematologic
Heavy-chain disease: Alpha, gamma
Hemolytic disease of newborn
Lymphocytic leukemia: Acute, chronic
Monocytic leukemia
Multiple myeloma
Myelocytic leukemia: Acute, chronic
Pernicious anemia
Waldenström's macroglobulinemia

Endocrine
Diabetes mellitus
Hyperthyroidism

Metabolic
Carcinoid syndrome

Cystic fibrosis
Diabetic acidosis
Hepatolenticular degeneration
Hyperlipoproteinemia: Types IIA, IIB
Lactosuria
Vitamin C deficiency

Infectious
Bacterial: Chlamydia, leprosy, leptospirosis
Fungal: Histoplasmosis
Parasitic: Leishmaniasis, malaria, schistosomiasis, trichinosis, trypanosomiasis
Rickettsial: Rocky Mountain spotted fever
Septicemia
Viral: Chickenpox, herpes zoster

Immunologic
Allergic purpura
Cranial arteritis and related conditions
Polyarteritis nodosa
Sjögren's syndrome
Systemic lupus erythematosus

Musculoskeletal
Osteomyelitis
Rheumatoid arthritis

Neuropsychiatric
Hepatic encephalopathy
Multiple sclerosis

Neoplastic
Benign neoplasm: Stomach
Lymphoma: Hodgkin's disease, lymphosarcoma, reticulum cell sarcoma
Malignant neoplasm: Bladder, breast, bronchus and lung corpus uteri, esophagus, kidney, large intestine, liver, pancreas, prostate, respiratory system, stomach
Secondary malignant neoplasm: Disseminated

Miscellaneous
Analbuminemia
Amyloidosis
Burns
Deficiency state: Unspecified
Eclampsia
Generalized dermatitis
Overhydration
Pemphigus
Pregnancy
Protein malnutrition
Sarcoidosis

Serum Sodium

Patient Preparation. Patient factors do not generally interfere.

Specimen Collection and Handling. Serum or heparinized plasma should be used, but avoid sodium salts of heparin. Significant hemolysis should be avoided since it will depress the serum sodium level due to a dilutional effect from red blood cell fluid. Lipemia can artifactually depress the serum sodium level, causing pseudohyponatremia. Serum sodium is stable for at least 2 weeks either at room or refrigerator temperature.

Methodology. A variety of methods are available. Most modern laboratories measure serum sodium by emission flame photometery or ion-selective electrode. Consult your laboratory for its methodology including in vitro drug interference.

Reference Interval. The reference interval for serum sodium is 136 to 142 mEq/liter. Consult your laboratory for its reference interval.

Agents Associated With Increased Levels of Serum Sodium in Vivo

Amino acids	Desoxycorticosterone	Mannitol	Prednisolone
Anabolic steroids	Diazoxide	Methandrostenolone	Prednisone
Androgens	Estrogens	Methoxyflurane	Progesterone
Angiotensin	Ethanol	Methyldopa	Prolactin
Carbenoxolone	Glucocorticoids	Methyltestosterone	Rauwolfia
Clonidine	Guanethidine	Oral contraceptives	Saline
Corticosteroids	Hydrocortisone	Oxyphenbutazone	Sodium bicarbonate
Corticotropin	Intra-amniotic saline	Phenelzine	Sodium sulfate
Cortisone	Isosorbide	Phenylbutazone	Tetracycline

Differential Diagnosis for Elevated Serum Sodium

Cardiovascular
Congestive heart failure

Respiratory
Usually no effect

Genitourinary
Chronic renal failure
Diuresis following relief of urinary tract obstruction
Diuretic phase of acute tubular necrosis
Hypercalcemic nephropathy
Hypokalemic nephropathy
Nephrogenic diabetes insipidus

Gastrointestinal
Bacillary dysentery
Cholera
Diarrhea
Gastroenteritis and colitis
Intestinal obstruction
Peritonitis
Vomiting

Pancreatic
Usually no effect

Hepatobiliary
Hepatic failure

Hematologic
Lymphocytic leukemia: Acute, chronic
Myelocytic leukemia: Acute, chronic

Endocrine
Acromegaly
Adrenal cortical hyperfunction
Diabetes insipidus
Ectopic ACTH production
Hypothalamic lesion
Ovarian hypofunction

Metabolic
Diabetic acidosis

Infectious
Usually no effect

Immunologic
Usually no effect

Musculoskeletal
Usually no effect

Neuropsychiatric
Bacterial meningitis
Cerebral embolism and thrombosis
Cerebral hemorrhage
Encephalomyelitis
Familial periodic paralysis

Neoplastic
Benign neoplasm: Central nervous system
Lymphoma: Lymphosarcoma, reticulum cell sarcoma
Malignant neoplasm: Brain, lung
Secondary malignant neoplasm: Brain

Miscellaneous
Dehydration
Diet: High-sodium
Excessive sweating

Agents Associated With Decreased Levels of Serum Sodium in Vivo

Ammonium chloride	Dichlorphenamide	Hydroflumethiazide	Quinethazone
Amphotericin B	Diuretics	Laxatives	Silver compounds
Bendroflumethiazide	Ethacrynic acid	Lithium	Spironolactone
Cathartics	Ethanol	Mannitol	Sulfonylureas
Chlorothiazide	Furosemide	Mercurial diuretics	Thiazides
Chlorpropamide	Glycerin	Mercury compounds	Urea
Chlorthalidone	Heparin	Metolazone	Vasopressin
Cyclophosphamide	Hydrochlorothiazide	Polythiazide	Vincristine
Cyclothiazide			

Differential Diagnosis for Decreased Serum Sodium

Cardiovascular
Acute myocardial infarction
Congestive heart failure
Essential hypertension

Respiratory
Pulmonary tuberculosis

Genitourinary
Medullary cystic disease
Nephrotic syndrome
Polycystic kidney disease
Renal failure: Acute, chronic
Renal tubular acidosis
Salt losing nephropathy

Gastrointestinal
Bacillary dysentery
Celiac disease
Diarrhea
Fistula of stomach and duodenum
Gastroenteritis and colitis
Malabsorption: Cause unspecified
Peptic ulcer: Site unspecified
Pyloric stenosis: Acquired
Regional enteritis
Ulcerative colitis
Vomiting

Pancreatic
Usually no effect

Hepatobiliary
Biliary cirrhosis
Cirrhosis: Cause unspecified
Hepatic failure
Laennec's or alcoholic cirrhosis
Reye's syndrome

Hematologic
Multiple myeloma

Endocrine
Adrenal cortical hypofunction

Anterior pituitary hypofunction
Diabetes mellitus
Hypothyroidism
Inappropriate antidiuretic hormone
Ovarian hyperfunction
Thyroiditis: Subacute

Metabolic
Acute intermittent porphyria
Cystic fibrosis
Diabetic acidosis
Hyperlipoproteinemia

Infectious
Bacterial: Disseminated tuberculosis
Parasitic: Malaria
Rickettsial: Brill's disease, endemic typhus, epidemic typhus, mite-borne typhus, rickettsialpox, Rocky Mountain spotted fever

Immunologic
Usually no effect

Musculoskeletal
Usually no effect

Neuropsychiatric
Meningitis: Bacterial, tuberculous

Neoplastic
Malignant neoplasm: Bronchus and lung

Miscellaneous
Burns
Eclampsia
Excessive sweating
Hyperlipidemia
Hyperglycemia
Hypothermia
Overhydration
Pemphigus
Pregnancy
Toxic effects: Non-medicinal metals

Serum Transaminase, Aspartate Amino (SGOT)

Patient Preparation. A fasting specimen is preferable because patients may show some elevation of the serum transaminase level after meals. An elevation has also been observed after intramuscular injections and muscular exercise.

Specimen Collection and Handling. A serum sample is satisfactory and hemolysis should be avoided because red blood cells contain 15 times more transaminase activity than serum. Specimens are best stored frozen if they are to be kept more than 3 to 4 days. Minimal loss of activity occurs at 0 to 4°C over 1 to 3 days.

Methodology. A number of different methods are available, both end-point and kinetic. Kinetic methods with continuous monitoring of the NADH/NAD+ reaction are preferable. Consult the laboratory for its methodology including in vitro drug interference.

Reference Interval. Reference intervals differ according to methodology. A generally used interval is 10 to 40 U/ml. Consult the laboratory for its reference interval.

Agents Associated With Increased Levels of SGOT in Vivo

Acetaminophen	Chlorpromazine	Ethionamide	Methimazole
Acetohexamide	Chlorpropamide	Ethosuximide	Methotrexate
Acetophenazine	Chlorprothixene	Ethyl chloride	Methoxyflurane
Allopurinol	Chlorzoxazone	Factor IX complex, human	Methyldopa
Aluminum nicotinate	Cholestyramine	Fenoprofen	Methyltestosterone
Amantadine	Cholinergics	Fibrinolysin	Metolazone
Aminocaproic acid	Cimetidine	Floxuridine	Metoprolol
Aminoglutethimide	Cinoxacin	Flucytosine	Minocycline
Aminosalicylic acid	Cisplatin	Fluorides	Mithramycin
Amitriptyline	Clindamycin	Fluoxymesterone	Monoamine oxidase
Amodiaquine	Clofibrate	Fluphenazine	inhibitors
Amphotericin B	Clonidine	Flurazepam	Morphine
Ampicillin	Cloxacillin	Gentamicin	Nafcillin
Anabolic steroids	Codeine	Glycopyrrolate	Nalidixic acid
Androgens	Colchicine	Gold	Nandrolone
Anesthetic agents	Copper	Griseofulvin	Naproxen
Anticonvulsants	Cortisone	Guanethidine	Narcotics
Antifungal agents	Coumarin derivatives	Haloperidol	Niacin
Antimony compounds	Cyclobenzaprine	Halothane	Niacinamide
Asparaginase	Cyclophosphamide	Hetacillin	Nicotinyl alcohol
Azathioprine	Cyclopropane	Hycanthone	Nitrofurantoin
Baclofen	Cycloserine	Hydrochlorothiazide	Norethandrolone
Barbiturates	Cyclothiazide	Hydroflumethiazide	Norethindrone
Bethanechol	Dantrolene	Hydroxyurea	Nortriptyline
Bismuth salts	Demeclocycline	Idoxuridine	Opiates
Bromocriptine	Dehydroemetine	Imipramine	Oral contraceptives
Butaperazine	Desipramine	Indandione derivatives	Oxacillin
Calcitriol	Dibenzoxazepine	Iron salts	Oxazepam
Capreomycin	Dicloxacillin	Isocarboxazid	Oxymetholone
Carbarsone	Dicumarol	Isoniazid	Oxyphenbutazone
Carbenicillin	Dienestrol	Kanamycin	Papaverine
Carbenoxolone	Diethylstilbestrol	Levodopa	Paraldehyde
Carmustine	Disopyramide	Lincomycin	Pargyline
Carphenazine	Doxycycline	Lomustine	Pemoline
Cefaclor	Enflurane	Mechlorethamine	Penicillamine
Cefoxitin	Epinephrine	Meclofenamate	Penicillin
Cephalosporins	Erythromycin	Melarsoprol	Phenacetin
Chenodeoxycholic acid	Estradiol	Meperidine	Phenazopyridine
Chloral hydrate	Estrogens	Meprobamate	Phenelzine
Chlorambucil	Estrone	Mercaptopurine	Phenindione
Chloramphenicol	Ethacrynic acid	Mesoridazine	Phenobarbital
Chlordiazepoxide	Ethambutol	Methacycline	Phenothiazines
Chlorophenothane	Ethanol	Methandrostenolone	Phenylbutazone
Chloroquine	Ethchlorvynol	Methdilazine	Piperacetazine
Chlorothiazide	Ether	Methenamine	Polythiazide

Probenecid
Procainamide
Prochlorperazine
Progesterone
Promazine
Promethazine
Propoxyphene
Propranolol
Propylthiouracil
Protriptyline
Pyrantel
Pyrazinamide
Pyridoxine

Quinacrine
Quinethazone
Quindine
Rifampin
Salicylates
Stanozolol
Streptokinase
Sulfadiazine
Sulfameter
Sulfamethizole
Sulfamethoxazole
Sulfisoxazole
Sulfonamides

Sulfones
Sulfonylureas
Testosterone
Tetracycline
Thiabendazole
Thiazides
Thiethylperazine
Thioguanine
Thioridazine
Thiosemicarbazones
Thiothixene
Ticarcillin

Tolazamide
Tolazoline
Tolbutamide
Trichlormethiazide
Trifluoperazine
Trimeprazine
Trimethadione
Trimethoprim
Trioxsalen
Vidarabine
X-ray therapy
Zomepirac

Differential Diagnosis for Elevated SGOT

Cardiovascular
Acute myocardial infarction
Acute myocarditis
Acute pericarditis
Arterial embolism and thrombosis
Cardiomyopathies
Chronic ischemic heart disease
Congestive heart failure
Dissecting aortic aneurysm
Essential hypertension
Phlebitis or thrombophlebitis
Rheumatic fever
Shock

Respiratory
Asthma
Influenza
Pneumonia: Bacterial, viral, resolving
Pulmonary embolism and infarction
Pulmonary tuberculosis

Genitourinary
Acute renal failure
Acute pylonephritis
Prostatitis
Renal infarction

Gastrointestinal
Celiac disease
Gastritis
Intestinal obstruction
Intestinal injury: Infarction, surgery
Mesenteric artery embolism
Regional enteritis
Ulcerative colitis

Pancreatic
Pancreatitis: Acute, chronic

Hepatobiliary
Biliary cirrhosis
Cholangitis
Cholecystitis: Acute
Chronic active hepatitis
Cirrhosis: Cause unspecified
Dubin-Johnson syndrome
Extrahepatic biliary obstruction
Granulomatous hepatitis
Hemochromatosis
Hepatic failure
Laennec's or alcoholic cirrhosis

Liver abscess
Necrosis of liver: Acute, subacute
Toxic hepatitis
Reye's syndrome
Viral hepatitis
Yellow fever

Hematologic
Hemolytic anemia
Hereditary spherocytosis
Infectious mononucleosis
Lymphocytic leukemia: Acute, chronic
Multiple myeloma
Myelocytic leukemia: Acute, chronic
Pernicious anemia
Thalassemia major

Endocrine
Diabetes mellitus
Hyperthyroidism
Hypoparathyroidism
Hypothyroidism
Thyroiditis: Subacute

Metabolic
Anderson's disease
Cystic fibrosis
Diabetic acidosis
Forbes' disease
Galactosemia
Gout
Hepatolenticular degeneration
Hereditary fructose intolerance
McArdle's disease
Metabolic acidosis
Niemann-Pick disease
Porphyria cutanea tarda

Infectious
Bacterial: Brucellosis, chlamydia, disseminated tuber-
culosis, leptospirosis, tetanus, typhoid fever
Fungal: Histoplasmosis
Parasitic: Amebiasis, hydatidosis, malaria, schistoso-
miasis, trichinosis
Rickettsial: Rocky Mountain spotted fever
Septicemia
Viral: Cytomegalic inclusion disease, herpes zoster

Immunologic
Dermatomyositis and polymyositis
Progressive systemic sclerosis
Systemic lupus erythematosus

Musculoskeletal
Crush injury following trauma
Familial progressive spinal muscular atrophy
Intramuscular injections
Juvenile rheumatoid arthritis
Muscle necrosis
Myoglobinuria
Myositis
Myotonia atrophica
Myotonia congenita
Osteoarthritis
Osteomyelitis
Progressive muscular dystrophy

Neuropsychiatric
Bacterial meningitis
Brain infarction
Cerebral embolism and thrombosis
Familial periodic paralysis
Metachromatic leukodystrophy
Paranoid states and other psychoses
Poliomyelitis: Acute

Neoplastic
Benign neoplasm: Cardiovascular tissue, central nervous
  system

Lymphoma: Hodgkin's disease, lymphosarcoma, reticulum cell sarcoma
Malignant neoplasm: Bone, brain, breast, bronchus and lung, esophagus, intrahepatic bile ducts, liver, pancreas, prostate, stomach, thyroid
Secondary malignant neoplasm: Liver, respiratory system

Miscellaneous
Alcoholism
Amyloidosis
Burns
Delirium tremens
Drug dependence: Opium and derivatives
Eclampsia
Effects of x-ray irradiation
Effects of electric current
Exercise
Gangrene
Heat stroke
Hematoma
Hypothermia
Postoperative state
Sarcoidosis
Toxic effects: Carbon monoxide, non-medicinal metals, venom

Agents Associated With Decreased Levels of SGOT in Vivo

Fluorides
Progesterone
Trifluoperazine

Differential Diagnosis for Decreased SGOT

Cardiovascular
Usually no effect

Respiratory
Usually no effect

Genitourinary
Chronic hemodialysis
Uremia

Gastrointestinal
Usually no effect

Pancreatic
Usually no effect

Hepatobiliary
Severe liver disease

Hematologic
Usually no effect

Endocrine
Usually no effect

Metabolic
Beriberi
Diabetic ketoacidosis

Infectious
Malaria

Immunologic
Usually no effect

Musculoskeletal
Usually no effect

Neuropsychiatric
Usually no effect

Neoplastic
Usually no effect

Miscellaneous
Pregnancy

Serum Urea Nitrogen (SUN)

Patient Preparation. The patient need not be fasting, but serum urea nitrogen (SUN) levels can vary greatly, secondary to the water and protein intake of the individual.

Specimen Collection and Handling. Serum or heparinized plasma may be used. Because urea may be lost through bacterial activity, the sample should be analyzed within several hours of collection or it should be preserved by refrigeration.

Methodology. A variety of methods are avail-able. They commonly depend on splitting urea with urease and measuring a product colorimetrically. Consult the laboratory for its methodology, including in vitro drug interference.

Reference Interval. A generally used reference interval for SUN is 8 to 23 mg/100 ml. However, the upper reference limit can be raised to 25 mg/100 ml in the presence of low water intake or high protein intake. Consult the laboratory for its reference intervals.

Agents Associated With Increased Levels of SUN in Vivo

Acetaminophen	Copper	Kanamycin	Phenazopyridine
Acetazolamide	Cyclothiazide	Levodopa	Phenformin
Alkaline antacids	Demeclocycline	Lipomul	Phenindione
Allopurinol	Diazepam	Meclofenamate	Phenylbutazone
Amantadine	Disopyramide	Mefenamic acid	Polymyxin
Amino acid infusion	Diuretics	Melphalan	Probenecid
Aminoglycosides	Doxapram	Mercurial diuretics	Propranolol
Amphotericin B	Doxycycline	Methacycline	Propylthiouracil
Anabolic steroids	Edetate	Methicillin	Protein
Androgens	Ergot preparations	Methotrexate	Quinethazone
Antimony compounds	Ethacrynic acid	Methoxyflurane	Quinine
Asparaginase	Ethambutol	Methyclothiazide	Radiographic agents
Benzthiazide	Ether	Methyldopa	Rifampin
Bismuth salts	Ethosuximide	Methysergide	Salicylates
Bromocriptine	Fibrinolysin	Metolazone	Silver compounds
Busulfan	Flucytosine	Metoprolol	Spectinomycin
Calcitriol	Fluorides	Minocycline	Spironolactone
Calcium salts	Furosemide	Minoxidil	Streptokinase
Capreomycin	Gentamicin	Mithramycin	Streptomycin
Carbamazepine	Gold	Mitomycin	Tartrates
Carbenoxolone	Griseofulvin	Nalidixic acid	Tetrachloroethylene
Carmustine	Guanethidine	Neomycin	Tetracyclines
Cefaclor	Halothane	Nitrofurantoin	Thiazides
Cefoxitin	Hydralazine	Oxacillin	Triamterene
Cephalosporins	Hydrochlorothiazide	Oxyphenbutazone	Trimethadione
Cinoxacin	Hydroflumethiazide	Paraldehyde	Trimethoprim
Cisplatin	Hydroxyurea	Pargyline	Urea
Clonidine	Imipramine	Paromomycin	Vancomycin
Clorazepate	Immune serum globulin	Penicillamine	Vitamin D
Codeine	Indomethacin	Penicillin	X-ray therapy
Colistimethate	Iron salts	Pentamidine	Zomepirac
Colistin	Isosorbide	Phenacetin	

Differential Diagnosis for Elevated SUN

Cardiovascular
Acute myocardial infarction
Arterial embolism and thrombosis
Arteriosclerosis
Bacterial endocarditis
Congestive heart failure
Essential hypertension
Hypotension
Malignant hypertension
Shock

Respiratory
Respiratory distress syndrome

Genitourinary
Azotemia
Benign prostatic hypertrophy
Glomerulonephritis: Acute poststreptococcal, membranous, memobranoproliferative, rapidly progressive
Hydronephrosis
Medullary cystic disease

Nephrotic syndrome
Polycystic kidney disease
Pyelonephritis: Acute, chronic
Renal failure: Acute, chronic

Gastrointestinal
Cholera
Diarrhea
Gastrointestinal hemorrhage
Intestinal obstruction
Mesenteric artery embolism
Peptic ulcer: Site unspecified
Peritonitis
Vomiting

Pancreatic
Acute pancreatitis

Hepatobiliary
Cirrhosis: Cause unspecified
Hepatic failure
Yellow fever

Hematologic
Acquired autoimmune hemolytic anemia
Heavy-chain disease: Gamma
Lymphocytic leukemia: Acute, chronic
Monocytic leukemia
Multiple myeloma
Myelocytic leukemia: Acute, chronic
Thrombotic thrombocytopenic purpura
Waldenström's macroglobulinemia

Endocrine
Adrenal cortical hyperfunction
Adrenal cortical hypofunction
Diabetes mellitus
Hyperthyroidism
Hyperparathyroidism
Hypothyroidism

Metabolic
Acute intermittent porphyria
Cystinosis
Diabetic acidosis
Gout
Hepatolenticular degeneration
Metabolic alkalosis
Milk-alkali syndrome

Infectious
Bacterial: Chlamydia, diphtheria, leptospirosis
Fungal: Actinomycosis, aspergillosis
Rickettsial: Epidemic typhus, Rocky Mountain spotted fever
Septicemia

Immunologic
Allergic purpura
Polyarteritis nodosa
Progressive systemic sclerosis
Systemic lupus erythematosus

Musculoskeletal
Rheumatoid arthritis

Neuropsychiatric
Bacterial meningitis

Neoplastic
Lymphosarcoma
Malignant neoplasm: Bladder

Miscellaneous
Amyloidosis
Dehydration
Diet: High-protein
Effects of electric current
Effects of x-ray irradiation
Exercise
Excessive sweating
Stress
Toxic effects: Carbon monoxide, lead and its compounds, non-medicinal metals, venom

Agents Associated With Decreased Levels of SUN in Vivo

| Enflurane | Glucose | Growth hormone | Paramethasone | Phenothiazines |

Differential Diagnosis for Decreased SUN

Cardiovascular
Usually no effect

Respiratory
Usually no effect

Genitourinary
Nephrotic syndrome

Gastrointestinal
Celiac disease

Pancreatic
Usually no effect

Hepatobiliary
Cirrhosis: Cause unspecified
Hepatic failure

Laennec's or alcoholic cirrhosis
Necrosis of liver: Acute, subacute
Toxic hepatitis

Hematologic
Usually no effect

Endocrine
Acromegaly
Inappropriate antidiuretic hormone secretion

Metabolic
Cystic fibrosis
Hepatolenticular degeneration

Infectious
Usually no effect

Immunologic
Usually no effect

Musculoskeletal
Usually no effect

Neuropsychiatric
Usually no effect

Neoplastic
Usually no effect

Miscellaneous
Diet: Low-protein
Eclampsia
Exercise
Overhydration
Pregnancy
Protein malnutrition

Serum Uric Acid

Patient Preparation. Patient factors do not generally interfere.

Specimen Collection and Handling. Serum or heparinized plasma may be used. Any of the common anticoagulants except potassium oxalate can usually be used. Uric acid is stable in serum for several days at room temperature and for longer periods if refrigerated. Since it is susceptible to destruction by bacterial action, the addition of thymol may increase the stability.

Methodology. A variety of methods, both endpoint and kinetic, are commonly used. Consult the laboratory for its methodology, including in vitro drug interference.

Reference Interval. The reference interval for serum uric acid is sex dependent: for males, 4.0 to 8.5 mg/100 ml; for females, 2.7 to 7.3 mg/100 ml. Consult the laboratory for its reference intervals.

Agents Associated With Increased Levels of Serum Uric Acid in Vivo

Acetazolamide	Dantrolene	Levodopa	Phenylbutazone
Aluminum nicotinate	Diazoxide	Lipomul	Polythiazide
Anabolic steroids	Diuretics	Mannose infusion	Prednisone
Androgens	Epinephrine	Mecamylamine	Probucol
Angiotensin	Ethacrynic acid	Mechlorethamine	Pyrazinamide
Antineoplastic agents	Ethambutol	Mercaptopurine	Quinethazone
Azathioprine	Ethanol	Mercurial diuretics	Radioactive compounds
Azathymine	Ethoxzolamide	Methazolamide	Rifampin
Bendroflumethiazide	Fluorides	Methicillin	Salicylates
Benzthiazide	Fructose infusion	Methotrexate	Spironolactone
Bromocriptine	Furosemide	Methoxyflurane	Thiazides
Busulfan	Gentamicin	Metolazone	Thioguanine
Capreomycin	Halothane	Mitomycin	Thiotepa
Chlorothiazide	Hydrochlorothiazide	Niacin	Triamterene
Chlorthalidone	Hydroflumethiazide	Nicotinic acid	Trichlormethiazide
Cisplatin	Hydroxyurea	Norepinephrine	Vincristine
Cyclothiazide	Levarterenol	Phenothiazines	X-ray therapy
Cytarabine			

Differential Diagnosis for Elevated Serum Uric Acid

Cardiovascular
Acute myocardial infarction
Angina pectoris
Arteriosclerosis
Chronic ischemic heart disease
Congestive heart failure
Essential hypertension
Renovascular hypertension

Respiratory
Asthma
Berylliosis
Pulmonary infarct
Pulmonary tuberculosis
Resolving pneumonia
Respiratory distress syndrome

Genitourinary
Benign prostatic hypertrophy
Glomerulonephritis: Focal, rapidly progressive
Nephrotic syndrome
Polycystic kidneys
Renal failure: Acute, chronic

Gastrointestinal
Celiac disease

Regional enteritis
Ulcerative colitis

Pancreatic
Usually no effect

Hepatobiliary
Cirrhosis: Cause unspecified
Laennec's or alcoholic cirrhosis
Viral hepatitis

Hematologic
Acquired autoimmune hemolytic anemia
Anemia due to disorder of glutathione metabolism
Erythroleukemia
Heavy-chain disease: Gamma
Hereditary spherocytosis
Lymphocytic leukemia: Acute, chronic
Monocytic leukemia
Multiple myeloma
Myelofibrosis
Myelocytic leukemia: Acute, chronic
Pernicious anemia, after treatment
Polycythemia: Vera, secondary
Sickle cell anemia

Endocrine
  Acromegaly
  Diabetes insipidus
  Diabetes mellitus
  Hyperparathyroidism
  Hypoparathyroidism
  Hypothyroidism

Metabolic
  Alkaptonuria
  Anderson's disease
  Asymptomatic hyperuricemia
  Calcinosis universalis and circumscripta
  Forbes' disease
  Diabetes acidosis
  Gout
  Hyperlipoproteinemia: Types IIA, IIB, III, IV, V
  Lesch-Nyhan syndrome
  McArdle's disease
  Maple syrup urine disease
  von Gierke's disease
  Xanthinuria

Infectious
  Leishmaniasis
  Septicemia

Immunologic
  Usually no effect

Musculoskeletal
  Rheumatoid arthritis

Neuropsychiatric
  Cerebral embolism and thrombosis
  Cerebral hemorrhage and infarction
  Convulsions

  Encephalomyelitis
  Manic depressive disorder
  Meningitis: Bacterial, tuberculous
  Paranoid states and other psychoses
  Transient cerebral ischemia

Neoplastic
  Benign neoplasm: Brain, central nervous system
  Lymphoma: Hodgkin's disease, lymphosarcoma, reticulum cell sarcoma
  Malignant neoplasm: Bladder, bone, breast, corpus uteri, esophagus, large intestine, pancreas, prostate, rectum, skin, stomach, testis
  Secondary malignant neoplasm: Respiratory system

Miscellaneous
  Alcoholism
  Amyloidosis
  Cancer chemotherapy
  Certain population groups: Blackfoot and Pima Indians, Filipinos, New Zealand Maoris
  Depressive neurosis
  Diet: High protein, high nucleoprotein (e.g., sweetbreads, liver)
  Down's syndrome
  Eclampsia
  Effects of x-ray irradiation
  Exercise
  Heat stroke
  Inflammation
  Pregnancy complicated by intrauterine death
  Protein malnutrition
  Psoriasis
  Sarcoidosis
  Tissue necrosis
  Toxic effects: Lead and its compounds

Agents Associated With Decreased Levels of Serum Uric Acid in Vivo

Acetohexamide	Corticotropin	Griseofulvin	Phenindione
Allopurinol	Cortisone	Halofenate	Phenolphthalein
Anticholinergics	Coumarin anticoagulants	Inandione anticoagulants	Phenothiazines
Azathioprine	Dicumarol	Indomethacin	Phenylbutazone
Chlorothiazide	Diethylstilbestrol	Lithium	Probenecid
Chlorpromazine	Estrogens	Mannitol	Salicylates
Chlorprothixene	Ethacrynic acid	Marihuana	Saline infusions
Clofibrate	Ethinyl estradiol	Mefenamic acid	Sulfamethoxazole
Contrast media, iodine containing	Fenoprofen	Mercurial compounds	Sulfinpyrazone
Corticosteroids	Glucose infusions	Methotrexate	Sulfonamides
	Glyceryl guaiacolate	Oxyphenbutazone	Vinblastine

Differential Diagnosis for Decreased Serum Uric Acid

Cardiovascular
  Usually no effect

Respiratory
  Usually no effect

Genitourinary
  Isolated defect in tubular transport of uric acid
  Renal tubular acidosis

Gastrointestinal
  Celiac disease

Pancreatic
  Usually no effect

Hepatobiliary
  Biliary cirrhosis
  Cirrhosis: Cause unspecified
  Laennec's or alcoholic cirrhosis

Hematologic
  Folic acid deficiency anemia
  Multiple myeloma
  Pernicious anemia

Endocrine
Acromegaly

Metabolic
Cystinosis
Hartnup disease
Hepatolenticular degeneration
Xanthinuria

Infectious
Usually no effect

Immunologic
Usually no effect

Musculoskeletal
Usually no effect

Neuropsychiatric
Familial periodic paralysis

Neoplastic
Hodgkin's disease
Malgiant neoplasm: Bronchus and lung

Miscellaneous
Burns
Diet: Low-protein
Overhydration
Pregnancy

REFERENCES

AMA Department of Drugs. AMA Drug Evaluations, ed 4. Chicago, AMA, 1980.

Brown SS, Mitchell FL, Young DS (eds): Chemical Diagnosis of Disease. New York, Elsevier North-Holland Biomedical Press, 1979.

Friedman RB, Anderson RE, Entine SM, Hirshberg SB: Effects of diseases on clinical laboratory tests. Clin Chem 26:1D–476D, 1980.

Gilman AG, Goodman LS, Gilman A, et al (eds): Goodman and Gilman's The Pharmacological Basis of Therapeutics, ed 6. New York, Macmillan Publishing Company, Inc, 1980.

Hansten PD: Drug Interactions, ed 4. Philadelphia, Lea & Febiger, 1979.

Henry JB (ed): Clinical Diagnosis and Management by Laboratory Methods, ed 16. Philadelphia, WB Saunders Company, 1979.

Henry RJ, Cannon DC, Winkelman JW (eds): Clinical Chemistry: Principles and Technics. Hagerstown, Md, Harper & Row, 1974.

Physicians Desk Reference, ed 36. Oradell, NJ, Medical Economics Company Inc, 1982.

Robbins SL, Cotran RS: Pathologic Basis of Disease, ed 2. Philadelphia, WB Saunders Company, 1979.

Teitz NW (ed): Fundamentals of Clinical Chemistry, ed 2. Philadelphia, WB Saunders Company, 1976.

Wallach J: Interpretation of Diagnostic Tests: A Handbook Synopsis of Laboratory Medicine, ed 3. Boston, Little, Brown & Company, 1978.

Williams WJ, Beutler E, Erslev AJ, Rundles, RW (eds): Hematology, ed 2. New York, McGraw-Hill Book Company, 1977.

Wolf PL: Interpretation of Biochemical Multitest Profiles: An Analysis of 100 Important Conditions. New York, Masson Publishing, Inc, 1977.

Wyngaarden JB, Smith LH (eds): Cecil Textbook of Medicine, ed 16. Philadelphia, WB Saunders Company, 1982.

Young DS, Pestaner LC, Gibberman V: Effects of drugs on clinical laboratory tests. Clin Chem 21:1D–432D, 1975.

Zimmerman HJ: Hepatotoxicity: The Adverse Effects of Drugs and Other Chemicals on the Liver. New York, Appleton-Century-Crofts, 1978.

REFERENCE INTERVALS (NORMAL RANGES)*

*These tables are adapted from Henry JB, Clinical Diagnosis and Management by Laboratory Methods, 16th ed, vol II. Philadelphia, WB Saunders Company, 1979, pp 2086–2103.

Table 1. WHOLE BLOOD, SERUM, AND PLASMA CHEMISTRY

COMPONENT	SYSTEM	TYPICAL REFERENCE INTERVALS		
		In Conventional Units	Factor*	In SI Units†
Acetoacetic acid:				
qualitative	Serum	Negative		Negative
quantitative	Serum	0.2–1.0 mg/dl	98	19.6–98.0 μmol/l
Acetone:				
qualitative	Serum	Negative		Negative
quantitative	Serum	0.3–2.0 mg/dl	172	51.6–344.0 μmol/l
Albumin:				
quantitative	Serum	3.2–4.5 g/dl (salt fractionation)	10	32–45 g/l
		3.2–5.6 g/dl (electrophoresis)	10	32–56 g/l
		3.8–5.0 g/dl (dye binding)	10	38–50 g/l
Alcohol, ethyl	Serum or whole blood	Negative—but presented as mg/dl	0.22	Negative—but presented as mmol/l
Aldolase	Serum:		7.4	
	adults	3–8 Sibley-Lehninger U/dl at 37°C.		22–59 mU/l at 37°C.
	children	Approximately 2 times adult levels		Approximately 2 times adult levels
	newborn	Approximately 4 times adult levels		Approximately 4 times adult levels
Alpha-amino acid nitrogen	Serum	3.6–7.0 mg/dl	0.714	2.6–5.0 mmol/l
δ-Aminolevulinic acid	Serum	0.01–0.03 mg/dl	76.3	0.76–2.29 μmol/l
Ammonia	Plasma	20–120 μg/dl (diffusion)	0.554	11.1–67.0 μmol/l
		40–80 μg/dl (enzymatic method)	0.554	22.2–44.3 μmol/l
		12–48 μg/dl (resin method)	0.554	6.7–26.6 μmol/l
Amylase	Serum	60–160 Somogyi units/dl	1.85	111–296 U/l
Argininosuccinic lyase	Serum	0–4 U/dl	10	0–40 U/l
Arsenic‡	Whole blood	<7 μg/dl	0.13	<0.91 μmol/l
Ascorbic acid (vitamin C)	Plasma	0.6–1.6 mg/dl	56.8	34–91 μmol/l
	Whole blood	0.7–2.0 mg/dl	56.8	40–114 μmol/l
Barbiturates	Serum, plasma, or whole blood	Negative	—	Negative
Base excess	Whole blood:			
	male	−3.3 to +1.2 mEq/l	1	−3.3 to +1.2 mmol/l
	female	−2.4 to +2.3 mEq/l	1	−2.4 to +2.3 mmol/l
Base, total	Serum	145–160 mEq/l	1	145–160 mmol/l
Bicarbonate	Plasma	21–28 mM	1	21–28 mmol/l
Bile acids	Serum	0.3–3.0 mg/dl	10	3.0–30.0 mg/l
Bilirubin:	Serum			
direct (conjugated)		Up to 0.3 mg/dl	17.1	Up to 5.1 μmol/l
indirect (unconjugated)		0.1–1.0 mg/dl	17.1	1.7–17.1 μmol/l
total		0.1–1.2 mg/dl	17.1	1.7–20.5 μmol/l
newborns total		1–12 mg/dl	17.1	17.1–205.0 μmol/l
Blood gases:	Whole blood			
pH		7.38–7.44 (arterial)	1	7.38–7.44
		7.36–7.41 (venous)	1	7.36–7.41

Constituent	Specimen	Conventional value	Factor	SI value
Pco₂	Whole blood	35–40 mm Hg (arterial)	0.133	4.66–5.32 kPa[a]
		40–45 mm Hg (venous)	0.133	5.32–5.99 kPa[a]
Po₂	Whole blood	95–100 mm Hg (arterial)	0.133	12.64–13.30 kPa[a]
Bromide	Serum	0–5 mg/dl	0.125	0–0.63 mmol/l
BSP (Bromosulphalein) (5 mg/kg)	Serum	less than 6% retention 45 min. after injection	0.01[b]	less than 0.06 retention 45 min after injection
Calcium: ionized	Serum	4–4.8 mg/dl	0.25	1.0–1.2
		2.0–2.4 mEq/l	0.5	1.0–1.2 mmol/l
total		30–58% of total	0.01[b]	0.30–0.58 of total
		9.2–11.0 mg/dl	0.25	2.3–2.8 mmol/l
		4.6–5.5 mEq/l	0.5	23–28 mmol/l
Carbon dioxide (CO₂ content)	Whole blood (arterial)	19–24 mM	1	19–24 mmol/l
	Plasma or serum (arterial)	21–28 mM	1	21–28 mmol/l
Carbon dioxide	Whole blood (venous)	22–26 mM	1	22–26 mmol/l
	Plasma or serum (venous)	24–30 mM	1	24–30 mmol/l
CO₂ combining power	Plasma or serum (venous)	24–30 mM	1	24–30 mmol/l
CO₂ partial pressure (Pco₂)	Whole blood (arterial)	35–40 mm Hg	0.133	4.66–5.32 kPa[a]
	Whole blood (venous)	40–45 mm Hg	0.133	5.32–5.99 kPa[a]
Carbonic acid (H₂CO₃)	Whole blood (arterial)	1.05–1.45 mM	1	1.05–1.45 mmol/l
	Whole blood (venous)	1.15–1.50 mM	1	1.15–1.50 mmol/l
	Plasma (venous)	1.02–1.38 mM	1	1.02–1.38 mmol/l
Carboxyhemoglobin (carbon monoxide hemoglobin)	Whole blood: suburban non-smokers	<1.5% saturation of hemoglobin	0.01[b]	<0.015 saturation of hemoglobin
	smokers	1.5–5.0% saturation	0.01	0.015–0.050 saturation
	heavy smokers	5.0–9.0% saturation	0.01	0.050–0.090 saturation
Carotene, beta	Serum	40–200 µg/dl	0.0186	0.74–3.72 µmol/l
Ceruloplasmin	Serum	23–50 µg/dl	10	230–500 mg/l
Chloride	Serum	95–103 mEq/l	1	95–103 mmol/l
Cholesterol total	Serum	150–250 mg/dl (varies with diet, sex, and age)	0.026	3.90–6.50 mmol/l
esters	Serum	65–75% of total cholesterol	0.01[b]	0.65–0.75 of total cholesterol
Cholinesterase (Pseudocholinesterase)	Erythrocytes	0.65–1.3 pH units	1	0.65–1.3 units[c]
	Plasma	0.5–1.3 pH units	1	0.5–1.3 units
	Serum or plasma	8–18 IU/l at 37°C.	1	8–18 U/l at 37°C.
Citrate		1.7–3.0 mg/dl	52	88–156 µmol/l
Copper	Serum, plasma: male	70–140 µg/dl	0.157	11.0–22.0 µmol/l
	female	80–155 µg/dl	0.157	12.6–24.3 µmol/l
Cortisol	Plasma: 8 a.m.–10 a.m.	5–23 µg/dl	27.6	138–635 nmol/l
	4 p.m.–6 p.m.	3–13 µg/dl	27.6	83–359 nmol/l

Table continued on following page

Table 1. WHOLE BLOOD, SERUM, AND PLASMA CHEMISTRY (Continued)

COMPONENT	SYSTEM	TYPICAL REFERENCE INTERVALS		
		In Conventional Units	Factor*	In SI Units†
Creatine as creatinine	Serum or plasma:			
	male	.1–.4 mg/dl	76.3	7.6–30.5 μmol/l
	female	.2–.7 mg/dl	76.3	15.3–53.4 μmol/l
Creatine kinase (CK)	Serum:			
	male	55–170 U/l at 37°C.	1	55–170 U/l at 37°C.
	female	30–135 U/l at 37°C.	1	30–135 U/l at 37°C.
Creatinine	Serum or plasma	0.6–1.2 mg/dl (adult)	88.4	53–106 μmol/l
		0.3–0.6 mg/dl (children < 2 yr.)	88.4	27–54 μmol/l
Creatinine clearance (endogenous)	Serum or plasma and urine:			
	male	107–139 ml/min.	0.0167	1.78–2.32 ml/s
	female	87–107 ml/min	0.0167	1.45–1.79 ml/s
Cryoglobulins	Serum	Negative	—	Negative
Electrophoresis, protein	Serum	per cent:		
Albumin		52–65% of total protein	0.01ᵇ	0.52–0.65 of total protein
Alpha-1		2.5–5.0% of total protein	0.01	0.025–0.05 of total protein
Alpha-2		7.0–13.0% of total protein	0.01	0.07–0.13 of total protein
Beta		8.0–14.0% of total protein	0.01	0.08–0.14 of total protein
Gamma		12.0–22.0% of total protein	0.01	0.12–0.22 of total protein
	Serum	Concentration		
Albumin		3.2–5.6 gm/dl	10	32–56 g/l
Alpha-1		0.1–0.4 gm/dl		1–4 g/l
Alpha-2		0.4–1.2 gm/dl		4–12 g/l
Beta		0.5–1.1 gm/dl		5–11 g/l
Gamma		0.5–1.6 gm/dl		5–16 g/l
Fats, neutral (see Triglycerides)				
Fatty acids:				
total (free and esterified)	Serum	9–15 mM	1	9–15 mmol/l
free (non-esterified)	Plasma	300–480 μEq/l	1	300–480 μmol/l
Fibrinogen	Plasma	200–400 mg/dl	0.01	2.00–4.00 g/l
Fluoride	Whole blood	<0.05 mg/dl	0.53	<0.027 mmol/l
Folate	Serum	5–25 ng/ml (bioassay)	2.27	11–56 nmol/l
		>2.3 ng/ml (radioassay)	2.27	>5.2 nmol/l
	Erythrocytes	166–640 ng/ml (bioassay)	2.27	376–1452 nmol/l
		>140 ng/ml (radioassay)	2.27	>318 nmol/l
Galactose	Whole blood:			
	adults	none	0.055	none
	children	<20 mg/dl	0.055	<1.1 mmol/l
Gamma globulin	Serum	0.5–1.6 gm/dl	10	5–16 g/l
Globulins, total	Serum	2.3–3.5 gm/dl	10	23–35 g/l
Glucose, fasting	Serum or plasma	70–110 mg/dl	0.055	3.85–6.05 mmol/l
	Whole blood	60–100 mg/dl	0.055	3.30–5.50 mmol/l

		Conventional	Factor	SI
Glucose tolerance				
oral	Serum or plasma:			
	fasting	70-110 mg/dl	0.055	3.85-6.05 mmol/l
	30 min.	30-60 mg/dl above fasting	0.055	1.65-3.30 mmol/l above fasting
	60 min.	20-50 mg/dl above fasting	0.055	1.10-2.75 mmol/l above fasting
	120 min.	5-15 mg/dl above fasting	0.055	0.28-0.83 mmol/l above fasting
	180 min.	Fasting level or below	0.055	Fasting level or below
intravenous	Serum or plasma:			
	fasting	70-110 mg/dl	0.055	3.85-6.05 mmol/l
	5 min.	Maximum of 250 mg/dl	0.055	Maximum of 13.75 mmol/l
	60 min.	Significant decrease	0.055	Significant decrease
	120 min.	Below 120 mg/dl	0.055	Below 6.60 mmol/l
	180 min.	Fasting level	0.055	Fasting level
Glucose 6-phosphate dehydrogenase (G6PD)	Erythrocytes	250-500 units/10^6 cells	1	250-500 units/10^6 cells
		1200-2000 mIU/ml packed erythrocytes	1	1200-2000 U/l packed erythrocytes
γ-Glutamyl transferase	Serum	5-40 IU/l	1	5-40 U/l at 37°C.
Glutathione	Whole blood	24-37 mg/dl	0.032	0.77-1.18 mmol/l
Growth hormone	Serum	<10 ng/ml	1	<10 µg/l
Guanase	Serum	<3 nM/ml/min	1	<3 U/l at 37°C.
Haptoglobin	Serum	60-270 mg/dl	.01	0.6-2.7 g/l
Hemoglobin	Serum or plasma:			
	qualitative	Negative	10	Negative
	quantitative	0.5-5.0 mg/dl	10	5-50 mg/l
	Whole blood:			
	female	12.0-16.0 g/dl	10	1.86-2.48 mmol/l
	male	13.5-18.0 g/dl	10	2.09-2.79 mmol/l
α-Hydroxybutyrate dehydrogenase	Serum	140-350 U/ml	1	140-350 kU/l
17-Hydroxycorticosteroids	Plasma:			
	male	7-19 µg/dl	10	70-190 µg/l
	female	9-21 µg/dl	10	9-21 µg/l
	after 24 USP units of ACTH I.M.	Serum	35-55 µg/dl	10	350-550 µg/l
Immunoglobulins:	Serum			
IgG		800-1801 mg/dl	0.01	8.0-18.0 g/l
IgA		113-563 mg/dl	0.01	1.1-5.6 g/l
IgM		54-222 mg/dl	0.01	0.54-2.2 g/l
IgD		0.5-3.0 mg/dl	10	5.0-30 mg/l
IgE		0.01-0.04 mg/dl	10	0.1-0.4 mg/l
Insulin	Plasma:			
	bioassay	11-240 µIU/ml[d]	0.0417	0.46-10.00 µg/l
	radioimmunoassay	4-24 µIU/ml	0.0417	0.17-1.00 µg/l
Insulin tolerance (0.1 unit/kg)	Serum:			
	fasting	Glucose of 70-110 mg/dl	0.055	Glucose of 3.85-6.05 mmol/l
	30 min.	Fall to 50% of fasting level	0.01[b]	Fall to 0.5 of fasting level
	90 min.	Fasting level		Fasting level

Table continued on following page

Table 1. WHOLE BLOOD, SERUM, AND PLASMA CHEMISTRY (Continued)

TYPICAL REFERENCE INTERVALS

COMPONENT	SYSTEM	In Conventional Units	Factor*	In SI Units†
Iodine:				
butanol-extraction (BEI)	Serum	3.5-6.5 µg/dl	0.079	0.28-0.51 µmol/l
protein bound (PBI)	Serum	4.0-8.0 µg/dl	0.079	0.32-0.63 µmol/l
Iron, total	Serum	60-150 µg/dl	0.179	11-27 µmol/l
Iron binding capacity	Serum	300-360 µg/dl	0.179	54-64 µmol/l
Iron saturation	Serum	20-55%	0.01^b	0.20-0.55 of total iron binding capacity
Isocitric dehydrogenase	Serum	50-240 units/ml at 25°C. (Wolfson-Williams Ashman units)	0.0167	0.83-4.18 U/l at 25°C.
Ketone bodies	Serum	Negative	—	Negative
17-Ketosteroids	Plasma	25-125 µg/dl	0.01	0.25-1.25 mg/l
Lactic acid (as lactate)	Whole blood:			
venous		5-20 mg/dl	0.111	0.6-2.2 mmol/l
arterial		3-7 mg/dl		0.3-0.8 mmol/l
Lactate dehydrogenase (LDH)	Serum	80-120 units at 30°C. (lactate → pyruvate)	0.48	38-62 U/l at 30°C. (lactate → pyruvate)
		185-640 units at 30°C. (pyruvate → lactate)	0.48	90-310 U/l at 30°C. (pyruvate → lactate)
		100-190 U/l at 37°C. (lactate → pyruvate)	1	100-190 U/l at 37°C. (lactate → pyruvate)
Lactate dehydrogenase isoenzymes:	Serum			
LDH$_1$ (anode)		17-27%	0.01^b	0.17-0.27 of total LDH
LDH$_2$		27-37%		0.27-0.37 of total LDH
LDH$_3$		18-25%		0.18-0.25 of total LDH
LDH$_4$		3-8%		0.03-0.08 of total LDH
LDH$_5$ (cathode)		0-5%		0.00-0.05 of total LDH
Lactate dehydrogenase (heat stable)	Serum	30-60% of total	0.01^b	0.3-0.6 of total LDH
Lactose tolerance	Serum	Serum glucose changes similar to glucose tolerance test	—	Serum glucose changes similar to glucose tolerance test
Lead	Whole blood	0-50 µg/dl	0.048	0-2.4 µmol/l
Leucine aminopeptidase (LAP)	Serum:			
male		80-200 U/ml (Goldbarg-Rutenberg)	0.24	19.2-48.0 U/l
female		75-185 U/ml (Goldbarg-Rutenberg)	0.24	18.0-44.4 U/l
Lipase	Serum	0-1.5 U/ml (Cherry-Crandall)	278	0-417 U/l
		14-280 mIU/ml	1	14-280 U/l
Lipids, total	Serum	400-800 mg/dl	0.01	4.00-8.00 g/l
cholesterol		150-250 mg/dl	0.026	3.9-6.5 mmol/l
triglycerides		10-190 mg/dl	0.109	1.09-20.71 mmol/l
phospholipids		150-380 mg/dl	0.01	1.50-380 g/l
fatty acids (free)		9.0-15.0 mM/l	1	9.0-15.0 mmol/l
		300-480 µEq/l	0.01	300-480 µmol/l
phospholipid phosphorous		8.0-11.0 mg/dl	0.323	2.58-3.55 mmol/l
Lithium	Serum	Negative	—	Negative
Therapeutic interval		0.5-1.4 mEq/l	1	0.5-1.4 mmol/l

Analyte	Specimen	Conventional value	Factor	SI value
Long-acting thyroid-stimulating hormone (LATS)	Serum	None	—	None
Lutenizing hormone (LH)	Serum:			
male		6-30 mIU/ml[f]	0.23	1.4-6.9 mg/l
female		Mid cycle peak: 3 times baseline value	0.23	Mid cycle peak: 3 times baseline value
		Premenopausal <30 mIU/ml	0.23	Premenopausal <5 times baseline value
		Postmenopausal >35 mIU/ml	0.23	Postmenopausal >5 times baseline value
Macroglobulins, total	Serum	70-430 mg/dl	0.01	0.7-4.3 g/l
Magnesium	Serum	1.3-2.1 mEq/l	0.5	0.7-1.1 mmol/l
		1.8-3.0 mg/dl	0.41	0.7-1.1 mmol/l
Methemoglobin	Whole blood	0-0.24 g/dl	10	0.0-2.4 g/l
		<3% of total hemoglobin	0.01[b]	<.03 of total hemoglobin
Mucoprotein	Serum or plasma	80-200 mg/dl	0.01	0.8-2.0 g/l
Non-protein nitrogen (NPN)	Serum or plasma	20-35 mg/dl	0.714	14.3-25.0 mmol/l
	Whole blood	25-50 mg/dl	0.714	17.9-35.7 mmol/l
5'Nucleotidase	Serum	0-1.6 units at 37°C.	1	0-1.6 units at 37°C.
Ornithine carbamyl transferase	Serum	8-20 mIU/ml at 37°C.	1	8-20 U/l at 37°C.
Osmolality	Serum	280-295 mOsm/kg	1	280-295 mOsm/l
Oxygen:				
pressure (PO_2)	Whole blood (arterial)	95-100 mm Hg	0.133	12.64-13.30 kPa[a]
content	Whole blood (arterial)	15-23 volume %	0.01[b]	0.15-0.23 of volume
saturation	Whole blood (arterial)	94-100%	0.01[b]	0.94-1.00 of total
pH	Whole blood (arterial)	7.38-7.44	1	7.38-7.44
	Whole blood (venous)	7.36-7.41	1	7.36-7.41
	Serum or plasma (venous)	7.35-7.45	1	7.35-7.45
Phenylalanine	Serum:			
adults		<3.0 mg/dl	0.061	<0.18 mmol/l
newborns (term)		1.2-3.5 mg/dl	0.061	0.07-0.21 mmol/l
Phosphatase				
acid phosphatase	Serum	0.13-0.63 U/l at 37°C. (paranitrophenyl phosphate)	16.67	2.2-10.5 U/l at 37°C. (p-nitrophenylphosphate)
				0.0-0.8 U/l at 37°C.
alkaline phosphatase	Serum	20-90 IU/l at 30°C. (paranitrophenylphosphate in AMP buffer)	1	20-90 U/l at 30°C. (p-nitrophenylphosphate)
				25-97 U/l at 37°C. (p-nitrophenylphosphate)
Phospholipid phosphorus	Serum	8-11 mg/dl	0.323	2.6-3.6 mmol/l
Phospholipids	Serum	150-380 mg/dl	0.01	1.50-3.80 g/l
Phosphorus, inorganic	Serum:			
adults		2.3-4.7 mg/dl	0.323	0.78-1.52 mmol/l
children		4.0-7.0 mg/dl	0.323	1.29-2.26 mmol/l
Potassium	Plasma	3.8-5.0 mEq/l	1	3.8-5.0 mmol/l
Prolactin	Serum	1-25 ng/ml (females)	1	1-25 µg/l
		1-20 ng/ml (males)	1	1-20 µg/l
Proteins:				
total	Serum	6.0-7.8 g/dl	10	60-78 g/l
albumin		3.2-4.5 g/dl	10	32-45 g/l
globulin		2.3-3.5 g/dl	10	23-35 g/l

Table continued on following page

Table 1. WHOLE BLOOD, SERUM, AND PLASMA CHEMISTRY (Continued)

COMPONENT	SYSTEM	TYPICAL REFERENCE INTERVALS		
		In Conventional Units	Factor*	In SI Units†
Protein fractionation		See electrophoresis		See electrophoresis
Protoporphyrin	Erythrocytes	15-50 μg/dl	0.018	0.27-0.90 μmol/l
Pyruvate	Whole blood	0.3-0.9 mg/dl	114	34-103 μmol/l
Salicylates	Serum	Negative	—	Negative
therapeutic interval		15-30 mg/dl	0.072	1.44-1.80 mmol/l
		150-300 μg/ml	0.0072	1.08-2.16 mmol/l
Sodium	Plasma	136-142 mEq/l	1	136-142 mmol/l
Sulfate, inorganic	Serum	0.2-1.3 mEq/l	0.5	0.10-0.65 mmol/l
		0.9-6.0 mg/dl as SO_4^{--}	0.104	0.09-0.62 mmol/l as SO_4^{--}
Sulfhemoglobin	Whole blood	Negative	—	Negative
Sulfonamides	Serum or whole blood	Negative	—	Negative
Testosterone	Serum or plasma:			
male	Serum	300-1200 ng/dl	0.035	10.0-42.0 nmol/l
female	Serum	30-95 ng/dl	0.035	1.1-3.3 nmol/l
Thiocyanate	Serum	Negative	—	Negative
Thymol flocculation	Serum	0-5 units^f	1	0-5 units
Thyroid hormone tests:				
a) Expressed as thyroxine:				
T_4 by column		5.0-11.0 μg/dl	13.0	65-143 nmol/l
T_4 by competitive binding—Murphy-Pattee		6.0-11.8 μg/dl	13.0	78-153 nmol/l
T_4 RIA		5.5-12.5 μg/dl	13.0	72-163 nmol/l
free T_4		0.9-2.3 ng/dl	13.0	12-30 pmol/l
b) Expressed as iodine:				
T_4 by column		3.2-7.2 μg/dl	79.0	253-569 nmol/l
T_4 by competitive binding—Murphy-Pattee		3.9-7.7 μg/dl	79.0	308-608 nmol/l
free T_4		0.6-1.5 ng/dl	0.01^b	47-119 pmol/l
T_3 resin uptake		25-38 relative % uptake	10	0.25-0.38 relative uptake
Thyroxine-binding globulin (TBG)	Serum	10-26 μg/dl	10	100-260 μg/l·
TSH	Serum	<10 μU/ml	1	<10^{-3} IU/l
Transferases				
aspartate amino transferase (AST or SGOT)	Serum	10-40 U/ml (Karmen) at 25°C. 16-60 U/ml (Karmen) at 30°C.	0.48	8-29 U/l at 30°C. 8-33 U/l at 37°C.
alanine amino transferase (ALT or SGPT)	Serum	10-30 U/ml (Karmen) at 25°C. 8-50 U/ml (Karmen) at 30°C.	0.48	4-24 U/l at 30°C. 4-36 U/l at 37°C.
gamma glutamyl transferase (GGT)	Serum	5-40 IU/l at 37°C.	1	5.40 U/l at 37°C.
Triglycerides	Serum	10-190 mg/dl	0.011^e	0.11-2.09 mmol/l
Urea nitrogen	Serum	8-23 mg/dl	0.357	2.9-8.2 mmol/l

Test	Specimen	Conventional value	Factor*	SI value
Urea clearance:	Serum and Urine			
maximum clearance		64-99 ml/min, or more than 75% of normal clearance	0.0167	1.07-1.65 ml/s
standard clearance		41-65 ml/min, or more than 75% of normal clearance	0.0167	0.68-1.09 ml/s or more than 0.75 of normal clearance
Uric acid	Serum: male	4.0-8.5 mg/dl	0.059	0.24-0.5 mmol/l
	female	2.7-7.3 mg/dl	0.059	0.16-0.43 mmol/l
Vitamin A	Serum:	15-60 µg/dl	0.035	0.53-2.10 µmol/l
Vitamin A tolerance	Serum: fasting 3 hr. or 6 hr. after 5000 units vitamin A/kg	15-60 µg/dl	0.035	0.53-2.10 µmol/l
	24 hrs.	200-600 µg/dl		7.00-21.00 µmol/l
		Fasting values or slightly above		Fasting values or slightly above
Vitamin B_{12}	Serum	160-950 pg/ml	0.74	118-703 pmol/l
Unsaturated vitamin B_{12} binding capacity	Serum	1000-2000 pg/ml	0.74	740-1480 pmol/l
Vitamin C	Plasma	0.6-1.6 mg/dl	56.8	34-91 µmol/l
Xylose absorption	Serum: normal	25-40 mg/dl between 1 and 2 hr.	0.067	1.68-2.68 mmol/l between 1 and 2 h
	in malabsorption	Maximum approximately 10 mg/dl		Maximum approximately 0.67 mmol/l
Dose: adult		25 g D-xylose	0.067	0.167 mol D-xylose
children		0.5 g/kg D-xylose	0.067	3.33 mmol/kg D-xylose
Zinc	Serum	50-150 µg/dl	0.153	7.65-22.95 µmol/l

*Factor = Number factor (note that units are not presented).

†Value in SI units = Value in conventional units × factor.

‡Usually not measured in blood (preferred specimen is urine, hair, or nails except in acute cases where gastric contents are used).

Table 2. URINE

COMPONENT	TYPE OF URINE SPECIMEN	TYPICAL REFERENCE INTERVALS		
		In Conventional Units	Factor	In SI Units
Acetoacetic acid	Random	Negative	—	Negative
Acetone	Random	Negative	—	Negative
Addis count	12 hr. collection	WBC and epithelial cells:		
		1,800,000/12 hr.	1	$1.8 \times 10^6/12$ h
		RBC 500,000/12 hr.	1	$0.5 \times 10^6/12$ h
		Hyaline casts: 0–5000/12 hr.	1	$5.0 \times 10^3/12$ h
Albumin:				
qualitative	Random	Negative	—	Negative
quantitative	24 hr.	15–150 mg/24 hr.	1	0.015–0.150 g/24 h
Aldosterone	24 hr.	2–26 μg/24 hr.	2.77	5.5–72.0 nmol/24 h
Alkapton bodies	Random	Negative	—	Negative
Alpha-amino acid nitrogen	24 hr.	100–290 mg/24 hr.	0.0714	7.14–20.71 mmol/24 h
δ-Aminolevulinic acid	Random:			
	adult	0.1–0.6 mg/dl	76.3	7.6–45.8 μmol/l
	children	<0.5 mg/dl	76.3	<38.1 μmol/l
	24 hr.	1.5–7.5 mg/24 hr.	7.63	11.15–57.2 μmol/24 h
Ammonia nitrogen	24 hr.	20–70 mEq/24 hr.		
	2 hr.	500–1200 mg/24 hr.	0.071	35.5–85.2 mmol/24 h
Amylase		35–260 Somogyi units/hr.	0.185	6.5–48.1 U/h
Arsenic	Random	<50 μg/l	0.013	<0.65 μmol/l
Ascorbic acid	24 hr.	1–7 mg/dl	0.057	0.06–0.40 mmol/l
	24 hr.	>50 mg/24 hr.	0.0057	>0.29 mmol/24 h
Bence Jones protein	Random	Negative	—	Negative
Beryllium	24 hr.	<0.05 μg/24 hr.	111	<5.55 nmol/24 h
Bilirubin, qualitative	Random	Negative	—	Negative
Blood, occult	Random	Negative	—	Negative
Borate	24 hr.	<2 mg/l	16	<32 μmol/l
Calcium:				
qualitative (Sulkowitch)	Random	1+ turbidity	1	1+ turbidity
quantitative	24 hr.:			
	average diet	100–240 mg/24 hr.	0.025	2.50–6.25 mmol/24 h
	low calcium diet	<150 mg/24 hr.	0.025	<3.75 mmol/24 h
	high calcium diet	240–300 mg/24 hr.	0.025	6.25–7.50 mmol/24 h
Catecholamines	Random	0–14 μg/dl	0.059	0–0.83 μmol/l
	24 hr.	<100 μg/24 hr. (varies with activity)	0.0059	<0.59 μmol/24 h
Epinephrine		<10 ng/24 hr.	5.46	<55 nmol/24 h
Norepinephrine		<100 ng/24 hr.	5.91	<590 nmol/24 h
Total free catecholamines		4–126 mcg./24 hr.	5.91	24–745 nmol/24 h
Total metanephrines		0.1–1.6 mg./24 hr.	5.07	0.5–8.1 μmol/24 h
Chloride	24 hr.	140–250 mEq/24 hr.	1	140–250 mmol/24 h
Concentration test (Fishberg):	Random—after fluid restriction			

Test	Specimen	Conventional	Factor	SI
Specific gravity		>1.025	1	>1.025
Osmolality		>850 mOsm/l	1	>850 mOsm/l
Copper	24 hr.	0–30 µg/24 hr.	0.016	0–0.48 µmol/24 h
Coproporphyrin	Random: adult	3–20 µg/dl	0.015	0.045–0.30 µmol/l
Creatine	24 hr.: adult	50–160 µg/24 hr.	0.0015	0.075–0.24 µmol/24 h
	children	0–80 µg/24 hr.	0.0015	0.00–0.12 µmol/24 h
	24 hr.: male	0–40 mg/24 hr.	0.0076	0–0.30 mmol/24 h
	female	0–100 mg/24 hr.	0.0076	0–0.76 mmol/24 h
		Higher in children and during pregnancy	0.0076	Higher in children and during pregnancy
Creatinine	24 hr.: male	20–26 mg/kg/24 hr.	0.0088	0.18–0.23 mmol/kg/24 h
		1.0–2.0 g/24 hr.	8.8	8.8–17.6 mmol/24 h
	female	14–22 mg/kg/24 hr.	0.0088	0.12–0.19 mmol/kg/24 h
		0.8–1.8 g/24 hr.	8.8	7.0–15.8 mmol/24 h
Cystine, qualitative	Random	Negative	—	Negative
Cystine and cysteine	24 hr.	10–100 mg/24 hr.	.0083[g]	0.08–0.83 mmol/24 h
Diacetic acid	Random	Negative	—	Negative
Epinephrine	24 hr.	0–20 µg/24 hr.	0.0055	0.00–0.11 µmol/24 h
Estrogens total	24 hr.: male	5–18 µg/24 hr.	1	5–18 µg/24 h
	female: ovulation	28–100 µg/24 hr.	1	28–100 µg/24 h
	luteal peak	22–80 µg/24 hr.	1	22–80 µg/24 h
	at menses	4–25 µg/24 hr.	1	4–25 µg/24 h
	pregnancy	Up to 45,000 µg/24 hr.	1	Up to 45,000 µg/24 h
	postmenopausal	Up to 10 µg/24 hr.	1	Up to 10 µg/24 h
fractionated	24 hr, non-pregnant, midcycle			
Estrone (E¹)	—	2–25 µg/24 hr.	3.7	7–93 nmol/24 h
Estradiol (E²)	—	0–10 µg/24 hr.	3.7	0–37 nmol/24 h
Estriol (E³)		2–30 µg/24 hr.	3.5	7–105 nmol/24 h
Fat, qualitative	Random	Negative	—	Negative
FIGLU (n-formiminoglutamic acid)	24 hr.	<3 mg/24 hr.	5.7	<17.0 µmol/24 h
	after 15 g of L-histidine	4 mg/8 hr.	5.7	23.0 µmol/8 h
Fluoride	24 hr.	<1 mg/24 hr.	0.053	0.053 mmol/24 h
Follicle-stimulating hormone (FSH)	24 hr.: adult	4–25 mIU/ml	1	6–50 Mouse uterine units (MUU) 24 h
	prepubertal	4–30 mIU/ml	1	<10 MUU/24 h
	postmenopausal	40–50 mIU/ml	1	>50 MUU/24 h
	midcycle	2+ baseline		
Fructose	24 hr.	30–65 mg/24 hr.	0.0056	0.17–0.36 mmol 24 h

Table continued on following page

367

Table 2. URINE (Continued)

COMPONENT	TYPE OF URINE SPECIMEN	TYPICAL REFERENCE INTERVALS		
		In Conventional Units	Factor	In SI Units
Glucose:				
qualitative	Random	Negative	—	Negative
quantitative:				
copper-reducing substances	24 hr.	0.5-1.5 g/24 hr.	1	0.5-1.5 g/24 h
total sugars		average 250 mg/24 hr.	1	average 250 mg/24 h
glucose		average 130 mg/24 hr.	0.0056	average 0.73 mmol/24 h
Gonadotropins, pituitary (FSH and LH)	24 hr.	10-50 MUU/24 hr.	1	10-50 MUU/24 h
Hemoglobin	Random	Negative	—	Negative
Homogentisic acid	Random	Negative	—	Negative
Homovanillic acid (HVA)	24 hr.	<15 mg/24 hr.	5.5	<83.0 μmol/24 h
17-Hydroxycorticosteroids	24 hr. male	5.5-14.5 mg/24 hr.	1	5.5-145 mg/24 h
	female	4.9-12.9 mg/24 hr.		4.9-12.9 mg/24 h
5-Hydroxyindoleacetic acid (5-HIAA)				
qualitative	Random	Negative	—	Negative
quantitative	24 hr.	<9 mg/24 hr.	5.2	<47 μmol/24 h
Ketone bodies	Random	Negative		Negative
17-Ketosteroids	24 hr. male	8-20 mg/24 hr.	1	8.0-20 mg/24 h
	female	4-15 mg/24 hr.		4.0-15 mg/24 h
Androsterone	24 hr. male	2.0-5.0 mg/24 hr.	3.44	6.9-17.2 μmol/24 h
	female	0.8-3.0 mg/24 hr.		2.8-10.3 μmol/24 h
Etiocholanolone	24 hr.: male	1.4-5.0 mg/24 hr.	3.44	4.8-17.2 μmol/24 h
	female	0.8-4.0 mg/24 hr.	3.44	2.8-13.8 μmol/24 h
Dehydroepiandrosterone	24 hr.: male	0.2-2.0 mg/24 hr.	3.46	0.7-6.9 μmol/24 h
	female	0.2-1.8 mg/24 hr.	3.46	0.7-6.2 μmol/24 h
11-Ketoandrosterone	24 hr.: male	0.2-1.0 mg/24 hr.	3.28	0.7-3.3 μmol/24 h
	female	0.2-0.8 mg/24 hr.	3.28	0.7-2.6 μmol/24 h
11-Ketoetiocholanolone	24 hr.: male	0.2-1.0 mg/24 hr.	3.28	0.7-3.3 μmol/24 h
	female	0.2-0.8 mg/24 hr.	3.28	0.7-2.6 μmol/24 h
11-Hydroxyandrosterone	24 hr.: male	0.1-0.8 mg/24 hr.	3.26	0.3-2.6 μmol/24 h
	female	0.0-0.5 mg/24 hr.	3.26	0.0-1.6 μmol/24 h
11-Hydroxyetiocholanolone	24 hr.: male	0.2-0.6 mg/24 hr.	3.26	0.7-2.0 μmol/24 h
	female	0.1-1.1 mg/24 hr.	3.26	0.3-3.6 μmol/24 h

		Normal value		SI value
Lactose	24 hr.	14-40 mg/24 hr.	2.9	41-116 μmol/24 h
Lead	24 hr.	<100 μg/24 hr.	0.0048	<0.48 μmol/24 h
Magnesium	24 hr.	6.0-8.5 mEq/24 hr.	0.5	3.0-4.3 mmol/24 h
Melanin, qualitative	Random	Negative	—	Negative
3-Methoxy-4-hydroxymandelic acid (VMA)	24 hr.:		5.05	
adults		1.5-7.5 mg/24 hr.		7.6-37.9 μmol/24 h
infants		83 μg/kg/24 hr.	0.0051	0.4 μmol/kg/24 h
Mucin	24 hr.	100-150 mg/24 hr.	1	100-150 mg/24 h
Myoglobin				
qualitative	Random	Negative	—	Negative
quantitative	24 hr.	<4 mg/l	1	<4 mg/l
Osmolality	Random	500-800 mOsm/kg water	1	500-800 mOsm/kg water
Pentoses	24 hr.	2-5 mg/kg/24 hr.	1	2-5 mg/kg/24 h
pH	Random	4.6-8.0	1	4.6-8.0
Phenolsulfonphthalein (PSP)	Urine timed after 6 mg PSP IV			
15 min.		20-50% dye excreted	0.01[b]	0.2-0.5 dye excreted
30 min.		16-24% dye excreted	0.01	0.16-0.24 dye excreted
60 min.		9-17% dye excreted	0.01	0.09-0.17 dye excreted
120 min.		3-10% dye excreted	0.01	0.03-0.10 dye excreted
Phenylpyruvic acid, qualitative	Random	Negative	—	Negative
Phosphorus	Random	0.9-1.3 g/24 hr.	32	29-42 mmol/24 h
Porphobilinogen:				
qualitative	Random	Negative	—	Negative
quantitative	24 hr.	0-1.0 mg/24 hr.	4.42	0-4.4 μmol/24 h
Potassium	24 hr.	40-80 mEq/24 hr.	1	40-80 mmol/24 h
Pregnancy tests	Concentrated morning specimen	Positive in normal pregnancies or with tumors producing chorionic gonadotropin	—	Positive in normal pregnancies or with tumors producing chorionic gonadotropin
Pregnanediol	24 hr.:			
male		0-1.5 mg/24 hr.	3.12	0-4.7 μmol/24 h
female		1-8 mg/24 hr.	3.12	3-25 μmol/24 h
peak		1 week after ovulation		1 week after ovulation
pregnancy		<50 mg/24 hr.	3.12	<156 μmol/24 h
children		Negative	3.12	Negative
Pregnanetriol	24 hr.:			
male		0.4-2.4 mg/24 hr.	2.97	1.2-7.1 μmol/24 h
female		0.5-2.0 mg/24 hr.	2.97	1.5-5.9 μmol/24 h
children		Up to 1 mg/24 hr.	2.97	Up to 3 μmol/24 h
Protein, qualitative	Random	Negative	—	Negative
Reducing substances, total	24 hr.	40-150 mg/24 hr.	1	40-150 mg/24 h
	24 hr.	0.5-1.5 mg/24 hr.	1	0.5-1.5 mg/24 h
Sodium	24 hr.	75-200 mEq/24 hr.	1	75-200 mmol/24 h
Solids, total	24 hr.	55-70 g/24 hr.	1	55-70 g/24 h
		Decreases with age to 30 gm/24 hr.	1	Decreases with age to 30 g/24 h
Specific gravity	Random	1.016-1.022 (normal fluid intake)	1	Relative Density (U 20°C./water 20°C.) 1.016-1.022 (normal fluid intake)
		1.001-1.035 (range)		1.001-1.034 (range)
Sugars (excluding glucose)	Random	Negative	—	Negative

Table continued on following page

Table 2. URINE (Continued)

COMPONENT	TYPE OF URINE SPECIMEN	TYPICAL REFERENCE INTERVALS		
		In Conventional Units	Factor	In SI Units
Titratable acidity	24 hr.	20-50 mEq/24 hr.	1	20-50 mmol/24 h
Urea nitrogen	24 hr.	6-17 g/24 hr.	0.0357	0.21-0.60 mol/24 h
Uric acid	24 hr.	250-750 mg/24 hr.	0.0059	1.48-4.43 mmol/24 h
Urobilinogen	2 hr.	0.3-1.0 Ehrlich Units	—	
	24 hr.	0.05-2.5 mg/24 hr. or	1.69	0.09-4.23 μmol/24 h
		0.5-4.0 Ehrlich units/24 hr.		
Uropepsin	Random	15-45 units/hr. (Anson)	7.37	111-332 U h
	24 hr.	1500-5000 units/24 hr. (Anson)	7.37	11-37 kU/h
Uroporphyrins:				
qualitative	Random	Negative	—	Negative
quantitative	24 hr.	10-30 μg/24 hr.	0.0012	0.012-0.037 μmol/24 h
Vanillylmandelic acid (VMA)	24 hr.	1.5-7.5 mg/24 hr.	5.05	7.6-37.9 μmol/24 h
Volume, total	24 hr.	600-1600 ml/24 hr.	0.001	0.6-1.61/24 h
Zinc	24 hr.	0.15-1.2 mg/24 hr.	15.3	2.3-18.4 μmol/24 h

Table 3. SYNOVIAL FLUID

| COMPONENT | TYPICAL REFERENCE INTERVALS | | |
	In Conventional Units	Factor	In SI Units
Blood-serum-synovial fluid glucose difference	$<$10 mg/dl	0.055	$<$0.55 mmol/l
Differential cell count	Granulocytes $<$ 25% of nucleated cells	0.01[b]	Granulocytes $<$ 0.25 of nucleated cells
Fibrin clot	Absent	—	Absent
Mucin clot	Abundant	—	Abundant
Nucleated cell count	$<$200 cells/μl	10^6	$<$2 $\times$ 10^8 cells/l
Viscosity	High	—	High
Volume	$<$3.5 ml	0.001	$<$0.0035 l

Table 4. SEMINAL FLUID

| COMPONENT | TYPICAL REFERENCE INTERVALS | | |
	In Conventional Units	Factor	In SI Units
Liquefaction	within 20 min.	1	within 20 min
Sperm morphology	$>$70% normal, mature spermatozoa	0.01[b]	$>$0.7 normal, mature spermatozoa
Sperm motility	$>$60%	0.01[b]	$>$0.6
pH	$>$7.0 (average 7.7)	1	$>$7.0 (average 7.7)
Sperm count	60-150 million/ml	10^3	60-150 $\times$ 10^9/l
Volume	1.5-5.0 ml	0.001	0.0015-0.005/1

Table 5. GASTRIC FLUID

| COMPONENT | TYPICAL REFERENCE INTERVALS | | |
	In Conventional Units	Factor	In SI Units
Fasting residual volume	$<$ 50 ml	0.001	$<$.05/1
pH (stimulated specimen)	$<$2.0	1	$<$2.0
Basal acid output (BAO)	0-6 mEq/hr.	1	0-6 mmol/h
Maximum acid output (MAO) (after histamine stimulation)	5-40 mEq/hr.	1	5-40 mmol/h
BAO/MAO ratio	$<$0.4	1	$<$0.4

Table 6. HEMATOLOGY

COMPONENT	TYPICAL REFERENCE INTERVALS			
	In Conventional Units		Factor	In SI Units
Red cell volume:				
male	25–35 ml/kg body weight		0.001	0.025–0.035 l/kg body weight
female	20–30 ml/kg body weight		—	0.020–0.030 l/kg body weight
Plasma volume:				
male	40–50 ml/kg body weight		0.001	0.040–0.050 l/kg body weight
female	40–50 ml/kg body weight		—	0.040–0.050 l/kg body weight
Coagulation tests:				
Bleeding time (Ivy)	1–6 minutes		1	1–6 min
Bleeding time (Duke)	1–3 minutes		1	1–3 min
Clot retraction	½ the original mass in 2 hr.		1	0.5 the original mass in 2 h
Dilute blood clot lysis time	Clot lysis between 6 and 10 hr at 37°C.		1	Clot lysis between 6 and 10 h at 37°C.
Euglobin clot lysis time	Clot lysis between 2 and 6 hr. at 37°C.		1	Clot lysis between 2 and 6 h at 37°C.
Partial thromboplastin time	60–70 seconds		1	60–70 s
Kaolin activated	35–50 seconds		1	35–50 s
Prothrombin time	12–14 seconds		1	12–14 s
Venous clotting time:				
3 tubes	5–15 minutes		1	5–15 min
2 tubes	5–18 minutes		—	5–8 min
Whole blood clot lysis time	None in 24 hr.		—	None in 24 h
Complete blood count (CBC)				
Hematocrit:				
male	40–54%		0.01^b	0.40–0.54
female	38–47%		—	0.38–0.47
Hemoglobin:				
male	13.5–18.0 g/dl		0.155	2.09–2.79 mmol/l
female	12.0–16.0 g/dl		—	1.86–2.48 mmol/l
Red Cell Count:				
male	$4.6–6.2 \times 10^6/\mu l$		0.155	$4.6–6.2 \times 10^{12}/l$
female	$4.2–5.4 \times 10^6/\mu l$		—	$4.2–5.4 \times 10^{12}/l$
White Cell Count	$4.5–11.0 \times 10^3/\mu l$		10^6	$4.5–11.0 \times 10^9/l$
Erythrocyte indices:				
Mean corpuscular volume (MCV)	80–96 cu. microns		1	80–96 fl
Mean corpuscular hemoglobin (MCH)	27–31 pg		1	27–31 pg
Mean corpuscular hemoglobin concentration (MCHC)	32–36%		0.01^b	0.32–0.36
White blood cell differential (adult):	Mean per cent	Range of absolute counts		Mean fraction* — Range of absolute count
Segmented neutrophils	56%	1800–7000/μl	10^6	0.56 — $1.8–7.0 \times 10^9/l$
Bands	3%	0–700/μl	10^6	0.03 — $0–0.70 \times 10^9/l$
Eosinophils	2.7%	0–450/μl	10^6	0.027 — $0–0.45 \times 10^9/l$
Basophils	0.3%	0–200/μl	10^6	0.003 — $0–0.20 \times 10^9/l$
Lymphocytes	34%	1000–4800/μl	10^6	0.34 — $1.0–4.8 \times 10^9/l$
Monocytes	4%	0–800/μl	10^6	0.04 — $0–0.80 \times 10^9/l$
Hemoglobin A_2	1.5–3.5% of total hemoglobin		0.01^b	0.015–0.035 of total hemoglobin
Hemoglobin F	<2%		0.01^b	<0.02

Table continued on opposite page

Table 6. HEMATOLOGY (Continued)

				TYPICAL REFERENCE INTERVALS				
COMPONENT	In Conventional Units			Factor		In SI Units		
Osmotic fragility	% NaCl	% Lysis		% NaCl—171 % Lysis—0.01[b]	NaCl mmol/l	Fractional Lysis		
		Fresh	24 hr. at 37°C.			Fresh	24 h at 37°C	
	0.2	—	95–100		34.2	—	0.95–1.00	
	0.3	97–100	85–100		51.3	0.97–1.00	0.85–1.00	
	0.35	90–99	75–100		59.8	0.90–0.99	0.75–1.00	
	0.4	50–95	65–100		68.4	0.50–0.95	0.65–1.00	
	0.45	5–45	55–95		77.0	0.05–0.45	0.55–0.95	
	0.5	0–6	40–85		85.5	0–0.06	0.40–0.85	
	0.55	0	15–70		94.1	0	0.15–0.70	
	0.6	—	0–40		102.6	—	0–0.40	
	0.65	—	0–10		111.2	—	0–0.10	
	0.7	—	0–5		119.7	—	0–0.05	
	0.75	—	0		128.3	—	0	
Platelet count	150,000–400,000/μl			10^6		$0.15–0.4 \times 10^{12}$/l		
Reticulocyte count	0.5–1.5%			0.01[b]		0.005–0.015		
	25,000–75,000 cells/μl			10^6		$25–75 \times 10^9$/l		
Sedimentation rate (ESR) (Westergren)								
Men under 50 yrs.	<15 mm/hr			1		<15 mm/h		
Men over 50 yrs.	<20 mm/hr			1		<20 mm/h		
Women under 50 yrs.	<20 mm/hr			1		<20 mm/h		
Women over 50 yrs.	<30 mm/hr			1		<30 mm/h		
Viscosity	1.4–1.8 times water			1		1.4–1.8 times water		
Zeta sedimentation ratio	41–54%			0.01[b]		0.41–0.54		

* All percentages are multiplied by 0.01[b] to give mean fraction.

Table 7. AMNIOTIC FLUID

		TYPICAL REFERENCE INTERVALS		
COMPONENT	In Conventional Units	Factor	In SI Units	
Appearance:				
early gestation	Clear	—	Clear	
term	Clear or slightly opalescent	—	Clear or slightly opalescent	
Albumin:				
early gestation	0.39 g/dl	10	3.9 g/l	
term	0.19 g/dl	10	1.9 g/l	
Bilirubin:				
early gestation	<0.075 mg/dl	17.1	<1.28 μmol/l	
term	<0.025 mg/dl	17.1	<0.43 μmol/l	
Chloride:				
early gestation	Approximately equal to serum chloride	—	Approximately equal to serum chloride	
term	Generally 1-3 mEq/l lower than serum chloride	1	Generally 1-3 mmol/l lower than serum chloride	
Creatinine:				
early gestation	0.8-1.1 mg/dl	88.4	70.7-97.2 μmol/l	
term	1.8-4.0 mg/dl (generally > 2 mg/dl)	88.4	159.1-353.6 μmol/l (generally > 176.8 μmol/l)	
Estriol:				
early gestation	<10 μg/dl	0.035	<0.35 μmol/l	
term	>60 μg/dl	0.035	>2.1 μmol/l	
Lecithin/sphingomyelin		1		
Early (immature)	<1:1	1	<1:1	
Term (mature)	>2:1	1	>2:1	

Table continued on following page

373

Table 7. AMNIOTIC FLUID (Continued)

COMPONENT	In Conventional Units	Factor	In SI Units
	TYPICAL REFERENCE INTERVALS		
Osmolality:			
early gestation	Approximately equal to serum osmolality	1	Approximately equal to serum osmolality
term	230-270 mOsm/l	1	<230-270 mOsm/l
P_{CO_2}:			
early gestation	33-55 mm Hg	0.133	4.39-7.32 kPa[a]
term	42-55 mm Hg (increases toward term)	0.133	5.59-7.32 kPa[a] (increases toward term)
pH:			
early gestation	7.12-7.38	1	7.12-7.38
term	6.91-7.43 (decreases toward term)	1	6.91-7.43
Protein, total:			
early gestation	0.60 ± 0.24 g/dl	10	6.0 ± 2.4 g/l
term	0.26 ± 0.19 g/dl	10	2.6 ± 1.9 g/l
Sodium:			
early gestation	Approximately equal to serum sodium	1	Approximately equal to serum sodium
term	7-10 mEq/l lower than serum sodium	1	7-10 mmol/l lower than serum sodium
Staining, cytologic:			
Oil red O:			
early gestation	<10%	0.01[b]	<0.1
term	>50%	0.01[b]	>0.5
Nile blue sulfate:			
early gestation	0	0.01[b]	0
term	>20%	0.01	>0.2
Urea:			
early gestation	18.0 ± 5.9 mg/dl	0.166	2.99 ± 0.98 mmol/l
term	30.3 ± 11.4 mg/dl	0.166	5.03 ± 1.89 mmol/l
Uric acid:			
early gestation	3.72 ± 0.96 mg/dl	0.059	0.22 ± 0.06 mmol/l
term	9.90 ± 2.23 mg/dl	0.059	0.58 ± 0.13 mmol/l
Volume:			
early gestation	450-1200 ml	0.001	0.45-1.2 l
term	500-1400 ml (increases toward term)	0.001	0.5-1.4 l (increases toward term)

Table 8. CEREBROSPINAL FLUID

COMPONENT	In Conventional Units	Factor	In SI Units
	TYPICAL REFERENCE INTERVALS		
Albumin	10-30 mg/dl	10	100-300 mg/l
Calcium	2.1-2.7 mEq/l	0.5	1.05-1.35 mmol/l
Cell count	0-5 cells/μl	10^6	$0-5 \times 10^6$/l
Chloride:			
adult	118-132 mEq/l	1	118-132 mmol/l
Colloidal gold curve	0001111000	—	0001111000
Glucose	50-80 mg/dl	0.055	2.75-4.40 mmol/l
Lactate dehydrogenase (LDH)	Approximately 10% of serum level	—	Approximately 0.1 of serum level
Protein:			
total CSF	15-45 mg/dl	10	150-450 mg/l
ventricular fluid	5-15 mg/dl	10	50-150 mg/l
Protein Electrophoresis:			
Prealbumin	2-7%	0.01[b]	0.02-0.07
Albumin	56-76%	0.01	0.56-0.76
Alpha-1 globulin	2-7%	0.01	0.02-0.07
Alpha-2 globulin	4-12%	0.01	0.04-0.12
Beta globulin	8-18%	0.01	0.08-0.18
Gamma globulin	3-12%	0.01	0.03-0.12
Xanthochromia	Negative	—	Negative

Table 9. MISCELLANEOUS

COMPONENT	SPECIMEN	TYPICAL REFERENCE INTERVALS		
		In Conventional Units	Factor	In SI Units
Bile, qualitative	Random stool	Negative in adults	—	Negative in adults
		Positive in children	—	Positive in children
Chloride	Sweat	4-60 mEq/l	1	4-60 mmol/l
Clearances:	Serum and urine (timed)			
creatinine, endogenous		115 ± 20 ml/min	0.0167	1.92 ± 0.33 ml/l
Diodrast		600-720 ml/min.	0.0167	10.02-12.02 ml/s
inulin		100-150 ml/min.	0.0167	1.67-2.51 ml/s
PAH		600-750 ml/min.	0.0167	10.02-12.53 ml/s
Diagnex blue (tubeless gastric analysis)	Urine	Free acid present	—	Free acid present
Fat:	Stool, 72 hr.			
total fat		<5 g/24 hr.	0.01[b]	<5 g/24 h
		10-25% of dry matter	0.01	0.1-0.24 of dry matter
neutral fat		1-5% of dry matter	0.01	0.01-0.05 of dry matter
free fatty acids		5-13% of dry matter	0.01	0.05-0.13 of dry matter
combined fatty acids		5-15% of dry matter	0.01	0.05-0.15 of dry matter
Nitrogen, total	Stool, 24 hr.	10% of intake	%—0.01[b]	0.1 of intake
		1-2 g/24 hr.	g/24 hr—0.071	0.071-0.142 mol/24 h
Sodium	Sweat	10-80 mEq/l	1	10-80 mmol/l
Trypsin activity	Random, fresh stool	Positive (2+ to 4+)	—	Positive (2+ to 4+)
Thyroid ^{131}I uptake		7.5-25% in 6 hr.	0.01[b]	0.075-0.25 in 6 h
Urobilinogen:				
qualitative	Random stool	Positive	—	Positive
quantitative	Stool, 24 hr	40-200 mg/24 hr.	0.00169	0.068-0.34 mmol/24 h
		80-280 Ehrlich units/24 hr.		

NOTES TO TABLES 1 THROUGH 9

a. It is recommended (World Health Organization, 1977) that the units mm Hg be retained for pressures (PCO_2, PO_2) at the present time.

b. Percentages are expressed as number fractions in the SI, where a number fraction is dimensionless quantity given by: the number of defined particles constituting a specified component divided by the total number of defined particles in the system.

c. Unit based on hydrogen ion concentration.

d. One (1) International Unit of insulin corresponds to 0.04167 mg of the 4th International Standard (a mixture of 52% beef insulin and 48% pig insulin).

e. Factor based on relative molecular mass of triolein (885.4)

f. One (1) International Unit of lutenizing hormone corresponds to 0.2296 mg of 2nd reference preparation (1964).

g. Factor based on the relative molecular mass of cysteine, 121.16.

INDEX

Numbers in *italics* refer to illustrations; numbers followed by t refer to tables.

Abell method, in measurement of serum cholesterol, 309
Absorption, failure of, in intestinal disease, 224t
Accuracy, in laboratory testing, 45
Acid phosphatase, prostatic, collection and handling of, 210–211
  secretion of, by prostatic carcinoma, 209
  serum, elevation of, causes of, 209
Acidosis, metabolic, computer-assisted interpretive report for, *99*
Action stub, of decision table, 62
Actions, defined, 60
Activated partial thromboplastin time (plasma) (APTT), possibilities for error in, 6
Acute myocardial infarction. See *Myocardial infarction, acute*.
Acute-phase protein(s), electrophoretic distribution of, 118, *118*
  measurement of, 114t, 115
Adrenal disease. See *Cushing's syndrome* and *Pheochromocytoma*.
Airway resistance, in COPD, 184
Albumin, serum, laboratory evaluation of, 343–344
Alkaline phosphatase (serum), diseases and disorders elevating, 144, 144t
  elevation of, clinical evaluation of, 142
    drug-metabolite interference and, 144
    due to improper testing procedure, 143, *143*
    inappropriate reference levels and, 143, *143*
    interpretation of, 142–145
    interpretive reporting in assessment of, 145, *146*
    pathophysiology of, 141–142
    significance of, 141
    test requests for evaluation of, 145
    unexplained, 141–145
      methodology in assessment of, 142
      strategy for evaluating, 142
      vs. baseline levels, 143–144
  in liver function studies, 242–243
  laboratory evaluation of, 144, 331–333
  levels of, and serum calcium levels, 150
  in evaluation of prostatic carcinoma, 209–211
  upper reference limits for, 143, 143t
ALP, serum. See *alkaline phosphatase, serum*.

Alpha$_1$-antitrypsin, deficiency of, 282–285
  clinical features of, 283
  common laboratory test results in, 284t
  diagnosis of, 283, 285, *286*
  interpretive reporting for, *287*
  laboratory evaluation of, interpretation of, 285
    strategy for, 283–284
    techniques for, 284–285
    test requests and reports in, 285
    test sequence in, 283–284
  pathophysiology of, 282–283
  presentation of, 282
  screening for, 283
  phenotypes of, 282–283, 283t
  serum, reference interval for, 285
  significance of, 282
Amniotic fluid, reference values for substances in, 373–374t
Amylase, 233
  serum, levels of, in evaluation of acute pancreatitis, 234
Amylase-creatinine clearance ratio, 233
  in differential diagnosis of acute pancreatitis, 234
Anacidity, definition of, 217
Analytes, 42
Anemia, hemolytic, 33–34, 34t
  iron-deficiency, diagnostic system for, 94
  pernicious, and gastric secretion, 216
    screening for, 217
    significance of, 216
Angiography, pulmonary, for suspected pulmonary embolism, 191
Anticoagulants, for blood cell measurement, 319–322, 327, 336
anti-HAV antibody, components of, in diagnosis of hepatitis A, 247, 249t, *249*
Anuria, in diagnosis of acute renal failure, 203
APTT. See *Activated partial thromboplastin time (plasma)*.
ARTEMIS, in computer-assisted management of hypertension, 178
Artificial intelligence, consultation systems based on, 77–78
Aspartate amino transaminase. See *Glutamic-oxaloacetic transaminase, serum*.

377